A Concise Guide to Understanding Suicide

Epidemiology, Pathophysiology, and Prevention

A Concise Guide to Understanding Suicide

Epidemiology, Pathophysiology, and Prevention

Edited by

Stephen H. Koslow

Science Consultant, Department of Psychiatry and Behavioral Sciences, Leonard M. Miller School of Medicine, University of Miami, Miami, FL;
current position Director, U.S. Medical Affairs, CNS Otsuka America Pharmaceutical, Inc., Princeton, NJ, USA

Pedro Ruiz

Professor, Executive Vice Chair and Director of Clinical Programs, Department of Psychiatry and Behavioral Sciences, Leonard M. Miller School of Medicine, University of Miami, Miami, FL, USA

Charles B. Nemeroff

Leonard M. Miller Professor and Chairman, Department of Psychiatry and Behavioral Sciences, Leonard M. Miller School of Medicine, University of Miami, Miami, FL, USA

CAMBRIDGE
UNIVERSITY PRESS

CAMBRIDGE
UNIVERSITY PRESS

University Printing House, Cambridge CB2 8BS, United Kingdom

One Liberty Plaza, 20th Floor, New York, NY 10006, USA

477 Williamstown Road, Port Melbourne, VIC 3207, Australia

314-321, 3rd Floor, Plot 3, Splendor Forum, Jasola District Centre, New Delhi - 110025, India

79 Anson Road, #06-04/06, Singapore 079906

Cambridge University Press is part of the University of Cambridge.

It furthers the University's mission by disseminating knowledge in the pursuit of education, learning and research at the highest international levels of excellence.

www.cambridge.org
Information on this title: www.cambridge.org/9781107033238

First published 2014
Reprinted 2015

A catalogue record for this publication is available from the British Library

Library of Congress Cataloging in Publication data
A concise guide to understanding suicide : epidemiology, pathophysiology, and prevention / edited by
Stephen H. Koslow, Pedro Ruiz, Charles B. Nemeroff.
p. ; cm.
Includes bibliographical references and index.
ISBN 978-1-107-03323-8 (hardback)
I. Koslow, Stephen H., editor of compilation. II. Ruiz, Pedro, 1936–
editor of compilation. III. Nemeroff, Charles B., editor of compilation.
[DNLM: 1. Suicide – psychology. 2. Self-Injurious Behavior – epidemiology.
3. Self-Injurious Behavior – physiopathology. 4. Suicide – prevention &
control. WM 165]
RC569
616.85′8445–dc23
2013046220

ISBN 978-1-107-03323-8 Hardback

Contents

Contributors

Michael H. Allen, MD, VA, VISN
19 Mental Illness Research Education and Clinical Center (MIRECC), Denver, CO, USA, and Department of Psychiatry, University of Colorado School of Medicine, Aurora, CO, USA, and Prophase, LLC, New York, NY, USA

Leora Amira, PhD
Child and Adolescent Psychiatry, New York State Psychiatric Institute, Columbia University, New York, NY, USA

Victoria Arango, PhD
Professor, Columbia University and The New York State Psychiatric Institute, New York, NY, USA

David W. Ayer, PhD
Centerstone Research Institute, Bloomington, IN, USA

Helene Bach, PhD
Assistant Professor, Columbia University and The New York State Psychiatric Institute, New York, NY, USA

Christopher R. Bailey, BA
Johns Hopkins University School of Medicine, Baltimore, MD, USA

Ross J. Baldessarini, MD, DSc
Department of Psychiatry, Harvard Medical School and International Consortium for Bipolar Disorder Research, McLean Hospital, Boston, MA, USA

Kelsey Ball
Graduate Student, Department of Psychology, Howard University, Washington, DC, USA

Alan L. Berman, PhD
Executive Director, American Association of Suicidology, Washington, DC, USA

Marian E. Betz, MD, MPH
Department of Emergency Medicine, University of Colorado School of Medicine, Aurora, CO, USA

Emily A. Biggs, MA
New York State Psychiatric Institute, New York, NY, USA

R. Warwick Blood
Emeritus Professor of Communication, News and Media Research Centre, University of Canberra, Australia

Kathleen T. Brady, MD, PhD
Distinguished University Professor, and Director, South Carolina Clinical and Translational Research Institute, Medical University of South Carolina and Ralh H. Johnson V. A. Medical Center, Charleston, SC, USA

David A. Brent, MD
University of Pittsburgh Medical Center, Western Psychiatric Institute and Clinic, Pittsburgh, PA, USA

Jeffrey A. Bridge, PhD
The Research Institute at Nationwide Children's Hospital and The Ohio State University College of Medicine, Columbus, OH, USA

Gregory K. Brown, PhD
Department of Psychiatry, Perelman School of Medicine of the University of Pennsylvania, Philadelphia, PA, USA

Anat Brunstein Klomek, PhD
Senior Lecturer, School of Psychology, Interdisciplinary Center, Herzilya, Israel, and Adjunct Associate Research Scientist, Division of Child and Adolescent Psychiatry, College of Physicians and Surgeons, Columbia University, New York, NY, USA

Jacqueline Buchanan, A.
Child & Adolescent Psychiatry, New York State Psychiatric Institute, Coloumbia University, New York, NY, USA

Michelle J. Chandley, PhD
Department of Biomedical Sciences, James H. Quillen College of Medicine, East Tennessee State University, Johnson City, TN, USA

Tim Coffey
Project Coordinator for the Eleventh Judicial Circuit Criminal Mental Health Project Miami, FL, USA

Jessica Coker, MD
Department of Psychiatry, University of Arkansas for Medical Sciences, Little Rock, AR, USA

Yeates Conwell, MD
Professor of Psychiatry, University of Rochester School of Medicine, Rochester, NY, USA

Scott J. Crow, MD
Professor of Psychiatry, University of Minnesota, Minneapolis, MN, USA

Collin L. Davidson, PhD
VAVISN, 19 Mental Illness Research Education and Clinical Center (MIRECC), Denver, CO, USA, and Department of Psychiatry University of Colorado School of Medicine, Aurora, CO, USA

Yogesh Dwivedi, PhD
Professor of Psychiatry and Pharmacology, Department of Psychiatry, University of Illinois at Chicago, Chicago, IL, USA

Stacey Espaillat, MD
Department of Psychiatry and Behavioral Sciences, University of Miami, Miller School of Medicine, Miami, FL, USA

Jan Fawcett, MD
Professor, Department of Psychiatry, The University of New Mexico, Albuquerque, NM, USA

Steven J. Garlow, MD, PhD
Division of Child and Adolescent Psychiatry, Department of Psychiatry and Behavioral Sciences, Emory University School of Medicine, Atlanta, GA, USA

Robert D. Gibbons, PhD
Professor of Biostatistics, Departments of Health Studies, Medicine and Psychiatry, University of Chicago, Chicago, IL, USA

Catherine R. Glenn, PhD
Department of Psychology, Harvard University, Cambridge, MA, USA

Deborah Goebert, DrPH
Professor of Psychiatry and Public Health Sciences, University of Hawaii, John A. Burns School of Medicine, Honolulu, Hawaii, USA

Erica Goldstein, BS
Child & Adolescent Psychiatry, New York State Psychiatric Institute, Columbia University, New York, NY, USA

Tina R. Goldstein, PhD
University of Pittsburgh Medical Center, Western Psychiatric Institute and Clinic, Pittsburgh, PA, USA

Madelyn S. Gould, PhD, MPH
Professor, Division of Child and Adolescent Psychiatry, College of Physicians and Surgeons, Columbia University; Professor, Department of Epidemiology, School of Public Health, Columbia University; and Research Scientist, New York State Psychiatric Institute, New York, NY, USA

Kelly L. Green, PhD
Department of Psychiatry, Perelman School of Medicine of the University of Pennsylvania, Philadelphia, PA, USA

Alison M. Greene, BA
New York University, New York, NY, USA

Philip D. Harvey, PhD
Professor, Department of Psychiatry and Behavioral Sciences, University of Miami Miller School of Medicine, Miami, FL, USA

Robert M. A. Hirschfeld, MD
Titus H. Harris Chair, Harry K. Davis Professor, Chair, Department of Psychiatry, The University of Texas Medical Branch, Galveston, TX, USA

Donna Holland Barnes, PhD
Director, Suicide Prevention Program, Howard University, Washington, DC, USA

Andres M. Kanner, MD
Director, Comprehensive Epilepsy Center; Head, Section of Epilepsy, Department of Neurology; and Professor of Clinical Neurology and Psychiatry, University of Miami, Miller School of Medicine, Miami, FL, USA

Gary J. Kennedy, MD
Professor of Psychiatry and Behavioral Sciences, Albert Einstein College of Medicine; Director, Division of Geriatric Psychiatry and the Leslie and Rosalyn Goldstein Fellowship Training Program in Geriatric Psychiatry, Montefiore Medical Center, Bronx, NY, USA

Stephen H. Koslow, PhD, FAMCI
Science Consultant, Department of Psychiatry and Behavioral Sciences, Leonard M. Miller School of Medicine, University of Miami, Miami, FL; current position Director, U.S. Medical Affairs, CNS Otsuka America Pharmaceutical, Inc., Princeton, NJ, USA

Benoit Labonté, BA
McGill Group for Suicide Studies, Department of Psychiatry, McGill University, Montreal, QC, Canada

Alison M. Lake, MA
Project Director, Division of Child and Adolescent Psychiatry, New York State Psychiatric Institute, New York, NY, USA

William B. Lawson, MD, PhD
Chair, Department of Psychiatry, Howard University, Washington, DC, USA

Steve Leifman
Associate Administrative Judge for the County Court, Criminal Division of the Eleventh Judicial Circuit of Florida, Miami, FL, USA

Adam Lesser, MSW
Child & Adolescent Psychiatry, New York State Psychiatric Institute, Columbia University, New York, NY, USA

Timothy W. Lineberry, MD
Department of Psychiatry and Psychology, Mayo Clinic, Rochester, MN, USA

Amanda L. McMillan, MD
Division of Child and Adolescent Psychiatry, Department of Psychiatry and Behavioral Sciences, Emory University School of Medicine, Atlanta, GA, USA

Herbert Y. Meltzer, MD
Department of Psychiatry and Behavioral Sciences, Northwestern Feinberg School of Medicine, Chicago, IL, USA

Michael Craig Miller, MD
Senior Editor, Mental Health Publishing, Harvard Health Publications, Harvard Medical School, Boston, MA, USA

Michael J. Miller, PsyD, LP
Assistant Professor of Psychiatry, Department of Psychiatry, University of Minnesota, Minneapolis, MN, USA

James A. Naifeh, PhD
Research Assistant Professor, Department of Psychiatry, Uniformed Services University of the Health Sciences, Bethesda, MD, USA

Katharine J. Nelson, MD
Assistant Professor of Psychiatry, Department of Psychiatry, University of Minnesota, Minneapolis, MN, USA

Charles B. Nemeroff, MD, PhD
Leonard M. Miller Professor and Chairman, Department of Psychiatry and Behavioral Sciences, Leonard M. Miller School of Medicine, University of Miami, Miami, FL, USA

Alexander Neumeister, MD
Professor of Psychiatry and Radiology and Director, Molecular Imaging Program for Anxiety and Mood Disorders, New York University School of Medicine, New York, NY, USA

Matthew K. Nock, PhD
Department of Psychology, Harvard University, Cambridge, MA, USA

Jennifer H. Olson-Madden, PhD
VA Veteran's Integrated Service Network, 19 Mental Illness Research Education and Clinical Center (MIRECC), 1055 Clermont St, Denver, CO, USA, and Department of Psychiatry University of Colorado School of Medicine, Autora, CO, USA

Gregory A. Ordway, PhD
Department of Biomedical Sciences, James H. Quillen College of Medicine, East Tennessee State University, Johnson City, TN, USA

Michael W. Otto, PhD
Department of Psychology, Boston University, Boston, MA, USA

Ghanshyam N. Pandey, PhD
Department of Psychiatry, University of Illinois at Chicago, Chicago, IL, USA

Giampaolo Perna, MD, PhD
Department of Clinical Neurosciences, Villa San Benedetto Hospital, Hermanas Hospitalarias, FoRiPsi, Albese con Cassano, Italy; Department of Psychiatry and Neuropsychology, Faculty of Health, Medicine and Life Sciences, University of Maastricht, The Netherlands; and Department of Psychiatry and Behavioral Sciences, Leonard M. Miller School of Medicine, University of Miami, Miami, FL, USA

Jane Pirkis, BA(Hons), MPsych, MAppEpid, PhD
Professor and Director, Centre for Mental Health, The University of Melbourne, Melbourne, Australia

Kelly Posner
Director, Center for Suicide Risk Assessment, New York State Psychiatric Institute, Associate Clinical Professor of Medical Psychology (in Psychiatry), Coloumbia University College of Physicians and Surgeons, New York, NY, USA

Anne Rohs, MD
Assistant Professor of Psychiatry, Montefiore Medical Center, Bronx, NY, USA

Pedro Ruiz, MD
Professor, Executive Vice Chair and Director of Clinical Programs, Department of Psychiatry and Behavioral Sciences, Leonard M. Miller School of Medicine, University of Miami, Miami, FL, USA

Molly Ryan, DO, MPH
Department of Psychiatry and Behavioral Sciences, Leonard M. Miller School of Medicine, University of Miami, Miami, FL, USA

Alan F. Schatzberg, MD
Professor of Psychiatry and Behavioral Sciences, Stanford University School of Medicine, Stanford, CA, USA

S. Charles Schulz, MD
Professor and Head of Psychiatry, Department of Psychiatry, University of Minnesota, Minneapolis, MN, USA

M. Katherine Shear, MD
Professor of Psychiatry, Columbia University School of Social Work, Columbia University College of Physicians and Surgeons, New York, NY, USA

Morton M. Silverman, MD
Assistant Clinical Professor of Psychiatry, The University of Colorado Denver School of Medicine, Aurora, CO, USA

April R. Smith, PhD
Assistant Professor, Department of Psychology, University of Miami, Miami, FL, USA

Marcus Sokolowski, MD, PhD
Professor of Immunology, National Center for Suicide Research and Prevention of Mental Ill-Health, Karolinska Institute, Stockholm, Sweden

Barbara Stanley, PhD
Professor of Clinical Psychology in Psychiatry and Director, Suicide Intervention Center, Columbia University College of Physicians and Surgeons, New York, NY, USA

Zachary N. Stowe, MD
Department of Psychiatry, Department of Pediatrics, and Department of Obstetrics and Gynecology, University of Arkansas for Medical Sciences, Little Rock, AR, USA

Sarah A. Struthers, MD
Department of Psychiatry, UT Southwestern Medical Center, Dallas, TX, USA; formerly Medical Student at UTMB Galveston, Galveston, TX, USA

Leonardo Tondo, MD, MSc
Department of Psychiatry, Harvard Medical School and International Consortium for Bipolar Disorder Research, McLean Hospital, Boston, USA; Lucio Bini Mood Disorder Centers, Cagliari and Rome, Italy

Gustavo Turecki, MD, PhD
McGill Group for Suicide Studies, Department of Psychiatry, McGill University, Montreal, QC, Canada

Robert J. Ursano, MD
Professor and Chair, Department of Psychiatry, Uniformed Services University of the Health Sciences, and Director, Center for the Study of Traumatic Stress, Bethesda, MD, USA

Kimberly Van Orden, PhD
Assistant Professor of Psychiatry, University of Rochester School of Medicine, Rochester, NY, USA

Anne C. Ward, BS
Department of Psychology, Boston University, Boston, MA, USA

Danuta Wasserman, MD, PhD
Professor of Psychiatry and Suicidology, Karolinska Institute, Stockholm, Sweden

Jerzy Wasserman, MD, PhD
Professor of Immunology, National Center for Suicide Research and Prevention of Mental Ill-Health, Karolinska Institute, Stockholm, Sweden

Melinda K. Westlund, BA
Department of Psychiatry, University of Minnesota, Minneapolis, MN, USA

Tracy K. Witte, PhD
Assistant Professor, Department of Psychology, Auburn University, Auburn, AL, USA

Kseniya Yershova, PhD
Child & Adolescent Psychiatry, New York State Psychiatric Institute, Columbia University, New York, NY, USA

Alexandra Zagoloff, PhD
Assistant Professor of Psychiatry, Department of Psychiatry, University of Minnesota, Minneapolis, MN, USA

Sidney Zisook, MD
Professor of Psychiatry, University of California San Diego, San Diego, CA, USA

The following authors wish to declare a conflict of interest:

Michael H. Allen has received support from the VISN 19 Mental Illness Research Education and Clinical Center, NIMH and the Military Suicide Research Consortium but has no conflict of interest relevant to this work. The views expressed do not necessarily represent those of the Veterans Administration or the Government.

Marian E. Betz has received a consulting honorarium and grant funding from the American Foundation for Suicide Prevention, but has no support that would pose a conflict of interest in this work.

David A. Brent currently works for the University of Pittsburgh School of Medicine and University of Pittsburgh Medical Center, Western Psychiatric Institute in Clinic. He also has research projects funded by the National Institute of Mental Health. Other potential conflicts include I have or will receive royalties from Guilford Press, I have or will receive royalties from the electronic self-rated version of the C-SSRS from ERT, Inc., UpToDate Psychiatry Editor, I receive honoraria from presentations for Continuing Medical Education events.

Steven J. Garlow receives research support from the Dana Foundation and Hope Foundation and has been on scientific advisory board and speaker bureau for Eli Lilly Inc, in 2010 and earlier. He was previously on speaker bureau for GSK and Pfizer also before 2010. He has received research support from Janssen Pharmaceuticals.

Robert D. Gibbons has been an expert witness on cases related to issues involving drugs and suicide for the US Department of Justice, Wyeth, and Pfizer over the past 10 years.

Deborah Goebert has a state suicide prevention grant from the Substance Abuse and Mental Health Services Administration and a behavioral health services grant from The Queen's Medical Center and has no conflict of interest.

Tina R. Goldstein is currently employed by the University of Pittsburgh School of Medicine and University of Pittsburgh Medical Center, Western Psychiatric Institute and Clinic. She has research projects funded by the National Institute of Mental Health, the National Institute on Drug Abuse, the National Institute on Child Health and Human Development, and The Pittsburgh Foundation. She has and will receive royalties from Guilford Press.

Madelyn S. Gould receives royalties as an author of the Columbia Suicide Severity Rating Scale (C-SSRS).

Philip D. Harvey has contract funding from Genentech. He also serves as a consultant/advisory board member for Abbvie, Boeheringer Ingelheim, Forest Labs, Genentech, Otsuka America, Roche, Shire, Sunovion, and Takeda.

Robert M. A. Hirschfeld has received royalties from Jones and Bartlett, has been a consultant for Grey Healthcare, Biostrategies, Merck Manual Editorial Board, Equinox Group and has received honorarium from Physicians Post Graduate Press, Health and Wellness Partners, Merck Manual Editorial Board, CME Outfitters, Letters & Sciences, Nevada Psychiatric Association, and CMEology.

Gary J. Kennedy has received grant support from Eli Lilly of less than $10 000 in the last 3 years but it has not influenced the content of his contribution to his chapter.

Timothy W. Lineberry is a Board Member of Institute for Clinical Symptoms Improvement and Government expert Military Suicide Prevention.

Herbert Y. Meltzer conflicts of interests include: *ownership/investment interests* – Suregene, ACADIA, and GlaxoSmithKline; *industry activities*, such as speaking, advising, consulting, providing educational programs with Janssen Pharmaceuticals, Lundbeck Inc., Sunovion Pharmaceuticals Inc (Dainippon Sumitomo Pharma Co., Ltd), TEVA, BiolineRx, BI (Boehringer Ingelheim Pharma GmbH & Co. KG), Envivo, Companion Diagnostics; and *expert testimony* – Janssen.

Charles B. Nemeroff has received research/grants from: National Institutes of Health (NIH), Agency for Healthcare Research and Quality (AHRQ); *consulting*: Xhale, Takeda, SK Pharma, Shire, Roche, Lilly, Allergan, Mitsubishi Tanabe Pharma Development America, Taisho Pharmaceutical Inc.; *stockholder*: CeNeRx BioPharma, PharmaNeuroBoost, Revaax Pharma, Xhale; *other financial interests*: CeNeRx BioPharma, PharmaNeuroBoost; *patents*: Method and devices for transdermal delivery of lithium (US 6 375 990B1), Method of assessing antidepressant drug therapy via transport inhibition of monoamine neurotransmitters by ex vivo assay (US 7,148,027B2); *scientific advisory boards*: American Foundation for Suicide Prevention (AFSP), CeNeRx BioPharma (2012), National Alliance for Research on Schizophrenia and Depression (NARSAD), Xhale, PharmaNeuroBoost (2012), Anxiety Disorders Association of America (ADAA), Skyland Trail, AstraZeneca Pharmaceuticals (2009); Board of Directors: AFSP, Mt. Cook Pharma (2010), NovaDel (2011), Skyland Trail, Gratitude America, ADAA; *income sources or equity of $10 000 or more*: AstraZeneca Pharmaceuticals, PharmaNeuroBoost, CeNeRx BioPharma, NovaDel Pharma, Reevax Pharma, American Psychiatric Publishing, Xhale; *honoraria*: various; *royalties*: various; *expert witness*; various.

Michael W. Otto has in the past 2 years served as a paid consultant for MicroTransponder Inc., Concert Pharmaceuticals, and ProPhase; and received royalty support for use of the SIGH-A from ProPhase.

Kelly Posner receives no remuneration from clinical practice users of the C-SSRS, as its use is free. She receives royalty payments from the e-CSSRS, which are distributed to her by her employer, the Research Foundation for Mental Hygiene.

Alan F. Schatzberg has been a consultant to Bay City Capital, CeNeRx, Cervel, Eli Lilly, Genentech, Gilead, Lunbeck/Takeda, McKinsey, Merck, MSI, Neuronetics, PharmaNeuroBoost, and Xhale. He has equity in Amnestix, BrainCells, Cervel, Corcept (co-founder), Delpor, Forest, Merck, Neurocrine, Pfizer, and Xhale. He is a named inventor on pharmacogenetic and antiglucocorticoid use patents on prediction of antidepressant response. He has received speaker honoraria from Merck.

S. Charles Schulz is reporting Grant/research support from: NIMH, Astra-Zeneca, Myriad/RBM, Otsuka; and Consultant for Eli Lilly, Genentech.

M. Katherine Shear has a book contract with Guilford Press for publication of a treatment manual for complicated grief. Other than that, she has no conflicts of interest to declare and no other financial relationships relevant to the subject of her chapter.

Zachary N. Stowe. Life time disclosure (no outside relationships since June 2008): he has received research support from GSK and Wyeth, served on advisory boards for Wyeth, BMS, and GSK, and received speakers' honoraria from Eli Lilly, GSK, Pfizer, and Wyeth.

Introduction

Looking to the future: how can research prevent suicide?

Stephen H. Koslow, Pedro Ruiz, and Charles B. Nemeroff

Suicide is a leading cause of mortality and morbidity. Suicide represents a major public health problem based on the fact that there are more than 1 000 000 suicides worldwide and approximately 40 000 in the United States per year. Many people throughout the world have therefore had direct experience with a suicide by having a relative, friend, or acquaintance solve their problems by taking their own life. This is a devastating experience, which on the surface is hard to understand and hard to recover from. Reducing the suicide rate and ultimately preventing suicide is a challenging task. The chapters in this Guide were developed to provide state of the art information on what is known about suicide, how we currently study it, and how we can reduce its frequency. The latter is the most important goal. Currently most preventive efforts are aimed at erecting physical barriers to suicide and/or hospitalization. None of these efforts are totally effective.

We designed this Guide for several audiences including clinicians and researchers but also others interested in this topic. The chapters that comprise this monograph are purposefully concise but are sufficiently comprehensive. It has been organized into sections on a common theme starting with a series of reports on understanding suicide that provide a context for the remainder of the book. This Guide goes on to provide information ranging from specific psychiatric disorders of unique "special" at risk populations highlighting the context of suicide and treatment within these illnesses and populations, through mediators and moderators of suicide from societal to biological mechanisms, including genomics, and ending with suicide prevention.

What makes suicide prevention and research so difficult? This theme is focused on throughout this volume. The answer is manifold and includes: (a) the incidence of suicide is low compared to other illnesses making subject availability low; (b) there is no accurate method to determine if any individual is going to take their own life in the next day(s) or year(s); and (c) potential suicide is based on a variety of factors which includes signs and symptoms and assessment of high-risk cognitive states or high-risk behavior, but there are obvious differences between suicide attempts and completed suicides. Studying the brains of subjects who have taken their life ensures that your sample is from a suicide; however whether the biology underlying suicide is transient or lasting and the debate as to whether there is a unique biology of suicide that cuts across diagnostic categories versus suicide as a symptom of various disorders with their own unique biology remain unresolved. One of the most important areas for research is obviously the development of an accurate, sensitive, and specific method to detect suicide potential. This can be a behavioral measure, clinical signs or symptoms, or a biological marker. All of these are active areas of research.

Promising data is offered from genetics research. Current major approaches, all with advantages and disadvantages, include Genome-Wide Association Studies (GWAS), candidate gene studies, and epigenetics. GWAS is an examination of many common genetic variants in large populations to determine if any variant is associated with a trait. GWAS typically focus on associations between single nucleotide polymorphisms (SNPs) and disease traits. Candidate gene studies focus on SNPs in systems previously implicated to be involved in the pathogenesis of suicide, such as serotonin. Epigenetics focuses on genes that are impacted and changed due to the environment. Both GWAS and epigenetics studies can be conducted from completed suicides. Here the biggest challenge again is the relative low incidence of suicide in the general population compared to, for example, diabetes or

A Concise Guide to Understanding Suicide, ed. Stephen H. Koslow, Pedro Ruiz, and Charles B. Nemeroff. Published by Cambridge University Press.

hypertension, rendering it difficult to get the large samples needed for GWAS. Similarly epigenetics reports are more often based on small numbers of subjects and use postmortem brain tissue. Additional research in this area is warranted given the paramount importance of identifying a biological marker for suicide. Clearly large sample GWAS studies, candidate gene studies, and more epigenetics studies on well-defined patient populations and controls are warranted.

Another major research goal is to integrate findings across high-risk populations including patients with mood and anxiety disorders, schizophrenia, personality disorders, substance abuse, eating disorders, epilepsy, and child and adolescent disorders as well as specific high-risk populations such as the armed forces, emergency room, bereavement and grief, college students, other medical illnesses, pregnancy, postpartum depression, LGBT, and older adults in order to distill core mediators and moderators leading to suicide and understand the biology underpinning these changes. To do this effectively and efficiently we need to develop and agree upon developed standard instruments to use in common in all these studies which are quantitative and objective. Subjective assessments are often biased and affected by the rater's experience and do not provide acceptable inter-rater reliability between individual raters. An excellent example of the ability to integrate among and between studies are the emerging imaging studies. These studies have different diagnostic groups; the selection of suicidal subject is based on various criteria including suicidal behavior, previous attempters, suicidal ideation, and seriousness of the attempt. Different imaging modalities have been employed including structural MRI, fMRI, DTI, SPECT, and PET. All of these are a rich source of direct brain data and we need to integrate these data across population and structure, function, neural circuitry and receptor/transporter binding which have yielded and will continue to yield new insights into the underlying neural suicide circuit. These could then be the groups studied for neuroregulatory systems and genomic expressions yielding both new information for understanding the processes involved in suicide, as well as new targets for pharmacological, genetic, or other interventions.

In this Guide specific sections focus on the behavioral assessments and clinical signs and symptoms currently used to assess suicidality in subjects who are deemed at risk. These include hopelessness, helplessness, described suicidal behaviors or intention to carry out suicide, comorbid substance abuse, and/or alcohol abuse as well as specific alterations in cognitive functions including decision-making. Understanding the neural network and processes involved in decision-making may start to provide insights into the altered thinking and decision-making that often occur in suicidal individuals. Other important risk factors discussed in this volume include age, trauma history, family history, past personal history of suicidality, and of most promise biological markers including genetics. It is paramount to develop a standardized objective assessment to be used in all studies. If this is accomplished we can begin to create databases to achieve adequate analytical statistical power.

Currently two drugs which appear efficacious in preventing suicide in specific populations are lithium and clozapine. Whether these drugs have specific antisuicidal properties or reduce suicide because of their superior efficacy remains unresolved. Should these drugs be used in other populations specifically for suicide prevention? To address this question requires a large-scale clinical trial of both drugs. The question of the dose required to produce an antisuicidal effect is important because at the doses they are currently clinically used they are often poorly tolerated and have unacceptable side effects. Low doses of either of these drugs may be effective in suicide prevention. Equally important is determining which psychotherapies are most likely to reduce suicide.

In summary and conclusion the research on suicide should focus on:

1. Development of a valid, easily usable algorithm predicting suicide risk with high sensitivity and specificity
2. Definition of biological markers that correlate with the predictor algorithm (1) above
3. Mapping the neural circuitry and the biological mechanisms involved in suicide
4. Development of effective and specific antisuicide treatments including pharmacological and/or psychotherapeutic
5. Establishment of an objective standardized assessment to be used in all studies on suicide.

Chapter 1

Brief history of suicide in Western cultures

Leonardo Tondo

Introduction

Western culture has never been completely indifferent toward those who take their own lives. Attitudes and beliefs concerning suicide have been complex and varied over the centuries. Some suicides were considered heroes, but mostly suicide was considered an offense against God, an insult to the state, or a particularly painful gesture toward those left behind after an an unexplained death. Yet, considerable tolerance toward suicide is evident in ancient times when death was more frequently encountered in everyday experience than in modern times. Nevertheless, suicide was punished as a criminal act in many cultures for centuries before becoming a medical-psychological issue in our current society and culture.

The contest between reason and passion

Since ancient Greece, suicide was not accepted, though most cases were not explicitly blamed for having committed a criminal act. Since the fourth century BCE, suicides usually were denied burial or traditional pre-burial preparation or cremation and were considered to have committed a greviously antisocial act. In Athens, for instance, the hand of a suicide was cut off and buried away from the rest of the body (Manson, 1899). Only suicides in which it was possible to find sufficient reason for self-destruction were deemed comprehensible; such reasons might include heroism, love-rejection, or serious and painful illness. Other suicides were considered to be unjustified and were punished; examples include soldiers who had deserted or criminals avoiding punishment or prison. The standard of "understanding" was – and largely still is – considered the key to assessing suicide as a justified action. Even nowadays, the suicide of a young healthy person is likely not to be "understood," whereas that of an elderly person with a terminal illness may seem more reasonable.

Judgments concerning suicide changed when ancient Greek philosophers became interested in the primacy of reason over the emotions. Their influence became dominant and continued to influence Western culture and the great religions to modern times. The dominant view has been that suicide was an immoral or criminal act. Early philosophers based their prohibition of suicide primarily on the basis of its incomprehensibility or irrationality. It was viewed as an aberration against the natural urge of the individual to survive, and became interpreted in the Jewish, Christian, and Moslem religions as an insult to God. Many cultures of ancient times as well as of today have tried to subject the emotional side of the individual to rational control. This fundamental principle has guided many laws and customs seeking to impose limits on the expression of emotion-driven behaviors. Religions borrowed the thinking of the Greek philosophers and transformed many passions into sins with the simple equation that rational behavior is directed by God, and the irrational by the Devil (Tondo, 2000).

Ancient cultures

A possibly first recorded suicide dates from the era of Egyptian Pharaoh Ramses II (1303–1213 BCE), in a written description of the story of two brothers who had committed suicide nearly two centuries previously. At that time, death was often actively sought for various reasons, to the point that groups gathered to discuss the least unpleasant ways to die, and it seems likely that was sufficiently frequent as often to pass unnoticed (Moron, 1976).

A Concise Guide to Understanding Suicide, ed. Stephen H. Koslow, Pedro Ruiz, and Charles B. Nemeroff. Published by Cambridge University Press.

The spirit of ancient Greece (mainly from the 5th and 4th centuries BCE) highlights a widespread melancholy toward life that encouraged appreciation for its end, in contrast with limited acceptance of suicide. A rejection of life, joined with a deep spirit of freedom characterized the Epicurean, Stoic, and Cynical philosophical schools to support decisions to die. Many celebrities of the time killed themselves, including the philosophers Empedocles, Democritus (to avoid old age), Diogenes, Zeno (held his breath after falling at the age of 98 years), Hegesias, Cleanthes (held deep contempt of life), Socrates (forced to kill himself), and poets including Sappho (love pain), Aristodemus (remorse), Cleomenes (honor), Demosthenes and Isocrates (both for patriotic reasons). Heroic suicide or self-sacrifice was almost unanimously approved in ancient Greece, and often was considered an example to follow. Kodros, the last legendary king of Athens, probably would have killed himself to avoid loss of a battle with the Dorians, as prophesied by the oracle of Delphi, but was killed by the Dorians. Themistocles, according to some historians, killed himself because of guilt resulting from his betrayal of Athens to join the service of the Persian king.

Plato (424–347 BCE), however, was opposed to suicide. He claimed that men are social individuals with responsibility to others and therefore property of a state that could not afford loss of its citizens. Along the same line, Aristotle (383–322 BCE) disapproved of suicide, seeing it as a transgression against a civic duty and an act of cowardice. He states (Moore, 1790):

> The law never commands a man to kill himself; but what it does not command, it forbids. Moreover, when any one hurts another contrary to law, having received no previous injury from him, he voluntarily commits an injury against that man ... Now when anyone, impelled by anger or resentment, kills himself, he does this voluntarily against right law, because the law does not permit it ... But [against] whom? Rather to the state than to himself ... To die only in order to avoid poverty, or [for] love, or uneasiness of any kind, is not the character of a brave, but rather of a servile spirit. For it is the part of an effeminate mind to fly from calamitous and laborious situations.

In ancient Rome, suicide was not a rare event. Grisé (1982) describes 314 suicides among prominent Romans between the 5th and 2nd centuries CE. For different reasons, but always with a character of integrity, many prominent politicians killed themselves rather than being subjected to Caesar; they included Cato Uticensis, Appius Claudius, Atticus, Crassus, Anthony, Brutus, Cassius, and Quintilio Publius Varus. Even the Roman emperors Marcus Cocceius Nerva and Nero killed themselves. In 69 CE, the year following the death of Emperor Nero, 32 politicians committed suicide. Suicides in Imperial Rome included many famous writers and philosophers, including Diodorus, Seneca, Petronius, Lucan, and Lucretius. The two prominent philosophical schools of ancient Rome, Epicureanism and Stoicism, approved of suicide for different reasons. The Epicureans stated that the goal of man was the pursuit of happiness and, when this could not be achieved, life lost its purpose. The Stoics placed reason, virtue, and morality above pleasures and common interests, sometimes to the point of reaching a state of detachment and a lack of interest in life. This philosophy influenced the laws so that weariness for life (*tædium vitæ*) leading to suicide was approved if it resulted from incurable diseases, accidents, deaths of others, or even from squalor or wounded pride (Manson, 1899).

Although suicide was culturally accepted, Seneca considered death as a refuge against the evils of life, but did not support suicide. He emphasized control of the emotions and submission to the will of superiors, according to the light of reason, but these principles led to his own suicide when ordered to do so by Emperor Nero for alleged treason.

The Neo-Platonic philosophers saw suicide as the result of a disturbance. However, Plotinus (204–270 CE), the most important leader of the movement, argued that this type of death prevented the soul from breaking away from the body, making it impossible to reach the Elysian Fields.

In general, in ancient Rome free men (but not slaves) could choose to commit suicide without problems. In fact suicide was praised for widows who followed their husbands after death, or had been raped (e.g., Lucretia), and for men who wanted to avoid dishonor or were becoming old (Minois 1999). Nevertheless, suicide was widely considered dishonorable or a crime from the 6th century, particularly by soldiers (as well as in feudal Japan), slaves, and embezzlers.

Despite several exceptions, the general attitude toward suicide in ancient Greece and Rome was relatively tolerant, and suicide was considered legitimate in many circumstances, especially when life was no longer considered worth living, based on philosophical principles or even individual judgment.

Early Christianity

Christianity spread easily, especially among the most wretched, offering hope for a better life, at least in the next world. At the same time, it had to stand against reaching them too early in order to avoid losing too many of the faithful too quickly. Initially, Church attitudes about death resulted in a propensity toward it so that for several centuries, religious writings counted enthusiastic stories of martyrs. However, in ca. 420, St. Augustine (353–430) forbade suicide in his *City of God*, considering it an act against God as an extension of the fifth Commandment to Moses (*Thou shalt not kill*). Suffering, rather than being deemed a reason to commit suicide, became a positive value that only increased the worthiness of those who would bear it (Manson, 1899).

With Roman Emperor Constantine (272–337), Christianity became the official religion of the Roman Empire, and was supported by law from the 4th century. Sanctions by the church and the state against suicide gradually became increasingly strict and punitive, including confiscation of property if suicide was a means of avoiding a legal trial (interpreted as an admission of guilt). It is likely that early legal and religious views were very similar – probably less spiritual and more practical, if not partly economic. It was important, even for the civil power of Rome, to encourage interest in life, given the high mortality of the times and life expectancy of less than 40 years, and concern about maintaining the population of a vast empire that needed an enormous amount of labor. In fact, in the year 374, infanticide was banned by Roman law, and soon suicide by servants or slaves also was outlawed, as well as for the military, who were considered property of their owners or of the state.

However, a problem of no small importance arose: how to punish criminal suicides after their death? Gradually increasingly imaginative and dramatic forms of brutality to the bodies of suicides arose, not only for a symbolically directly punitive effect, but also for a spectacular and hopefully deterrent effect upon onlookers. Legal authorities collected the assets of suicides, and the Church increasingly attempted to avoid the loss of the faithful by discouraging the practice of voluntary martyrdom. It is also surely not a coincidence that, in the same era, the Church emphasized the sacredness of marriage, the blessing of procreation of many children, as well as the repression of all non-procreative sexuality as a sin.

Hebraism

Old Testament (probably written between the 9th and 5th centuries BCE) reports on five suicides not associated with a sinful judgment. However, it required that the body of a suicide could not be buried until sunset and without the usual rites. Laws and customs had been continued through oral tradition, and were transcribed by rabbinical scholars in the Mishnah between the 2nd and 3rd centuries. It taught that a suicide's body should not receive respect from family and friends. However, this prohibition was enforced only if the act was intentional and without external pressure, whereas suicide was considered as natural death if the act was induced by a mental illness or by the fear of a terrible torture.

The Committee of Jewish Law and Standards (1998) affirmed the prohibition of suicide, but supported an obligation of understanding why some people think of suicide, so as to ameliorate those circumstances. Even for terminally ill patients, increased pain control is recommended.

Despite that suicide is forbidden in Judaism through the same arguments proposed by Christians, there may be some extreme circumstances where a choice other than suicide is impossible. Such was the case in the mass suicide at the siege of Masada (73–74 CE) when more than 900 Jews killed themselves instead of falling prisoner to the Romans.

Islamism

As in the other Abrahamic, monotheistic religions, for Islam suicide is one of the worst possible sins. Unlike the Old Testament in which there is no explicit condemnation of suicide, the Koran warns: "Do not kill yourselves, certainly Allah will be more merciful with you." In several other passages of the holy Islamic text, there are warnings against suicide. In fact, most early Islamic scholars forbade suicide even in the case of terroristic attacks, citing that Koranic verse. This prohibition seems not to have prevented Islamic fundamentalists from killing themselves through the ages as well as currently, sometimes while killing scores of other persons.

Muhammad (570–632) taught that it is necessary to submit to divine will under any circumstance. For this same reason, the Islamic religion does not allow any form of euthanasia. Suicide is so sinful in Islamic countries that it would explain why official data on it are lacking or extremely low – much lower than among Muslims living in Western countries.

Middle Ages

Mass suicides occasionally occurred at the end of banquets in Scandinavia as a means of gaining entry to Valhalla, possibly close to Odin's seat – normally, a concession granted only to those who had died violently but courageously in battle, but then extended even to those who self-inflicted death (Moore, 1790). The Gauls and Visogoths sometimes elected suicide to avoid being enslaved by the Romans and to reach heaven (Moron, 1976). Yet, through their contact with the Romans, these northern peoples eventually absorbed Roman laws regarding voluntary death (Manson, 1899).

Perhaps in part to avoid legal penalties, suicide was replaced by medieval knights with violent and dangerous practices, such as tournaments or duels. Indeed, the Church synods of 813 (Châlons), 829 (Paris), and 855 (Valence) in France declared that duel to death was prohibited.

Theodore of Tarsus (602–690 CE), Archbishop of Canterbury, acknowledged the Roman tradition of legal non-liability in cases involving obvious lack of rationality at the time of suicide. This tradition was incorporated into English law and later accepted by the Church of England following the reign of King Henry VIII (1491–1547). Early English laws against suicide are attributed to King Edgar I of England (943–975) and were promulgated in 967 CE, including the distinction maintained over the centuries between those who committed suicide when of sound mind or were insane (*non compos mentis*). That is, suicide was not considered a sinful or criminal act in cases of insanity. English laws of that time also included the provision that the goods of a suicide had to be forfeited to the state, and did not exclude other forms of punishment or defilement carried out on the dead bodies of suicides.

During the brief Viking conquest of England (1013–1042), the Danish rulers supported the confiscation of goods from suicides. In *De Legibus et Consuetidinibus Angliae* (*Treatise on the Laws and Customs of the Kingdom of England*; ca. 1188), Henry of Bracton formulated the relationship between crime and intent in suicide by importing Roman law as interpreted by the school of Bologna. He stated that: (a) a suicide could not have heirs, and his goods were to be confiscated by the Crown because his act was an admission of criminal guilt; (b) this measure could not be implemented if the suicide had not been accused of crimes, (c) movable assets were confiscated from those who suicided for apparent weariness of life, severe physical pain or grief, but the family would inherit their real estate. In the same document, a difference was drawn between suicides resulting from *felo de se* (crime against himself) versus *non compos mentis*. In England, consideration of the issue of confiscating the property of suicides became increasingly sophisticated following its first application (MacDonald & Murphy, 1990).

MacDonald and Murphy (1990) report evidence from the King's Bench which show a steady increase in suicides in England from 1510 to 1590, and an initial criminal (*felo de se*) judgment in 95% of such cases. There was an evident conflict of interest in the certification of suicide. It is quite likely that this increase reflected payment of a fee to coroners in the case of a verdict of voluntary or criminal suicide resulting in the confiscation of goods by the Crown. However, coroners could sometimes be persuaded to make judgments of mental illness after receiving bribes greater than their "commission," and these were gladly paid by the families of many suicides. With the passing of centuries, English laws gradually were interpreted less strictly and mental illness was recognized more frequently among suicides, to the point of recognizing the very act of suicide as an indication of mental illness after 1600.

Laws concerning confiscation of property of suicides gradually spread across Europe and were applied unless the suicide was associated with insanity. Starting in about 1600, attitudes in European legal systems toward suicide became more indulgent and less punitive. In the 1700s, the majority of suicides were judged to be based on mental illness (*non compos mentis*). It is also likely that the accuracy, recording, and reporting of data from the English courts since the Middle Ages led to increased awareness of the issues surrounding suicide, and may have contributed to the steady decrease in suicides from about 1700 to modern times. Even today, the English suicide rate is far less than that in other European countries, although suicide rates vary markedly among countries, within regions, and over time (Baldessarini et al., 2007).

Throughout Europe between the 18th and 20th centuries, many ordinary people entangled hopelessly in wretched living conditions committed suicide, evidently in despair (Minois, 1999). Hanging was a prevalent method among both commoners and aristocrats. If they were publicly acknowledged at all, such acts committed by aristocrats might be considered honorable. However, for the poor, suicide usually was considered cowardly and a way of avoiding responsibility, calling for selective and furious punishment and retribution. It was also deemed noble and understandable when Christians who did not want to fall into Ottoman hands carried out collective suicides, or for a woman to take her life in order to avoid sexual assault. In addition, deaths in war were considered heroic even when preceded by the killing of many other human beings.

The clergy could arrange for suicides to avoid punishments or refusal of burial in consecrated ground by ascribing suicide to physical or mental illnesses, again often citing suicide itself as evidence of mental illness (Minois, 1999). In addition, many Christians enacted mystical forms of suicide with their isolation from the world until dying of starvation or thirst.

MacDonald and Murphy (1990) reported that suicide rates among the rich in early modern England (18th and 19th centuries) were much lower than in the lower classes, which increased during periods of poor harvest, hunger, and disease. Ironically, people who were punished for suicide most often were laborers or peasants with little property to confiscate, leaving their families impoverished even further.

The Italian Dominican priest, Thomas Aquinas (1225–1274) adduced several reasons to condemn suicide: it was an act against nature and against the benevolence we should have toward ourselves, and therefore considered a mortal sin. It was also an insult against the community to which we belong and to which we have duties. Finally, it represents an act of usurpation of the laws of God who gave us life and is the only one who may decide to take it back (Manson, 1899). Aquinas concluded that, *Whoever kills himself sins against God* (Clark, 2000).

Following strong ecclesiastical condemnations of suicide from the 12th century onwards, jurists viewed suicide as requiring punishment in addition to the eternal damnation expected by canon law. This view led to severe sanctions concerning disposition of the bodies of suicides: often they were not buried, were dismembered or left as food for the animals, exposed at crossroads, buried under large boulders, dragged through the streets face-down, taken out of the house through a window or a passage under the threshold of the house, or nailed to a barrel and left to drift at sea (Minois, 1999). It was believed that the body of a suicide could contaminate the land, lakes or rivers, that if a pregnant woman approached the burial site of a suicide, her offspring would follow the same fate. The spirits of suicides were considered vengeful and able to evoke anger and despair in those who came in contact with them. Of note, it was believed that suicide was a result of anger (more than melancholy), which could be aimed at the survivors (Kushner 1989).

In France, suicides were hanged by their feet and dragged through the streets as a warning to others (Minois, 1999). Similar procedures were followed in Germany, and included exposure of the unburied corpse, as well as removal of stones on which a suicide had walked. In Zurich, the Swiss stipulated, precisely, that a person who had stabbed himself was to have an awl driven into his head, those who had drowned were to be buried in the sand two meters from the lake shore, and those who had died by jumping off a cliff should be buried under a pile of stones.

Although spectacular, the retributions inflicted on the bodies of suicides apparently did not have a desired deterrent effect. Nevertheless, such fury continued for centuries. The last known abuse of the bodies of suicides occurred in Paris in 1749 and London as recently as 1823 (Minois, 1999).

Renaissance and Enlightenment

During the Renaissance (14th to 17th centuries) living conditions and culture improved markedly, and there was a renewed interest in the teachings of the classical Mediterranean world. This renewal of scholarship and learning was greatly facilitated by rapid adoption of the printing press in the 16th century. This process brought reminders that suicides had included many prominent ancient leaders or philosophers, as reviewed above, and their popularization tended again to cast doubt about the sinful or criminal nature of suicide.

Growing interest in humanism resulted in frank admiration for suicide in which intellectuals found an implicit message of freedom. The revaluation of suicide in that period manifested itself in the appreciation for Lucretia (in the early Roman Republic, 5th century BCE), whose suicide after being raped was featured in *De Claris Mulieribus* (*Of Famous Women*) by Giovanni Boccaccio (1313–1375), in the *Divina Commedia* (*Divine Comedy*) by Dante Alighieri (1265–1321) among the noble spirits of Limbo, and in more than one hundred paintings produced between the 1360s and the early 20th century (Cutter, 1983).

In addition, the Protestant Reformation stimulated growth of individual thinking and efforts to set aside the rules and rigidity of the Catholic Church, as notably manifested in the Inquisition.

This development strongly favored a more liberal and questioning attitude toward suicide. Civil and religious convictions resisted acceptance of suicide, but one could discuss the matter more openly and relatively freely.

Sebastian Brant (1457–1521) in his poem *The Ship of Fools* (1494) justifies suicide as a means of eliminating the suffering of life. Desiderius Erasmus of Rotterdam (1466–1536) in his *Praise of Folly* (1511) expressed sympathy for suicide as a way out of a life full of problems and evils, although he still considered suicide an insane act.

In this period a high number of suicides were recorded throughout Europe. Nevertheless, doubts remain about the accuracy of the reports since estimated rates of suicide were easily distorted or misrepresented, including being inflated, perhaps in response to increased attention afforded to the phenomenon by philosophers, writers, and moralists.

In 1594, William Shakespeare (1564–1616) wrote the poem *The Rape of Lucretia*, which stresses the political effect of her suicide during the transition from monarchy to republic in ancient Rome. In the following 40 years in the early 1600s, more than 200 suicides of characters appeared in British theatrical works. The dramatic effect of suicide fits very well in a play associated with special events, often romantic in nature, and suicide was sometimes used for the conclusion of a drama, with cathartic effect. In Shakespeare's plays, suicides involved famous characters of the classical world (Anthony and Cleopatra), or were for love (Romeo and Juliet), blame (Othello) or despair (Ophelia), and Hamlet debated whether to live or die. These works anticipated an association between suicide and melancholy.

The most intense expression of the English debate on suicide was by clergyman John Donne (1572–1631) in an essay on the topic, *Biathanatos* (*Violent Death*), where he wrote about the "paradox" that self-murder is not a sin against nature (1647). Donne, despite being an Anglican clergyman and the Dean of Saint Paul's Cathedral in London, justified suicide. Nevertheless, evidently owing to its controversial content, his book initially was shown only to close friends and finally published 16 years after Donne's death. In it, he argued that suicide was not contrary to nature, as there were other ways of mortification of human nature imposed by civilization. Human nature was guided by rationality and it could be considered appropriate to commit suicide and not contrary to reason. Moreover, Roman law had not condemned it for a long time. Donne also rejected the persisting argument that suicide deprives the army of a soldier, since soldiers could retire from military life without being condemned. A further point concerned the development of the divine law. Donne had no difficulty in arguing that the Bible did not condemn suicide, though murder was deemed sinful. A further irony is that many more men die during wars and are considered patriotic or even heroic than those who die by their own hand.

English political philosopher, Thomas Hobbes (1588–1679) saw suicide as a destructive act against natural law, and therefore should not be allowed. However, suicide could not be considered illegal, even accepting the Platonic position on the loss of an individual belonging to the community. Also the relatively moderate French philosopher, René Descartes (1596–1650) argued against suicide pragmatically, in considering that leaving the safe for the uncertain did not make sense, that life is not always happy but often offers consolation, and that good things may be even more frequent than bad ones. He rejected the idea of sin and punishment with regard to suicide. He believed these considerations to be unnecessary, since suicide is a punishment by itself. Finally, in a letter, Descartes expressed doubts about the mental health of suicides (Minois, 1999).

Robert Burton (1577–1640) of Oxford, in his *Anatomy of Melancholy* (1621) saw suicide in a much more modern view than his contemporaries. For the first time, he suggested the presence of mental illness behind suicidal behavior, considering melancholy of the Hippocratic and Galenic traditions. He put suicide in a non-religious, contemporary perspective and described conditions contributing to suicide, including agitation, hopelessness, and impulsivity. Nevertheless, most writers of the next century continued to oppose suicide, supported by ecclesiastical powers (Brown, 2001).

In 1788 English physician William Rowley (1742–1806) wrote *A Treatise on Female, Nervous, Hysterical, Hypocondriacal, Bilious, Convulsive Diseases; Apoplexy and Palsy with Thoughts on Madness, Suicide, et cetera, in Which the Principal Disorders are Explained from Anatomical Facts, and the Treatment Formed on Several New Principles.* It reiterated the views of previous centuries, arguing that suicide was an act against religion and so a crime against civil society because it deprived others of expected physical and mental services, and was immoral for being contrary to the individual's duties to maintain relational ties. Following such thinking, Rowley attacked the ideas of Jean-Jacques Rousseau (1712–1778) as expressed in *Julie, la Nouvelle Héloïse* (*Julie, The New Eloise*; 1761):

> Seeking good and avoiding evil when you do not cause harm to others, it is a law of nature. When life becomes bad for us and it is not good for anyone, we can get rid of it.

Rowley's position was mainly utilitarian in seeing only the duties of men toward one another. However, he introduced advanced ideas concerning *remote* causes of suicide, which might include mental illness (*insania*) or bodily pain. In addition, he described *proximate* causes, including not being sufficiently brave or balanced as to endure misfortunes, or basically, not being of sound mind (*non compos mentis*). He noted that, "In every violent passion there is a degree of madness." He concluded that, when an individual contemplates suicide, his mental status must necessarily be compromised.

Rowley's condemnation of suicide was out of keeping with contrary trends that had been evolving on the Continent. For example, two centuries earlier, French Renaissance writer, Michel Eyquem de Montaigne (1533–1592) spoke in his *Essais* (*Essays*; 1580) quite favorably about suicide: "death makes life precious, but at the same time decrees its vanity." Following the footsteps of suicides in the classical period, he argued that "the wise man lives as much as he ought to, not as much as he can" and even if he thought that "death . . . is the remedy for every illness." Nevertheless, in his essays, Montaigne did not encourage anyone to commit suicide, and moreover, although he became very ill and was in a constant pain, he did not hasten his own end. His point of view is close to that of those who must deal with a person at risk of suicide: understanding the wish to die, but at the same time making all efforts to avoid it. Charles-Louis Baron de Montesquieu (1689–1755) in his *Lettres Persanes* (*Persian Letters*; 1721) spoke of legal convictions for suicide as an injustice because, "if the gift of life is a blessing, it is justifiable to give it up when it seems no longer to be a blessing." French Enlightenment philosopher Voltaire (François-Marie Arouet [1694–1778]), more than many other writers influenced thinking about suicide in the direction of liberalism, defending self-destruction in cases of extreme necessity.

Another tolerant view of suicide was expressed by Scottish Enlightenment philosopher David Hume (1711–1776) in his *Essays on Suicide and the Immortality of the Soul* (1755). He stated that suicide could not be seen as an offense against God. It was not condemned in the Bible and he considered the Augustinian interpretation of suicide as homicide and therefore against the fifth Commandment, as not justified. He noted that the commandment, *Thou shalt not kill* "evidently has sense only to exclude the killing of others over whose lives we have no authority and that many precepts derived from the Scriptures should be changed by reason and common sense."

During the 17th and 18th centuries, suicide was sufficiently common in England as to be called *la maladie anglaise* (the English disease) by the French, evidently following the still-present tendency for each country to attribute eccentric, outrageous, or distasteful customs to the other. It is likely that suicide was not at all more common in London than in Paris, although the British press reported on suicides more frequently. The first weekly publication, *The Gentleman's Magazine*, appeared in London in 1731, and frequently reported news about suicides. In contrast, in France the subject was considered private or shameful and not often reported in publications. Later, however, evidence was uncovered that the suicide in France was nearly three times higher than in England at the same time (Minois, 1999).

A particularly harsh position against suicide was taken by Prussian philosopher Immanuel Kant (1724–1804) who, in his *Metaphysics of Ethics* (1786), reasoned that suicide is contrary to the love we owe to ourselves. In addition, he claimed that suicide could not be considered an act of free choice since it limited the universal duty of acting as if individual actions belonged to the universal law of nature.

English clergyman Charles Moore (1771–1826) wrote a treatise, *A Full Inquiry on the Subject of Suicide* (1790). The introduction of his comprehensive book on the topic states:

> Though many excellent sermons and short essays have been written on the guilt of suicide, yet it has never been treated (as far as the author's knowledge extends) on a large and comprehensive scale, so as to unite all its several parts branches in one and the same work.

Moore leaned toward then prevalent religious ideas, but added that "the usual arguments brought in favor of suicide will be proposed and answered." He discussed Donne's *Biathanatos*, Hume's *Essay on Suicide*, and "the book of most pernicious influence, called *The Sorrows of Young Werther*" (*Die Leiden des jungen Werthers*; 1774) by German writer-politician Johann Wolfgang von Goethe (1749–1842), as well as works of famous philosophers of his time, including Beccaria, Montaigne, Montesquieu, More, Rousseau, and Voltaire.

Nineteenth century

A court case in London in the early 19th century shook prevailing moral opinion. It involved the suicide in 1822 of Robert Stewart (Lord Castlereagh, Second Marquis of Londonderry [1769–1822]), a very powerful and conservative man. The London coroner had to decide between the act as a crime or the product of an unsound mind. If the death were adjudged to be a crime, a member of the ruling class had to be buried ignominiously under a crossroad; if it was considered the product of mental illness, that information would become public. The coroner decided in favor of mental illness, noting his recent expression of suicidal thoughts and persecutory ideas, and Lord Castlereagh was granted a funeral at Westminster Abbey. His funeral provoked angry reactions from the public and many of his colleagues, but also consideration that suicide could be a noble act. The debate raised a range of considerations about suicide, prominent among which was the frequent connection of suicide with mental disorder.

In the following year (1823), Abel Griffiths, a 22-year-old law student, clad only in underwear, socks and a winding sheet, was interred at the crossroads formed by Eaton Street, Grosvenor Place, and the King's Road in London. His bloodied, unwashed body was quickly dropped into a hole following removal of a stake driven into his chest. The young man had killed himself after killing his father. A neighbor reported that he had suffered "depression in the brain." Nevertheless, despite this and other evidence, a jury decided that Griffiths had been in a sound state of mind. Remarkably, there was no public resistance to this outcome. However, in the same year, a law was promulgated to prohibit further burials under crossroads (Gates, 2013).

In the British colonies in America, laws pertaining to suicide were the same as in England. For instance, in Massachusetts, Chief Justice Samuel Sewall (1652–1730) was unconditionally opposed to suicide and applied full sanctions against people who attempted or committed suicide (Kushner, 1989). For the Justice it was the worst kind of murder and melancholy – even when recognized – instead of being considered a defense added culpability because it made one vulnerable to Satan's temptation of suicide. Puritans insisted that suicide was an individual act and punishments had to be directed to the individual suicide and not to their families so that, contrary to English custom, there was no confiscation of goods (Kushner, 1989). Also in colonial New England, attempted suicides were punished with whipping and incarceration.

Puritan values in the British colonies resisted the evolution of thought in 17th century England that viewed melancholy as a disease. Even the recognition of a *non compos mentis* was left to interpretation. The English county Justice Michael Dalton (1564–1644) stated in 1619: "If a lunatike person killeth himselfe" while lucid "he shall forfeit his goods" (Dalton, 1618). Although there were isolated cases in which the law against suicide was strictly enforced, in other colonial jurisdictions such as Providence Plantantions (today part of Rhode Island), Pennsylvania, New Jersey, Maryland, North Carolina, and Virginia, as well as in some coroners' juries in Massachusetts, suicide associated with melancholy was considered a mental illness and not punished. However, in most cases a suicide was still a sinner and thus denied religious burial.

The 19th century German philosopher Arthur Schopenhauer (1788–1860) was not in favor of suicide and argued that it did not really offer a plausible escape from difficulties intrinsic to an essentially irrational world. Suicides indeed want to live, but not on terms that are offered; they need to give up life because they are unable to give up the will to live better. Schopenhauer's suggested solution in his book, *On Suicide, in The World as Will and Representation* (1818), was to reach a negation of life through asceticism.

The French Enlightenment philosopher Paul-Henri Thiry (Baron of Holbach [1723–1789]) even more vigorously proclaimed the legitimacy of suicide, considering it neither an act against nature nor an act of cowardice. At the same time, he rejected the idea of philosophical suicide to be attributed to moral or physical suffering, whether conscious or unconscious.

During the 19th century, while old ideas were still present, the prevailing attitude seemed to be that suicide was a result of an altered mental state. Modern studies of suicide were about to appear, and views of suicide as either noble self-sacrifice or escape from responsibilities were less and less often associated with voluntary death. In England, reports of suicides were often included in published reports of the news, with varied interpretations of the persons involved and their decisions to end their lives. Prevalent were stories of women (including Virginia Woolf [1882–1941]) throwing themselves into the sea or a river, or of men who hanged or shot themselves. Female suicide was usually related to emotional delusions or loss of chastity which were repented, whereas suicides in men were often ascribed to financial difficulties. Apparent attempts to avoid punishment or shame were sometimes offered as rational conclusions and proof of sanity. In addition, an association was being suspected between suicide and alcohol abuse; by 1877 alcoholism was granted the dignified status of being a disease (Harrison, 1971). In the late 19th and early 20th centuries, magazines included engravings in stories (mainly about women) of persons who threw themselves from bridges or were pulled out of the water, often barely clad. By contrast, on the Continent, most news reports excluded suicides.

The publication by Belgian mathematician and statistician-sociologist Adolphe Quetelet (1796–1874) of a book, *Sur l'Homme et le Développement de ses Facultés, ou Essai de Statistique Social* (*About Man and the Development of His Facultes, or an Essay on Social Statistics*; 1835) began a phase of intense statistical study of suicide. This tradition was continued by the work of Professor of Psychiatry at Turin, Enrico Morselli (1852–1929), in his book *Il Suicidio. Saggio di Statistica Morale Comparata* (*Suicide. Essay of Moral Comparative Statistics*; 1879) and by French sociologist Emile Durkheim (1857–1919) in his *Suicide: un Essai Sociologique* (*Suicide: A Sociological Study*; 1897). In these texts, the central point was to look for possible causes of suicide outside the individual, though from differing perspective. Their most important contribution was the initiation of modern epidemiological, sociological, psychological, and medical investigations aimed at describing, understanding, and preventing voluntary death.

Conclusions

Throughout the centuries there has been enormous tension in the perception of suicide as a sin or a criminal act versus a socially acceptable or tolerable behavior associated with an illness or with an extreme life condition. Nowadays, a similar dichotomous tension contrasts social determinants of suicide allegedly related to environmental factors versus a medical perspective viewing suicide as the consequence of psychiatric illness, mainly mood disorders. The social view would require complex intervention on the environment of potential suicides that, in most cases, is not practicable. A psychological-medical approach has the advantage of leading to feasible interventions aimed at preventing suicidal behavior.

Acknowledgments

Supported by Aretaeus Association, by a grant from the Bruce J. Anderson Foundation, and by the McLean Private Donors Research Fund. The author is deeply grateful to Professor Ross J. Baldessarini, M.D., of Harvard Medical School for his comments and suggestions during the preparation of this chapter.

Disclosures

The author and immediate family members have no financial relationships with commercial organizations that might present the appearance of potential conflicts of interest in the material presented.

References

Baldessarini, R. J., Tondo, L., Strombom, I., et al. (2007). Analysis of ecological studies of relationships between antidepressant utilization and suicidal risk. *Harvard Review of Psychiatry*, **15**, 133–145.

Brown, R. M. (2001). *The Art of Suicide*. London: Reaktion Books.

Clark, M. T. (Ed.). (2000). *An Aquinas Reader: Selections from the Writings of Thomas Aquinas*. New York: Fordham University Press.

Committee of Jewish Law and Standards. (1998). Teshuvah on assisted suicide. *Conservative Judaism*, **50**, 3–24

Cutter, F. (1983). *Art and the Wish to Die*. Chicago: Nelson Hall.

Dalton, M. (1618). *The Countrey Justice: Conteyining the Practice of the Justice of the Peace out of their Sessions, Gathered for the Better Helpe of Such Justices of Peace as have not beene much Conversant in the Studie of the Laws of this Realme*. London: Societie of Stationers.

Gates, B.T. Verdicts. Available at: http://www.victorianweb.org/books/suicide/01.html (accessed: February 2, 2013).

Grisé, Y. (1982). *Le Suicide dans la Rome Antique*. Paris: Belles Lettres.

Harrison, B. (1971). *Drink and the Victorians: The Temperance Question in England, 1815–1872*. Pittsburgh: University of Pittsburgh Press.

Kushner, H. I. (1989). *Self-destruction in the Promised Land*. New Brunswick and London: Rutgers University Press.

MacDonald, M. & Murphy, T. R. (1990). *Sleepless Souls: Suicide in Early Modern England*. Oxford: Clarendon Press.

Manson, E. (1899). Suicide as a crime. *Journal of the Society of Comparative Legislation*, **1**, 311–319.

Minois, G. (1999). *History of Suicide: Voluntary Death in Western Culture*. Baltimore: Johns Hopkins University Press.

Moore, C. (1790). *A Full Inquiry Into the Subject of Suicide: To which are Added (as Being Closely Connected with the Subject) Two Treatises on Duelling and Gaming*, Vol **1**. London: J.F. and C. Rivington.

Moron, P. (1976). *Il Suicidio*. Garzanti: Milan.

Tondo, L. (2000). *Prima del Tempo. Conoscere e Prevenire il Suicidio*. Roma: Carocci.

Chapter 2

Global epidemiology of suicide

Pedro Ruiz

Introduction

Suicidal behavior certainly presents a major challenge to humanity in all regions of the world. For centuries, the phenomenon of suicide has been studied and examined at all levels of sciences, and still is a major dilemma for scientists and researchers (Nock et al., 2012a). Over the years, suicidal behavior has definitely called the attention of researchers, clinicians, and philosophers (Durkeim, 1951; World Health Organization, 2009). Recently, the World Health Organization (WHO) has decided to look at this phenomenon and is currently attempting to understand it, and address it from a comprehensive point of view. Indeed, suicide worldwide has already become a major player as an important contributor to the global burden of disease in every respect.

It is within this context that we decided to assess the phenomenon of suicide from a global point of view, focusing on an epidemiological perspective.

A United States perspective

In the USA alone, 11 persons in every 100 000 complete suicide annually; additionally, in the USA 193 persons suffering from bipolar and other mood disorders also kill themselves in every 100 000 persons (Simon & Hales, 2006). There is no evidence that "suicide contracts" are honored by the patients and, thus, it has no impact on the number of suicides that take place (Simon, 2006). Several factors are well known to increase suicide, among them, the presence of personality disorders (Linelman et al., 2000); in this population group, there is a seven times greater risk for suicide than in the general population (Harris & Barraclough, 1997). In the USA, there are significant racial differences with respect to suicidal behavior: Native Americans have the highest rates of completed suicide, followed by Whites. African Americans have the lowest suicide rates; however, in recent years the African American suicide rate, particularly among the African American youth, is increasing (Gould et al., 2003). The focus on "youth" in the USA is more intense than the focus on older adults. The predominant cultural values are youth, beauty, and a vigorous lifestyle; however, the highest rate of suicide is observed among older adults (US Public Health Service, 2001).

Males commit suicide at a rate three to four times greater than females (Simon, 2006), and the highest suicide rates for women occur among White females in the age range 40 to 44 years old (Moscicki, 1999). Despite the low rates of suicide among women in the USA, they tend to have two of the most significant suicide risk factors, that is, depression and suicide attempts.

A worldwide perspective

More than one million people died in 2000 worldwide due to suicide. Despite the fact that most people who commit suicide suffer from a mental illness, suicide tends to occur during periods of social, economic, family, and individual crisis (Horton, 2006). On many occasions, even if persons who commit suicide suffer from mental illness, especially depression and/or substance abuse, the basic issues related to the suicidal behavior are tied to social, cultural, economic, family, and/or individual crisis (Delgado & Ruiz, 1985; GAP, 1989).

Unquestionably, suicidal behavior is a leading cause of injury and death at a worldwide level and, thus, addressing the epidemiology of such behavior is very important from a policy-making viewpoint. Approximately one million people worldwide die by suicide, thus making it one of the leading causes of death (Nock et al., 2012b).

Worldwide, suicide was ranked the 14th leading cause of death globally in 2002, and is projected to increase by 50% and become the 12th leading cause of death by year 2030 (Mathers & Loncar, 2006). Despite the fact that an association between early childhood

A Concise Guide to Understanding Suicide, ed. Stephen H. Koslow, Pedro Ruiz, and Charles B. Nemeroff. Published by Cambridge University Press.

abuse and later suicidal behavior has been reported in several studies (Stein et al., 2012), this assumption has not been confirmed as yet (Bradsky & Stanley, 2008).

With respect to Latin America and the Caribbean, it has been historically reported that the level of suicide is lower than that in the rest of the world, especially when compared with European countries. It is important to note that the suicide rate data for Latin America are recent. Levels of suicide tend to fluctuate among the countries of Latin America (Kohn & Friedman, 2009), and thus, additional research efforts are needed in this area.

It should be noted, however, that quite a few studies on migration and suicide that focus on Mexican and Mexican-American populations have been conducted in recent years (Ruiz, 1995, 1996a, b). In general, the suicide rate is lower in Mexico but it increases among Mexican-American migrants who settle in the USA as they become acculturated to the prevailing Anglo-Saxon culture.

One recent publication has focused on the topic of suicide in Latin America. It focuses on all key aspects of suicide in Latin American (Martinez et al., 2009),

A recent publication in Latin America primarily focuses on suicide among Latin American women, addressing important areas such as the role of the Hispanic family, the evolution from childhood to adulthood, and preventive aspects with regard to suicidal behavior among Latin American women. Cultural aspects, the impact of substance abuse, the role of psychotherapy, and family dynamics are discussed (Zayas, 2011).

Another recent book published in 2009 (Wasserman & Wasserman, 2009) offers an extensive "global perspective" on suicide and suicide prevention. This text offers a worldwide understanding of the most important aspects of suicidal behavior and suicide prevention, discussing the role of religion and culture, and includes theories of suicidal behavior, its political determinants, socioeconomic aspects, clinical and biological measures, public health components, and preventive strategies.

Another recent book focuses on the preventive aspects of suicide, including its clinical assessment and management (Simon, 2011).

An epidemiological perspective

In accordance with the World Health Organization (WHO) 2011 suicide data, the rates of suicide per 100 000 persons, by country, year, and sex are as follows (World Health Organization, 2011):

Country	Year	Males	Females
Albania	2003	4.7	3.3
Antigua and Barbuda	1995	0.0	0.0
Argentina	2008	12.6	3.0
Armenia	2008	2.8	1.1
Australia	2006	12.8	3.6
Austria	2009	23.8	7.1
Azerbaijan	2007	1.0	0.3
Bahamas	2005	1.9	0.6
Bahrain	2006	4.0	3.5
Barbados	2006	7.3	0.0
Belarus	2007	48.7	8.8
Belgium	2005	28.8	10.3
Belize	2008	6.6	0.7
Bosnia and Herzegovina	1991	20.3	3.3
Brazil	2008	7.7	2.0
Bulgaria	2008	18.8	6.2
Canada	2004	17.3	5.4
Chile	2007	18.2	4.2
China (Selected Rural & Urban Areas)	1999	13.0	14.8
China (Hong Kong)	2009	19.0	10.7
Colombia	2007	7.9	2.0
Costa Rica	2009	10.2	1.9
Croatia	2009	28.9	7.5
Cuba	2008	19.0	5.5
Cyprus	2008	7.4	1.7
Czech Republic	2009	23.9	4.4
Denmark	2006	17.5	6.4
Dominican Republic	2005	3.9	0.7
Ecuador	2009	10.5	3.6
Egypt	2009	0.1	0.0
El Salvador	2008	12.9	3.6
Estonia	2008	30.6	7.3
Finland	2009	29.0	10.0
France	2007	24.7	8.5
Georgia	2009	7.1	1.7
Germany	2006	17.9	6.0
Greece	2009	6.0	1.0

Country	Year	Males	Females
Grenada	2008	0.0	0.0
Guatemala	2008	5.6	1.7
Guyana	2006	39.0	13.4
Haiti	2003	0.0	0.0
Honduras	1978	0.0	0.0
Hungary	2009	40.0	10.6
Iceland	2008	16.5	7.0
India	2009	13.0	7.8
Iran	1991	0.3	0.1
Ireland	2009	19.0	4.7
Israel	2007	7.0	1.5
Italy	2007	10.0	2.8
Jamaica	1990	0.3	0.0
Japan	2009	36.2	13.2
Jordan	2008	0.2	0.0
Kazakhstan	2008	43.0	9.4
Kuwait	2009	1.9	1.7
Kyrgyzstan	2009	14.1	3.6
Latvia	2009	40.0	8.2
Lithuania	2009	61.3	10.4
Luxembourg	2008	16.1	3.2
Maldives	2005	0.7	0.0
Malta	2008	5.9	1.0
Mauritius	2008	11.8	1.9
Mexico	2008	7.0	1.5
Netherlands	2009	13.1	5.5
New Zealand	2007	18.1	5.5
Nicaragua	2006	9.0	2.6
Norway	2009	17.3	6.5
Panama	2008	9.0	1.9
Paraguay	2008	5.1	2.0
Peru	2007	1.9	1.0
Philippines	1993	2.5	1.7
Poland	2008	26.4	4.1
Portugal	2009	15.6	4.0
Puerto Rico	2005	13.2	2.0
Republic of Korea	2009	39.9	22.1
Republic of Moldova	2008	30.1	5.6
Romania	2009	21.0	3.5
Russian Federation	2006	53.9	9.5

Country	Year	Males	Females
Saint Kitts and Nevis	1995	0.0	0.0
Saint Lucia	2005	4.9	0.0
Saint Vincent and the Grenadines	2008	5.4	1.9
Sao Tome and Principe	1987	0.0	1.8
Serbia	2009	28.1	10.0
Seychelles	2008	8.9	0.0
Singapore	2006	12.9	7.7
Slovakia	2005	22.3	3.4
Slovenia	2009	34.6	9.4
South Africa	2007	1.4	0.4
Spain	2008	11.9	3.4
Sri Lanka	1991	44.6	16.8
Suriname	2005	23.9	4.8
Sweden	2008	18.7	6.8
Switzerland	2007	24.8	11.4
Syrian Arab Republic	1985	0.2	0.0
Tajikistan	2001	2.9	2.3
Thailand	2002	12.0	3.8
Tfyr Macedonia	2003	9.5	4.0
Trinidad and Tobago	2006	17.9	3.8
Turkmenistan	1998	13.8	3.5
Ukraine	2009	37.8	7.0
United Kingdom	2009	10.9	3.0
United States of America	2005	17.7	4.5
Uruguay	2004	26.0	6.3
Uzbekistan	2005	7.0	2.3
Venezuela	2007	5.3	1.2
Zimbabwe	1990	10.6	5.2

Conclusion

We addressed many important aspects of "suicidal behavior" and its "prevention". In so doing, we focused this very important clinical topic from a global point of view. This approach addresses key issues, such as cultural aspects, as well as religious, ethnic, racial, language, and other culturally related factors; additionally, socio-economic factors; age aspects; gender differences; clinical considerations, preventive approaches, public health perspectives, educational interventions, factors related to families, health-related factors, and political considerations. Additional details are featured in the following sections of this book.

In so doing, we focused on the most relevant and recent literature related to this topic, with an emphasis on the global aspects of suicidal behavior and suicide prevention. It is our expectation that this chapter will positively add to our efforts in preventing suicidal behavior and effectively address suicide attempts.

References

Bradsky, B. S. & Stanley, B. (2008). Adverse childhood experiences and suicidal behavior. *Psychiatric Clinics of North America*, **31**(2), 223–235.

Delgado, A. & Ruiz, P. (1985). Suicide and hispanic americans. In P. Pichet et al. (Eds.) *Psychiatry: The State of the Art* (pp. 433–437). New York: Plenum Press.

Durkeim, E. (1951). *Suicide: A Study in Sociology*. New York: Free Press.

Gould, M. S., Greenberg, I., Velting, D. M., et al. (2003). Youth suicide risk and preventive interventions: a review of the past 10 years. *Journal of the American Academy of Child and Adolescent Psychiatry*, **42**, 386–405.

Group for the Advancement of Psychiatry (GAP) (1989). *Suicide and Ethnicity in the United States*, Report No. 128 (pp. 72–94). New York: Brunner/Mazel Publishers.

Harris, C. E. & Barraclough, B. (1997). Suicide as an outcome for mental disorders. *British Journal of Psychiatry*, **170**, 205–328.

Horton, L. (2006). Social, cultural, and demographic factors in suicide. In R. I. Simon & R. E. Hales (Eds.) *Textbook of Suicide Assessment and Management* (pp. 107–137). Washington, DC: American Psychiatric Publishing, Inc.

Kohn, R. & Friedman, H. (2009). La Epidemiologia del Suicidio, los Intentos y las Ideaciones Suicidas en América Latina y el Caribe. In J. J. Rodriguez, R. Kohn, S. Aguilar-Gaxiola (Eds.) *Epidemiologia de los Trastornos Mentales en América Latina y el Caribe, Organización Panamericana de la Salud*. Publicación Científico y Técnica No. 632. Washington, DC.

Linelman, M. M., Rizvi, S. L., Welch, S. S., et al. (2000). Psychiatric aspects of suicidal behavior: personality disorders. In K. Hawton & K. Van Heeringen (Eds.) *The International Handbook of Suicide and Attempted Suicide* (pp. 147–178). New York: Wiley.

Martinez, J. C., Saad, E. & Forero, J. (2009). *Suicidio: Una Realidad en Latinoamérica*. Ecuador: Asociación Psiquiátrica de América Latina (APAL).

Mathers, C. D. & Loncar, D. (2006). Projections of global mortality and burden of disease from 2002 to 2030. *PLoS Medicine*, **3**(11), e. 442.

Moscicki, E. K. (1999). Epidemiology of suicide. In D. G. Jacob (Ed.) *Harvard Medical School Guide to Suicide Assessment and Intervention* (pp. 40–51). San Francisco, CA: Jossey-Bass.

Nock, M. K., Borges, G., & Ono, Y. (2012a). Introduction: global perspectives on suicidal behavior. In M. K. Nock, G. Borges & Y. Ono (Eds.) *Suicide: Global Perspectives from the WHO World Mental Health Surveys* (pp. 1–4). New York: Cambridge University Press.

Nock, M. K., Borges, G. Bromet, E. J., et al. (2012b). The epidemiology of suicide and suicide behavior. In *Suicide: Global Perspectives from the WHO World Mental Health Surveys* (pp. 5–32). New York: Cambridge University Press.

Ruiz, P. (1995). Impacto cultural y migratorio en el fenómeno del suicidio. In *La Psiquiatría en la Década del Cerebro* (pp. 329–334). Madrid, Spain: Grupo Aran.

Ruiz, P. (1996a). Aspectos Culturales del Suicidio Entre los México-Americanos. *Medico Interamericano*, **15**(1), 75–78.

Ruiz, P. (1996b). Suicide and acculturation: a Mexican American perspective. *Psychline*, **1**(2), 26–28.

Simon, R. I. (2006). *Assessing and Managing Suicide Risk: Guidelines for Clinically Based Risk Management*. Washington, DC: American Psychiatric Publishing.

Simon, R. I. (2011). *Preventing Patient Suicide: Clinical Assessment and Management*. Washington, DC: American Psychiatric Publishing, Inc.

Simon, R. I. & Hales, R. E. (2006). *Textbook of Suicide Assessment and Management*. Washington, DC: American Psychiatric Publishing, Inc.

Stein, D. J., Chiu, W. T., Hwang, I., et al. (2012). Traumatic events and suicidal behavior. In M. K. Nock, G. Borges, Y. Ono (Eds.) *Suicide: Global Perspectives from the WHO World Mental Health Surveys* (pp. 131–147). New York: Cambridge University Press.

US Public Health Service (2001). *National Strategy for Suicide Prevention: Goals and Objectives for Action*. Rockville, MD: US Department of Health and Human Services, US Public Health Service.

Wasserman, D. & Wasserman, C. (eds.) (2009). *Oxford Textbook of Suicidology and Suicide Prevention: A Global Perspective*. Oxford, UK: Oxford University Press.

World Health Organization. (2009). *Data and Statistics: Causes of Death*. World Health Organization.

World Health Organization (2011). *Suicide Rates per 100,000 by Country, Year and Sex*. World Health Organization.

Zayas, L. H. (2011). *Latinas Attempting Suicide: When Cultures, Families, and Daughters Collide*. New York: Oxford University Press.

Chapter 3

Identification and screening of suicide risk

Kelly Posner, Jacqueline Buchanan, Leora Amira, Kseniya Yershova, Adam Lesser, and Erica Goldstein

Introduction

Suicide remains one of the world's greatest public health crises; however, the magnitude of its public health impact and global disease burden is under-recognized (Insel, 2010). Suicide recently became the number one cause of injury mortality in the USA (Rockett et al., 2012), surpassing motor vehicle crashes. Every 15 minutes an adult dies by suicide (Centers for Disease Control and Prevention, 2010), and seemingly no population is spared. Suicide has been shown to be a leading cause of death among law enforcement officers (Clark et al., 2012) and in correctional facilities (Hayes, 2010). Within an average corporation of 100 000 employees, every 7 days one employee or family member will die by suicide, and each day there will be three suicide attempts. (Paul, 2005). Approximately 8% of high school students report having attempted suicide in the past year (Eaton et al., 2012). Most often suicide occurs with no clear warning signs and its economic burden is staggering. The annual global disease burden of suicide is nearly $141 billion (John & Ross, 2010). In the USA alone, non-fatal suicide attempts cost $6 billion a year. (Centers for Disease Control and Prevention, 2010).

Identification is the first necessary element of any prevention effort – ability to treat is contingent upon the ability to find at risk individuals or those suffering in silence. However, a large proportion of individuals who later die by suicide go undetected due to lack of querying and inadequate methods to do so, especially in non-mental health settings. Forty-five percent of suicides across all age groups have contact with their primary care providers within 1 month prior to their death; 77% across all age groups will see their primary care provider within 1 year of their death (Luoma et al., 2002). Nearly 90% of suicidal youth were also seen for a medical appointment within a 12-month period (McCarty et al., 2011). Yet, less than 3% of primary care patient appointment records prior to suicide reflect a comment about suicide risk (Appleby et al., 1996). Among approximately 1500 individuals admitted to Walter Reed Army Medical Center between 2001 and 2006, 11% were admitted for serious suicidal ideation and 12% with suicide attempt, yet no documentation of past suicidal behaviors was noted. There was no suicide screening or assessment measure administered in a single case. It was later strongly recommended that military providers be trained in the use of screening or assessment tools (Posner et al., 2013). One in five adolescents who screened positive for suicidal ideation and/or attempts in an emergency department presented for non-psychiatric reasons (King et al., 2009); thus, without general screening, suicidal individuals will be missed. 20–25% of adolescents who die by suicide have had contact with mental health professionals within a year of their death (Gould et al., 2003). Only 19% of primary care providers relative to 59% of psychiatric practitioners knew about the suicidal intentions of their patients who died by suicide (Isometsa et al., 1994). Individuals at high-risk for suicide will not be adequately detected if screening is not done routinely and relies on those who self-identify. All of this is to suggest that screening should be a first-line prevention strategy and that screening for suicide should be as common as monitoring for blood pressure.

Screening for suicide has been shown to be effective in identifying at risk individuals and connecting them with treatment. Local depression screening programs

A Concise Guide to Understanding Suicide, ed. Stephen H. Koslow, Pedro Ruiz, and Charles B. Nemeroff. Published by Cambridge University Press.

are known to increase the number of individuals treated for depression and to decrease suicide rates (Mann et al., 2005) and administering screening instruments for depression, suicidal ideation, or suicidal acts to high school students more than doubled the proportion of identified at risk individuals relative to those identified by school professionals (Scott et al., 2009). Studies show that use of a standardized screening tool can result in a 600% increase in detection of suicidal ideation (Bryan et al., 2008). Screening programs such as *The College Screening Project* of the American Foundation for Suicide Prevention encouraged high-risk students to enter treatment for the first time and resulted in a 67% reduction in suicides during the 4-year screening program relative to the previous 4 years (Haas et al., 2008). In addition, continuous monitoring for suicide, especially in high-risk populations, can be an intervention in and of itself with a strong impact on reducing suicide attempts. Research has shown that monitoring suicidal symptoms alone for 1 year reduced attempts from the previous year by 80% (Stanley, 2006).

While identification of high-risk individuals is critical to prevention, inquiry about suicide has been complicated by the historical lack of clear definitions for suicidal ideation and behavior, concern over whether asking about suicide can be iatrogenic or harmful, and confusion about how to ask such questions. Research has shown that inquiring about suicide-related phenomena does not, in fact, cause suicidal thinking or distress in youth (Gould et al., 2005). On the contrary, asking questions about suicidal ideation and behavior improves risk identification (Posner et al., 2011).

Gaps in suicide risk management and physician training are responsible for some of these misconceptions (Sudak et al., 2007; Goldman et al., 1999; Milton et al., 1999; Smith & Scoullar, 2001). The implementation of training programs such as the Skills Training on Risk Management (STORM) project significantly improve physician suicide assessment practices (Appleby et al., 2000; Nutting et al., 2005).

Traditional methods of relying upon open-ended questions in assessing suicide risk have been problematic. Clinicians who perform routine intakes identify only 25% of patients with history of suicide attempt compared to structured instruments (Hawton, 1987). When clinicians were trained to ask two open-ended questions about suicide they over-detected suicidal ideation and under-detected suicidal behavior in adolescent patients (Holi et al., 2008). Structured or semi-structured tools improve detection in routine clinical assessments. Use of a structured questionnaire detected 29.7% of patients with suicidal ideation and 18.7% of patients with a history of a suicide attempt that went undetected by an open-ended clinician interview (Bongiovi-Garcia et al., 2009). In medical emergency department screening, a phone-administered suicide questionnaire (Columbia-Suicide Severity Rating Scale (C-SSRS)) increased suicide attempt detection by more than 40% compared to chart reviews (Arias et al., 2014).

Furthermore, utilizing research-supported instruments facilitates clinical decision-making and fosters confidence in the determination of next steps for individuals identified with various levels of suicide risk. Using a scale with stratified thresholds in conjunction with triage protocols may enable the reduction of burden on limited mental health services and the subsequent redirection of scarce resources (Peñta & Caine, 2006).

Assessment of suicidal ideation and behavior

The prevailing diathesis-stress model of suicidal behavior suggests that such behavior occurs when an individual with a pre-existing vulnerability such as a family history of suicide or impulsivity experiences a precipitating stressor (Mann et al., 1999; Oquendo et al., 2003). Having any psychiatric diagnoses is also a well-documented risk factor for suicidal ideation and behavior (Petronis et al., 1990; Shaffer et al., 1996; Gould et al., 1998; Vijayakumar & Rajkumar, 1999; Kessler et al., 1999; Borges et al., 2010); more than 90% of those who die by suicide meet criteria for at least one psychiatric disorder (American Psychiatric Association, 2003). Specifically, major depressive disorder is a strong risk factor for suicide (Harris & Barraclough, 1997; Kessler et al., 1999), and alcohol disorders are also known to raise risk (Harris & Barraclough, 1997). Screening for depression is recommended in primary care settings and can lead to improved identification of high-risk individuals (Mann et al., 2005). Referral and subsequent treatment of individuals with these disorders may be helpful in diminishing suicide rates (Mann et al., 2005).

Suicidal ideation and a history of suicidal behavior are among the most salient short- and long-term risk factors for suicide (Nordström et al., 1995; Beck et al., 1999; Brown et al., 2000; Kuo et al., 2001).

The clinical concern associated with a suicide attempt also necessitates its status as an outcome along with suicide. For these reasons, and because many individuals die from their first suicide attempt (Isomets, 1998), it is important to identify suicidal ideation and behavior risk factors. Identification of short-term risk necessarily requires identification and differentiation of symptoms of suicidal ideation and behavior.

The identification of suicidal ideation and behavior is challenged by inadequate standardization of definitions. The US Institute of Medicine concluded that absence of consistent definitions for suicidal phenomena is one of the major impediments to suicide prevention: "research on suicide is plagued by many methodological problems...definitions lack uniformity...[and] reporting of suicide is inaccurate" (Goldsmith et al., 2002). Inconsistent or ambiguous terminology for identical suicidal phenomena (O'Carroll et al., 1996; Posner et al., 2007) has contributed to confusion about how to label discrete instances of suicidal ideation or behavior, with a multitude of terms often referring to the same occurrence. Terms that carry value judgments such as "failed attempt," "suicide gesture," "manipulative act," and "suicide threat" (Crosby & Melanson, 2011) further inhibit identification. Historically, the ambiguity in definitions has resulted in over- (e.g., a clinician labeled a slap in the face a suicide attempt) and under-identification (e.g., a patient hung himself after a fight with his father, which was incorrectly attributed to his schizophrenia) of high-risk individuals, increasing both false positive and false negative cases. Numerous international agencies, including the US Centers for Disease and Control (CDC), the World Health Organization (WHO), and the US Food and Drug Administration (FDA), have undertaken initiatives to standardize definitions and classification of suicidal ideation and behavior.

Suicide screening instruments should strive to make multiple distinctions within suicide ideation and behavior risk factors for more precise determination of suicide risk. There are several elements that are critical to the identification of high-risk individuals, including the assessment of: (1) the full range of suicidal behaviors, (2) intent to die, a necessary component of suicidal behavior that distinguishes it from non-suicidal self-injurious behavior, (3) suicidal ideation and suicidal behavior as separate entities, and (4) the wish to die and intent to act as components of suicidal ideation.

The full range of suicidal behaviors

Traditionally, suicide screening instruments and other assessment tools queried about suicide attempts only. Consequently, behaviors in which steps are taken imminently before a suicide attempt or suicide would have otherwise occurred (e.g., putting a noose around one's neck and changing one's mind, being rescued by another before jumping from the roof of a building) and behaviors in preparation of suicide (e.g., buying a gun, collecting pills, writing a suicide note) have been left undetected. In the effort to establish a meaningful common language for suicidal behavior, the CDC has adopted terminology that distinguishes between the following suicidal behaviors: (1) suicide, (2) suicide attempt, (3) interrupted attempt, (4) self-interrupted/aborted attempt, and (5) preparatory acts or behavior (Crosby & Melanson, 2011) (See Figure 3.1 for definitions). A suicide assessment instrument should ideally assess for the full range of behavior and have distinct definitions with corresponding probes.

In addition to an abundance of extant research demonstrating the potent risk of a suicide attempt for future suicide attempts or death by suicide (Steer et al., 1988; Fawcett et al., 1990; Malone et al., 1995; Harris & Barraclough, 1997; Brown et al., 2000), recent data support the predictive properties of other suicidal behaviors for high risk of future suicidal behavior. These other suicidal behaviors – interrupted attempt, self-interrupted/aborted attempt, or preparatory acts or behavior – also confer significant risk, with odds ratios similar to that of suicide attempts (Posner, Greist et al., 2013). Moreover, the very behaviors that have historically been overlooked constitute the majority of suicidal behaviors that individuals engage in (Mundt et al., 2011). Extant research suggests that interrupted attempts are predictive of suicide (Steer, 1988), aborted attempts increase risk for suicide attempts (Marzuk et al., 1997; Barber et al., 1998), and individuals who engage in preparatory behavior are more likely to die by suicide than those who do not report such behavior (Steer et al., 1988; Marzuk et al., 1997; Beck et al., 1999). While suicidal behavior is a rare occurrence, more precise identification of high-risk individuals is paramount to prevention efforts.

Intent to die

Research supports the use of an intent-based definition of suicidal behavior (Brent et al., 1993;

Definitions

Self-directed violence (analogous to self-injurious behavior)

Behavior that is self-directed and deliberately results in injury or the potential for injury to oneself.

This does not include behaviors such as parachuting, gambling, substance abuse, tobacco use or other risk taking activities, such as excessive speeding in motor vehicles. These are complex behaviors some of which are risk factors for SDV but are defined as behavior that while likely to be life-threatening is not recognized by the individual as behavior intended to destroy or injure the self. (Farberow, N. L. (Ed.) (1980). *The Many Faces* of Suicide. New York: McGraw-Hill Book Company). These behaviors may have a high probability of injury or death as an outcome but the injury or death is usually considered unintentional. Hanzlick R, Hunsaker JC, Davis GJ. *Guide for Manner of Death Classification.* National Association of Medical Examiners. Available at: http//www.charlydmiller.com/LIB03/2002NAMEmannerofdeath.pdf. Accessed 1 Sept 2009.

Self-directed violence is categorized into the following:

Non-suicidal (as defined below)

Suicidal (as defined below).

Non-suicidal self-directed violence

Behavior that is self-directed and deliberately results in injury or the potential for injury to oneself.

There is no evidence, whether implicit or explicit, of suicidal intent. Please see appendix for definition of implicit and explicit.

Suicidal self-directed violence

Behavior that is self-directed and deliberately results in injury or the potential for injury to oneself.

There is evidence, whether implicit or explicit, of suicidal intent.

Suicide attempt

A non-fatal self-directed potentially injurious behavior with any intent to die as a result of the behavior.

A suicide attempt may or may not result in injury.

Interrupted self-directed violence - by self or by other

By other-A person takes steps to injure self but is stopped by another person prior to fatal injury. The interruption can occur at any point during the act such as after the initial thought or after onset of behavior.

By self (in other documents may be termed "aborted*suicidal behavior) - A person takes steps to injure self but is stopped by self prior to fatal injury.

Source: Posner K, Oquendo MA, Gould M, Stanley B, Davies M. Columbia Classification Algorithm of Suicide Assessment (C-CASA): Classification of Suicidal Events in the FDA's Pediatric Suicidal Risk Analysis of Antidepressants. *Am J Psychiatry.* 2007; 164:1035-1043.
http://cssrs.columbia.edu/

Other suicidal behavior including preparatory acts

Acts or preparation towards making a suicide attempt, but before potential for harm has begun. This can include anything beyond a verbalization or thought, such as assembling a method (e.g., buying a gun, collecting pills) or preparing for one's death by suicide (e.g., writing a suicide note, giving things away). Posner et al, 2007.

Suicide

Death caused by self-directed injurious behavior with any intent to die as a result of the behavior.

Figure 3.1. CDC definitions of self-directed violence. Reproduced with permission.)

Fergusson et al., 2005; Clark et al., 2012), yet suicide screening instruments often do not adequately assess for the intent of the self-injurious behavior. Individuals engaging in suicidal behavior frequently have mixed motives (Andriessen, 2006). The degree of intent to die is often difficult to discern and there is rarely a single intent or a desire for a single outcome accompanying a suicidal act (Marzuk et al., 1997; Silverman, 2006). Thus, it is recommended that screening instruments assess for *any* or "non-zero" intent to die (Posner et al., 2011). The behavior is considered suicidal unless one engages in the act entirely for reasons other than to end one's life. Additionally, intent to die must be causally linked to the suicidal behavior such that the behavior is executed partially or wholly to fulfill this intent. Historically, suicide scales have asked whether a person tried to kill themselves; however this omission of the ascertainment of intent to die can result in non-suicidal behavior being called suicidal. Thus, asking whether "any part" of a person wanted to die is preferable to simply asking whether a person wanted to die or whether they tried to kill themselves.

Frequently, intent is not explicitly stated or is overtly denied, rendering the ability to infer intent essential to identification (Oquendo et al., 2003). For example, a loved one may bring a family member to the emergency department and the patient denies suicidal thoughts, but the family member shares with the clinician that he has been talking about suicide for the past 2 weeks and wrote a suicide note the day before. Intent can be inferred from (1) outside sources of information (e.g., psychological assessments or informant interviews) (Pfeffer et al., 1993) or (2) clinical circumstances surrounding the lethality (Wichstrom, 2000) or potential lethality of an act as well as an individual's beliefs about the behavior. Acts of impressive circumstances, including behavior that is highly lethal (e.g., jumping from the roof of a tall building) or potentially lethal (e.g., the gun failing to fire when attempting to shoot oneself in the heart), may warrant an inference of intent to die. Additionally, if an individual denies intent to die but admits to the possibility of death from the behavior, intent to die can be inferred. An individual's beliefs about the lethality or potential lethality of an act are integral in the ascertainment of intent to die (e.g., jumping from a tall building due to the delusion that one can fly would not warrant an inference of intent to die) (Conwell & Thompson, 2008).

Distinction of suicidal ideation and behavior

Historically, suicidal ideation and behavior were conceived as a unidimensional construct, with ideation and behavior and their respective distinctions existing along a continuum (Posner et al., 2007; Silverman, 2006), and the definition of suicidal ideation overlapped with that of suicidal behavior (Beck et al., 1973). The separation of ideation and behavior is supported, however, based on extant literature that suggests that suicidal ideation and behavior do not always co-occur (Fawcett, 1992) and suicidal ideation is predictive of or a precursor to suicidal behavior (Kessler et al., 1999; Posner et al., 2011), in a manner that may depend on other factors, such as age (Brent et al., 1993; Pfeffer et al., 1993; Lewinsohn et al., 1994; Brown et al., 2000; Wichstrom, 2000; Fergusson et al., 2005; Vannoy et al., 2007; Conwell & Thompson, 2008; King et al., 2012). Current consensus on criteria for the utility of risk assessment instruments includes separate assessment of suicidal ideation and suicidal behavior (Meyer et al., 2010). Yet, existing instruments typically assess either suicidal ideation alone or suicidal behavior alone, or conflate suicidal ideation and behavior in a single item. Table 3.1 displays a representative sample of screening instruments and accompanying suicide-specific risk factors.

Suicidal ideation

The National Institute of Mental Health (NIMH) Developing Centers for Intervention and Prevention of Suicide determined that wish to die, thoughts of killing oneself, and intent to kill oneself constitute types of suicidal ideation (Brown et al., 2008). Thoughts of killing oneself may also include methods for killing oneself or intent to act with a specific plan.

Existing scales vary considerably in how they measure passive ideation, from thoughts of death to feelings that life is not worth living. The National Institute of Mental Health (NIMH) Developing Centers for Intervention and Prevention of Suicide consensus conference determined that passive suicidal ideation includes any internal experience that indicates a wish or desire to die ("wish to die") and excludes thoughts of being better off dead, thoughts of one's own death, or that life is not worth living

Table 3.1 Select screening instruments: measured suicidal ideation and suicidal behavior characteristics

Measure		Administration Method	# of items*	Ideation				Behavior				
			min–max	Wish to be dead	Thoughts of killing self	Thoughts with intent to act	Thoughts with intent to act and plan	Attempt	Interrupted/ aborted attempt	Preparatory acts or behavior	Intent to die	Lethality
ASQ	Ask Suicide-Screening Questions (ASQ) Horowitz et al., 2012	SR	4	x	x			x				
BSI	Beck Scale for Suicide Ideation (BSI) (self report) Beck et al., 1979	SR	6–21	x	x			x		x		
CHS	Columbia Health Screen (CHS) Shaffer et al., 2004	SR	14	x	x			x			x	x
C-SSRS**	Columbia-Suicide Severity Rating Scale (C-SSRS), Adolescent/Adult Version Posner et al., 2009	RA or SR	6–15	x	x	x	x	x	x	x	x	x
C-SSRS Screen*	Columbia-Suicide Severity Rating Scale (C-SSRS) Screen Version Posner et al., 2009	RA or SR	3–6	x	x	x	x	x	x	x	x	

MSSI	Modified Scale for Suicide Ideation (MSSI) Miller et al., 1986	RA	4–18	x	x		x		
P4	P4 Suicidality Screener (Past History, Plan, Probability, and Preventive Factors) Dube et al., 2010	SR	1–5						
PANSI	Positive and Negative Suicide Ideation Inventory (PANSI) Osman et al., 1998	SR	14						
PSS	Paykel Suicide Scale (PSS) Paykel et al., 1974	RA	5	x	x	x			
RSQ	Risk of Suicide Questionnaire (RSQ) Horowitz et al., 2001	RA	4		x				
SASII	Linehan Suicide Attempt-Self-Injury Interview (SASII) – Short Version Linehan et al., 2006	RA	5–46			x		x	x

Table 3.1 (cont.)

Measure		Administration Method	# of items*	Ideation				Behavior				
			min–max	Wish to be dead	Thoughts of killing self	Thoughts with intent to act	Thoughts with intent to act and plan	Attempt	Interrupted/ aborted attempt	Preparatory acts or behavior	Intent to die	Lethality
SBQ-14	Suicidal Behaviors Questionnaire Linehan, 1996	SR	14–90		x			x			x	
SBQ-R	Suicide Behavior Questionnaire-Revised Osman et al., 2001	SR	4		x			x			x	
SIQ-JR	Suicide Ideation Questionnaire – Junior (SIQ-JR) Reynolds, 1988	SR	15	x	x							
SIS	Suicide Ideation Scale (SIS) Rudd, 1989	SR	10	x				x				
SITBI-L	Self-Injurious Thoughts and Behaviors Interview (SITBI) Long Form Nock et al., 2007	RA	24–189		x			x	x		x	x

SITBI-S	Self-Injurious Thoughts and Behaviors Interview (SITBI) Short Form Nock et al., 2007	RA	18–92		x		x	x		x	x
SPS	Suicide Probability Scale (SPS) Cull & Gill, 1988	SR	36		x						
SSI	Scale of Suicidal Ideation (SSI) Beck et al., 1979	RA	19	x					x		
Single item in depression scales											
BDI-II	Beck Depression Inventory-II (BDI-II) Beck & Steer, 1988; Beck et al., 1996	SR	21		x	x					
HRSD	Hamilton Rating Scale for Depression (Suicide Item) (HRSD) Hamilton, 1960	RA	21	x			x				
IDS	Inventory of Depressive Symptomatology (IDS-SR, IDS-C) Rush et al., 1986	SR or RA	28				x				

Table 3.1 (cont.)

Measure		Administration Method	# of items*	Ideation						Behavior		
			min–max	Wish to be dead	Thoughts of killing self	Thoughts with intent to act	Thoughts with intent to act and plan	Attempt	Interrupted/ aborted attempt	Preparatory acts or behavior	Intent to die	Lethality
MADRS	The Montgomery–Åsberg Depression Rating Scale (MADRS) Montgomery & Åsberg, 1979	RA	10		x					x		
PHQ-9	The Patient Health Questionnaire – 9 (PHQ-9) Spitzer et al., 1999	SR	9–10									
Single item in general clinical scales												
SCL-90	Symptom Check-List-90 (SCL-90) Derogatis, 1975	SR	90		x							

* Maximum number of items refers to the total number of items on the scale and may include questions extraneous to the suicide-specific risk factors covered in the table.

** The C-SSRS and C-SSRS Screen can incorporate multiple sources of information and be used across all ages. Mental health training is not required to administer the scale and it has been used by all types of providers and gatekeepers.

(Brown et al., 2008). Individuals with a high wish to die/wish to live index have been found to be six times more likely to end their life in a 20-year follow-up study on the Scale for Suicide Ideation (SSI) (Brown et al., 2005). Additionally, non-suicidal and suicidal self-injurious thoughts or behaviors are often conflated. For example, a well-established measure of depression, the PHQ-9, includes one item that assesses thoughts of self-injurious behavior ("Thoughts of. . .huting yourself"), which may confound thoughts of non-suicidal self-injurious behavior (NSSIB) with thoughts of suicide. Moreover, "thoughts...of hurting yourself" is blended with what has been traditionally mistaken for passive ideation ("thoughts that you would be better off dead"). Both of these result in identification of cases that should not be considered suicidal (i.e., high rate of false positive cases). At Cleveland Clinic, this PHQ-9 item resulted in 23.8% positive screens versus 6.2% with the C-SSRS Screener, while the C-SSRS identified cases that were missed (Katzan et al., 2013).

Intent to act

Thoughts of killing oneself are thoughts, beliefs, images, voices, or other cognitions about intentionally ending one's own life (suicide), and may include the intent to act on such thoughts. Intent to act is having any intention of acting on one's thoughts of killing oneself. This contrasts with having thoughts but never intending to do anything about them. While intent to act on suicidal thoughts is an integral component of the definition of suicidal ideation, it was historically unacknowledged as a separate entity (Bagley, 1975; Beck et al., 1979). However, there has been an increasing trend of recognizing ideation with intent to act as a distinct type of suicidal ideation (Hawton, 1987; Silverman et al., 2007; Posner et al., 2011). The presence of intent to act confers higher risk for subsequent suicidal behavior (Currier et al., 2009; Posner et al., 2011, Mundt et al., 2013).

Clinical utility of instruments

The use of a research-supported and evidence-based tool for screening can help guide appropriate care to those who need it by redirecting scarce resources. In order to determine whether a particular instrument is optimal for screening, assessment, or monitoring, the following parameters should be considered: administration time, type of raters and administration methods, and level of training required for administration.

Short administration time

Screening instruments should be brief. Brief administration time may be enabled by the structure of an instrument, such as streamlined decision tree and skip patterns.

Multiple sources of information

Ability to obtain or integrate information from different informants gives users the necessary flexibility. First responders may not be able to obtain information directly from the victim but could collect it from relatives.

Format of delivery

Suicide screening instruments may be available in a variety of paper and electronic mediums (e.g., telephone, tablet, smartphone). Innovative and feasible delivery methods can facilitate screening of a greater number of individuals resulting in more blanketed screening implementation. Format of delivery is especially crucial post-discharge when patients are at a very high risk. Research indicates an increased risk for suicide in the first few weeks after discharge from psychiatric inpatient hospitalization (Goldacre et al., 1993; Qin & Nordentoft, 2005). With electronic methods, post-discharge patients can be monitored over time from their home at designated time intervals.

Multiple administration methods

Self-report measures and interviews administered by an individual or rater are typical methods for screening for suicide risk. Self-report instruments may have the advantage of higher sensitivity by eliciting more accurate self-disclosure for sensitive issues (Greist et al., 1973; Levine et al., 1989; Hesdorffer et al., 2013). Self-reports can be instrumental to the disclosure of suicide-related phenomena, which may be denied face-to-face, including in adolescents (Shain, 2007; Vitiello et al., 2009). The availability of rater-administered and self-report screening methods are optimal for providing maximum flexibility in administration. A brief suicide questionnaire (C-SSRS) administered over the phone has shown improved detection by approximately 40% of suicide attempts compared to hospital chart reviews in medical emergency departments (Arias et al., 2014).

Gatekeepers

Screening settings are arguably countless, including primary care, schools, religious centers, and legal and forensic settings. Training in the administration of a screening method provided for those outside mental health professions may enhance implementation efforts. It is critical that non-mental health professionals be able to ask the questions; non-clinicians have demonstrated strong inter-rater reliability using the C-SSRS in a juvenile justice system (Kerr, et al., 2014). For example, the ability to screen by non-professional gatekeepers is important in rural communities where the nearest mental health practitioner may be hours away and over-burdened.

Generalizability to multiple populations

Similarly, it is important to use screening instruments that can be effectively used across many varied populations (Peñta & Caine, 2006). Some instruments offer additional questions for specific populations. Other scales have versions for different age groups.

Triage capacity

It is important that scales have operationalized criteria or thresholds that distinguish higher levels of risk so that next steps can be determined. These may include referrals to mental health professionals for further evaluation, hospitalization, or suicide watch protocols for high risk. Without that, providers will be unable to triage patients and will remain anxious about everyone. This over-estimation of risk may cause clinicians to think they need more one-to-ones than they have staff to cover, which wastes resources and ultimately reduces the quality of care.

Furthermore, for screening in schools, using a scale with stratified thresholds that allow for the identification of the most at risk individuals and others who are less at risk can help triage students and reduce the burden on the limited number of mental health professionals who will need to follow-up (Peñta & Caine, 2006).

Conclusion

Suicide prevention is a topic of high national and international importance and identification of at risk individuals is the first necessary step toward prevention. Screening for suicidal ideation and behavior should be integrated across public health settings and made as routine as monitoring for blood pressure. Knowledge of the full range of suicidal behaviors and key criteria for differentiating suicidal and non-suicidal events are paramount to the advancement of screening efforts. Feasible, brief, and research-supported screening tools can identify individuals at increased risk for suicide. Effectiveness of screening tools should be measured in terms of their relation to suicide prevention efforts.

References

American Psychiatric Association. (2003). *Practice Guideline for the Assessment and Treatment of Patients with Suicidal Behaviors*. American Psychiatric Association.

Andriessen, K. (2006). On "intention" in the definition of suicide. *Suicide and Life-Threatening Behavior*, **36**(5), 533–538.

Appleby, L., Amos, T., Doyle, U., et al. (1996). General practitioners and young suicides: a preventive role for primary care. *The British Journal of Psychiatry*, **168**(3), 330–333.

Appleby, L., Morriss, R., Gask, L., et al.(2000). An educational intervention for front-line health professionals in the assessment and management of suicidal patients (The STORM Project). *Psychological Medicine*, **30**(4), 805–812.

Arias, S. A., Zhang, Z., Hillerns, C., et al. (2014). Using structured telephone follow-up assessments to improve suicide-related adverse event detection. *Suicide and Life-Threatening Behavior*. doi: 10.1111/sltb.12088.

Bagley, C. R. (1975). Suicidal behavior and suicidal ideation in adolescents: problem for counselors in education. *British Journal of Guidance and Counselling*, **3**(2), 190–208.

Barber, M. E., Marzuk, P., Leon, A., & Portera, L. (1998). Aborted suicide attempts: a new classification of suicidal behavior. *American Journal of Psychiatry*, **155**(3), 385–389.

Beck, A., Davis, J. H., Frederick, C. J., et al. (1973). Classification and nomenclature. In H. L. P. Resnick & B. C. Hathorne (Eds). *Suicide Prevention in the Seventies* (pp. 7–12). Washington, DC: US Government Printing Office.

Beck, A. T., Kovacs, M., & Weissman, A. (1979). Assessment of suicidal intention: the Scale for Suicide Ideation. *Journal of Consulting and Clinical Psychology*, **47**(2), 343–352.

Beck, A. T., Brown, G. K., Steer, R. A., et al. (1999). Suicide ideation at its worst point: a predictor of eventual suicide in psychiatric outpatients. *Suicide and Life-Threatening Behavior*, **29**(1), 1–9.

Bongiovi-Garcia, M. E., Merville, J., Almeida, M., et al. (2009). Comparison of clinical and research assessments of diagnosis, suicide attempt history and suicidal ideation in major depression. *Journal of Affective Disorders*, **115** (1–2), 183–188.

Borges, G., Nock, M., Abad, J., et al. (2010). Twelve month prevalence of and risk factors for suicide attempts in the WHO World Mental Health Surveys. *The Journal of Clinical Psychiatry*, **71**(12), 1617.

Brent, D. A., Perper, J. A., Moritz, G., et al. (1993). Psychiatric risk factors for adolescent suicide: a case-control study. *Journal of the American Academy of Child & Adolescent Psychiatry*, **32**(3), 521–529.

Brown, G. K., Beck, A. T., Steer, R. A., & Grisham, J. R. (2000). Risk factors for suicide in psychiatric outpatients: a 20-year prospective study. *Journal of Consulting and Clinical Psychology*, **68**(3), 371–377.

Brown, G. K., Steer, R. A., Henriques, G. R., & Beck, A. T. (2005). The internal struggle between the wish to die and the wish to live: a risk factor for suicide. *American Journal of Psychiatry*, **162**(10), 1977–1979.

Brown, G. K., Currier, G., & Stanley, B. (2008). Suicide Attempt Registry Pilot Project. In *National Institute of Mental Health Annual Meeting of the Developing Centers for Intervention and Prevention of Suicide*, September 2008, Canandaigua, NY.

Bryan, C., Corso, K., David, R., & Cordero, L. (2008). Improving identification of suicidal patients in primary care through routine screening. *Primary Care and Community Psychiatry*, **13**(4), 143–147.

Centers for Disease Control and Prevention: National Center for Injury Prevention and Control. (2010). Web-based Injury Statistics Query and Reporting System (WISQARS) Available at:. http://www.cdc.gov/injury/wisqars/index.html

Clark, D., White, E., & Violanti, J. (2012). Law enforcement suicide: current knowledge and future directions. *The Police Chief*, **LXXIX**(5), 48–51.

Conwell, Y., & Thompson, C. (2008). Suicidal behavior in elders. *Psychiatric Clinics of North America*, **31**(2), 333–356.

Crosby, A. O. L., & Melanson, C. (2011). *Self-directed Violence: Uniform Definitions and Recommended Data Elements, Version 1.0.* Atlanta, GA: Centers for Disease Control and Prevention.

Currier, G., Brown, G., & Stanley, B. (2009). *Unpublished Data: Scale For Suicide Ideation Total Score by Level of C-SSRS Severity of Ideation.* American Foundation for Suicide Prevention.

Eaton, D. K., Kann, L., Kinchen, S., et al. (2012). Youth risk behavior surveillance – United States, 2011. *MMWR Surveillance Summary*, **61**(4), 1–162.

Fawcett, J. (1992). Suicide risk factors in depressive disorders and in panic disorder. *Journal of Clinical Psychiatry*. **53** (Suppl), 9–13.

Fawcett, J., Scheftner, W., Fogg, L., & Clark, D. (1990). Time-related predictors of suicide in major affective disorder. *The American Journal of Psychiatry*, **147**(9), 1189–1194.

Fergusson, D., Doucette, S., Glass, K. C., et al. (2005). Association between suicide attempts and selective serotonin reuptake inhibitors: systematic review of randomised controlled trials. *BMJ*, **330** (7488), 396.

Goldacre, M., Seagroatt, V., & Hawton, K. (1993). Suicide after discharge from psychiatric inpatient care. *The Lancet*, **342**(8866), 283–286.

Goldman, L. S., Nielsen, N. H., & Champion, H. C. (1999). Awareness, diagnosis, and treatment of depression. *Journal of General Internal Medicine*, **14**(9), 569–580.

Goldsmith, S. K., Pellmar, T. C., Kleinman, A. M., & Bunney, W. E. (Eds.) (2002). *Reducing Suicide: A National Imperative*. Washington, DC: The National Academies Press.

Gould, M. S., King, R., Greenwald, S., et al. (1998). Psychopathology associated with suicidal ideation and attempts among children and adolescents. *Journal of the American Academy of Child & Adolescent Psychiatry*, **37**(9), 915–923.

Gould, M. S., Greenberg, T., Velting, D., et al. (2003). Youth suicide risk and preventive interventions: A review of the past 10 years. *Journal of the American Academy of Child & Adolescent Psychiatry*, **42**(4), 386–405.

Gould, M. S., Marrocco, F. A., Kleinman, M., et al. (2005). Evaluating iatrogenic risk of youth suicide screening programs: A randomized controlled trial. *JAMA*, **293** (13), 1635–1643.

Greist, J. H., Gustafson, D., Stauss, F., et al. (1973). A computer interview for suicide-risk prediction. *American Journal of Psychiatry*, **130**(12), 1327–1332.

Haas, A., Koestner, B., Rosenberg, G., et al. (2008). An interactive web-based method of outreach to college students at risk for suicide. *Journal of American College Health*, **57**(1), 15–22.

Harris, E. C., & Barraclough, B. (1997) Suicide as an outcome for mental disorders. A meta-analysis. *The British Journal of Psychiatry*, **170**(3),205–228.

Hawton, K. (1987). Assessment of suicide risk. *British Journal of Psychiatry*, **150**, 145–153.

Hayes, L. M. (2010). *National Study of Jail Suicide: 20 Years Later*. Washington, DC: US Department of Justice, National Institute of Corrections.

Hesdorffer, D. C., French, J., Posner, K., et al. (2013). Suicidal ideation and behavior screening in intractable focal epilepsy eligible for drug trials. *Epilepsia*, **54**(5), 879–887.

Holi, M., Pelkonen, M., Karlsson, L., et al. (2008). Detecting suicidality among adolescent outpatients: evaluation of trained clinicians' suicidality assessment against a structured diagnostic assessment made by trained raters. *BMC Psychiatry*, **8**(1), 97.

Insel, T. (2010). The Under-recognized Public Health Crisis of Suicide. In National Institute of Mental Health Director's Blog. http://www.nimh.nih.gov/about/director/2010/the-under-recognized-public-health-crisis-of-suicide.shtml

Isometsa, E. (1998). Suicide attempts preceding completed suicide. *The British Journal of Psychiatry*, 1998, **173**(6), 531–535.

Isometsa, E., Aro, H., Henriksson, M., & Lonnqvist, J. (1994). Suicide in major depression in different treatment settings. *Journal of Clinical Psychiatry*, **55**(12), 523–527.

John, R. & Ross, H., (2010). *The Global Economic Cost of Cancer*. Atlanta, GA: American Cancer Society and LIVESTRONG.

Katzan, I., Viguera, A., Burke, T., Buchanan, J., & Posner, K. (2013). Improving Suicide Screening at the Cleveland Clinic through Electronic Self-Reports: PHQ-9 and the Columbia-Suicide Severity Rating Scale (C-SSRS). 1st Annual Meeting of the International Academy for Suicide Research, Montreal, Canada.

Kerr, D.C., Gibson, B., Leve, L.D., & DeGarmo, D.S. (2014). Young adult follow-up of adolescent girls in juvenile justice using the Columbia Suicide Severity Rating Scale. *Suicide and Life-Threatening Behavior*, **44** (2), 113–129.

Kessler, R. C., Borges, G., & Walters, E. E. (1999). Prevalence of and risk factors for lifetime suicide attempts in the National Comorbidity Survey. *Archives of General Psychiatry*, **56**(7), 617–626.

King, C. A., O'Mara, R., Hayward, C., et al. (2009). Adolescent suicide risk screening in the emergency department. *Academic Emergency Medicine*, **16**(11), 1234–1241.

King, C., Gipson, P., Agarwala, P., & Opperman, K. (2012). Using the C-SSRS to Assess Adolescents in Psychiatric Emergency Settings Predictive Validity Across a One-Year Period. May 2012. 52nd Annual NCDEU Meeting, Phoenix, AZ.

Kuo, W.-H., Gallo, J. J., & Tien, A. (2001). Incidence of suicide ideation and attempts in adults: the 13-year follow-up of a community sample in Baltimore, Maryland. *Psychological Medicine*, **31**(7), 1181–1191.

Levine, S., Ancill, R. J., & Roberts, A. P. (1989). Assessment of suicide risk by computer-delivered self-rating questionnaire: preliminary findings. *Acta Psychiatrica Scandinavica*, **80**(3), 216–220.

Lewinsohn, P. M., Rohde, P., & Seeley, J. R. (1994). Psychosocial risk factors for future adolescent suicide attempts. *Journal of Consulting and Clinical Psychology*, **62**(2), 297–305.

Luoma, J. B., Martin, C. E., & Pearson, J. L. (2002). Contact with mental health and primary care providers before suicide: a review of the evidence. *American Journal of Psychiatry*, **159**(6), 909–916.

Malone, K. M., Szanto, K., Corbitt, E. M., & Mann, J. J. (1995). Clinical assessment versus research methods in the assessment of suicidal behavior. *American Journal of Psychiatry*, **152**(1), 1601.

Mann, J. J., Waternaux, C., Haas, G. L., & Malone, K. M. (1999). Toward a clinical model of suicidal behavior in psychiatric patients. *American Journal of Psychiatry*, **156**(2), 181–189.

Mann, J., Apter, A., Bertolote, J., et al. (2005). Suicide prevention strategies: A systematic review. *JAMA*, **294**(16), 2064–2074.

Marzuk, P., Tardiff, K., Leon, A., Portera, L., & Weiner, C. (1997). The prevalence of aborted suicide attempts among psychiatric inpatients. *Acta Psychiatrica Scandinavica*,. **96**(6), 492–496.

McCarty, C. A., Russo, J., Grossman, D., et al. (2011). Adolescents with suicidal ideation: health care use and functioning. *Academic Pediatrics*, **11**(5), 422–426.

Meyer, R. E., Salzman, C., Youngstrom, E., et al. (2010). Suicidality and risk of suicide – definition, drug safety concerns, and a necessary target for drug development: a consensus statement. *The Journal of Clinical Psychiatry*, **71**(8), e1–e21.

Milton, J., Ferguson, B., & Mills, T. (1999). Risk assessment and suicide prevention in primary care. *Crisis: The Journal of Crisis Intervention and Suicide Prevention*. **20**(4), 171–177.

Mundt, J., Greist, J., Jefferson, J., Federico, M., Mann, J., & Posner, K. (2013). Prediction of suicidal behavior in clinical research by lifetime suicidal ideation and behavior ascertained by the electronic Columbia-Suicide Severity Rating Scale. *Journal of Clinical Psychiatry*, **74**(9), 887–893.

Nordström, P., Samuelsson, M., & Åsberg, M. (1995). Survival analysis of suicide risk after attempted suicide. *Acta Psychiatrica Scandinavica*, **91**(5), 336–340.

Nutting, P. A., Dickinson, L. M., Rubenstein, L. V., et al. (2005). Improving detection of suicidal ideation among depressed patients in primary care. *The Annals of Family Medicine*, **3**(6), 529–536.

O'Carroll, P. W., Berman, A. L., Maris, R. W., et al. (1996). Beyond the Tower of Babel: a nomenclature for suicidology. *Suicide and Life Threatening Behavior*, **26**(3), 237–252.

Oquendo, M. A., Halberstam, B., & Mann, J. J. (2003). Risk factors for suicidal behavior. *Standardized Evaluation in Clinical Practice*, **22**, 103–129.

Paul, R. (2005). *A Workplace Strategy for Preventing Suicide*. SPRC Teleconference.

Peñta, J. B., & Caine, E. D. (2006). Screening as an approach for adolescent suicide prevention. *Suicide and Life-Threatening Behavior*, **36**(6), 614–637.

Petronis, K. R., Samuels, J. F., Moscicki, E. K., et al. (1990). An epidemiologic investigation of potential risk factors for suicide attempts. *Social Psychiatry and Psychiatric Epidemiology*, **25**(4), 193–199.

Pfeffer, C. R., Klerman, G. L., Hurt, S. W., et al. (1993). Suicidal children grow up: rates and psychosocial risk factors for suicide attempts during follow-up. *Journal of the American Academy of Child & Adolescent Psychiatry*, **32**(1), 106–113.

Posner, K., Oquendo, M. A., Gould, M., Stanley, B., & Davies, M. (2007). Columbia Classification Algorithm of Suicide Assessment (C-CASA): classification of suicidal events in the FDA's pediatric suicidal risk analysis of antidepressants. *American Journal of Psychiatry*, **164**(7), 1035–1043.

Posner, K., Brown, G. K., Stanley, B., et al. (2011). The Columbia-Suicide Severity Rating Scale: initial validity and internal consistency findings from three multisite studies with adolescents and adults. *American Journal of Psychiatry*, **168**(12), 1266–1277.

Posner, K., Brown, M., Walsh, A., Apperson, C., & Martin, A. (2013a). Dissemination of a suicide risk assessment tool, the Columbia Suicide Severity Rating Scale, across numerous branches of national and international militaries and VAs. 1st Annual Meeting of the International Academy for Suicide Research, June 10–13 2013, Montreal, Canada.

Posner, K., Greist, J., Mundt, J., et al. (2013b). The full range of suicidal behaviors, its total number, and suicidal ideation predict short-term risk of suicidal behavior in clinical trials, Autumn Conference of the International Society for CNS Clinical Trials and Methodology, Sept 30–Oct 2 2013, Philadelphia, Pennsylvania.

Qin, P., & Nordentoft, M. (2005). Suicide risk in relation to psychiatric hospitalization: Evidence based on longitudinal registers. *Archives of General Psychiatry*, **62**(4), 427–432.

Rockett, I. R., et al. (2012). Leading causes of uninterntional and intentional injury mortality: United States, 2000–2009. *American Jouranl of Public Health*, **102**(11), e84–e92.

Scott, M., Wilcox, H., Schonfeld, I., et al. (2009). School-based screening to identify at-risk students not already known to school professionals: the Columbia Suicide Screen. *American Journal of Public Health*, **99**(2), 334–339.

Shaffer, D., Gould, M. S., Fisher, P., et al. (1996). Psychiatric diagnosis in child and adolescent suicide. *Archives of General Psychiatry*, **53**(4), 339–348.

Shain, B. N. (2007). Suicide and suicide attempts in adolescents. *Pediatrics*, **120**(3), 669–676.

Silverman, M. M. (2006). The language of suicidology. *Suicide & Life-Threatening Behavior*, **36**(5), 519–532.

Silverman, M. M., Berman, A. L., Sanddal, N. D., O'Carroll, P. W., & Joiner, T. E. (2007). Rebuilding the Tower of Babel: A revised nomenclature for the study of suicide and suicidal behaviors. Part 1: Background, rationale and methodology. *Suicide & Life-Threatening Behavior*, **37**(3), 248–263.

Smith, D. I., & Scoullar, K. M. (2001). How well informed are Australian general practitioners about adolescent suicide? Implications for primary prevention. *International Journal of Psychiatry in Medicine*, **31**(2), 169–182.

Stanley, B., (2006). *Fluoxetine and dialectical behavior therapy for borderline personality disorder*. Paper presented at the 46th Annual Meeting of the New Clinical Drug Evaluation Unit, June 12–15, Boca Raton, FL.

Steer, R. A. (1988). Use of the Beck Depression Inventory, Hopelessness Scale, Scale for Suicidal Ideation, and Suicidal Intent Scale with adolescents. *Advances in Adolescent Mental Health*, **3**, 219–231.

Steer, R. A., Beck, A., Garrison, B., & Lester, D. (1988). Eventual suicide in interrupted and uninterrupted attempters: a challenge to the cry-for-help hypothesis. *Suicide and Life-Threatening Behavior*, **18** (2), 119–128.

Sudak, D., Roy, A., Sudak, H., et al. (2007). Deficiencies in suicide training in primary care specialties: a survey of training directors. *Academic Psychiatry*, **31**(5), 345–349.

Vannoy, S. D., Duberstein, P., Cukrowicz, K., et al. (2007). The relationship between suicide ideation and late-life depression. *American Journal of Geriatric Psychology*, **15**(12), 1024–1033.

Vijayakumar, L., & Rajkumar, S. (1999). Are risk factors for suicide universal? A case-control study in India. *Acta Psychiatrica Scandinavica*, **99**(6), 407–411.

Vitiello, B., Silva, S., Rohde, P., et al. (2009). Suicidal events in the Treatment for Adolescents with Depression Study (TADS). *The Journal of Clinical Psychiatry*, **70**(5), 741.

Wichstrom, L. (2000). Predictors of adolescent suicide attempts: a nationally representative longitudinal study of Norwegian adolescents. *Journal of the American Academy of Child & Adolescent Psychiatry*, **39**(5), 603–610.

Chapter 4

Rethinking suicide risk assessment and risk formulation

Alan L. Berman and Morton M. Silverman

Introduction

Approximately one in three American, and one in four British, citizens contact a mental health care provider or service in the year prior to dying by suicide (Luoma et al., 2002; Appleby et al., 2012). About one in ten patients are seen in emergency departments within 2 months of dying by suicide (Knesper, 2010). A conservatively estimated 31.3% of individuals who died by suicide were receiving mental health treatment at the time of their death (Centers for Disease Control and Prevention, 2012).

Clearly, health care providers have significant opportunity to identify at risk individuals and engage them in treatment to reduce the risk of suicidal behavior, yet many lack the requisite training and skills to appropriately assess for suicide risk (Schulberg et al., 2004; Schmitz et al., 2012). Tragically, the Joint Commission's Sentinel Event Report denotes failures in conducting an assessment to be the leading root cause of hospital-based suicides, associated with 84% (N = 502) of the 600 suicides reported between 2004 and 2011(www.jointcommission.org).

We see the assessment process as encompassing two key steps: first to determine whether an individual is at risk for suicide; second to determine the level of risk. These steps then inform appropriate interventions (ideally evidence-based) to reduce the level of risk and clinical judgments about modifying or tailoring interventions to the specific individual and setting.

This chapter addresses suicide risk assessment (SRA) and suicide risk formulation (SRF) commonly employed by mental health practitioners. We will challenge the current thinking and the lack of an evidence base that appear to guide these processes.

An SRA involves the collection of data, of observable and reported factors associated with suicide risk and ascertained by mental health interview, collateral information gathering, screening tools, and/or scales. A thorough SRA is a necessary precursor to an SRF. The SRF is a more abstruse process forged by clinical judgment about the dynamic contributions of this data to determine the patient's level of risk that, then, dictates safety planning, triage decisions, and treatment planning and management.

Suicide risk assessment

No method of SRA has been empirically tested for reliability and validity (Busch et al., 2003) or has sufficient sensitivity and specificity to be effective (Simon, 2012). Yet, the standard of care[1] requires mental health professionals to recognize and foresee the possibility that a patient might engage in suicidal behavior, hence to conduct an SRA and make an SRF sufficient to guide triage and treatment planning.

The SRA, ideally, incorporates separate but integrated components, the first two of which are:

1. Identifying perpetuating (non-modifiable), predisposing (modifiable), acute (warning signs), precipitating (triggering), contributing, and protective risk factors (see www.suicidology.org)
2. Exploring the presence/absence of suicidal ideation, motivations, intent, planning, and behavior.

A focus on suicide ideation

The presence of communicated SI has traditionally been the gateway to the investigation of whether an individual might be "suicidal." Hence the normative approach to an SRA is to first inquire about the presence of SI. The unfortunate corollary has been the clinical assumption that the absence of SI is

[1] The standard of care is generally defined as that duty to exercise that degree of skill and care ordinarily employed in similar circumstances by members of the same profession.

A Concise Guide to Understanding Suicide, ed. Stephen H. Koslow, Pedro Ruiz, and Charles B. Nemeroff. Published by Cambridge University Press.

tantamount to the absence of any suicide risk, hence no need to pursue a line of questioning that might reveal the presence of other factors that help define presence of risk. As noted by Simon (2012), "the extent of suicide risk assessment usually is no more than the statement 'Patient denies HI, SI, CFS (homicidal ideation, suicidal ideation, contracts for safety).'"

If a patient states that SI is present, the clinician is obligated to explore SI further regarding questions of intent, content (active thoughts of suicide versus passive wishes for death; planning), duration, frequency, intensity, controllability, etc. Received wisdom has dictated that if SI is deemed to be active and with intent or plans, risk should be judged to be greater than if SI is chronic, passive and/or without intent (Rudd et al., 2006).

The reality is the following:

- Among those who die by suicide, SI is more likely to be denied than admitted to upon clinical inquiry conducted reasonably proximate to the date of death (see below).
- Active SI is no more associated with death by suicide than is passive SI (Simon, 2006).
- The association between currently expressed SI and subsequent death by suicide is less clear (Beck et al., 1999).

Determining the presence of suicide ideation

Determining the presence of suicide ideation depends upon how the question is asked, how the respondent understands the question, and whether the respondent feels safe in providing an honest answer.

SI in the past year

The prevalence of SI in the past 12 months in the general population (18 years of age or older) varies from 3.3% to 3.8% (Kessler et al., 2005; www.samhsa.gov/data/NSDUH/2k10State/NSDUHsae2010). However, how the question gets asked determines what responses are given. Asking questions that are imprecise, vague, and non-specific does not help identify those at risk for suicidal behaviors in the long- or near-term. For example, the response to the question, "Have you seriously considered ending your life?" will be determined by how a respondent interprets the term "seriously."

SI across the lifespan

Kessler et al. (1999) reported that the lifetime prevalence of suicide ideation in the general population (aged 15–54) was 13.5%. The probability of transitioning from SI to plan was 34%, from a plan to an attempt was 72%, and from SI to an unplanned attempt, 26%. Identifying which persons with SI are at greatest risk of progressing to a suicide attempt, however, has been elusive (May et al., 2012).

Does the presence of suicide ideation predict anything?

Hence,

- the majority of individuals reporting SI do not go on to make a plan (~66%)
- SI with plan is no more predictive of a suicide attempt than is SI without a plan (~19–25%)
- the majority of individuals reporting SI do not go on to attempt suicide (~66%). However, within a year of onset of SI, there is an increased risk for suicide attempts.

Fawcett et al. (1990) followed a mostly inpatient sample of over 950 patients for 10 years and found that hopelessness and SI were significantly associated with suicide in those patients who died by suicide (N = 32), *but more than a year after the intake evaluation.* Hence, it appears that acknowledgment of SI is a more significant *chronic* risk factor for eventual death by suicide than it is an acute (near-term) risk factor (Rudd et al., 2006).

Moreover, the presence of current SI may not be the most important focus in an SRA. Beck et al. (1999) found that a retrospective report of SI at the worst point in a patient's life was a better predictor of eventual death by suicide than was current SI or hopelessness.

Does the denial of suicide ideation predict death by suicide?

It is common sense to believe that suicidal behavior must be preceded by SI – and it may well be – but in fact the majority of patients who die by suicide actually *deny* having suicidal thoughts when last asked prior to their death (or communicate their risk behaviorally) (Isometsa et al., 1995; Hall et al., 1999; Busch et al., 2003). As but one example, the US National Violent Death Reporting System informs us that only 28.3% of almost 10 000 persons who died by suicide disclosed their intent to die by suicide (Karch et al., 2012).

For the clinician, inquiring about SI is seen as the key data point in the decision to admit or discharge a patient, extend hospitalization, or refer a patient to specialized mental health treatment. But, for the patient, denying SI may be seen as essential to maintaining autonomy and control over one's life and choices, avoiding hospitalization, facilitating discharge, and a consequent freedom to act on a desire and intent to die by suicide, etc.

Similarly, taking active precautions against discovery during an attempt is an important predictor for eventual death by suicide (Wenzel et al., 2011).

Accordingly, it is incumbent upon the clinician to go beyond a cursory exploration of SI to be reassured about the level of risk. Quite simply stated, a "No" response to a clinical query regarding the presence of SI does not suffice to constitute an SRA (Simon, 2012).

Is there a difference between "active" and "passive" SI? If there is, does the difference make a difference?

SI may be described as passive ("I wonder what it would be like if I were dead") to active ("I'm thinking of killing myself"). Nevertheless, there are no clear definitions or guidelines to differentiate active vs. passive SI.

When SI extends to suicide planning and/or preparation, the level of risk is presumed to be greater, i.e., the more detailed and specific the plan, the greater the risk (American Psychiatric Association, 2003). However, this guideline has developed an unintended corollary, i.e., when passive ideation is expressed, clinicians see less risk than when active ideation is expressed, often minimizing the risk altogether.

This thinking carries over to often used scales. The HAM-D, for example, has a suicide item that scales "suicidal ideas" (whatever these may be) at a score of "3," hence more significant than "wishes he were dead" at a score of "2," which is more significant than "feels life is not worth living" at a score of "1" (Hamilton, 1960).

There is simply no empirical support for this supposition, hence the difference between active and passive suicide ideation has no clinical utility (Szanto et al., 1996).

SI in the primary care setting and emergency department

The primary care physician is typically the first, and often the last, medical provider visited by those who die by suicide (Luoma et al., 2002; Schulberg et al., 2004).

Although SI is present in 2–7% of all primary care patients (Olfson et al., 1996), the rate of inquiry and detection of SI in primary care is abysmally low (cf. Schulberg et al., 2004). Rates of inquiry about SI, even when the patient presents with symptoms of major depression, remain low (Feldman et al., 2007).

Similarly, Claassen & Larkin (2005) found that SI was common in emergency department (ED) patients who present for medical disorders. In a study of 1590 ED patients, 11.6% reported SI. However, there is wide variance between and within EDs surrounding suicide risk screening and assessment and most patients who present to the ED are not assessed for suicide risk, due to time constraints, inadequate training, and a lack of screening instruments (Larkin et al., 2009).

In summary, simply inquiring about SI does not constitute an adequate SRA. Terminating the SRA or indicating that risk is low because SI is denied are tragic mistakes too often made by clinicians. Correspondingly, the presence of SI does not indicate high-risk for suicide and active SI is no more associated with risk for death by suicide than is passive SI.

A note about screening

Both the Joint Commission and the American Academy of Pediatrics have called for suicide screening for all patients in health care settings (www.jointcommission.org; American Academy of Child and Adolescent Psychiatry, 2009). Screening is not synonymous with assessment. As commented upon by Simon (2009, p. 292), "forms tend to be an event, whereas clinical assessment is a process."

A screening tool is a brief instrument, typically consisting of a list of evidence-based risk (and, possibly, protective) factors, designed to provide a short-cut to identify patients at risk for suicide. Because these tools are brief, they, by necessity, must exclude a large number of chronic and acute factors associated with elevated risk for suicide. Most often, their focus is on the presence of suicide ideation and behavior, with little, if any, attention paid to the variety of symptoms, behaviors, and other signs of increased and acute risk. They are rarely tested for reliability and validity; too often are scored, as if the derived score has some validated relationship to a reasonable judgment of risk; and are widely variable, institution to institution, as there is no universally accepted instrument.[2]

[2] The Joint Commission makes each facility responsible for developing its own screening protocol (www.jointcommission.org/assets/1/18/NPSG_Chapter_Jan2013_HAP.pdf)

The function of a positive score on a screening instrument is solely to alert the clinician to the need for a more extensive SRA. A negative score on a screening instrument should not alleviate the need for an SRA, if there is any indication of potential risk for suicide. In short, clinicians need to have a working understanding of and sensitivity to acute risk factors for suicide that should automatically trigger an SRA, regardless of how someone "scores" on a screening instrument.

Moreover, screening instruments can generate false negatives, in part because they rely on the individual to self-report responses to often ill-defined, undefined, and/or idiosyncratically defined terms; in part because individuals at risk may not respond with full and accurate disclosure because of their pathology, their embarrassment, etc. Of course, these same barriers may present in a face-to-face SRA, but the clinician has the advantage of a trained eye and ear to discern and question non-verbal cues, to gently confront denials, etc. in the face of other available evidence of possible risk.

The Suicide Ideation Questionnaire (SIQ; Reynolds, 1998) and, more recently, a variation on the SIQ, the Ask Suicide Screening Questions (ASQ) (Horowitz et al., 2012), are two examples of such rapid screening tools, the former developed with the intent to measure the severity of SI and the latter, mostly a briefer version of the former, suggesting that it has predictive value regarding risk for suicide. This claim, however, has been questioned, essentially, again, on the limited available data on the relationship between SI and death by suicide (Wintersteen et al., 2013).

Other screening instruments, primarily developed for the *retrospective* classification of suicidal events in clinical trials increasingly have been widely promoted as *prospective* clinical measures of suicide risk. Two examples of these are the Sheehan Suicidality Tracking Scale (Sheehan-STS: Coric et al., 2009) and the Columbia-Suicide Severity Rating Scale (C-SSRS: Posner et al., 2011).

The STS was designed to track treatment-emergent suicide ideation and behavior and has been found to be more sensitive at this than the screen for these observations that historically served this function, item 3 from the HAM-D.

The C-SSRS, similarly, was developed to track changes in SI and behavior in the Treatment of Adolescent Suicide Attempters (TASA) study (Brent et al., 2009). Predictive validity data (for suicide attempts) essentially hinge on worst-point lifetime suicide ideation and lifetime history of severe suicide ideation (Posner et al., 2011). As these measures of SI are strongly correlated with suicide attempts, these findings are expected. Notably, the C-SSRS makes no claims to predict risk for death by suicide.

The C-SSRS risk assessment version is a checklist of empirically based risk and protective factors, typical of many other checklists. The C-SSRS screening tool is entirely based on past week and lifetime observations of SI (rated on a 1–5 scale with active SI scoring as more severe than passive SI) and suicidal behavior. Of interest, the screen differentiates suicidal behavior into classifications inclusive of actual attempts, interrupted or aborted attempts, preparatory behaviors, and non-suicidal self-injurious behaviors. The categories of recent preparatory behaviors, interrupted, and aborted attempts are claimed to be associated, empirically, with increased risk (http://www.commondataelements.ninds.nih.gov/doc/CSSRS%20Additional%20Information.pdf), but upon closer examination are based on studies with very small Ns (recent preparatory behaviors: N = 4 cases out of 30 [G. Brown, personal communication, January 3, 2013]; interrupted attempts: N = 6 cases out of 41 [Steer et al., 1988]; and aborted attempts: N = 22 cases out of 71 [Barber et al., 1998]). Clearly, more research with larger datasets is called for in this regard.

Simon (2009) has written forcefully about the pitfalls of screening, arguing, appropriately we believe, that assessment forms and checklists cannot – and should not – replace a face-to-face clinical risk assessment. Moreover, the US Preventive Services Task Force has found insufficient evidence that screening for suicide risk in the primary care setting reduces suicide attempts or deaths by suicide (O'Connor et al., 2013).

A brief guide to a better assessment of suicide ideation

First: Ask about SI:

- Always frame and ask (and document) at least two different questions regarding the presence of SI and ask patients to explain their responses.
- Always ask about SI at the worst point in the patient's life.
- Refrain from using vague temporal references such as "recently."

- Be specific about what you are asking the patient. Define what you mean by "suicidal thoughts" or "thinking of killing yourself."
- Explore, understand, and document expressed SI – its frequency, intensity, duration, temporality, intent, controllability, context, motivation for, etc.
- Explore the patient's history of impulsivity or predisposition to be poorly controlled (e.g., alcoholic). Any type of SI, in the context of poor impulse control, may be just as lethal as SI with resolved plans and preparations.
- If you choose to categorize SI as passive versus active, do not assume that one is more, versus less, indicative of future suicidal behavior.

Second: If SI is denied:

- If motivation (unfulfilled need states) for leaving life is present, continue to conduct an SRA.
- Use multiple screening methods, ranging from self-report scales to computer-administered screens to direct psychiatric interview.
- Ask, "When you were at your worst point psychologically, did you have any thoughts of suicide? If so, what was going on at that time and what kind of thoughts did you have?"
- Confront (gently) the denial of SI, when other signs of acute risk are present.
- It is only appropriate to accept a denial of SI as a sufficient SRA when there is no presence of predisposing risk factors or acute risk factors, independent reports of suicide-related activities, and/or potential motivation for suicide.

Suicide risk formulation

The data collected via an SRA informs an SRF. The SRF requires an understanding of how risk factors interact, exacerbate, and otherwise fuel heightened or lowered risk for suicide, no less how they inform a clinical formulation about level of risk.

The clinical literature abounds with reference to an SRF as an intuitive enterprise. Motto (1992) wrote about formulating suicide risk, "...there is no avoiding subjectivity...leaving us with what I have referred to above as an intuitive judgment" (p. 633). Maltsberger (1992) wrote, "Because no one knows how to do this [integrate a large mass of data] precisely and with empirical certainty, the clinician is forced to rely on clinical experience and on inductive reasoning. He does not know how important each datum may be in comparison to the others that have been collected" (p. 38).

Surprisingly, there is little in the clinical literature that offers a model for an SRF, i.e., a guideline for establishing levels of risk. What was noted by Motto in 1989 remains true almost a quarter of a century later:

> "...to date we have no established and generally accepted procedure to guide us ... Innumerable decisions regarding risk are made and implemented every day – the job gets done – but how it gets done is determined primarily by the skills and philosophy of the individual clinician."
>
> (Motto, 1989, p. 245).

The detection of suicide risk (SRA) and formulation of suicide risk (SRF), and the consequent triage and treatment decisions that are dependent on these procedures are, perhaps, the most significant actions a clinician must make. The failure to reasonably accomplish these tasks has the potential for significant negative outcomes for both the patient (a possibly preventable death by suicide) and the clinician (the premature death of a patient; a preventable tort action). It is time to move beyond the intuition and philosophy of the clinician and to develop and train to models for conducting an SRA and SRF.

What is meant by "level of suicide risk"?

Traditionally, the clinician evaluates a patient's risk on an ordinal scale ranging from No Risk to High-Risk; and, within this last category, determines whether "High-Risk" might be "Imminent." Standardized, operational definitions of these levels of risk do not exist, and some question the concept of "Imminent Suicide" (Simon, 2006). What is generally understood by the clinician is merely that higher versus lower levels of judged risk carry more significant demands for aggressive treatment planning, triage, and intervention (and potentially civil commitment).

Imminent risk. Imminent risk determinations are clinical and temporally related predictions of behavior in the ill-defined near future.

In the USA, statutes for assisted treatment (involuntary hospitalization) vary considerably, but, typically, employ language to guide the clinician as follows:

- *Real and present threat of substantial harm*
- *Likely to injure if not thwarted*
- *...in the reasonable future*

As Simon (2006) wrote, this near-term prediction of imminent risk "imposes an illusory time frame on an unpredictable act" (p. 296).

Just how reliable are judgments of risk? Cahill and Rakow (2011) presented 35 hypothetical case examples to seven practitioners and found all but two potential risk factors were related to risk and priority judgments. They noted that "low risk" might be particularly subject to variability in its interpretation, noting that the term "risk" could reflect "the probability of occurrence for some," and "the severity of occurrence to others." It should come as no surprise that Appleby et al. (2012) reported that more than 80% of patients who die by suicide are seen by their clinical teams as having no or low risk.

Suicide risk scales

Beginning in the early 1960s, clinical researchers began developing suicide potential scales to help evaluate a patient or caller who identified him/herself as suicidal. For example, Tuckman and Youngman (1968) developed a scale for differentiating high versus low suicide risk among those who had made an attempt, defining high-risk operationally as a predicted death from suicide within 1 year of the attempt. Perhaps, the most significant contribution to developing a SRF was offered by suicide researchers at the NIMH in the early 1970s, who developed sophisticated models for formulating risk among four demographic groups defined by age and gender (old–young, male–female). Weighted items and associated ratings of risk were established, with scaled scores indicating high-risk equating to the likelihood of being dead by suicide within 2 years (Beck et al., 1974). None of these early efforts to predict suicide were ever replicated or validated.

Given the low base rate of suicide, predictive scales will produce far more false positives than could be clinically tolerated. Indeed, attempts to actuarially integrate suicide risk factors into some sort of formula for judging level of risk have been shown to have poor specificity (Haney et al., 2012). There is a need for clinical models to inform clinical judgments about levels of risk. Moreover, questions remain as to whether clinical judgments of risk are to be based reasonably on science, intuition, or both, and whether good clinical judgment regarding a patient's relative level of suicide risk can be trained.

Current models for suicide risk formulation

The National Suicide Prevention Lifeline (www.suicidepreventionlifeline.org/crisiscenters/bestpractices) has offered a guide to determine imminent risk, as follows:

> *Imminent risk may be determined if an individual states (or is reported to have stated by a person believed to be a reliable informant) both a desire and intent to die and has the capability of carrying through his/her intent.*
>
> (Joiner et al., 2007).

This model asserts that desire, intent, and acquired capability, in a context of low buffers or connectedness, are associated with imminent risk. While the individual components of these factors have support for their association with greater lifetime risk for suicide, no test of the asserted combination of desire, intent, and capability and imminent or even near-term risk has yet been made.

An alternative model is outlined in The American Association of Suicidology's *Recognizing and Responding to Suicide Risk* (www.suicidology.org) clinical training program. This model asserts that the presence of warning signs (acute risk factors) (Rudd et al., 2006)[3] in the context of the patient's vulnerability to be suicidal across his/her lifetime (chronic risk) informs imminent risk. Although no actuarial statement is made about cut-off scores, the presence of three or more acute risk factors has been shown to describe the majority of 55 suicidal decedents on whom a psychological autopsy was conducted (Berman, 2011). Unfortunately, current warning signs (Rudd et al., 2006) are associated with suicide *over the subsequent 12 months*, not the next 30 or 7 days or, for that matter, 48 hours. There is an important need for research on observable risk factors in the last days of life of those who die by suicide.

A third model is offered by the SAFE-T pocket card (www.sprc.org/library/safe_t_pcktcrd_edc.pdf). The downside to the SAFE-T model is that it maintains a focus on current SI or behavior as integral to informing that judgment of level of risk.

The outcome of an SRF is a disposition, for example in an emergency department: release without follow-up or recommendation for further treatment, release with recommendation for follow-up outpatient care, release with crisis management and safety planning interventions, release with arranged outpatient interventions (psychotherapy and/or medications), or hospitalization (for safety and further assessment). In this case, triage decisions would have to include an assessment of the patient's support system, evidence of

[3] see www.suicidology.org for an extensive list of chronic and acute risk factors.

controls over SI and/or subsequent attempt, ability to cooperate, and degree of resolution of life crises that prompted the presentation to the ED, in addition to an assessment of current acute risk factors and warning signs. These same variables might be considered in an outpatient setting to help guide dispositional decision-making about the need for hospitalization.

A final note on clinical judgment

As noted, there is a need for research to inform an SRF:

- On risk factors associated with very near-term risk
- On which of the many components of the SRA – and to what degree the frequency, duration, intensity, timing, etc., of each of these components, as well as their combinations and permutations – informs the appropriate level of risk in an SRF
- On validating models for an SRF
- On evaluating the appropriateness of interventions linked to an SRF.

Clinicians deserve a better roadmap or clinical tool to assist in assigning a level of suicide risk to an individual. Without such a guide, the clinician is left to his/her education, training, intuition, judgment, and prior experience to determine how best to intervene and manage the patient. Clinical judgments and intuitions are influenced by knowledge and experience (Bittner & Tobin, 1998), but greater experience does not necessarily equate to better judgment. Clinical "expertise" adds little to the accuracy of clinical judgment (Hilton et al., 2006).

Clinical errors are both universal and inevitable in clinical practice. Clinical judgments, particularly those made under the stress of seeking to be life-saving, may be especially prone to error. As noted by Karthikeyan and Pais (2010), "clinical judgment conjures up visions of the archetypal clinician endowed with infinite wisdom and breathtaking clairvoyance." We recognize that creating clinicians in this mold is an unattainable goal. No doubt that sound clinical judgment must be brought to the task of formulating risk, but the questions of whether good clinical judgment can be improved upon, no less trained, remain outstanding.

Moreover, despite the obvious appeal, it remains dangerous and unpredictable to rely on "clinical intuition" in arriving at a judged risk level for an individual, when life or death hangs in the balance. In the end actuarial models for predicting a patient's risk of violence, in contrast to clinical judgment, may not be superior (Litwack, 2001). The need now is to bring as much science into this process as is possible to arrive at the best possible approach to risk formulation. Indeed, evidence that this is possible exists (Swets et al., 2000).

Conclusion

An SRA is a data gathering enterprise that may be approached initially by asking questions regarding the presence of SI, but must not be limited to inquiries about SI. Suicide risk may exist and may even be imminent with or without communicated SI. Moreover, SI has an inconclusive association with death by suicide; it is a better predictor of suicide attempt, but, again, is neither necessary, nor sufficient, for the assessment of that risk. SI comes in a variety of forms and little to no research has been conducted to assure clinicians that one or another form, such as passive versus active SI, is more, versus less, associated with near-term or long-term risk of death by suicide.

An SRF is akin to a recipe to piece together the ingredients developed from an SRA. The types and amounts of the ingredients will dictate the final product. Clinical intuition and judgment will always be necessary to an SRF, as purely actuarial models will never attain the level of specificity and sensitivity desired. That said, models for an SRF and guidelines to better inform clinical judgment are called for and need to be empirically tested. It is time to establish empirically whether good clinical judgment in the assessment and formulation of suicide risk can be trained. Additionally we need to better understand how decisions about dispositions are made based on the SRF.

References

American Academy of Child and Adolescent Psychiatry, Committee on Health Care Access and Economics Task Force on Mental Health (2009). Improving mental health services in primary care: reducing administrative and financial barriers to access and collaboration. *Pediatrics*, **123**(4), 1248–1251.

American Psychiatric Association (2003). Practice guidelines for the assessment and treatment of patients with suicidal behaviors. *American Journal of Psychiatry*, **160**(Suppl 11), 1–60.

Appleby, L., Kapur, N., Shaw, J., et al (2012). The National Confidential Inquiry into Suicide and Homicide by People with Mental Illness Annual Report, July 2012, London: Department of Health.

Barber, M. E., Marzuk, P. M., Leon, A. C., & Portera, L. (1998). Aborted suicide attempts: A new classification of suicidal behavior. *American Journal of Psychiatry*, **155**(3), 385–389.

Beck, A. T., Resnik, H. L., & Lettieri, D. J. (1974). *The Prediction of Suicide*. Philadelphia, PA: Charles Press.

Beck, A. T., Brown, G. K., Steer, R. A., Dahlsgaard, K. K., & Grisham, J. R. (1999). Suicide ideation at its worst point: A predictor of eventual suicide in psychiatric outpatients. *Suicide & Life-Threatening Behavior*, **29**(1), 1–9.

Berman, A. L. (2011). *Countermeasures to Reduce Suicides on Railway Rights-of-Way in the United States*. Washington, DC: American Association of Suicidology.

Bittner, M. P., & Tobin, E. (1998). Critical thinking: Strategies for clinical practice. *Journal for Nurses Staff Development*, **14**(6), 267–272.

Brent, D. A., Greenhill, L. L., Compton, S., et al. (2009). The Treatment of Adolescent Suicide Attempters Study (TASA): Predictors of suicidal events in an open treatment trial. *Journal of the American Academy of Child and Adolescent Psychiatry*, **48**(10), 987–996.

Busch, K. A., Fawcett, J., & Jacobs, D. G. (2003). Clinical correlates of inpatient suicide. *Journal of Clinical Psychiatry*, **64**, 14–19.

Cahill, S., & Rakow, T. (2011). Assessing risk and prioritizing referral for self-harm: When and why is my judgment different from yours? *Clinical Psychology & Psychotherapy*, **19**(5), 399–410.

Centers for Disease Control and Prevention (2012). Surveillance for violent deaths – National Violent Death Reporting System, 16 states, 2009. *Morbidity and Mortality Weekly*, **61**(6), 1–43.

Claassen, C. A., & Larkin, G. L. (2005). Occult suicidality in an emergency department population. *British Journal of Psychiatry*, **186**, 352–353.

Coric, V., Stock, E. G., Pultz, J., & Marcus, R. (2009). Sheehan Suicidality Tracking Scale (Sheehan-STS). *Psychiatry*, **6**(1), 26–31.

Fawcett, J., Scheftner, W., Fogg, L., et al. (1990). Time-related predictors of suicide in major affective disorder. *American Journal of Psychiatry*, **147**, 1189–1194.

Feldman, M. D., Frank, P., Duberstein, P. R., et al. (2007). Let's not talk about it: Suicide inquiry in primary care. *Annals of Family Medicine*, **5**(5), 412–418.

Hall, R. C., Platt, D. E., & Hall, R. C. (1999). Suicide risk assessment: a review of risk factors for suicide in 100 patients who made severe suicide attempts. Evaluation of suicide risk in a time of managed care. *Psychosomatics*, **40**(1), 18–27.

Hamilton, M. (1960). A rating scale for depression. *Journal of Neurology, Neurosurgery and Psychiatry*, **2**, 56–62

Haney, E. M., O'Neil, M. E., Carson, S., et al. (2012). *Suicide risk factors and risk assessment tools: A systematic review*. VA-ESP Project #05-225 (ESP=Evidence-based Synthesis Program).

Hilton, N. Z., Harris, G. T., & Rice, M. E. (2006). Sixty-six years of research on the clinical versus actuarial prediction of violence. *The Counseling Psychologist*, **34**(3), 400–409.

Horowitz, L. M., Bridge, J. A., Teach, S. J., et al. (2012). Ask Suicide-Screening Questions (ASQ): A brief instrument for the pediatric emergency department. *Archives Pediatric and Adolescent Medicine*, **166**(12), 1170–1176.

Isometsa, E. T., Heikkinen, M. E., Marttunen, M. J., et al. (1995). The last appointment before suicide: Is suicide intent communicated? *American Journal of Psychiatry*, **152**(6), 919–922.

Joiner, T. E., Kalafat, J., Draper, J., et al. (2007). Establishing standards for the assessment of suicide risk among callers to the National Suicide Prevention Lifeline. *Suicide and Life-Threatening Behavior*, **37**(3), 353–365.

Karch, D. L., Logan, J., McDaniel, D., Parks, S., & Patel, N. (2012). Surveillance for violent deaths – National Violent Death Reporting System, 16 States, 2009. *Morbidity and Mortality Weekly Report (MMWR)*, **61** (6), 1–43.

Karthikeyan, G., & Pais, P. (2010). Clinical judgment and evidence-based medicine: Time for reconciliation. *Indian Journal of Medical Research*, **132**(5), 623–626.

Kessler, R. C., Borges, G., & Walters, E. E. (1999). Prevalence of and risk factors for lifetime suicide attempts in the National Comorbidity Survey. *Archives of General Psychiatry*, **56**(7), 617–626.

Kessler, R. C., Berglund, P., Borge, G., Nock, M., & Wang, P. S. (2005). Trends in suicide ideation, plans, gestures, and attempts in the United States, 1990–92 to 2001–03. *Journal of the American Medical Association*, **293**, 2487–2495.

Knesper, D. J. (2010): *Continuity of Care for Suicide Prevention and Research: Suicide Attempts and Suicide Deaths Subsequent to Discharge from the Emergency Department or Psychiatry or Psychiatry Inpatient Unit*. Newton, MA: Education Development Center, Inc.

Larkin, G. L., Beautrais, A. L., Spirito, A., et al. (2009). Mental health and emergency medicine: a research agenda. *Academic Emergency Medicine*, **16**(11), 1110–1119.

Litwack, T. R. (2001). Actuarial versus clinical assessments of dangerousness. *Psychology, Public Policy, and Law*, **7**(2), 409–443.

Luoma, J., Martin, C., & Pearson, J. (2002). Contact with mental health and primary care providers before suicide: A review of the evidence. *American Journal of Psychiatry*, **159** (6), 909–916.

Maltsberger, J. T. (1992). The psychodynamic formulation: An aid in assessing suicide risk. In R. W. Maris, A. L. Berman,

J. T. Maltsberger, & R. I. Yufit (Eds.) *Assessment and Prediction of Suicide* (pp.25–49). New York: Guilford.

May, A. M., Klonsky, E. D., & Klein, D. N. (2012). Predicting future suicide attempts among depressed ideators: A 10-year longitudinal study. *Journal of Psychiatric Research*, **46**(7), 946–952.

Motto, J. A. (1989). Problems in suicide risk assessment. In D. Jacobs & H. N. Brown (Eds.) *Suicide: Understanding and Responding* (pp. 129–142). Madison, CT: International Universities Press.

Motto, J. A. (1992). An integrated approach to estimating suicide risk. In R. W. Maris, A. L. Berman, J. Maltsberger, & I. Yufit, R. (Eds) *Assessment and Prediction of Suicide* (pp. 625–639). New York: Guilford.

O'Connor, E., Gaynes, B. N., Burda, B. U., Soh, C., & Whitlock, E. P. (2013). Screening for and treatment of suicide risk relevant to primary care: A systematic review for the U.S. Preventive Services Task Force. *Annals of Internal Medicine*, **158**(10), 741–754.

Olfson, M., Weissman, M. M., Leon, A. C., Sheehan, D. V., & Farber, L. (1996). Suicidal ideation in primary care. *Journal of General and Internal Medicine*, **11**, 447–453.

Posner, K., Brown, G. K., Stanley, B., et al. (2011). The Columbia-Suicide Severity Rating Scale: Initial validity and internal consistency findings from three multisite studies with adolescents and adults. *American Journal of Psychiatry*, **168**(12), 1266–1277.

Reynolds, W. (1998). *Suicidal Ideation Questionnaire*. Odessa, FL: Psychological Assessment Resources.

Rudd, M. D., Berman, A. L., Joiner, T. E., et al. (2006). Warning signs for suicide: Theory, research and clinical applications. *Suicide and Life Threatening Behavior*, **36**, 255–262.

Schmitz, W. M., Allen, M. H., Feldman, B. N., et al. (2012). Preventing suicide through improved training in suicide risk assessment and care: An American Association of Suicidology Task Force report addressing serious gaps in U.S. mental health training. *Suicide and Life-Threatening Behavior*, **42**(3), 292–304.

Schulberg, H. C., Bruce, M. L., Lee, P. W., Williams, J. W., & Dietrich, A. J. (2004). Preventing suicide in primary care patients: The primary care physician's role. *General Hospital Psychiatry*, **26**, 337–345.

Simon, R. I. (2006). Imminent suicide: The illusion of short-term prediction. *Suicide and Life Threatening Behavior*, **36**, 296–301.

Simon, R. I. (2009). Suicide risk assessment forms: Form over substance. *The Journal of the American Academy of Psychiatry and the Law*, **37**, 290–293.

Simon, R. I. (2012). Suicide risk assessment: gateway to treatment and management. In R. I. Simon & R. E. Hales (Eds.) *The American Psychiatric Publishing Textbook of Suicide Assessment and Management*, 2nd edn (pp. 3–28). Washington, DC: American Psychiatric Publishing.

Steer, R. A., Beck, A. T., Garrison, B., & Lester, D. (1988). Eventual suicide in interrupted and uninterrupted attempters: A challenge to the cry-for-help hypothesis. *Suicide and Life-Threatening Behavior*, **18**(2), 119–128.

Swets, A., Dawes, R. M., & Monahan, J. (2000). Psychological science can improve diagnostic decisions. *Psychological Science in the Public Interest*, **1**, 1–26.

Szanto, K., Reynolds, C. F., Frank, E., et al. (1996). Suicide in elderly depressed patients: Is active vs. passive suicidal ideation a clinically valid distinction? *American Journal of Geriatric Psychiatry*, **4**(3), 197–207.

Tuckman, J., & Youngman, W. (1968). A scale for assessing suicide risk of attempted suicides. *Journal of Clinical Psychology*, **24**(1), 17–19.

Wenzel, A., Berchick, E. R., Tenhave, T., et al. (2011). Predictors of suicide relative to other deaths in patients with suicide attempts and suicide ideation: A 30-year prospective study. *Journal of Affective Disorders*, **132**(3), 375–382.

Wintersteen, M. B., Berman, A. L., & Silverman, M. M. (2013). What is meant by "Increased risk for suicide?" *JAMA Pediatrics*, **167**(7), 675–676.

Chapter 5

High-risk cognitive states

Gregory K. Brown and Kelly L. Green

High-risk cognitive states

A middle-aged man is brought to the emergency room via ambulance after his wife comes home early to discover him unconscious with empty bottles of whisky and prescription medication lying next to him. His stomach is pumped and doctors are able to stabilize him. He admits to a psychiatrist the next morning that he attempted to kill himself and wanted to die and is subsequently admitted to an inpatient psychiatric unit. A critical question that his treatment team will be asking over the course of his stay is: "What was he thinking?" Understanding the types of thoughts, beliefs, and cognitive processes that were experienced before, during and following the suicidal crisis is critical for formulating a treatment plan that is tailored to the patient's individual needs. In this chapter, cognition and its role in suicide attempts and death by suicide will be discussed by examining high-risk states for suicide, particularly suicidal ideation, attentional fixation, hopelessness, problem solving deficits, perfectionism, and homicidal ideation. The state of the literature for each of these risk factors will be briefly summarized and recommendations for future research in this area will be outlined.

Suicidal ideation

The most important cognitive risk factor to consider in determining an individual's risk of making a suicide attempt or dying by suicide is suicidal ideation. Although the field has yet to reach consensus on a standard nomenclature for suicide-related constructs, suicidal ideation is commonly defined as thinking about, contemplating, or planning for suicide (Crosby et al., 2011). Suicidal ideation may include thoughts, beliefs, images, voices, or other cognitions reported by the individual about intentionally ending one's own life. According to the recent World Health Organization (WHO) Surveys, the 12-month prevalence rate for suicidal ideation across 21 different countries is 2% (Borges et al., 2010). Results from the National Comorbidity Study in the United States suggest a lifetime prevalence rate of 13.5% for suicidal ideation among individuals between the ages of 15 and 54 (Kessler et al., 1999).

The construct of suicidal ideation can be thought of as a continuum of increasing severity. The least severe type of suicidal ideation occurs when an individual wishes for death, but has no specific thoughts about wanting to kill him- or herself. For example, a patient experiencing these types of thoughts might say things like "I wish I could go to sleep and not wake up." The next level of severity may include thoughts of killing oneself, but without any intent to act on the thoughts or any specific plan to carry out these thoughts. An example of this type of ideation would be a patient who says "I think about killing myself, but I haven't worked out a way to do it and I don't think that I could ever go through with it." More severe forms of suicidal ideation are those that involve an intent to act on these thoughts with or without a specific plan to do so. An individual who has suicidal ideation with a plan but no intent might describe thinking about killing themselves via overdose, but then state that they have no intention to act on their plan in the immediate future. Conversely, an example of suicidal ideation that involves intent with no plan would be a patient who states that they are going to kill themselves in the next week, but that they do not know how they will do it yet. The most severe form of suicidal ideation includes both a specific plan and intent. That is, a patient has worked out the steps that they will need to take in order to bring about their death and intends to follow through on their plan in the near future.

While the association between suicidal ideation and suicidal behavior (including suicide and suicide attempts) has been well established by correlational

A Concise Guide to Understanding Suicide, ed. Stephen H. Koslow, Pedro Ruiz, and Charles B. Nemeroff. Published by Cambridge University Press.

studies, longitudinal studies have further demonstrated that suicidal ideation is a major risk factor for subsequent suicidal behavior. Suicidal ideation consistently predicts later suicide attempts in diverse samples of adults and adolescents across many studies (Larzelere et al., 1996; Kuo et al., 2001; Fergusson et al., 2005; Reinherz et al., 2006; Wong et al., 2008; Britton & Conner, 2010; Posner et al., 2011; Mundt et al., 2013; O'Connor et al., 2013). Further, suicidal ideation has also been found to prospectively predict death by suicide in both inpatient and outpatient samples (Beck et al., 1999; Brown et al., 2000; Joiner et al., 2003; Sani et al., 2011; Wenzel et al., 2011; Mundt et al., 2013).

The measurement of suicidal ideation varies widely across studies with some studies using a single question (e.g., "Are you thinking about suicide?") to other studies using more comprehensive self-report questionnaires or interviews to assess ideation. Although there are numerous reliable and valid measures of suicidal ideation, we have found only three measures with demonstrated predictive validity for suicidal behavior: (1) Scale for Suicide Ideation (SSI), (2) Columbia-Suicide Severity Rating Scale (C-SSRS), and (3) Suicide Probability Scale (SPS). The SSI is a 19-question structured interview that assesses both current suicidal ideation (i.e., over the past week) and suicidal ideation when it was at its worst in an individual's lifetime (Beck et al., 1997). It is the only measure of suicide ideation that has demonstrated predictive validity for death by suicide in a sample of psychiatric outpatients (Brown et al., 2000). The C-SSRS is also an interview-based measure that assesses current suicidal ideation as well as the worst point of suicidal ideation in one's life (Posner et al., 2011). This predictive validity of the worst-point suicidal ideation subscale has been established for suicide attempts in a population of adolescents involved in outpatient treatment (Posner et al., 2011). In a subsequent study, individuals who endorsed lifetime suicide ideation with intent to act on the C-SSRS were five times more likely to report suicidal behavior during follow-up than those who did not (Mundt et al., 2013). Finally, the SPS is a self-report inventory comprised of 36 items that measure suicidal ideation and related constructs such as hopelessness (Cull & Gill, 1982). Like the C-SSRS, one study supported the predictive validity of the SPS for suicide attempts in adolescents (Larzelere et al., 1996).

When considering suicidal ideation in the context of risk assessment, the literature suggests that it is important to not only assess for current suicidal ideation, but that past suicidal ideation at its worst point is also an important indicator for future risk. In a landmark longitudinal study, death records of over 3500 outpatients seen consecutively over the course of an almost 20-year period were collected in order to determine those patients who later died by suicide (Beck et al., 1999). This study revealed that scores on the worst-point SSI at intake were much more predictive of death by suicide than scores on the current SSI as well as the Beck Hopelessness Scale. A similar result was found for the worst-point suicidal ideation severity score on the C-SSRS in the prediction of future suicide attempts in outpatient adolescents (Posner et al., 2011).

As discussed previously, the particular content involved in an individual's suicidal thinking may also confer differential risk. Two of the most important components of suicidal ideation to consider when conducting a risk assessment are the determination of whether an individual has a plan for suicide as well as the intent to act on a plan to kill oneself. Patients with suicide intent and/or plan have been found much more likely to attempt suicide than those with no intent or plan (Borges et al., 2006; Posner et al., 2011). Further, those with high intent are much more likely to eventually die by suicide than those without high intent (Suominen et al., 2004; Stefansson et al., 2012). The presence of a plan to kill oneself is also able to distinguish between groups of individuals who have made recent suicide attempts versus those who have not (Joiner et al., 1997; Pettit et al., 2009). Similar to suicidal ideation in general, the extent of a suicide plan at its worst point in one's lifetime is also particularly predictive of death by suicide (Joiner et al., 2003).

It is important to note that individuals who think about suicide do not necessarily wish for death all the time (or alternately have no wish for life). Rather, most individuals who experience suicidal thinking vacillate between wishing to live and wishing to die, in a conflict that has been coined an "internal debate" (Kovacs & Beck, 1977; Harris et al., 2010). It is estimated that around half of suicidal individuals experience this ambivalent state between wanting to live and wanting to die and that patients who endorse this conflict demonstrate lower levels of suicide intent (Kovacs & Beck, 1977). Follow-up studies have suggested that the magnitude of difference between the wish to die versus the wish to live is an independent risk factor for eventual suicide and that classifying patients into typologies based on the degree of conflict (i.e., ambivalent, mostly wishes to live, mostly wishes to die) may relate to future suicide risk (Brown et al., 2005; O'Connor et al., 2012).

Although research involving the assessment of suicidal ideation on the risk of suicidal behavior has yielded useful results, there are a number of research advances that are recommended for further study. First, most of the studies conducted have generally included samples of adults or adolescents. Less is known about whether current results are replicable in populations of older adults. Given that older adults represent a particularly high-risk group for suicide, research with suicidal elders is especially warranted. Additionally, although greater attention to operational definitions has been given in recent years, a standard nomenclature for suicidal ideation has yet to be adopted by researchers. The lack of standard definitions can limit the ability to compare results across studies and can cause confusion when discussing these constructs. Thus, it is also recommended that standard operational definitions for types of suicidal ideation are tested and agreed upon by consensus in the field. Finally, while we have evidence to suggest that suicidal ideation waxes and wanes over time, our current methodology for measuring ideation is unable to fully capture this phenomenon. Ecological momentary assessment (EMA) is a novel method that allows for assessing changes in suicidal ideation over time and is a promising approach for collecting more detailed information about how a suicidal crisis develops in real time (Shiffman & Stone, 1998). It is recommended that future research incorporate EMA and other novel assessment methods in order to gain more accurate knowledge about the course of suicidal ideation over time.

Attentional fixation

A concept that has received increasing attention over recent years is the idea that not only do high-risk individuals think about and desire suicide, but in fact these individuals may have cognitive biases toward suicide. For example, cognitive theory of suicide posits that individuals at risk for suicide may have an attentional bias toward suicide, such that they may fixate on the idea of suicide to the exclusion of other thoughts when experiencing negative emotions or a crisis (Wenzel et al., 2009).

Researchers have investigated this phenomenon using modified versions of the Stroop Test. This measure typically involves showing the subject a list of words in different colors (e.g., blue, red, green, etc.) and recording how quickly the subject can verbally identify the color of the words (Stroop, 1935). The specific content of the words may lead to longer response delays because the subject diverts their attention to the specific content of the word rather than its color. That is, specific types of words may interfere with a subject's ability to perform the task, as evidenced by the subject taking longer to identify the colors of the word types.

Indeed, individuals who attempted suicide had longer responses to words with emotional content than neutral words compared to psychiatric controls (Williams & Broadbent, 1986). Additionally, suicide attempters have been found to take longer to respond to suicide-specific words versus other types of negative words compared to psychiatric patients who did not attempt suicide as well as to control subjects (Becker et al., 1999; Cha et al., 2010). Additionally, performance on this task has been found to predict the incidence of a repeat suicide attempt over a 6-month follow-up period above and beyond common clinical indicators of risk, such as severity of suicide ideation, psychiatric diagnosis, and clinician prediction (Cha et al., 2010).

While only a few studies have examined attentional fixation as it relates to suicide, this is an area that deserves increased attention. Additional prospective studies of attentional fixation are warranted to determine if current results are replicable and generalizable. This is another area in which novel assessment methods such as EMA could be particularly helpful. Given that it is theorized that attentional fixation is mood state-dependent (Wenzel et al., 2009), it is especially important to be able to examine attentional fixation in the context of a suicidal crisis.

Hopelessness

Negative attitudes and pessimistic expectancies about the future are also a significant risk factor for suicidal behavior. A common misconception about the construct of hopelessness is that it describes a feeling and thus falls into the domain of emotion rather than cognition. However, hopelessness is fundamentally a belief (i.e., cognition) that involves making negative predictions about the future.

Hopelessness is a unique construct in that it can be both a state (i.e., something that can change) and a trait (i.e., something that is relatively stable and consistent over time). For example, some individuals may have stable, ongoing hopelessness that occurs independently of negative affect or an episode of mental illness. Some studies suggest that trait hopelessness may be particularly important as they have found that it predicts suicidal behavior beyond state hopelessness (Young et al., 1996; Goldston et al., 2006). Thus, it is important to not only assess for levels of hopelessness when a patient is in distress, but also to determine the degree of hopelessness when the individual is not experiencing an extreme mood state.

Hopeless cognitions are a significant predictor of future death by suicide, such that individuals with stronger beliefs that things are hopeless are at greater risk for suicide (Beck et al., 1985, 1989, 1990; Clayton, 1993). In a landmark study on hopelessness with psychiatric outpatients, death records were obtained for nearly 2000 outpatients who had been seen over the course of 6 years in an outpatient clinic (Beck et al., 1990). In this study, hopelessness was assessed using the Beck Hopelessness Scale (BHS) which is a 20-item self-report measure that asks an individual to answer either true or false to a variety of statements involving expectancies about the future (Beck & Steer, 1988). The higher the score on the BHS, the higher the level of hopelessness an individual is currently experiencing. The Beck et al. (1990) study found that individuals who died by suicide had significantly higher levels of hopelessness at intake than those who did not.

Additional studies have also found evidence that hopeless beliefs confer risk for suicidal behavior across diverse samples of patients (Henriques et al., 2004; Valtonen et al., 2006; Klonsky et al., 2012; Links et al., 2012; O'Connor et al., 2013). Some studies have found that hopelessness is a very robust predictor of suicide attempts, conferring risk above and beyond highly predictive constructs such as a history of suicide attempts and may be a particularly important factor for individuals who have already made suicide attempts (Goldston et al., 2001; Chandrasekaran & Gnanaselane, 2008; Klonsky et al., 2012). Hopelessness has also been studied as an explanatory construct and has been found to mediate the relationship between depressive symptoms and suicidal ideation and behaviors (Minkoff et al., 1973; Beck et al., 1975, 1993; Dieserud et al., 2001).

Future research on hopelessness should include populations of older adults, who are not well-represented in existing studies. Further research is recommended that better measures and disentangles state and trait hopelessness and their contribution to both near- and long-term risk in the prediction of suicide and suicide attempts.

Problem solving deficits

A deficit in an individual's ability (and perception of their ability) to solve problems is also a cognitive risk factor for suicidal behavior. Problem solving is a process by which an individual generates adaptive solutions to life problems (D'Zurilla & Chang, 1995). Problem solving is theorized to consist of two primary domains: problem orientation and problem solving skills (D'Zurilla & Nezu, 1990). Problem orientation is the set of responses (based on past experience) that an individual brings to their problems. Problem solving skills usually include four tasks: defining the problem, generating alternative solutions, choosing a solution, and finally implementing the solution and evaluating its outcome.

Although problem solving is a construct that has received much attention in the suicide literature, few prospective studies have been done to examine the effect of problem solving skills on suicide and suicide attempts. Poor problem solving has been shown to prospectively predict suicide attempts in two different populations of adults (McAuliffe et al., 2002; Dieserud et al., 2003). Most research studies in this area are cross-sectional and involve comparing groups of individuals (e.g., controls, individuals with suicidal ideation, individuals who made suicide attempts) in order to identify the effects of problem solving on suicidal behavior. Problem solving has been found to be associated with suicidal ideation and attempts in a range of studies with adults, older adults, and adolescents (Linehan et al., 1987; McLeavey et al., 1987; Schotte & Clum, 1987; Clum & Febbraro, 1994; Rudd et al., 1994; D'Zurilla et al., 1998; Howat & Davidson, 2002; Pollock & Williams, 2004; Williams et al., 2005; Gibbs et al., 2009; Dour et al., 2011). Some studies further suggest that individuals with an overgeneralized autobiographical memory are particularly prone to poor problem solving (Pollock & Williams, 2001; Williams et al., 2005). That is, individuals who tend to recall nonspecific general memories as opposed to specific events tend to have greater difficulty solving problems, as it may be more difficult for them to generalize from specific past experiences.

Although there are a variety of instruments that have been created to measure problem solving, the three most commonly used measures include: (1) Problem Solving Inventory (PSI), (2) Means Ends Problem Solving Task (MEPS), and (3) Social Problem Solving Inventory-Revised (SPSI-R). The PSI is a 35-item self-report inventory designed to measure the five components of problem solving described earlier (Heppner & Petersen, 1982). The MEPS is a task that presents a series of scenario vignettes to the subject and the subject is asked to describe the best strategy to solve the problem presented (Platt & Spivack, 1975). The subject's performance is then scored via the number of effective problem solving steps generated, as well as with an overall effectiveness score, and a score for how specific the generated solution was. The SPSI-R, the most widely used measure, is a 25-item self-report inventory that contains five subscales: Positive Problem Orientation, Negative Problem Orientation, Rational Problem Solving, Impulsivity/Carelessness Style, and Avoidance Style (D'Zurilla et al., 2002). Positive problem orientation refers to viewing a problem as an opportunity rather than a threat (as in Negative Problem Orientation). Rational problem solving measures the degree to which an individual possesses effective problem solving skills. The impulsivity scale measures the degree to which an individual solves problems impulsively and the avoidance scale measures to what degree a person avoids active problem solving.

Given that much of the current research on problem solving is cross-sectional, further research on problem solving should focus on examining this construct using prospective methods in order to determine its unique contribution to the prediction of suicidal behavior.

Perfectionism

Cognitions involving perfectionism have also been studied for their role in suicide risk. Perfectionism is often comprised of numerous unrealistic beliefs that perfection of oneself or others is necessary for success and that the lack of perfection will result in failure. One theory of perfectionism purports to have three components: (1) self-oriented perfectionism, (2) socially prescribed perfectionism, and (3) other-oriented perfectionism (Hewitt & Flett, 1991). Self-oriented perfectionism involves strict self-evaluation and the setting of very high personal standards. Socially prescribed perfectionism is the belief that one must attain the high standards that others have for them. Other-oriented perfectionism involves setting high standards for others and negative evaluative beliefs of individuals who do not meet the standards. Perfectionism is most commonly measured using the Multidimensional Perfectionism Scale (MPS). The MPS is a 45-item self-report scale that is designed to measure the three components of perfectionism (Hewitt & Flett, 1991).

Like problem solving deficits, limited prospective research has been conducted to examine the effect of perfectionism on suicide and suicide attempts. One prospective study found that perfectionism at baseline predicted suicidal ideation over a 6-month follow-up period (Beevers & Miller, 2004). Much of the data on the relationship between perfectionism and suicide risk involves cross-sectional studies. Perfectionism has been found to be associated with suicidal ideation and intent (Hewitt et al., 1992, 1994, 1997; Hamilton & Schweitzer, 2000; Blankstein et al., 2007; Flamenbaum & Holden, 2007). Further, the literature suggests that self-oriented and socially prescribed perfectionism may be particularly associated with suicidal ideation (Hewitt et al., 1992, 1994, 1997; Blankstein et al., 2007). Additionally, studies have found that individuals who attempt suicide may evidence higher levels of perfectionism than those who have not attempted suicide (Hewitt et al., 1998; Hunter & O'Connor, 2003). Although such research shows promise for establishing a link between perfectionism and suicide risk, longitudinal studies of perfectionism and suicidal behavior are warranted.

Homicidal ideation

Homicidal and suicidal thinking are related via their shared content of aggression and violence, and there is anecdotal evidence to suggest that, for a subset of individuals, homicidal and suicidal behaviors are associated with each other (e.g., murderers who kill themselves after the act of homicide). However, there is a paucity of research on the association between homicidal ideation and suicidal behavior. To date, we are aware of only one study on this topic that was conducted in a sample of approximately 500 psychiatric outpatients, who were assessed for homicidal and suicidal ideation and attempts (Asnis et al., 1994). This study found that 91% of the patients who had made past homicide attempts also made suicide attempts in the past. Given this association, it has been recommended that the assessment of homicidal ideation should be included in any suicide risk assessment (Wenzel et al., 2009). More research in this area is greatly needed and encouraged as there are no prospective studies examining the role of homicidal ideation or attempts in suicide risk.

Additional recommendations for future research

Future research should seek to address methodological shortcomings that exist in the current literature. For example, while adult and adolescent populations are heavily represented, older adults and special populations such as Veterans and Military Service Members are understudied with regard to high-risk cognitive states. There is also a pressing need for longitudinal research, as cross-sectional studies are limited in identifying causative pathways between cognitive variables and suicidal behavior. More research should be conducted to develop and test theoretical models of how cognitive risk factors might interact or otherwise work together to confer risk for suicide. Additionally, further studies are needed to examine how cognitive states are associated with both near-term and long-term risk for suicide. Many of the important studies that have found predictive validity for cognitive states (e.g., suicidal ideation and hopelessness) have focused on long periods of follow-up over many years. Less is known about short-term risk, especially over shorter durations of time (i.e., days and weeks). It is especially important to gather more information about acute short-term risk, as this is the most important time period for clinicians assessing the safety of their patients in clinical settings. Additionally, there is limited information available about subtypes of individuals and their corresponding risk levels with regard to cognitive states. For example, do fluctuations of cognitive states, such as suicidal ideation or hopelessness, confer more or less risk than chronically high levels of such states?

An important consideration for future research is the ethical obligation to maintain patient safety over the course of a longitudinal research study. Learning that a patient is at risk for suicide may necessitate intervention to reduce the risk of suicide. This is particularly important to consider for studies using EMA during which patients may be responding to assessments at several points during a day or week. For these studies, it is imperative that they include a plan for monitoring patient responses and intervening as clinically appropriate.

Additionally, there are many cognitive risk factors that are emerging in the literature that warrant further prospective study to assess their association with future suicidal behavior. For example, the cognitive factors in Joiner's Interpersonal-Psychological Theory of suicide have been gaining increasing research attention and should be further studied. These factors are perceived burdensomeness, the belief that one is a burden to others, and thwarted belongingness, the belief that one does not have meaningful relationships with other people (Van Orden et al., 2005). Additionally, Shneidman's concept of psychache, or psychological pain that is believed to be intolerable or unbearable, is another understudied cognitive state (Shneidman, 1993). Similarly, helplessness (i.e., the belief that one cannot escape negative situations), which has been extensively studied for its role in depression (Seligman, 1975) should be further examined for its potential role in suicide risk.

In addition to these cognitive states, there are also other cognitive processes that should be further examined for their role in suicide. Cognitive rigidity, or an inflexible style of perceiving and interacting with the world, might be particularly applicable to suicide and could perhaps be a potential underlying cognitive process for problem solving deficits (Patsiokas et al., 1979). Memory is also an important cognitive process that may have important effects on cognitive states and therefore the risk for suicide and should be more explicitly studied. Similarly, implicit associations have recently gained attention in the literature and more research should be done to elucidate their role in suicide risk (Nock et al., 2010). A final important area for further research is to begin to identify how cognitive states are related to potential biomarkers for suicide in order to elucidate the biological underpinnings that characterize suicide risk.

In conclusion, the suicide literature contains important findings on high-risk cognitive states for suicide such as identifying measures of suicidal ideation and hopelessness that have demonstrated predictive validity for suicide. This chapter also describes other cognitive states and cognitive processes, such as perfectionism, problem solving deficits, homicidal ideation, and attentional fixation, which clearly warrant further research using prospective research designs for understanding suicide risk. Other cognitive processes, such as cognitive rigidity, memory, psychological pain and implicit associations for suicide, also show promise for conferring risk.

References

Asnis, G. M., Kaplan, M. L., van Praag, H. M., & Sanderson, W. C. (1994). Homicidal behaviors among psychiatric outpatients. *Hospital & Community Psychiatry*, **45**(2), 127–132.

Beck, A. T., & Steer, R. A. (1988). *Manual for the Beck Hopelessness Scale*. San Antonio, TX: Psychological Corporation.

Beck, A. T., Kovacs, M., & Weissman, A. (1975). Hopelessness and suicidal behavior: An overview. *JAMA*, **234**(11), 1146–1149.

Beck, A. T., Steer, R. A., Kovacs, M., & Garrison, B. (1985). Hopelessness and eventual suicide: A 10-year prospective study of patients hospitalized with suicidal ideation. *The American Journal of Psychiatry*, **142**(5), 559–563.

Beck, A. T., Brown, G., & Steer, R. A. (1989). Prediction of eventual suicide in psychiatric inpatients by clinical ratings of hopelessness. *Journal of Consulting and Clinical Psychology*, **57**(2), 309–310.

Beck, A. T., Brown, G., Berchick, R. J., Stewart, B. L., & Steer, R. A. (1990). Relationship between hopelessness and ultimate suicide: A replication with psychiatric outpatients. *The American Journal of Psychiatry*, **147**(2), 190–195.

Beck, A. T., Steer, R. A., Beck, J. S., & Newman, C. F. (1993). Hopelessness, depression, suicidal ideation, and clinical diagnosis of depression. *Suicide and Life-Threatening Behavior*, **23**(2), 139–145.

Beck, A. T., Brown, G. K., & Steer, R. A. (1997). Psychometric characteristics of the scale for suicide ideation with psychiatric outpatients. *Behaviour Research and Therapy*, **35**(11), 1039–1046.

Beck, A. T., Brown, G. K., Steer, R. A., Dahlsgaard, K. K., & Grisham, J. R. (1999). Suicide ideation at its worst point: A predictor of eventual suicide in psychiatric outpatients. *Suicide and Life-Threatening Behavior*, **29**(1), 1–9.

Becker, E. S., Strohbach, D., & Rinck, M. (1999). A specific attentional bias in suicide attempters. *Journal of Nervous and Mental Disease*, **187**(12), 730–735.

Beevers, C. G., & Miller, I. W. (2004). Perfectionism, cognitive bias, and hopelessness as prospective predictors of suicidal ideation. *Suicide and Life-Threatening Behavior*, **34**(2), 126–137.

Blankstein, K. R., Lumley, C. H., & Crawford, A. (2007). Perfectionism, hopelessness, and suicide ideation: Revisions to diathesis-stress and specific vulnerability models. *Journal of Rational-Emotive & Cognitive-Behavior Therapy*, **25**(4), 279–319.

Borges, G., Angst, J., Nock, M. K., et al. (2006). A risk index for 12-month suicide attempts in the National Comorbidity Survey Replication(NCS-R). *Psychological Medicine*, **36**(12), 1747–1757.

Borges, G., Nock, M. K., Haro Abad, J. M., et al. (2010). Twelve-month prevalence of and risk factors for suicide attempts in the World Health Organization World Mental Health Surveys. *Journal of Clinical Psychiatry*, **71** (12), 1617–1628.

Britton, P. C., & Conner, K. R. (2010). Suicide attempts within 12 months of treatment for substance use disorders. *Suicide and Life-Threatening Behavior*, **40**(1), 14–21.

Brown, G. K., Beck, A. T., Steer, R. A., & Grisham, J. R. (2000). Risk factors for suicide in psychiatric outpatients: a 20-year prospective study. *Journal of Consulting and Clinical Psychology*, **68**(3), 371–377.

Brown, G. K., Steer, R. A., Henriques, G. R., & Beck, A. T. (2005). The internal struggle between the wish to die and the wish to live: A risk factor for suicide. *The American Journal of Psychiatry*, **162**(10), 1977–1979.

Cha, C. B., Najmi, S., Park, J. M., Finn, C. T., & Nock, M. K. (2010). Attentional bias toward suicide-related stimuli predicts suicidal behavior. *Journal of Abnormal Psychology*, **119**(3), 616–622.

Chandrasekaran, R., & Gnanaselane, J. (2008). Predictors of repeat suicidal attempts after first-ever attempt: A two-year follow-up study. *Hong Kong Journal of Psychiatry*, **18** (4), 131–135.

Clayton, P. I. (1993). Suicide in panic disorder and depression. *Current Therapeutic Research*, **54**(6), 825–831.

Clum, G. A., & Febbraro, G. A. R. (1994). Stress, social support, and problem solving appraisal/skills: Prediction of suicide severity within a college sample. *Journal of Psychopathology and Behavioral Assessment*, **16**(1), 69–83.

Crosby, A., Ortega, L., & Melanson, C. (2011). *Self-directed Violence Surveillance: Uniform Definitions and Recommended Data Elements, Version 1.0.* Atlanta, GA: Centers for Disease Control and Prevention, National Center for Injury Prevention and Control.

Cull, J. G., & Gill, W. (1982). *Suicide Probablity Scale*. Los Angeles, CA: Western Psychological Services.

D'Zurilla, T. J., & Chang, E. C. (1995). The relations between social problem solving and coping. *Cognitive Therapy and Research*, **19**(5), 547–562.

D'Zurilla, T. J., & Nezu, A. M. (1990). Development and preliminary evaluation of the Social Problem Solving Inventory. *Psychological Assessment: A Journal of Consulting and Clinical Psychology*, **2**(2), 156–163.

D'Zurilla, T. J., Chang, E. C., Nottingham, E. J., & Faccini, L. (1998). Social problem solving deficits and hopelessness, depression, and suicidal risk in college students and psychiatric inpatients. *Journal of Clinical Psychology*, **54**(8), 1091–1107.

D'Zurilla, T. J., Nezu, A. M., & Maydeu-Olivares, A. (2002). *Manual for the Social Problem Solving Inventory-Revised*. North Tonawanda, NY: Multi-Health Systems.

Dieserud, G., Røysamb, E., Ekeberg, Ø., & Kraft, P. (2001). Toward an integrative model of suicide attempt: A cognitive psychological approach. *Suicide and Life-Threatening Behavior*, **31**(2), 153–168.

Dieserud, G., Røysamb, E., Braverman, M. T., Dalgard, O. S., & Ekeberg, Ø. (2003). Predicating repetition of suicide attempt: A prospective study of 50 suicide attempters. *Archives of Suicide Research*, **7**(1), 1–15.

Dour, H. J., Cha, C. B., & Nock, M. K. (2011). Evidence for an emotion-cognition interaction in the statistical prediction of suicide attempts. *Behaviour Research and Therapy*, **49**(4), 294–298.

Fergusson, D. M., Horwood, L. J., Ridder, E. M., & Beautrais, A. L. (2005). Suicidal behaviour in adolescence and subsequent mental health outcomes in young adulthood. *Psychological Medicine*, **35**(7), 983–993.

Flamenbaum, R., & Holden, R. R. (2007). Psychache as a mediator in the relationship between perfectionism and suicidality. *Journal of Counseling Psychology*, **54**(1), 51–61.

Gibbs, L. M., Dombrovski, A. Y., Morse, J., et al. (2009). When the solution is part of the problem: Problem solving in elderly suicide attempters. *International Journal of Geriatric Psychiatry*, **24**(12), 1396–1404.

Goldston, D. B., Daniel, S. S., Reboussin, B. A., et al. (2001). Cognitive risk factors and suicide attempts among formerly hospitalized adolescents: A prospective naturalistic study. *Journal of the American Academy of Child & Adolescent Psychiatry*, **40**(1), 91–99.

Goldston, D. B., Reboussin, B. A., & Daniel, S. S. (2006). Predictors of suicide attempts: State and trait components. *Journal of Abnormal Psychology*, **115**(4), 842–849.

Hamilton, T. K., & Schweitzer, R. D. (2000). The cost of being perfect: Perfectionism and suicide ideation in university students. *Australian and New Zealand Journal of Psychiatry*, **34**(5), 829–835.

Harris, K. M., McLean, J. P., Sheffield, J., & Jobes, D. (2010). The internal suicide debate hypothesis: Exploring the life versus death struggle. *Suicide and Life-Threatening Behavior*, **40**(2), 181–192.

Henriques, G. R., Brown, G. K., Berk, M. S., & Beck, A. T. (2004). Marked increases in psychopathology found in a 30-year cohort comparison of suicide attempters. *Psychological Medicine*, **34**(5), 833–841.

Heppner, P. P., & Petersen, C. H. (1982). The development and implications of a personal problem solving inventory. *Journal of Counseling Psychology*, **29**(1), 66–75.

Hewitt, P. L., & Flett, G. L. (1991). Perfectionism in the self and social contexts: Conceptualization, assessment, and association with psychopathology. *Journal of Personality and Social Psychology*, **60**(3), 456–470.

Hewitt, P. L., Flett, G. L., & Turnbull-Donovan, W. (1992). Perfectionism and suicide potential. *British Journal of Clinical Psychology*, **31**(2), 181–190.

Hewitt, P. L., Flett, G. L., & Weber, C. (1994). Dimensions of perfectionism and suicide ideation. *Cognitive Therapy and Research*, **18**(5), 439–460.

Hewitt, P. L., Newton, J., Flett, G. L., & Callander, L. (1997). Perfectionism and suicide ideation in adolescent psychiatric patients. *Journal of Abnormal Child Psychology*, **25**(2), 95–101.

Hewitt, P. L., Norton, R., Flett, G. L., Callander, L., & Cowan, T. (1998). Dimensions of perfectionism, hopelessness, and attempted suicide in a sample of alcoholics. *Suicide and Life-Threatening Behavior*, **28**(4), 395–406.

Howat, S., & Davidson, K. (2002). Parasuicidal behaviour and interpersonal problem solving performance in older adults. *British Journal of Clinical Psychology*, **41**(4), 375–386.

Hunter, E. C., & O'Connor, R. C. (2003). Hopelessness and future thinking in parasuicide: The role of perfectionism. *British Journal of Clinical Psychology*, **42**(4), 355–365.

Joiner, T. E., Jr., Rudd, M. D., & Rajab, M. H. (1997). The Modified Scale for Suicidal Ideation: Factors of suicidality and their relation to clinical and diagnostic variables. *Journal of Abnormal Psychology*, **106**(2), 260–265.

Joiner, T. E., Jr., Steer, R. A., Brown, G., et al. (2003). Worst-point suicidal plans: A dimension of suicidality predictive of past suicide attempts and eventual death by suicide. *Behaviour Research and Therapy*, **41**(12), 1469–1480.

Kessler, R. C., Borges, G., & Walters, E. E. (1999). Prevalence of and risk factors for lifetime suicide attempts in the National Comorbidity Survey. *Archives of General Psychiatry*, **56**(7), 617–626.

Klonsky, E. D., Kotov, R., Bakst, S., Rabinowitz, J., & Bromet, E. J. (2012). Hopelessness as a predictor of attempted suicide among first admission patients with psychosis: A 10-year cohort study. *Suicide and Life-Threatening Behavior*, **42**(1), 1–10.

Kovacs, M., & Beck, A. T. (1977). The wish to die and the wish to live in attempted suicides. *Journal of Clinical Psychology*, **33**(2), 361–365.

Kuo, W.-H., Gallo, J. J., & Tien, A. Y. (2001). Incidence of suicide ideation and attempts in adults: The 13-year follow-up of a community sample in Baltimore, Maryland. *Psychological Medicine*, **31**(7), 1181–1191.

Larzelere, R. E., Smith, G. L., Batenhorst, L. M., & Kelly, D. B. (1996). Predictive validity of the suicide probability scale among adolescents in group home treatment. *Journal of the American Academy of Child & Adolescent Psychiatry*, **35**(2), 166–172; discussion 172–174.

Linehan, M. M., Camper, P., Chiles, J. A., Strosahl, K., & Shearin, E. (1987). Interpersonal problem solving and parasuicide. *Cognitive Therapy and Research*, **11**(1), 1–12.

Links, P., Nisenbaum, R., Ambreen, M., et al. (2012). Prospective study of risk factors for increased suicide ideation and behavior following recent discharge. *General Hospital Psychiatry*, **34**(1), 88–97.

McAuliffe, C., Keeley, H. S., & Corcoran, P. (2002). Problem solving and repetition of parasuicide. *Behavioural and Cognitive Psychotherapy*, **30**(4), 385–397.

McLeavey, B. C., Daly, R. J., Murray, C. M., O'Riordan, J., & Taylor, M. (1987). Interpersonal problem solving deficits in self-poisoning patients. *Suicide and Life-Threatening Behavior*, **17**(1), 33–49.

Minkoff, K., Bergman, E., Beck, A. T., & Beck, R. (1973). Hopelessness, depression, and attempted suicide. *The American Journal of Psychiatry*, **130**(4), 455–459.

Mundt, J. C., Greist, J. H., Jefferson, J. W., et al. (2013). Prediction of suicidal behavior in clinical research by lifetime suicidal ideation and behavior ascertained by the Electronic Columbia-Suicide Severity Rating Scale. *Journal of Clinical Psychiatry*, **74**(9), 887–893.

Nock, M. K., Park, J. M., Finn, C. T., et al. (2010). Measuring the suicidal mind: Implicit cognition predicts suicidal behavior. *Psychological Science*, **21**(4), 511–517.

O'Connor, R. C., Smyth, R., Ferguson, E., Ryan, C., & Williams, J. M. G. (2013). Psychological Processes and Repeat Suicidal Behavior: A Four-Year Prospective Study. *Journal of Consulting and Clinical Psychology*, **81** (6), 1137–1143.

O'Connor, S. S., Jobes, D. A., Yeargin, M. K., et al. (2012). A cross-sectional investigation of the suicidal spectrum: Typologies of suicidality based on ambivalence about living and dying. *Comprehensive Psychiatry*, **53**(5), 461–467.

Patsiokas, A. T., Clum, G. A., & Luscomb, R. L. (1979). Cognitive characteristics of suicide attempters. *Journal of Consulting and Clinical Psychology*, **47**(3), 478–484.

Pettit, J. W., Garza, M. J., Grover, K. E., et al. (2009). Factor structure and psychometric properties of the Modified Scale for Suicidal Ideation among suicidal youth. *Depression and Anxiety*, **26**(8), 769–774.

Platt, J. J., & Spivack, G. (1975). *Manual for the Means-End Problems Solving (MEPS): A Measure of Interpersonal Problem Solving Skill.* Philadelphia, PA: Hahnemann Medical College and Hospital.

Pollock, L. R., & Williams, J. M. G. (2001). Effective problem solving in suicide attempters depends on specific autobiographical recall. *Suicide and Life-Threatening Behavior*, **31**(4), 386–396.

Pollock, L. R., & Williams, J. M. G. (2004). Problem solving in suicide attempters. *Psychological Medicine*, **34**(1), 163–167.

Posner, K., Brown, G. K., Stanley, B., et al. (2011). The Columbia-Suicide Severity Rating Scale: Initial validity and internal consistency findings from three multisite studies with adolescents and adults. *The American Journal of Psychiatry*, **168**(12), 1266–1277.

Reinherz, H. Z., Tanner, J. L., Berger, S. R., Beardslee, W. R., & Fitzmaurice, G. M. (2006). Adolescent suicidal ideation as predictive of psychopathology, suicidal behavior, and compromised functioning at age 30. *The American Journal of Psychiatry*, **163**(7), 1226–1232.

Rudd, M. D., Rajab, M. H., & Dahm, P. F. (1994). Problem solving appraisal in suicide ideators and attempters. *American Journal of Orthopsychiatry*, **64**(1), 136–149.

Sani, G., Tondo, L., Koukopoulos, A., et al. (2011). Suicide in a large population of former psychiatric inpatients. *Psychiatry and Clinical Neurosciences*, **65**(3), 286–295.

Schotte, D. E., & Clum, G. A. (1987). Problem solving skills in suicidal psychiatric patients. *Journal of Consulting and Clinical Psychology*, **55**(1), 49–54.

Seligman, M. E. P. (1975). *Helplessness: On Depression, Development, and Death*: New York, NY: W H Freeman/ Times Books/ Henry Holt & Co.

Shiffman, S. M., & Stone, A. A. (1998). Ecological momentary assessment: A new tool for behavioral medicine research. In *Technology and Methods in Behavioral Medicine* (pp. 117–131). Mahwah, NJ: Lawrence Erlbaum Associates.

Shneidman, E. S. (1993). *Suicide as Psychache: A Clinical Approach to Self-Destructive Behavior*. Lanham, MD. Jason Aronson.

Stefansson, J., Nordström, P., & Jokinen, J. (2012). Suicide Intent Scale in the prediction of suicide. *Journal of Affective Disorders*, **136**(1–2), 167–171.

Stroop, J. R. (1935). Studies of interference in serial verbal reactions. *Journal of Experimental Psychology*, **18**(6), 643–662.

Suominen, K., Isometsä, E., Ostamo, A., & Lönnqvist, J. (2004). Level of suicidal intent predicts overall mortality and suicide after attempted suicide: A 12-year follow-up study. *BMC Psychiatry*, **4**, 11.

Valtonen, H. M., Suominen, K., Mantere, O., et al. (2006). Prospective study of risk factors for attempted suicide among patients with bipolar disorder. *Bipolar Disorders*, **8**(5 pt 2), 576–585.

Van Orden, K. A., Merrill, K. A., & Joiner, T. E., Jr. (2005). Interpersonal-psychological precursors to suicidal behavior: A theory of attempted and completed suicide. *Current Psychiatry Reviews*, **1**(2), 187–196.

Wenzel, A., Brown, G. K., & Beck, A. T. (2009). *Cognitive Therapy for Suicidal Patients: Scientific and Clinical Applications*: Washington, DC: American Psychological Association.

Wenzel, A., Berchick, E. R., Tenhave, T., et al. (2011). Predictors of suicide relative to other deaths in patients with suicide attempts and suicide ideation: A 30-year prospective study. *Journal of Affective Disorders*, **132**(3), 375–382.

Williams, J. M., & Broadbent, K. (1986). Distraction by emotional stimuli: Use of a Stroop task with suicide attempters. *British Journal of Clinical Psychology*, **25**(2), 101–110.

Williams, J. M., Barnhofer, T., Crane, C., & Beck, A. T. (2005). Problem solving deteriorates following mood challenge in formerly depressed patients with a history of suicidal ideation. *Journal of Abnormal Psychology*, **114**(3), 421–431.

Wong, J. P. S., Stewart, S. M., Claassen, C., et al. (2008). Repeat suicide attempts in Hong Kong community adolescents. *Social Science & Medicine*, **66**(2), 232–241.

Young, M. A., Fogg, L. F., Scheftner, W., et al. (1996). Stable trait components of hopelessness: Baseline and sensitivity to depression. *Journal of Abnormal Psychology*, **105**(2), 155–165.

Chapter 6

Suicide clusters and suicide contagion

Alison M. Lake and Madelyn S. Gould

Introduction

Suicide contagion is defined as the direct or indirect transmission of suicidal behavior from one person to another, after the manner of an infectious disease (Gould, 1990). Exposure, whether direct or mediated, to another person's suicide is unlikely to generate suicide risk where none existed previously (Gould & Davidson, 1988); however, a growing body of research indicates that such exposure can confer additional risk on already vulnerable persons. Adolescents have been shown to be more susceptible to suicide contagion than adults (Gould et al., 1990b). With this exception, the characteristics of people at risk of engaging in suicidal behavior in the context of a suicide cluster appear to be consistent with those at risk of engaging in suicidal behavior outside a cluster (Haw et al., 2013). While suicide contagion can be a factor in producing statistically significant clusters of suicide attempts and/or suicide deaths (see e.g., Gould et al., 1990a), the risk conferred by suicide contagion inevitably operates in concert with many other suicide risk factors (Brent, 1995; Gould et al., 1996; Hawton & van Heeringen, 2009). This chapter will review research findings on suicide clusters of various kinds, while considering the role of suicide contagion in each. It will then consider the evidence for person-to-person transmission of suicidal behavior outside suicide clusters. It will conclude by reviewing risk factors for susceptibility to suicide contagion, possible mechanisms underlying suicide contagion, and strategies to prevent the spread of suicide.

Suicide clusters

A suicide cluster is comprised of an excessive number of suicides occurring in close temporal and/or geographical proximity (Gould et al., 1989). Because there are no standard definitions of what constitutes temporal or geographical closeness, researchers have determined the intervals they wish to examine on a study by study basis. Statistical techniques such as Kulldorff's spatial scan technique (Kulldorff, 1997), the time–space Scan statistic (Wallenstein et al., 1989), the Knox procedure (Knox, 1964), Yule-Walker estimation, and Poisson distribution modeling have been used to locate suicide clusters and to verify that observed clustering is not likely to be due to chance. The three types of suicide clusters to be covered here are spatial or geographic suicide clusters, temporal or "mass" suicide clusters, and space–time or "point" suicide clusters.

Geographic suicide clusters

Recent epidemiological analyses of geographic suicide clustering have used retrospective review of national or regional mortality data to identify areas with higher than expected suicide rates, and have then proceeded to investigate what socioeconomic, historical, cultural, or demographic features may be associated with the elevated rates. Contagion is not generally offered as an explanation for suicides that cluster in space but not time. For example, an examination of rates of suicide deaths among 18- to 44-year-olds in small areas of Scotland over three distinct 3-year periods identified consistent geographical clustering of suicide deaths in an area characterized by economic deprivation (Exeter & Boyle, 2007). When economic deprivation was controlled for, the geographic clustering of suicide during these periods became insignificant. The authors conclude that the association of economic deprivation with higher suicide rates is adequate to account for this geographic clustering of suicides, without implicating a contagion effect. An examination of rates of suicide deaths in neighborhoods of São Paulo, Brazil over a 10-year period identified neighborhoods with uncharacteristically high and low rates

A Concise Guide to Understanding Suicide, ed. Stephen H. Koslow, Pedro Ruiz, and Charles B. Nemeroff. Published by Cambridge University Press.

of suicide deaths (Bando et al., 2012). Within the higher risk neighborhood, higher suicide risk was associated with being single, being Catholic (a less socially cohesive group), recent migration, and higher income, whereas lower risk was associated with being married and being Evangelical (a more socially cohesive group). The authors conceptualize their findings in terms of an association between suicide and low social cohesion, with poverty playing a protective role within a sociocultural context where "low life standards are compensated by a solidarity response" (Bando et al., 2012). Neither of these studies assessed whether those who died by suicide may have been aware of or exposed to the other suicides in their localities over time. However, a study of the contextual effects of community poverty in high school communities in Iceland indicates that community-level household poverty can increase adolescent suicide risk independently of the effects of individual-level household poverty (Bernburg et al., 2009). The authors found this contextual effect to be mediated by the more frequent exposure to others' suicidal behavior experienced by adolescents in less affluent school districts over time. This finding suggests that the effects of social and economic factors on a locality's suicide rates can be compounded by the co-occurring effects of suicide contagion.

Temporal suicide clusters: media effects

Statistically significant temporal fluctuations in suicide rates following media reports on suicide support the idea that media reporting can facilitate the transmission of suicidal behavior from one person to others (see Gould, 1990 and Gould, 2001 for earlier reviews). Suicide rates have been observed to rise for a period of time following the publication of fictional (cf. Goethe's *Sorrows of Young Werther*) and non-fictional (cf. newspaper reporting on Marilyn Monroe's suicide) stories about suicide. Extensive research has been done in an attempt to determine whether this relationship is causal or merely correlational.

A ground-breaking analysis of the impact of newspaper reporting about suicide deaths on suicide rates in the USA and Britain over a 20-year period found that suicide rates increased in the month of and the month following publication of a suicide story; that the increase was greater when the story spent more days on the front page; and that the increase was greater in the region where the newspaper was distributed (Phillips, 1974). The same author subsequently found that, over a seven-year period, teenage suicide rates increased in the eight days following television news stories about suicide, with a greater increase when more programs carried the story (Phillips & Carstensen, 1986). This study also found that the peak suicide rate in the 8 days following a suicide story was followed by no compensatory drop in the 16 days thereafter, making it unlikely that the excess suicides would have happened anyway and were merely displaced in time. Furthermore, the study found no increase in teenage suicide rates after television news stories about well-known individuals dying by other means than suicide, making it improbable that the excess suicides were motivated by grief or loss. A later extension of this study to cover an additional 5-year period and a larger number of television news programs failed to replicate a number of its findings (Kessler et al., 1988). This study of a 12-year period found that teenage suicide rates did not significantly rise in the 8 days following a television news story about suicide, and that stories to which more teenagers were exposed did not yield greater increases in suicide rates. However, when news stories were broken down by type, significant increases in teenage suicide rates were found to follow stories about the suicide deaths of adult celebrities, although not of non-celebrity adults or of teens.

The argument for the impact of media stories has been strengthened by the repeated demonstration of a dose–response relationship between newspaper reporting on suicide and suicide rates. For example, greater increases in suicide rates have been observed in regions with higher distribution of the newspaper carrying the suicide story (Etzersdorfer, 2001). Moreover, suicide rates have been shown to go down following a decrease in the frequency of stories about suicide. For example, suicide rates among women decreased significantly during a 9-month newspaper blackout in Detroit, and rose again when the blackout ended (Motto, 1970). Suicide rates in Austria went down following the implementation of media guidelines for reporting on suicide, with greater decreases in areas of higher distribution of guideline-compliant media (Niederkrotenthaler & Sonneck, 2007).

Although some findings have been mixed, therefore, evidence for media effects on suicide rates is convincing and supports the conclusion that, at least under certain circumstances, indirect exposure to the suicidal behavior of a model can trigger suicidal behavior in others. One explanation for mixed findings may be that studies have grouped together media items which are more and less likely to produce a contagion effect, and have often not specified the audience most likely to be affected. Ongoing research into the impact of the media on suicide rates has sought to fine-tune our understanding of this transmission by identifying characteristics of stories that are more likely to be followed by increased suicide rates, and characteristics of suicide models whose deaths are more likely to be followed by increased suicide rates. In addition, protective characteristics have been sought.

Meta-analysis of research into media effects has determined that non-fictional stories about suicide are more likely than fictional stories, newspaper reports are more likely than television reports, and reports of female suicides are more likely than reports of male suicides to be followed by increased suicide rates (Stack, 2005). News stories that characterize suicide in a negative light are less likely to be followed by increased suicide rates (Stack, 2005). Celebrity suicides are more likely and the suicides of criminals are less likely to be followed by increased suicide rates (Niederkrotenthaler et al., 2009); reports of non-celebrity suicides do impact suicide rates, but to a lesser degree than suicides of political and entertainment celebrities (Stack, 1990a). Repetitive reporting on the same suicide and definitive labeling of the death as a suicide have each been associated with greater increases in subsequent suicide rates (Niederkrotenthaler et al., 2009, 2010). On the other hand, media stories about individuals with suicidal ideation who used adaptive coping strategies to handle adverse events and did not attempt suicide have been negatively associated with subsequent suicide rates (Niederkrotenthaler et al., 2010).

A limitation of the ecological studies described above is that they are unable to demonstrate that individuals who engaged in suicidal behavior following a media report were in fact exposed to and influenced by the media report. A handful of extant individual-level studies have addressed these questions directly, and have contributed evidence to support the specificity of the media effect. Hawton and colleagues (1999) conducted a study in EDs in the UK examining the pattern of suicide attempts before and after a fictional character took an overdose of paracetamol (a.k.a., acetaminophen) in an episode of a popular weekly TV drama. Presentations for self-poisoning increased by 17% in the first week after the broadcast and 9% in the second week. Increases in overdoses using the specific drug used by the model were more marked than increases in other types of overdoses. The most compelling evidence of modeling from this study was that among overdose patients who were viewers of the drama, use of the specific drug used by the model doubled after the episode in question, compared to before. Among overdose patients presenting at one of 25 hospitals in the first week after the episode, 18% reported having seen the episode, and 20% of these reported that the episode had influenced their decision to overdose. In a more recent study, 63 individuals who attempted suicide in Taipei City following the suicide of a young female pop singer were assessed for exposure to media reporting about her death. Forty-three (68%) respondents had been exposed to the media reporting, of whom 37% reported that the media stories influenced their suicide attempts (Chen et al., 2010). This study also demonstrated a positive modeling effect on the chosen method of suicide (burning charcoal inside a closed car), with an adjusted odds ratio of 7.3 (see also Chen et al., 2012; Cheng et al., 2007c; Etzersdorfer et al., 2004 and Tousignant et al., 2005 for additional evidence of a modeling effect based on choice of suicide method).

Space–time suicide clusters

Space–time or "point" suicide clusters occur within localized communities such as schools, towns, psychiatric hospitals or companies, where community members may be expected to know or to know of one another. Although the existence of a space–time suicide cluster can be verified statistically, they are often first identified through the alarm experienced by community members. Space–time suicide clusters are likely to arise from a confluence of multiple causes.

Statistical analysis of the outbreak of suicides at the Foxconn Company in China found support for a temporal clustering effect (Cheng et al., 2011). Both the occurrence of a Foxconn suicide or suicide attempt and the publication of a national (but not local) newspaper report on the suicides were associated with elevated chances of an additional suicide 3 days later, demonstrating the potential impact of both media exposure and community membership on the transmission of suicide within the Foxconn company.

A space–time cluster of eight suicides of inpatients in a psychiatric clinic in Finland over a span of 3 months sparked an investigation by clinic researchers

(Taiminen et al., 1992; Taiminen & Helenius, 1994). The cluster was statistically verified as unlikely to have occurred by chance. It was found to have taken place at a time of organizational instability at the clinic, with major administrative changes and an unusually high number of inexperienced employees contributing to an atmosphere of insecurity. Qualitative review of the patients' clinical records revealed that the suicide deaths of two patients seemed to provide models for four additional suicides by patients who personally knew and identified with the models and, in three cases, copied their model's method and location of suicide. The suicides of the two remaining patients appeared unrelated on these grounds. The authors conclude that the influence of temporary, microsocial conditions within the clinic and a contagion or modeling effect each contributed to the emergence of the suicide cluster.

An analysis of a youth suicide epidemic on the island nation of Guam has also proposed multiple contributing causal factors (Booth, 2010). Ecological factors which may have contributed to the spike in youth suicide rates in the 1990s on Guam include social disruption due to large-scale economic development beginning in the mid-1980s, and rising immigration rates, with a particular influx of an ethnic group itself characterized by a higher suicide rate. As a compounding factor, the author points to the highly visible and highly publicized suicide of a prominent politician in 1990. This death seems to have had strong short-term effects on suicide rates among teenagers and among adults over 50, the politician's age group, with rates increasing by factors of 3.6 and 3.8 respectively in those age groups that year. By a year later, rates for adults over 50 had returned to earlier levels, while youth suicide rates remained unusually high. Finally, youth suicide rates on Guam in the 1990s were inflated by the cultural phenomenon of suicide "friendship pacts" which originated on the west coast of the USA and spread via the Internet. By the early 2000s, following the implementation of suicide prevention programming, youth suicide rates on Guam had returned to 1980s levels. It can be concluded that suicide contagion, working through internet communication about teen suicide pacts and through exposure to a local celebrity suicide, accounted for some portion of the excess of youth suicides at this time and place.

A study of space–time suicide clusters in 90 prisons in England and Wales over a 10-year period found statistical evidence for significant space–time clustering of deaths by suicide, while not of deaths from natural causes (McKenzie & Keane, 2007). The expected number of suicides was subtracted from the number of observed close pairs to calculate the maximum number of imitative suicides. A model simulation was used to derive an estimate of 5.8% (95% CI 1%–11%) for imitative suicides as a percentage of all prison suicides in that period.

Space–time suicide clusters occur most frequently among teenagers and young adults, with between 1% and 5% of teen suicides occurring in clusters (Gould, 1990; see also Gould et al., 1990a, b). A case–control study of two teen suicide clusters in Texas indicated that the clusters included teens who had close personal relationships with others in the cluster, as well as teens from the same community who were not directly acquainted with one another (Davidson et al., 1989). All decedents subsequent to the two suicides that initiated the clusters were aware of the preceding suicide(s), and parents of five of 11 of those teens believed their child's suicide to have been modeled after an earlier suicide or suicide attempt. When compared with matched living controls, teens who died in these space–time suicide clusters were more likely to have pre-existing vulnerabilities (to be discussed in detail under "Risk Factors" below), but were no more likely than controls to have been exposed to media reports about suicide. The authors conclude that in the context of these clusters, suicide contagion may have triggered suicidal behavior in adolescents who were already vulnerable, but who nonetheless may not have died by suicide without the added impetus of exposure to the suicide of a peer.

Direct exposure to another's suicide

Suicide contagion may also play a role in instigating individual suicides or suicide attempts, outside the context of suicide clusters. Studies of the individual-level impact of direct exposure to the suicide of a friend or acquaintance have largely focused on adolescents, and have produced mixed results (see Insel & Gould, 2008). One extant study of the effects of direct exposure to suicide on adults found that adults exposed to the suicide of a friend or acquaintance within the previous 12 months were more likely to endorse suicidal ideation, suicide plans, and a suicide attempt than adults with no such exposure (Crosby & Sacks, 2002). In a multivariate analysis including young age, male sex, and unmarried status, this finding lost significance, perhaps due to the study's small sample size. A case–control study of nearly lethal suicide attempts among 13- to 34-year-olds (a mixed age group) found that attempters were no more likely than non-attempters to have been exposed to the suicidal behavior of friends or acquaintances over their lifetimes, in a model also including depression, alcoholism, and having moved within the past year (Mercy et al., 2001). When examining the effects of frequency, recency, and emotional proximity, moreover, exposure to the suicidal behavior of a friend or acquaintance more than a year earlier, or of a friend or acquaintance with whom the subject was not close, appeared to have a protective effect, in that more non-attempters than attempters reported these kinds of exposure. A study of friends and acquaintances of adolescent suicides found case subjects to be at increased risk of major depression, generalized anxiety disorder, and post-traumatic stress disorder (PTSD) at 3-year follow-up, but not at increased risk of suicide attempt, compared with matched controls with no exposure; the researchers' clinical impressions also indicated a potential protective effect of exposure to the negative consequences of a peer's suicide (Brent et al., 1996). However, these findings are inconsistent with other robust results. Analysis of data on a nationally representative sample of over 10 000 US high school students from the National Longitudinal Study of Adolescent Health (ADD Health) found that "teens who know friends or family members who have attempted suicide are about three times more likely to attempt suicide than are teens who do not know someone who attempted suicide" (Cutler et al., 2001). In a further analysis of this same data, an effect was also found for exposure to a friend's completed suicide (Feigelman & Gorman, 2008). Having lost a friend to suicide within the previous 12 months increased the odds of a suicide attempt by 2.47 at Wave 1, and by 2.54 at Wave 2, a year later, but this effect was no longer significant at Wave 3, 6 years after that. Of 16 studies reviewed by Insel and Gould (2008) on the impact on adolescents of exposure to a suicidal peer, the majority found a significant association between exposure to the suicidal behavior of an adolescent peer and a subsequent adolescent suicide attempt. Odds ratios ranged from 2.8 to 11.0 for the effects of exposure to attempted suicide, which appeared to confer greater risk than exposure to completed suicide. As with research on media effects, mixed results on the effects of direct exposure to suicidal behavior may indicate that researchers have yet to isolate the conditions (including factors such as age group, recency and lethality of the model behavior, pre-existing vulnerability, and emotional proximity to the model) which facilitate direct suicide contagion from those which inhibit it.

Risk factors

Apart from the finding that adolescents and young adults are more susceptible to suicide clustering than other age groups (Gould et al., 1990b), the risk factors for dying in a suicide cluster identified by research to date do not differ appreciably from those for dying by suicide in general, as noted in a recent review (Haw et al., 2013). Decedents in the two teenage suicide clusters analyzed by Davidson and colleagues (1989) were found to be more likely than controls to have threatened or attempted suicide previously, to have been hospitalized for a mental illness or substance abuse problem, to have a recent or anticipated relationship break-up, and to have had experiences that familiarized them with violence or the use of force, such as physical self-injury and physical violence toward others. Students who manifested serious suicidal ideation or suicidal behavior as part of the high school suicide cluster described by Brent and colleagues (1989) were more likely than non-suicidal students to have been suicidal in the past, or to have experienced a past or current episode of major depression. Prior and current psychopathology predicted suicidality after exposure better than a student's relationship with the deceased, or funeral attendance. Some students who were close friends with the deceased were observed to become suicidal in the absence of prior or current affective disorder; however, the suicidality of these students was limited to ideation that was not acted upon.

As with cluster suicide risk, the most commonly identified risk factors for susceptibility to suicide contagion via the media appear to mirror those for suicide in general: namely, affective disorder and a history of suicide attempts. Two studies of attempted suicide in the wake of extensive media reporting on a celebrity suicide found that among psychiatric outpatients with depressive diagnoses, those who had made prior suicide attempts within the past month and those in current major depressions were most likely to make a suicide attempt following media exposure (Cheng et al., 2007a); similarly, among suicide attempters referred for medical treatment at two community mental health clinics in the 2 months after the celebrity suicide, the self-reported impact of the media reports was greatest among repeat attempters who had made a prior suicide attempt within the past year (Cheng et al., 2007b).

It has been theorized that a similarity in gender, age, nationality, or life circumstance to an observed suicide may also present a risk factor for suicide contagion. The theory of differential identification, wherein people are more likely to imitate the suicidal behavior of models they identify with, was recently tested in an ecological study of 179 newspaper-reported suicides (Niederkrotenthaler et al., 2009). There was an increase in similar suicides, defined on the combined basis of sex, age group, and suicide method, following celebrity suicides, suicides in the 30- to 64-year-old age group, and suicides definitively labeled as such by the media report; increases in dissimilar suicides were not found for any condition. A limitation of this study is that it does not allow for disaggregation of the effects of age, sex, and suicide method. In all, very few studies have been done which match the age and sex of the suicide model with the age and sex of the observer, or which control for other bases of identification, such as nationality and marital status (Stack, 2003). One ecological study of newspaper suicide reports in Japan did find that the media effect on Japanese suicide rates was restricted to stories about Japanese suicides (Stack, 1996). A study of increases in suicide rates among the elderly following media reports on suicide found that the effect was doubled when only stories about elderly suicides were considered; however, the effect of stories about celebrity suicides was greater for elderly women than for elderly men, despite the fact that all celebrity suicides in the study period were male (Stack, 1990b). In the two individual-level studies of the impact of a Taiwanese celebrity suicide described in the previous paragraph, effects of identification with the gender of the celebrity suicide were inconsistent. Among the psychiatric outpatients, women were more likely than men to attempt suicide in the wake of the male celebrity's suicide; however, in both studies, men who attempted suicide were more likely than women to say that the media reports had influenced their attempts. Among suicide attempters exposed to suicide reporting about a young female pop star, those who self-reported that her suicide influenced their suicide attempt were more likely to be male and under 30, a group the authors identify as the pop star's primary fan base (Chen et al., 2010).

Possible mechanisms underlying suicide contagion

Cutler and colleagues (2001) suggest that in suicide contagion, "a 'social multiplier' may amplify the effects" of other suicidogenic factors (p.233). In a review of possible mechanisms underlying suicide contagion, Blood and Pirkis (2001) identify social learning theory as providing the most convincing explanation (see also Gould, 2001; Gould et al., 1989). According to this theory, a subject's previously instigated but inhibited behavior is disinhibited when the subject witnesses the behavior modeled by another, with the effect mediated by identification, either vertical (with an admired or superior person, such as a celebrity) or horizontal (with someone like oneself). Citing social psychology research by Wheeler and Bandura, David Levy defines disinhibitory contagion "as a case of social contagion in which a recipient, who is in an approach–avoidance conflict, experiences a reduction in restraints as a consequence of observing an initiator perform the desired act" (Levy & Nail, 1993). This type of behavioral contagion is seen as mediated by restraint reduction. Individuals who were not already instigated to perform the behavior in question would not be susceptible to contagion. In fact, "the occurrence of behavioral contagion is greatest when the avoidance gradient is just slightly higher than the approach gradient. If the restraints are barely sufficient to prevent overt expression of the approach tendency, a small reduction in fear will be sufficient to produce the approach behavior" (Wheeler, 1966). In studies of the contagion of aggression and of other forbidden behaviors, such as smoking in class, observing a model perform the behavior was enough to produce this incremental reduction in restraint (Levy & Nail, 1993).

The idea that many suicidal individuals experience an approach–avoidance conflict regarding suicide is supported by research on the "internal suicide debate," which indicates that for a majority of suicidal people, the wish to die coexists in tension with a wish to live (Brown et al., 2005; Harris et al., 2010). The more the wish to die outweighs the wish to live, the greater the risk of suicidal behavior (Brown et al.,

2005). Individuals experiencing internal conflict regarding suicide can be conceptualized as instigated to suicide (by their reasons for dying) but psychologically restrained from acting (by their reasons for living). Notably, when surveyed about their reasons for living, non-suicidal individuals are more likely to endorse "the importance of family, beliefs, a strong self, and enjoyable things," whereas individuals at high-risk of suicide are more likely to endorse "fear (of suicide or death), fear of burdening others (by completing suicide), and responsibility," reasons which suggest an avoidance tendency with regard to suicide, rather than an approach tendency with regard to life (Harris et al., 2010). It is therefore plausible that, for an at risk individual, learning of another's decision to choose suicide could have the effect of reducing internal restraints against suicide, thereby tipping the approach–avoidance balance in the direction of approach.

Three studies to date have presented insight into the mechanisms underlying suicide contagion from the point of view of individuals either attempting (Cheng et al., 2007a, b) or completing (Tousignant et al., 2005) suicide under the self-reported influence of a celebrity model. Interviews with suicide attempters who reported having been influenced by the suicide of a Taiwanese television actor suggested that news of that suicide gave them either information about how to commit suicide, a sense of the positive consequences of suicide ("People care about you more after you kill yourself than when staying alive"), a sense of the admirable qualities of the model ("a big star has gone, why not me?") or of his death ("Suicide can be a glorious act like his became"), an identification with the model's circumstances ("All my sorrows will be over just like him, a man with loss of love and career"), or a heightened sense of hopelessness ("The end of depression is suicide, treatment is useless") (Cheng et al., 2007b, p.864). Coroners' reports describing suicide notes and comments from individuals who completed suicide in the month following the suicide of a Canadian television reporter included references to distress at the reporter's death, the stated intention to imitate his methods, an identification with the model's unhappiness ("Mister Girouard [must] have been desperate like me"), an interpretation of his death as a meaningful statement ("His gesture is not more serious than mine, this is sure"), and a sense of having been given permission to act ("Mentioned that if he, who had two young girls could do it, she could also do the same") (Tousignant et al., 2005, p.1923).

Strategies to prevent suicide contagion

A number of evidence-based interventions capable of combatting suicide contagion have been developed. Studies have shown that it is possible to mitigate media effects on suicide rates by implementing media guidelines for suicide reporting (see Pirkis & Nordentoft, 2011). Media guidelines can interrupt the transmission of suicidality by identifying the types of media reporting through which suicidality is likely to be transmitted, and by modifying the volume and content of media reporting, with resultant decreases in suicide rates. For example, suicides in the Vienna subway system decreased by approximately 75% in 1987 following implementation of media guidelines for reporting on subway system suicides (Etzersdorfer et al., 1992).

Screening for suicide risk can also interrupt the transmission of suicidality, by identifying in advance individuals who may be at risk of suicide, and therefore also susceptible to suicide contagion (Gould et al., 2009). Screening can help to alleviate that susceptibility by enabling preventive services to be directed to at risk individuals identified by the screen. Key settings for suicide screening include schools and primary care practices. A range of school- and community-based psychosocial programs may also work to alleviate susceptibility to suicide contagion by, for example, changing adolescent peer norms through positive messaging (Wyman et al., 2010), or educating and empowering parents to communicate with teens (Toumbourou & Gregg, 2002). Finally, research suggests that coordinated postvention/crisis intervention efforts following a death by suicide may minimize and contain the effects of suicide contagion within a community (Poijula et al., 2001; Hacker et al., 2008).

Conclusion

While the complex etiology of suicidal behavior is recognized (Gould et al., 2003), it has become increasingly apparent that suicide contagion exists and contributes to suicide risk along with other factors. Strategies to prevent suicide contagion are essential and require ongoing evaluation.

References

Bando, D. H., Moreira, R. S., Pereira, J. C. R., & Barrozo, L. V. (2012). Spatial clusters of suicide in the municipality of Sao Paulo 1996–2005: an ecological study. *BMC Psychiatry*, **12**, 124–139.

Bernburg, J. G., Thorlindsson, T., & Sigfusdottir, I. D. (2009). The spreading of suicidal behavior: The contextual effect of community household poverty on adolescent suicidal behavior and the mediating role of suicide suggestion. *Social Science and Medicine*, **68**, 380–389.

Blood, R. W., & Pirkis, J. (2001). Suicide and the media: Part III: Theoretical issues. *Crisis*, **22(4)**, 163–169.

Booth, H. (2010). The evolution of epidemic suicide on Guam: Context and contagion. *Suicide and Life-Threatening Behavior*, **40(1)**, 1–13.

Brent, D. A. (1995). Risk factors for adolescent suicide and suicidal behavior: mental and substance abuse disorders, family environmental factors, and life stress. *Suicide and Life-Threatening Behavior*, **25** (Suppl), 52–63.

Brent, D. A., Kerr, M. M., Goldstein, C., et al. (1989). An outbreak of suicide and suicidal behavior in a high school. *Journal of the American Academy of Child and Adolescent Psychiatry*, **28(6)**, 918–924.

Brent, D. A., Moritz, G., Bridge, J., Perper, J., & Conobbio, R. (1996). Long-term impact of exposure to suicide: a three-year controlled follow-up. *Journal of the American Academy of Child and Adolescent Psychiatry*, **35(5)**, 646–653.

Brown, G. K., Steer, R. A., Henriques, G. R., & Beck, A. T. (2005). The internal struggle between the wish to die and the wish to live: a risk factor for suicide. *American Journal of Psychiatry*, **162**, 1977–1979.

Chen, Y. Y., Tsai, P. C., Chen, P. H., et al. (2010). Effect of media reporting of the suicide of a singer in Taiwan: the case of Ivy Li. *Social Psychiatry Psychiatric Epidemiology*, **45**(3), 363–369.

Chen, Y. Y., Liao, S. F., Teng, P. R., et al. (2012). The impact of media reporting of the suicide of a singer on suicide rates in Taiwan. *Social Psychiatry Psychiatric Epidemiology*, **47(2)**, 215–221.

Cheng, A. T., Hawton, K., Chen, T. H., et al. (2007a). The influence of media reporting of a celebrity suicide on suicidal behavior in patients with a history of depressive disorder. *Journal of Affective Disorders*, **103**, 69–75.

Cheng, A. T., Hawton, K., Chen, T. H., et al. (2007b). The influence of media coverage of a celebrity suicide on subsequent suicide attempts. *Journal of Clinical Psychiatry*, **68**(6): 862–866.

Cheng, A. T., Hawton, K., Lee, C. T., & Chen, T. H. (2007c). The influence of media reporting of the suicide of a celebrity on suicide rates: a population-based study. *International Journal of Epidemiology*, **36**, 1229–1234.

Cheng, Q., Chen, F., & Yip, P. S. (2011). The Foxconn suicides and their media prominence: is the Werther Effect applicable in China? *BMC Public Health*, **11**, 841.

Crosby, A., & Sacks, J. (2002). Exposure to suicide: incidence and association with suicidal ideation and behavior: United States, 1994. *Suicide and Life-Threatening Behavior*, **32**(3), 321–328.

Cutler, D. M., Glaesen, E. L., & Norberg, K. E. (2001). Explaining the rise in youth suicide. In J. Gruber (Ed.) *Risky Behavior Among Youths: An Economic Analysis* (pp. 219–269). Chicago: University of Chicago Press.

Davidson, L. E., Rosenberg, M. L., Mercy, J. A., Franklin, J., & Simmons, J. T. (1989). An epidemiologic study of risk factors in two teenage suicide clusters. *The Journal of the American Medical Association*, **262**(19), 2687–2692.

Etzersdorfer, E. (2001). A dose-response relationship of imitational suicides with newspaper distribution. *Australian and New Zealand Journal of Psychiatry*, **35**, 249–252.

Etzersdorfer, E., Sonneck, G., & Nagel-Kuess, S. (1992). Newspaper reports and suicide. *New England Journal of Medicine*, **327**(7), 502–503.

Etzersdorfer, E., Voracek, M., & Sonneck, G. (2004). A dose-response relationship between imitational suicides and newspaper distribution. *Archives of Suicide Research*, **8** (2), 137–145.

Exeter, D. J., & Boyle, P. J. (2007). Does young adult suicide cluster geographically in Scotland? *Journal of Epidemiological and Community Health*, **61**, 731–736.

Feigelman, W., & Gorman, B. S. (2008). Assessing the effects of peer suicide on youth suicide. *Suicide and Life-Threatening Behavior*, **38**(2), 181–194.

Gould, M. S. (1990). Suicide clusters and media exposure. In S. J. Blumenthal & D. J. Kupfer (Eds.) *Suicide Over the Life Cycle*. Washington, DC: American Psychiatric Press.

Gould, M. S. (2001). Suicide and the media. *Annals of the New York Academy of Science*, **932**, 200–221; discussion 221–24.

Gould, M. S., & Davidson, L. (1988). Suicide contagion among adolescents. In A. R. Stiffman & R. A. Felman (Eds.) *Advances in Adolescent Mental Health, Vol. III: Depression and Suicide*. Greenwich, CT: JAI Press.

Gould, M. S., Wallenstein, S., & Davidson, L. (1989). Suicide clusters: a critical review. *Suicide and Life-Threatening Behavior*, **19**(1), 17–29.

Gould, M. S., Wallenstein, S., & Kleinman, M. (1990a). Time-space clustering of teenage suicide. *American Journal of Epidemiology*, **131**(1), 71–78.

Gould, M. S., Wallenstein, S., Kleinman, M. H., O'Carroll, P., & Mercy, J. (1990b). Suicide clusters: an examination of age-specific effects. *American Journal of Public Health*, **80**(2), 211–212.

Gould, M. S., Fisher, P., Parides, M., Flory, M., & Shaffer, D. (1996). Psychosocial risk factors of child and adolescent completed suicide. *Archives of General Psychiatry*, **53**(12), 1155–1162.

Gould, M. S., Greenberg, T., Velting, D. M., & Shaffer, D. (2003). Youth suicide risk and preventive interventions: a review of the past 10 years. *Journal of the American Academy of Child and Adolescent Psychiatry*, **42**(4), 386–405.

Gould, M. S., Marrocco, F. A., Hoagwood, K., et al. (2009). Service use by at risk youths after school-based suicide screening. *Journal of the American Academy of Child and Adolescent Psychiatry*, **48**(12), 1193–1201.

Hacker, K., Collins, J., Gross-Young, L., Almeida, S., & Burke, N. (2008). Coping with youth suicide and overdose: one community's efforts to investigate, intervene, and prevent suicide contagion. *Crisis*, **29**(2), 86–95.

Harris, K. M., McLean, J. P., Sheffield, J., & Jobes, D. (2010). The internal suicide debate hypothesis: exploring the life versus death struggle. *Suicide and Life-Threatening Behavior*, **40**(2), 181–192.

Haw, C., Hawton, K., Niedzwiedz, C., & Platt, S. (2013). Suicide clusters: a review of risk factors and mechanisms. *Suicide and Life-Threatening Behavior*, **43**(1), 97–108.

Hawton, K., & van Heeringen, K. (2009). Suicide. *Lancet*, **373**, 1372–1381.

Hawton, K., Simkin, S., Deeks, J. J., et al. (1999). Effects of a drug overdose in a television drama on presentations to hospital for self-poisoning: time series and questionnaire study. *British Medical Journal*, **318**(7189), 972–977.

Insel, B. J., & Gould, M. S. (2008). Impact of modeling on adolescent suicidal behavior. *Psychiatric Clinics of North America*, **31**(2), 293–316.

Kessler, R. C., Downey, G., Milavsky, J. R., & Stipp, H. (1988). Clustering of teenage suicides after television news stories about suicides: a reconsideration. *American Journal of Psychiatry*, **41**(11), 1379–1383.

Knox, G. (1964). The detection of space–time interactions. *Applied Statistics*, **3**, 25–29.

Kulldorff, M. (1997). A spatial scan statistic. *Communications in Statistics: Theory and Methods*, **26**, 1481–1496.

Levy, D. A., & Nail, P. R. (1993). Contagion: A theoretical and empirical review and reconceptualization. *Genetic, Social & General Psychology Monographs*, **19**(2), 235–285.

McKenzie, N., & Keane, M. (2007). Contribution of imitative suicide to the suicide rate in prisons. *Suicide and Life-Threatening Behavior*, **37**(5), 538–542.

Mercy, J. A., Kresnow, M., O'Carroll, P. W., et al. (2001). Is suicide contagious? A study of the relation between exposure to suicidal behavior of others and nearly lethal suicide attempts. *American Journal of Epidemiology*, **154** (2), 120–127.

Motto, J. A. (1970). Newspaper influence on suicide. *Archives of General Psychiatry*, **23**, 143–148.

Niederkrotenthaler, T., & Sonneck, G. (2007). Assessing the impact of media guidelines for reporting on suicides in Austria: interrupted time series analysis. *Australian and New Zealand Journal of Psychiatry*, **41**, 419–428.

Niederkrotenthaler, T., Till, B., Kapusta, N. D., et al. (2009). Copycat effects after media reports on suicide: a population-based ecologic study. *Social Science and Medicine*, **69**(7), 1085–1090.

Niederkrotenthaler, T., Voracek, M., Herberth, A., et al. (2010). Role of media reports in completed and prevented suicide: Werther v. Papageno effects. *British Journal of Psychiatry*, **197**(3), 234–243.

Phillips, D. P. (1974). The influence of suggestion on suicide: substantive and theoretical implications of the Werther effect. *American Sociological Review*, **39**(3), 340–354.

Phillips, D. P., & Carstensen, L. L. (1986). Clustering of teenage suicides after television news stories about suicide. *New England Journal of Medicine*, **315**(11), 685–689.

Pirkis, J. E., & Nordentoft, M. (2011). Media influences on suicide and attempted suicide. In R. C. O'Connor, S. Platt, & J. Gordon (Eds.) *International Handbook of Suicide Prevention: Research, Policy and Practice* (pp. 531–544). Oxford: Wiley-Blackwell.

Poijula, S., Wahlberg, K. E., & Dyregrov, A. (2001). Adolescent suicide and suicide contagion in three secondary schools. *International Journal of Emergency Mental Health*, **3**(3), 163–168.

Stack, S. (1990a). A reanalysis of the impact of non-celebrity suicides. *Social Psychiatry and Psychiatric Epidemiology*, **25**, 269–273.

Stack, S. (1990b). Audience receptiveness, the media, and aged suicide, 1968–1980. *Journal of Aging Studies*, **4**(2), 195–209.

Stack, S. (1996). The effect of the media on suicide: Evidence from Japan, 1955–1985. *Suicide and Life-Threatening Behavior*, **26**(2), 132–142.

Stack, S. (2003). Media coverage as a risk factor in suicide. *Journal of Epidemiology and Community Health*, **57**(4), 238–240.

Stack, S. (2005). Suicide in the media. A quantitative review of studies based on nonfictional stories. *Suicide and Life-Threatening Behavior*, **35**(2), 121–133.

Taiminen, T. J., & Helenius, H. (1994). Suicide clustering in a psychiatric hospital with a history of a suicide epidemic: a quantitative study. *American Journal of Psychiatry*, **151**, 1087–1088.

Taiminen, T., Salmenpera, T., & Lehtinen, K. (1992). A suicide epidemic in a psychiatric hospital. *Suicide and Life-Threatening Behavior*, **22**(3), 350–363.

Toumbourou, J. W., & Gregg, M. E. (2002). Impact of an empowerment-based parent education program on the reduction of youth suicide risk factors. *Journal of Adolescent Health*, **31**(3), 277–285.

Tousignant, M., Mishara, B. L., Caillaud, A., Fortin, V., & St-Laurent, D. (2005). The impact of media coverage of the suicide of a well-known Quebec reporter: the case of Gaetan Girouard. *Social Science and Medicine*, **60**, 1919–1926.

Wallenstein, S., Gould, M. S., and Kleinman, M. (1989). Use of the scan statistic to detect time-space clustering. *American Journal of Epidemiology*, **130**(5), 1057–1064.

Wheeler, L. (1966). Toward a theory of behavioral contagion. *Psychological Review*, **73**(2), 179–192.

Wyman, P. A., Brown, C. H., LoMurray, M., et al. (2010). An outcome evaluation of the Sources of Strength suicide prevention program delivered by adolescent peer leaders in high schools. *American Journal of Public Health*, **100**(9), 1653–1661.

Chapter 7

Ethnicity

How much of our understanding of suicide is applicable across ethnic cultures?

Donna Holland Barnes, William B. Lawson, and Kelsey Ball

Introduction

How do you sort people? Attempts to communicate suicide prevention and intervention messages to diverse populations can be complicated. What are the primary constructs? Do we consider color of skin, shared heritage, cultural beliefs, and religious beliefs? In fact, there are various belief systems, religious practices, and behavioral patterns that must be considered for each ethnic population. Because suicide prevention and intervention initiatives focus on behavioral change – i.e., developing practices to minimize suicidality – the primary construct should be behavioral. It is important to be clear on the targeted behavior to be changed, and to understand what controls such behavior, such as attitude, perceived norms, or personal agency (Institute of Medicine, 2002).

Maharajh and Abdool (2005) discuss cultural-bound syndromes as it applies to aberrant behavior and troubling experiences that can sometimes be linked to diagnostic categories. These syndromes are generally related to a cultural emphasis or a stress situation or more specifically suicidal behavior. For example, does the culture or ethnic group view suicide as a criminal act or a symptom of a mental disorder? Some cultures may even view it as an honorable act when publically disgraced. It is imperative to understand how suicide is viewed among various ethnic groups to understand better prevention measures. How a population views the world, others, and themselves is key in understanding their views of suicide.

According to David Lester (Lester, 2007) any research findings on suicide prevention and intervention with recommendations need to establish if the findings are cross-cultural or apply specifically to one culture. Lester studied 17 industrialized nations and attempted to predict their rates of suicide using five variables common to American dominant culture. He found that "*Western theories of suicide do not apply to nonwestern cultures.*" There were too many differences in genetic make-up, differences in the prevalence of psychological and psychiatric factors, and social variables.

Suicide is multidimensional and therefore efforts to understand suicide and prevention and intervention should be multilayered. The differences in suicidal behavior can be explained partly by differences in psychiatric disorders.

Mental illness and cultural differences

Mental disorders and substance abuse are major risk factors for suicide. Yet these disorders are often under-recognized or undertreated in many communities of color, mainly African Americans. For a host of reasons, depression is under-recognized; one being that depression in other cultures is presented differently than mainstream benchmarks and commonly known systems from the dominant populations. Anger in Black males should be viewed as a symptom but is often dismissed as a typical reaction among Black males in general. Stigma is also attached to the diagnosis. For many young men discussing sadness is proposed as a sign of weakness and suicidal thoughts are not discussed. As a result, their depression or mental disorder is internalized and it manifests itself in other ways such as striking out at others or they may arrange their own death such as engaging in homicidal behavior in an effort to be killed simply by putting themselves in harms-way or suicide-by-cop. Other disorders like bipolar is well recognized as being underdiagnosed especially in African Americans. It is

A Concise Guide to Understanding Suicide, ed. Stephen H. Koslow, Pedro Ruiz, and Charles B. Nemeroff. Published by Cambridge University Press.

the number one disorder associated with suicide attempts (depression being number one with completed suicides). In addition, African Americans are often misdiagnosed with schizophrenia and thought to be antisocial and therefore they are mistreated or not treated. Post-traumatic stress disorder is more likely in African Americans in the inner city or combat. It too is often misdiagnosed and not treated.

When cultural factors have a predominant influence

Clearly there is an unmet need to address suicide among various ethnic groups. The need parallels the disparities in treatment seen for other disorders. The Surgeon General's Report (Satcher, 2001) clearly documents that African Americans are only half as likely to receive depression treatment. Moreover treatment often is not evidence based. Similarly bipolar disorder is often not diagnosed or treated. Post-traumatic stress disorder is frequently treated with benzodiazepines alone, which has been shown to be ineffective. Schizophrenia is often treated with antipsychotics alone and in excessive doses. All of these disorders are associated with an excessively high risk of suicide. More creative approaches are necessary as African Americans, for instance, have different illness demographics and receive treatment in different settings than the general population. Suicide risk increases with age for Whites and Asians but peak in the 20s for African American males. Thus interventions useful for the rest of the population may not be applicable for African Americans. Moreover the clinician may not be aware of the idioms of distress for the African American community. The Surgeon General and other reports show that African Americans are less likely to seek treatment from specialized mental health providers when in distress. Rather they are more likely to seek help from friends, ministers, traditional healers (Garlow et al., 2005), and if they seek professional help, from primary care providers, who often may screen but not intervene with suicidal individuals, there are higher levels of untreated mental health problems, and low levels of compliance as well as satisfaction with the services.

While some of the common risk factors for suicide among the dominant population rest with social isolation, unemployment, untreated mental disorders, means availability, substance abuse and psychiatric illnesses, risk factors in various ethnic groups may differ. On an individual level, racism, acculturation, culture clash with parents, loss of religious affiliation, difficulty with identity formation, and loss of community support can have effects on suicide risk (McKenzie et al., 2003; Barnes, 2003; Guzman et al., 2009). These risk factors have much to do with the influence of the socioeconomic situation, immigration, moving from a traditional community to a more mainstream environment, and its culture and history.

One of the major defining issues within groups is acculturation – an appreciation for (and contact with) the dominant culture and a form of assimilation. While most ethnic groups work at assimilating with the dominant culture, and are encouraged to do so because it helps maintain positive relationships, more attention needs to be focused on conflictive issues that develop once acculturation has occurred. For example, many individuals in certain groups who are proficient in English tend to disassociate from, or leave behind, family members who are not. This can lead to loss of family bonds and support. Similarly, studies have shown a correlation between acculturation and elevated suicide rates among young Black males (Willis et al., 2003). The lack of a strong sense of identity in relation to the dominant group can become a key risk factor for suicidal behavior.

There are also critical questions associated with race, ethnicity, and culture. Should populations be sorted by skin color, by religious practices, or by lifestyles? Getting various ethnic groups involved in traditional preventive intervention programs takes planning. Programmers must (1) know who is in the community, (2) identify the influential leaders, (3) create the right environment by inviting members of the community to the planning table and listening to what they have to offer, and (4) recognize the value of their alternative ways of preventive intervention procedures.

Furthermore, individuals who are biracial and/or assimilated must decide for themselves which culture they will follow when seeking treatment for mental disorders. Do they seek treatment through the system of the dominant culture or do they use the approaches of their ethnic traditions? And, which ethnic practice should be used for a multi-racial individual, for example, one who is part Japanese, part Hawaiian, and part American Indian? Internal complexities are widespread among minority groups and should be recognized and discussed when approaching a community of color.

Finally, successful suicide prevention interventions in diverse communities require a sophisticated understanding of the complex dynamics of "otherness," or feelings of "outsiderness" and "insiderness." Unless this understanding is combined with a deep appreciation of the political, social, and psychological phenomena, even very sincere and well-intentioned efforts to promote social change or healing are easily thwarted.

Conclusion: a global perspective

African American males aged 20–24 have the highest rate of suicide compared to Whites with males ages 45–64 having the highest rates within their population. However, the suicide rate for Blacks of all ages is slightly half the overall US rate. In the latest report from the Centers for Disease Control on suicides in the USA, Blacks are listed as having the lowest rates out of all populations. However, one of the major risk factors that need more attention for our young Black males is "no hope for the future." When we focus on that risk factor, we may not see completed suicides in the traditional manner, but life-threatening behavior: behavior that puts one in harm's way almost on a daily basis, e.g., engaging in violence that could cause one to be killed, smoking harmful cigarettes with chemicals in them that can cause brain disorders, or driving recklessly. Once you do not care about life anymore, perhaps because it no longer has any meaning, an attitude of unresponsiveness sets in.

Many studies have found that among ethnic groups, risk for suicide is low among immigrants prior to migration in comparison to the US born immigrants, and equalizes over time after migration (Borges et al., 2012)

Worldwide, suicide rates have increased by 60% in the last 45 years (WHO, 2007). The highest rates of suicide are found in Eastern Europe – a group of countries that have similar historical and sociocultural characteristics, mainly Lithuania and Kazakhstan (<25 per 100 000), and to a lesser degree the Russian Federation and Hungary (>25 per 100 000) (Figure 7.1). Also, the lowest rate of suicide for many years has been in the Eastern Mediterranean region which is generally made up of countries of Islamic traditions (Bertolote & Fleischmann, 2002) as well as Christian traditions. These countries include Cyprus, the State of Palestine, Lebanon, Syria, Jordan, and Israel. This low rate is most likely due to homogeneity where the majority of the populations have the same practices and lifestyle with very little diversity; and they are more observant of traditions and customs. Traditional theories of suicide indicate that populations with high rates of integration and regulation generally have low rates of suicide (Durkheim, 1951).

It is believed that many of the traditions in various ethnic cultures provide protective factors, such as religiosity, sweat lodges, or meditation and in some cultures singing or dancing. As we advance and create benchmarks for healing in the traditional way, many coping skills are forgotten and lost.

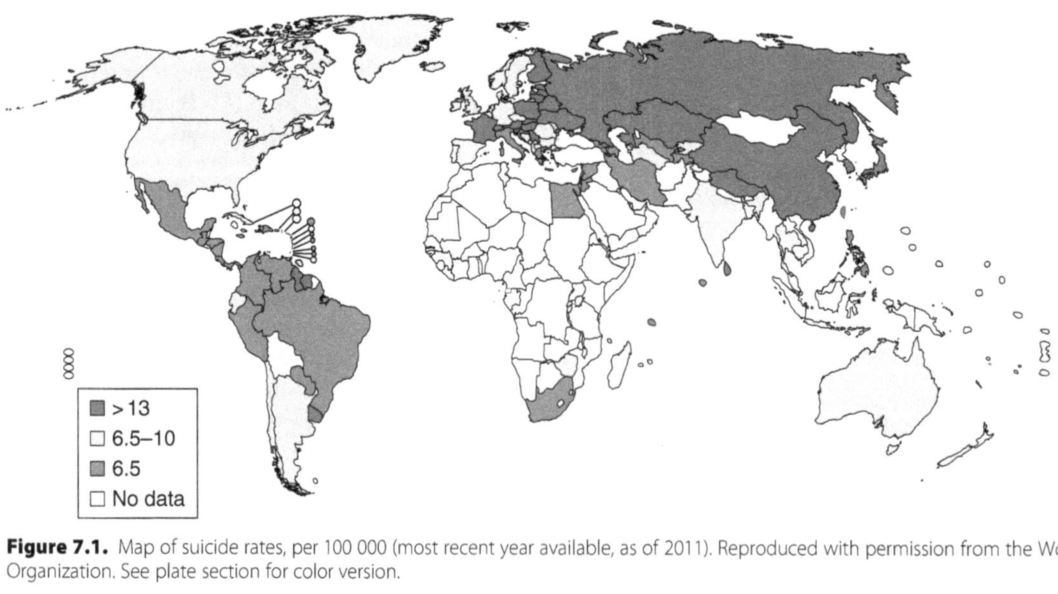

Figure 7.1. Map of suicide rates, per 100 000 (most recent year available, as of 2011). Reproduced with permission from the World Health Organization. See plate section for color version.

References

Barnes, D. H. (Ed.) (2003). Cultural Competency: Developing strategies to engage minority populations in suicide prevention. (Online) Available at: www.sprc.org/library_resources/items/cultural-competency-developing-strategies-engage-minority-populations-suicid

Bertolote, J. M., & Fleischmann, A., (2002). A global perspective in the epidemiology of suicide. *Suicidologi*, 7(2).

Borges, G., Orozco, R., Rafful, C., Miller, E., & Breslau, J. (2012). Suicidality, ethnicity, and immigration in the USA. *Psychological Medicine*, **42**, 1115–1184.

Durkheim, E. (1951). *Suicide*. Glencoe, Illinois: The Free Press.

Garlow, S. J., Purselle, D., & Heninger, M. (2005). Ethnic differences in patterns of suicide across the life cycle. *The American Journal of Psychiatry*, **162**(2), 319–323.

Guzman, A., Koons, A., & Postolache, T. (2009). Suicidal behavior in Latinos: focus on the youth. *International Journal of Adolescent Medicine and Health*, **21**(4), 431–439.

Institute of Medicine (2002). *Reducing Suicide: A National Imperative*. Washington, DC: The National Academies Press.

Lester, D. (2007). Theories of suicide. In F. Leong & M. Leach (Eds) *Suicide Among Racial and Ethnic Minority Groups: Theory, Research and Practice*, Chapter 3. Danvers, MA: Brunner-Routledge.

Maharajh, H. D., & Abdool, P. S. (2005). Cultural aspects of suicide. *The Scientific World Journal*, **5**, 736–746.

McKenzie, K., Serfaty, M., & Crawford., M. (2003). Suicide in ethnic minority groups. *The British Journal of Psychiatry*, **183**, 100–101.

Satcher, D. (2001). *Mental Health: Culture, Race, and Ethnicity: A Supplement to Mental Health: A Report of the Surgeon General*. Rockville, MD: Office of the Surgeon General (US), Center for Mental Health Services (US), National Institute of Mental Health (US).

Willis, L. A., Coombs, D. W., Drentea, P., & Cockerham, W. C. (2003). Uncovering the mystery: Factors of African American suicide. *Suicide and Life-Threatening Behavior*, **33**(4), 412–429.

World Health Organization (WHO). (2007). http://www.who.int/mediacentre/news/statements/2007/s16/en/

Chapter 8

Suicide-related bereavement and grief

M. Katherine Shear and Sidney Zisook

Introduction

The decision to take one's own life is incomprehensible to most people and yet suicide is a fact of life. Statistics document that more than a million people die each year, around the world, and it is likely that recorded statistics underestimate the actual rate of suicide deaths. The effects of a suicide death almost always extend to a wide range of people, including close attachments of the deceased, other immediate and extended family, friends and acquaintances, health and mental health professionals, clergy, police, firefighters, funeral directors, coroner's office, and others who may be involved in discovery or processing activities related to the death. In a famous and widely cited book, Schneidman made the claim that there are an average of six survivors affected by each suicide. Since then, there have been scores of papers discussing the ways that the lives of survivor-victims of suicidal deaths are changed forever. These authors concur with Schneidman in the view that the largest public health problem related to suicide is alleviation of effects of stress in these survivors, whose numbers are far larger than the suicide decedents themselves (Dyregrov, 2011) In recognition of this need, a Special Interest Group on suicide bereavement was proposed at the XXVI International Association for Suicide Prevention (IASP) World Congress in Beijing China in September 2011. Yet as of 2013, only 20 of 46 member countries list suicide bereavement services.

Bereavement is one of life's most difficult experiences, and one that seems all the more challenging when a loved one dies by suicide. For many, it is difficult to shake the idea that such a death could have been prevented, and/or to lay blame at the feet of survivors who might have failed to prevent the suicide, or might even seem to have caused it. The perspective that suicide presents a unique ordeal for survivors is shared by most clinicians and documented in numerous publications. Recently, though, the validity of this perspective has been challenged and methodological problems with existing studies brought to the fore (Murphy et al., 2003; Sveen and Walby, 2008; Bolton et al., 2013; Floyd et al., 2013). Notwithstanding the questions about whether or not suicide bereavement differs in severity or quality from other kinds of losses, there is no question that losing a loved one to suicide is a very intense and disruptive experience. The purpose of this chapter is to provide a framework for understanding suicide-related grief and mourning in the larger context of bereavement more generally, to highlight issues commonly seen in association with suicide loss, and to summarize thinking about optimal professional support for suicide bereaved individuals. We begin by defining terms to facilitate clear communication.

Definitions

Terminology is imprecise in both thanatology and suicidology and key concepts lack consensus definitions. For this reason we begin with definitions of terms used in this paper. The terms bereavement, grief, and mourning are often used interchangeably and/or in ways different from how we use them. We use the term bereavement to refer to the situation of having lost someone close. We note that in most studies, people simply self-identify as bereaved by responding to the question of whether they have lost "someone important" where this designation is not defined and open to a range of interpretations. As a result, there is little methodologically rigorous data regarding the epidemiology of bereavement.

We use the term *grief* to refer to the response to loss and further characterize grief as acute, integrated, and complicated. Acute grief is the initial response to bereavement that is often intense and disruptive, especially when the loss is untimely, unexpected, or violent. *Integrated grief* is a permanent form of grief that is not

A Concise Guide to Understanding Suicide, ed. Stephen H. Koslow, Pedro Ruiz, and Charles B. Nemeroff. Published by Cambridge University Press.

disruptive and that emerges as the loss is assimilated, the acute anguish subsides, and the individual begins acclimating to life without his or her lost loved one; *complicated grief* is the condition that results when transformation from acute to integrated grief does not occur. The term complicated is used here in the medical sense of a superimposed condition that influences the course of another condition.

We use the term *mourning* as Bowlby did, to refer to the range of psychological processes set in motion by a loss in order to facilitate adjustment to the myriad of changes that accompany the loss. Mourning typically proceeds in concert with social, spiritual, and cultural rituals. Put another way, mourning is the process by which acute grief is transformed to integrated grief. This transformation typically entails acknowledging the finality and consequences of the loss, finding a way to maintain a sense of connection to the deceased, and re-envisioning a life with purpose and meaning and the possibility for joy and satisfaction, even without the lost loved one.

Definitions of suicide and suicide survivor are also somewhat ambiguous. *Suicide* is the act of taking one's own life on purpose; however intention is not always clear-cut and not operationally defined. Confirmation of suicide often falls to a process that involves medical or legal professionals, eyewitnesses, and family and friends of the deceased. The conclusion of this process is not emotionally or morally neutral for those involved. Interpretation of information is socially influenced such that there may be a systematic bias against a suicide verdict, and this may differ within or between judicial districts, countries, or cultures (e.g., Timmermans, 2005; Chapple et al., 2012) We therefore note that any research related to suicidal deaths begins with a level of uncertainty about the dependent variable. We additionally note that in most research suicide is treated as a unitary phenomenon, whereas not all suicide deaths are the same. Some are expected and some are not (Wojtkowiak et al., 2012). Some are more violent than others and some occur against a background of strife and conflict whereas others occur in a setting of severe physical pain, and still others seem to come out of the blue. In one study, age of the deceased played a role in survivor's response (Schneider et al., 2011).

The definition of *suicide survivor* is even more problematic. Dyregrov (2011) claims that this term, used widely in North and South America, is synonymous with suicide bereaved as applied in other parts of the world. However, the term survivor is often used to designate someone who was not especially close to the deceased person. Further, it is clear that there are many people who survive the suicide who are affected by it in some way, who might not be considered bereaved (Clark, 2001; Jordan & McIntosh, 2011). Dyregrov further notes that the term suicide survivor includes three important ideas; it refers to the behavior of someone else (suicide), to the death of that person, and to the impact on the surviving person. However, none of these concepts has been consistently operationalized. Moreover, Berman (2011) points out that there is no consensus regarding the definition of suicide survivor. Definitions may entail degree of kinship, degree of impact of the death, defined as either life changing or symptom evoking or degree of exposure. Berman concludes that there is a need for a clear and consensual definition of survivorship. This could also be said of bereavement more generally. However, the work reported in this chapter is not based on such a consensus. Given the vagaries, there are still some useful observations about grief in general and suicide-related grief in particular. In this paper we focus primarily on *suicide bereavement* defined as the loss of someone close who dies by suicide. We discuss the effects of larger social groups being impacted by the suicide.

A framework for understanding bereavement and grief

It is a truism that each person's grief is unique. Moreover, grief related to each loss is unique. However, in spite of this, there are commonalities among bereaved people that are useful to consider. In order to understand the response to loss we need to understand what it is that was lost. While again there are unique answers to this question for every relationship, researchers have learned a lot about our closest relationships and what they provide. In particular, secure attachment relationships help regulate a myriad of psychological and physiological functions on a day-to-day basis. In essence our loved ones help define who we are and how we function. Not surprisingly, loss of such a person causes great disruption, regardless of how they die.

John Bowlby introduced the idea that humans, like many other animals, are biologically motivated to seek, form, and maintain close relationships with a small number of people across the lifespan, and further, that we instinctively respond to their loss. Bowlby (1980) described the acute response to the loss of a loved one as one that typically entails intense, unfamiliar emotions, as well as preoccupying thoughts and memories of the person who died. He observed that a bereaved person naturally resists accepting the reality that the loved one is gone forever, and incorporates this painful information slowly, oscillating between registering the unwanted news and blocking it out. Bowlby further noted that during acute grief, the bereaved person faces a dilemma. The question of whether to reject or to find a way to accept the reality entails an avoid–avoid dilemma as either option forebodes pain. However, he argued that only by resolving the dilemma in a way that enables the bereaved person to acknowledge the finality and consequences of the loss, reconfigure the mental representation of the deceased, and find a way to envision life going forward without the deceased in a positive way, can acute grief be transformed and healed.

The natural healing process is thus fundamentally a learning process requiring assimilation of painful, unwanted information about the finality of the loss, its personal meaning, and its implications for the future. Memories of close attachments are thought to be stored in an internal working model that contains representations of aspects of the other person, the self, and the relationship. These include both explicit and implicit memory systems. Among the implicit memories are conditioned reward responses that must be extinguished as mourning proceeds. The marked increase in yearning and longing for a deceased loved one that typically occurs in early bereavement might be seen as a manifestation of an extinction burst. If so, willingness to continue to engage with cues that trigger this desire for the loved one may be an important part of the healing process.

Emotion regulation is important in order to successfully assimilate information about the death, and is usually achieved during mourning by a combination of processes. Among them are oscillating attention between engaging with, and defensively excluding, this painful information, experiencing positive emotions, drawing upon supportive companionship, and engaging in reappraisal. The learning and emotion regulation processes usually progress in fits and starts that are not predictable or controllable. This experience, though healing in the long run, is often unfamiliar, uncomfortable, and disconcerting for bereaved people. Observing the process of acute grief can also be unsettling and difficult for others who are needed to bear witness and provide comfort and support. Most people do not heal well when left completely on their own.

What makes a grief response unique

Within the overall framework of acute grief and its transformation over time, there is considerable variability in the specific content, intensity, frequency, and duration of grief symptoms. This variability is related to a number of factors, among them are characteristics of the bereaved person, and the nature of the relationship she or he had with the deceased. The closeness of the relationship is important, and there are some commonalities within different relationships, for example among people who have lost a child, a life partner, a parent or someone else with whom they were close. Additionally, each person has his or her unique personal history and psychobiological make-up and each love relationship is unique. Acute grief symptoms are also influenced by the circumstances of the death, including the manner of the death, its timing, the degree to which it is expected, and the manner of notification of the death. The aftermath of the loss is also an important determinant of the features and course of acute grief, including the consequences and implications of the death and the context in which the bereaved person mourns. Suicide death has some commonalities in each of these areas, and also some variability. The commonalities can guide us in understanding what to expect following suicide bereavement, and the variability suggests that there will also be differences in the quality, intensity, and duration of acute grief among a group of suicide bereaved people. Research to date supports the idea that there are some common issues that suicide bereaved people are likely to confront (Bailley et al., 1999; Begley & Quayle, 2007), and also that there is enough variability that, similar to acute grief following other losses, people grieving a suicide experience grief in their own unique way. Overall, when control groups are included in studies of suicide bereavement, there are few differences based on the manner of death.

Complicated grief

Complicated grief occurs when there is a co-occurring problem that interrupts the natural healing process, in a manner analogous to an infection that complicates wound healing or pneumonia that complicates healing of a myocardial infarction. In the case of healing after loss, these complications usually entail ruminative preoccupying thoughts, excessive avoidance, or other interfering behaviors and/or ineffective emotion regulation. These complicating processes can usually be traced to the bereaved person's history, personal traits,

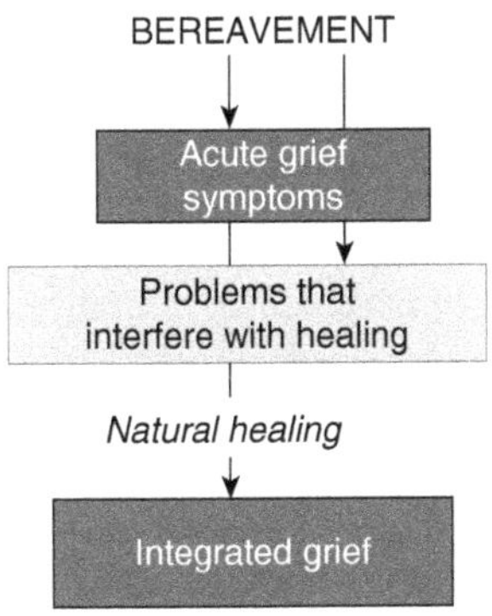

Figure 8.1. Model of bereavement, grief, and healing.

or relationship with the deceased, to aspects of the circumstances or consequences of the death or the context in which the bereaved person mourns. Figure 8.1 illustrates a model of complicated grief. Suicide bereavement is associated with an increased rate of complicated grief (Mitchell et al., 2004, 2005), likely contributed to by some group differences in each of these areas. Somewhat counter-intuitively, though, the increased rates of complicated grief appear to be modest. Personal growth and resilience is also seen with suicide bereavement but is less often a focus of attention (Feigelman et al., 2009)

Suicide bereavement and grief

One of the most impactful features of suicide is that most people intuitively feel that the death was preventable. More than any other kind of death, suicide seems to be a poor decision on the part of the deceased. This perception opens the door to a range of blaming thoughts and feelings, focusing on counterfactual thinking about how things could have, and should have, gone differently. Many suicide bereaved people struggle with questions about how they, the deceased person or someone else, might have acted differently. It can be easy for a bereaved person to imagine that she or he missed or ignored an important cue, that she or he failed to provide needed expressions of love or support, or that they could have interrupted or prevented the death in some other way. Questions such as these can be difficult to resist. Guilty, self-blaming thoughts and feelings can be accompanied by angry, other-blaming thoughts including ideas that a caregiver, health or mental health professional, colleague or co-worker, or other professional could and should have prevented the death. Sometimes, too, these thoughts focus on the deceased person him- or herself. Why could not the person stop this behavior? Why didn't they understand how terrible it would be for those left behind? These thoughts are often accompanied by painful feelings of rejection by the deceased loved one.

Suicide has been described throughout human history (Cvinar, 2005). In some cultures and historical periods, little stigma was attached to taking one's own life, and at times, such an act has even been perceived as honorable or heroic. However, during the Middle-Ages, Western culture began to view suicide as anathema, the effects of which extended to the family of the suicide decedent. Scocco et al (Scocco et al., 2012) note that while the more extreme forms of stigmatization have been discontinued, informal social disapproval, isolation, and shunning are still sometimes seen. Since modern suicide is almost always associated with mental illness, stigma related to mental disorders also infects suicide. Internalization of stigma also occurs and this can be an important obstacle to healing. Interestingly, Sudak et al. (Sudak et al., 2008) point to the fact that, unlike mental disorders, there is some reason not to destigmatize suicide. Gould and Shaffer (Gould et al., 1988) found that fictional portrayal of suicide resulted in an increase in suicidal behavior in some locations. Sudak et al. suggest this could possibly be attributed, in part, to normalization of this behavior. Clearly, though, there is a need to reduce stigma that interferes with support for the suicide bereaved (Scocco et al., 2012).

Cvinar (2005) highlights the fact that self-stigmatization and perception of stigma may be more problematic after suicide than actually being the object of stigma, and there is some support for this idea. There is also some indication in the literature that suicide loss is not more stigmatized than some other losses – in particular drug overdose and HIV-AIDS-related deaths. To some degree, there is a strong aversion to death in our culture that tends to limit the ability of many people to provide support, regardless of the cause of death. Bereaved people often feel that there is a very short period of time in which others are empathic and supportive of a loss, after which they are expected to "stop wallowing and move on." This very harmful attitude is beginning to be addressed. One very promising approach is the emergence of "Death Cafes" in which people gather to discuss attitudes and beliefs about death.

In addition to stigma, there are other social and cultural procedures that occur with suicide and are more unusual with other deaths. One of these is involvement of the media. Media interest in suicide can be damaging to survivors as it can intrude on their privacy and create opportunities for negative judgments. Media involvement is also thought to be a potential focus of imitation suicidal behavior. As a consequence guidelines for media coverage of suicide have been developed by the American Foundation for Suicide Prevention (AFSP) and other national organizations. Involvement of police, fire, and/or medical examiners' offices is also more common with suicide than most other kinds of death. Witnessing suicide, finding the body, or insensitive death notification procedures can all occur and be a focus of traumatic stress for a bereaved person. Recent work by the AFSP as well as The Association for Death Education and Counseling (ADEC) has addressed support and education for these service providers in an effort to reduce the trauma associated with suicide.

Postvention for suicide bereaved individuals

Schneidman (1973) coined the term "postvention" to refer to the act of providing clinical care after a suicide, a period roughly equivalent to tertiary prevention or rehabilitation. Suicidologists have taken up this idea, emphasizing that what is needed is activities to facilitate healing and resolve problems that can lead to adverse outcomes. Most believe that these activities need to be developed in collaboration with survivors themselves. Several authors have suggested that the great majority of suicide bereaved people believe they need professional help. In spite of this need relatively few organizations include a focus on providing assistance to survivors. Those who are active in devising programs for suicide bereaved point to a need for improved attitudes of mental health professions, including being less patronizing and judgmental, having more compassion, knowledge and understanding, and being more willing to listen respectfully (Grad et al., 2004)

Dyregov and colleagues (Dyregrov et al., 2010) outline a useful approach to help for suicide bereavement. They stress the importance of openness as a coping strategy, defining this concept as sincerity, candor and directly speaking about the suicide, the pain of the loss, the need for support and the experience of the attitudes of others. Somewhat surprisingly, this kind of openness can be very difficult to achieve. It requires a deep level of trust, a willingness to accept and show vulnerability, and a commitment to integrity in the face of possible social ostracism. These authors note that some bereaved people understand from an early stage that it is sometimes necessary to instruct and train the people in their surroundings regarding how to relate to them. In our experience, bereaved people can feel resentful of this need, and helping them to accept it can be an important step in healing.

Effective postvention includes peer support, social network support, and professional help. Existing surveys suggest that bereaved individuals desire more help from professionals than they typically receive (e.g., Provini et al., 2000; Dyregrov, 2002). They ask for assistance early and for outreach from professionals, preferring not to be required to proactively request assistance. This assistance entails information and practical assistance, as well as therapeutic help with difficult emotions and maladaptive thinking. Suicide survivors also believe they need long-term follow-up. The natural social environment often has expectations of a steep trajectory of improvement in grief symptoms, to a degree that may not be realistic. Certainly many people require a prolonged period of time to adjust to the suicide death of a loved one. Support from peers, social network, and professionals is needed throughout this period.

Professionals might encourage activities that help integrate the deceased person into daily life, such as rituals, ceremonies, candle lighting, review of pictures and momentos, or even finding new information about the deceased person or the death. Some people find artistic expression is helpful, including writing, painting, drawing, listening to or playing music, or engaging in watching or participating in dance or theater performances. Religious and spiritual activities are helpful to many people. Interestingly, a recent paper reports that a high proportion of suicide bereaved people who attended a support group experience personal growth as a result of their bereavement experiences. Personal growth was associated with religious membership as well as voting, thought to be an indicator of civic involvement (Feigelman et al., 2009) Other helpful strategies include regular physical activity, good nutrition and sleep hygiene, and taking "time out" from grief. Also important early in bereavement is recognition, diagnosis, and treatment of co-occurring mental disorders. Major depression and post-traumatic stress disorder are among the most common of these, though by no means do all suicide bereaved people experience these disorders. The recent decision to remove the bereavement exclusion for major depression from the psychiatric diagnostic

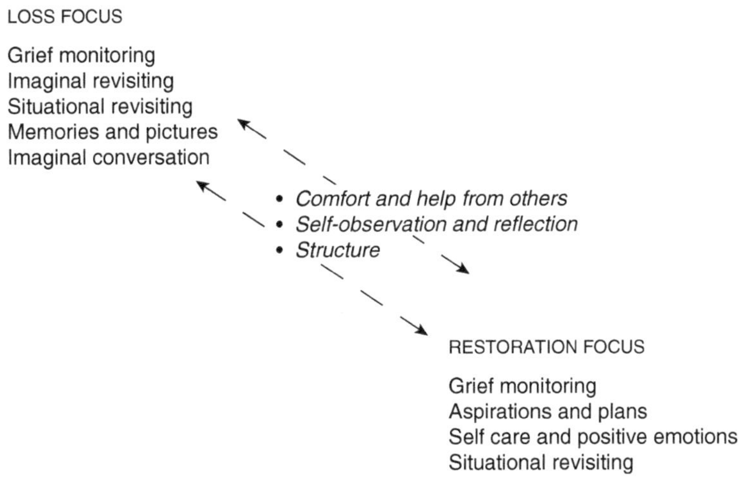

Figure 8.2. Summary of CGT.

system was made in recognition that not all bereaved people are depressed, and when they are, they may benefit from treatment.

Identification and treatment of complicated grief among suicide bereaved

Complicated grief (CG) occurs in about 20% of suicide bereaved individuals, a rate approximately twice that seen after natural death. CG can be recognized using a brief 5-item screening instrument (Shear et al., 2006) or the 19-item self-report Inventory of Complicated Grief (ICG) (Prigerson et al., 1995). Either of these instruments can identify people who are experiencing a persistent period of acute grief, longer than 6 months after the loss of a loved one. These people are at risk for increased rates of suicidal ideation, sleep disturbance, functional impairment, and new-onset physical illness. The distress and impairment caused by CG warrants treatment and several studies suggest that standard psychotherapy and/or grief counseling is not optimal for treating CG. We have developed and tested a treatment that is efficacious for these symptoms (Shear et al., 2005; Shear et al., submitted for publication). Early results from our ongoing trial suggest suicide bereaved individuals with CG respond equally well as those bereaved in other ways.

Complicated grief treatment (CGT) is based on the attachment theory model of grief and mourning described above. The treatment is a 16-session manualized approach that uses a set of specific procedures to achieve two main goals: to find and resolve grief complications and to facilitate the natural healing process. Core procedures (see Figure 8.2) include a grief monitoring diary, psychoeducation about bereavement, grief and mourning, imaginal revisiting exercises that entail repeated retelling of the story of the death, and situational revisiting that entails deliberately confronting situations that evoke painful reminders of the loss, personal aspiration and goals work, work with memories and pictures, and imaginal conversation with the deceased person. Work with suicide bereaved people usually also includes in depth discussion of what is known about suicide, from the perspective of a stress diathesis model. We often use a metaphor of suicide as a "heart attack of the brain." As noted above, it is usually necessary to work with feelings of guilt and responsibility, and sometimes with feelings of anger or rejection or shame. Any of these feelings can be associated with troubling ruminations and/or excessive avoidance behavior that need to be resolved in order to free the natural healing process. However the overall framework of CGT appears to be effective in helping people who are suicide bereaved, as it is with other bereaved individuals.

Summary and conclusion

Suicide survivors face a number of challenges that often accompany the normal grieving process (Tal Young et al., 2012), putting survivors at increased risk for developing complicated grief. Suicide is virtually the only kind of loss where a bereaved family may decide not to report the true cause of death. Because of shame and internalized stigma associated with suicide, some survivors feel reluctant to seek support from friends or family. Attending support groups with other survivors who share the experience of suicide may be especially helpful for this group to feel safe and understood. However, at least one recent study found that for the minority who are struggling with complicated grief, support groups have lower satisfaction ratings and less positive impact (Johnsen et al., 2012). For this group, complicated grief treatment, a focused, manualized brief psychotherapeutic approach, has been demonstrated to be effective and address troubling symptoms should they occur. Studies document an important need of suicide bereaved people for support from peers, family, social network, and community. The right intervention, at the right time, promotes healing, reduces suffering, and optimizes long-term outcomes.

References

Bailley, S. E., Kral, M. J., & Dunham, K. (1999). Survivors of suicide do grieve differently: Empirical support for a common sense proposition. *Suicide and Life-Threatening Behavior*, **29**, 256–271.

Begley, M., & Quayle, E. (2007). The lived experience of adults bereaved by suicide: A phenomenological study. *Crisis*, **28**, 26–34.

Berman, A. L. (2011). Estimating the population of survivors of suicide: Seeking an evidence base. *Suicide and Life-Threatening Behavior*, **41**, 110–116.

Bolton, J. M., AU, W., Leslie, W. D., et al. (2013). Parents bereaved by offspring suicide: A population-based longitudinal case-control study. *JAMA Psychiatry*, **70**, 158–167.

Chapple, A., Ziebland, S., & Hawton, K. (2012). A proper, fitting explanation?: Suicide bereavement and perceptions of the coroner's verdict. *Crisis*, **33**, 230–238.

Clark, S. (2001). Bereavement after suicide: how far have we come and where do we go from here? *Crisis*, **22**, 102–108.

Cvinar, J. G. (2005). Do suicide survivors suffer social stigma: A review of the literature. *Perspectives in Psychiatric Care*, **41**, 14–21.

Dyregrov, K. (2002). Assistance from local authorities versus survivors' needs for support after suicide. *Death Studies*, **26**, 647–668.

Dyregrov, K. (2011). What do we know about needs for help after suicide in different parts of the world? A phenomenological perspective. *Crisis*, **32**, 310–318.

Dyregrov, K., Plyhn, E., & Dieserud, G. (2010). *After the Suicide*. London and Philadelphia: Jessica Kingsley Publishers.

Feigelman, W., Jordan, J. R., & Gorman, B. S. (2009). Personal growth after a suicide loss: Cross-sectional findings suggest growth after loss may be associated with better mental health among survivors. *Omega (Westport)*, **59**, 181–202.

Floyd, F. J., Mailick Seltzer, M., Greenberg, J. S., & Song, J. (2013). Parental bereavement during mid-to-later life: Pre- to postbereavement functioning and intrapersonal resources for coping. *Psychology and Aging*, **28**, 402–413.

Gould, M. S., Shaffer, D., & Kleinman, M. (1988). The impact of suicide in television movies: Replication and commentary. *Suicide and Life-Threatening Behavior*, **18**, 90–99.

Grad, O. T., Clark, S., Dyregrov, K., & Andriessen, K. (2004). What helps and what hinders the process of surviving the suicide of somebody close? *Crisis*, **25**, 134–139.

Johnsen, I., Dyregrov, A., & Dyregrov, K. (2012). Participants with prolonged grief: how do they benefit from grief group participation? *Omega (Westport)*, **65**, 87–105.

Jordan, J. R., & McIntosh, J. L. 2011. *Grief After Suicide: Understanding the Consequences and Caring for the Survivors*. New York: Routledge.

Mitchell, A. M., Kim, Y., Prigerson, H. G., & Mortimer-Stephens, M. (2004). Complicated grief in survivors of suicide. *Crisis*, **25**, 12–18.

Mitchell, A. M., Kim, Y., Prigerson, H. G., & Mortimer, M. K. (2005). Complicated grief and suicidal ideation in adult survivors of suicide. *Suicide and Life-Threatening Behavior*, **35**, 498–506.

Murphy, S. A., Johnson, L. C., & Lohan, J. (2003). Challenging the myths about parents' adjustment after the sudden, violent death of a child. *Journal of Nursing Scholarship*, **35**, 359–364.

Prigerson, H. G., Maclejewski, P. K., Reynolds, C. F., 3rd, et al. (1995). Inventory of Complicated Grief: a scale to measure maladaptive symptoms of loss. *Psychiatry Research*, **59**, 65–79.

Provini, C., Everett, J. R., & Pfeffer, C. R. (2000). Adults mourning suicide: self-reported concerns about bereavement, needs for assistance, and help-seeking behavior. *Death Studies*, **24**, 1–19.

Schneider, B., Grebner, K., Schnabel, A., & Georgi, K. (2011). Do suicides' characteristics influence survivors' emotions? *Suicide and Life-Threatening Behavior*, **41**, 117–125.

Scocco, P., Castriotta, C., Toffol, E., & Preti, A. (2012). Stigma of Suicide Attempt (STOSA) scale and Stigma of Suicide and Suicide Survivor (STOSASS) scale: two new assessment tools. *Psychiatry Research*, **200**, 872–878.

Shear, K., Frank, E., Houck, P. R., & Reynolds, C. F., 3rd (2005). Treatment of complicated grief: a randomized controlled trial. *JAMA*, **293**, 2601–2608.

Shear, K. M., Jackson, C. T., Essock, S. M., Donahue, S. A., & Felton, C. J. (2006). Screening for complicated grief among Project Liberty service recipients 18 months after September 11, 2001. *Psychiatric Services*, **57**, 1291–1297.

Sudak, H., Maxim, K., & Carpenter, M. (2008). Suicide and stigma: a review of the literature and personal reflections. *Academic Psychiatry*, **32**, 136–142.

Sveen, C. A., & Walby, F. A. (2008). Suicide survivors' mental health and grief reactions: a systematic review of controlled studies. *Suicide and Life-Threatening Behavior*, **38**, 13–29.

Timmermans, S. (2005). Death brokering: constructing culturally appropriate deaths. *Sociology of Health and Illness*, **27**, 993–1013.

Wojtkowiak, J., Wild, V., & Egger, J. (2012). Grief experiences and expectance of suicide. *Suicide and Life-Threatening Behavior*, **42**, 56–66.

Young, T., et al. (2012). Suicide bereavement and complicated grief. *DialoguesClinNeuroscience*, **14**, 177.

Chapter 9

Statistics

Robert D. Gibbons

One of the greatest recent controversies in the safety of pharmaceuticals is the question of whether certain classes of medications (e.g., antidepressants) increase the risk of suicidal thoughts, behavior, and completion. In 2004, the US FDA placed a black box warning on all antidepressants with respect to concern that such medications increased risk of suicidal thoughts and behavior in children and in 2006, extended the warning to young adults. It should be noted that these warnings are not limited to antidepressants, but have also been placed on anti-epileptics, smoking cessation drugs (varenicline), acne medications such as isotretinoin, beta blockers, reserpine, and drugs for weight loss (FDA, 2012). For antidepressants, FDA based their black box warning on meta-analyses of randomized clinical trials (RCTs) conducted in pediatric and adult psychiatric and non-psychiatric populations; whereas in the case of the anti-smoking medication varenicline the black box warning was based largely on spontaneous reports of neuropsychiatric events and suicide.

In the following sections I review a variety of approaches for studying the question of whether pharmaceuticals increase suicide risk, ranging from spontaneous reports to ecological studies to analysis of medical claims databases to meta-analyses of RCTs. This review (which focuses the more general reviews provided by Gibbons et al. (Gibbons et al., 2010; Gibbons & Mann, 2011) to the problems and solutions specific to suicide and related events) describes both design and analytic issues, highlights strengths and limitations, and is illustrated with examples of the relationship between antidepressants and suicide.

Spontaneous reports

Spontaneous reports are made by patients, doctors, pharmaceutical companies, and plaintiff attorneys. They are both primary or secondary reports of an adverse event (AE) and a listing of one or more medications a patient was taking at the time of the event. While spontaneous reporting systems (SRSs) have been used extensively for drug safety, they represent the least rigorous form of data for this purpose. They are riddled with problems, including: (1) confounding by indication (i.e., patients taking a particular drug may have a disease that is itself associated with a higher incidence of the AE (e.g., antidepressants, depression and suicide)), (2) systematic underreporting, (3) questionable representativeness of patients, (4) effects of publicity in the media on numbers of reports, (5) extreme duplication of reports, (6) attribution of the event to a single drug when patients may be exposed to multiple drugs, and (7) extensive amounts of missing data. These limitations degrade the capacity for optimal data mining and analysis (Hauben et al., 2007). Despite these known limitations, these are the data that regulatory agencies around the world primarily rely upon for the purpose of post-marketing surveillance.

Several statistical methods have been proposed for analysis of SRS data. They can be grouped into two categories: numerator-based methods and denominator-dependent methods; the former category makes no adjustments for the population at risk (e.g., number of prescriptions sold for each drug) whereas the latter category makes direct or indirect adjustments. Spontaneous reporting centers and drug safety research units routinely use various numerator-based methods such as empirical Bayes screening (EBS) (a variant of which is used by FDA), Bayesian Confidence Propagation Neural Network (BCPNN used by WHO), and proportional reporting ratio (PRR). Denominator-based methods include Cumulative Sum, Time Scan, and Poisson methods.

Proportional reporting ratio

Proportional reporting ratio is the simplest method available for signal detection. Its computational form

A Concise Guide to Understanding Suicide, ed. Stephen H. Koslow, Pedro Ruiz, and Charles B. Nemeroff. Published by Cambridge University Press.

is similar to the well-known relative risk calculation for 2×2 tables in epidemiology (Evans et al., 2001). It is the ratio of the number of reports of a specific AE to all AEs for a particular drug. Of concern is that large numbers of AE reports of a particular kind effectively inflate the denominator for that drug and thereby reduce sensitivity for detecting other signals associated with that drug. PRRs have large numbers of false positive signals because they provide no adjustment for multiple comparisons.

Empirical Bayes screening

Empirical Bayes screening (EBS) (DuMouchel, 1999) computes the baseline (expected) frequency under a row (drug) and column (event) independence assumption for multiple two way tables. If the drug and event are independent, the proportional representation of that event for a specified drug should be the same as the proportional representation of that event in the entire database.

Cumulative sum method

The cumulative sum (CUSUM) method is based on the cumulative sum of differences between observations and their expected values. A signal is detected if the signal statistics exceed the threshold value (Sonesson and Bock, 2003). The threshold is determined by average run length (ARL) based on the mean and variance of the background incidence. The method requires a background comparison time interval and may therefore limit the timely identification of safety problems.

Poisson method

The Poisson method is a denominator-based method that requires some estimate of the population at risk (e.g., national prescription rates). Gibbons et al. (2008) developed a random-effects Poisson regression model for the simultaneous analysis of large numbers of spontaneous reports of possible ADRs. Parameters are estimated using marginal maximum likelihood, and individual drug–AE rate ratios are estimated using either empirical Bayes or parametric or non-parametric full Bayes methods. Confidence (posterior) intervals that do not include 1.0 provide evidence for either significant protective or harmful associations of the drug and the adverse effect.

Illustration

Gibbons et al. (2008) analyzed data from the FDA AERS from 1998 to 2004 for all antidepressants and completed suicide. The dataset consisted of a total of 28 317 382 records which included all reported AEs and drug combinations. The denominator for the analyses was based on national prescription rates for each antidepressant by year.

Figure 9.1 presents a plot of the empirical Bayes (EB) rate multiplier estimates and their confidence limits for each drug, for all ages combined.

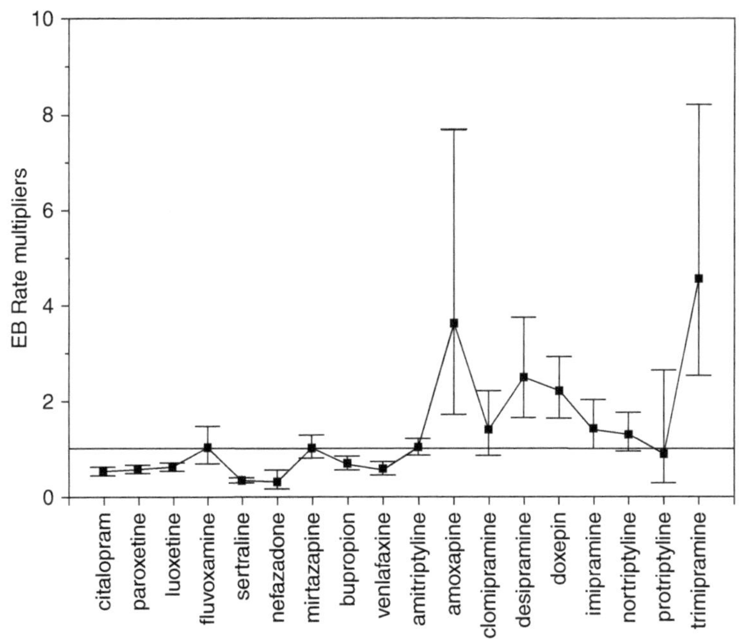

Figure 9.1. Rate multipliers – Bayes estimates and confidence intervals – all ages.

Figure 9.1 reveals that as a class, selective serotonin reuptake inhibitors (SSRIs) (drugs 1–5) and serotonin and norepinephrine reuptake inhibitors (SNRIs – drugs 6–9) have rate multipliers that are significantly less than 1.0, which means lower than the national average suicide AE report rate for antidepressants. By contrast, as a class tricyclic antidepressants (TCAs) (drugs 10–18) have rate multipliers that are significantly above the national average suicide rate for antidepressants. TCAs have significantly higher risk of suicide AE reports as compared to SSRIs and SNRIs, although these data do not support a causal inference due to potential confounding by indication. This is striking because one might predict an increase in reports related to SSRIs given the highly publicized concern over a possible link between suicide and use of SSRIs.

Ecological methods for rare adverse events

For very rare events (e.g., death by suicide) that occur at rates on the order of 1 in 10 000 or less, there may be few options for routine drug surveillance. One approach is to use ecological data that relate changes in drug prescription rates to suicide rates. These more global associations do not support causal inferences, but the availability of large denominators and close to complete enumeration of events such as suicides, can be hypothesis generating and help support inferences drawn from other studies. In some cases, natural experiments such as a black box warning that the FDA placed on antidepressants because of their potential link to suicide attempts, provide an opportunity to evaluate the positive or negative consequences of decreased access to the drug on the event of interest. Here we may compare national suicide rates before and after the public health warning, to determine if the warning has had the anticipated effect. If the warning is specific to a stratum of the population, comparison of changes in that stratum versus those for which the warning did not apply provides stronger inferences.

Traditional approaches

The traditional approach to ecological analysis typically involves either log-linear or Poisson regression analysis of rates over time, using exposure based on prescription rates during the same time period. Serial correlation can be accommodated using Huber-White robust standard errors that allow for an arbitrary autocorrelation pattern (Huber, 1967). Where data from multiple countries are combined, both fixed-effects and random-effects models (Hedeker & Gibbons, 2006) can be used to allow each country to have its own linear time trend. For the fixed-effects log-linear model, weighted least squares can be used to adjust for heterogeneity in the residual errors, using each country's population as a weight. A similar approach can be taken using a mixed-effects Poisson regression model where each country's population is used as an offset (see Hedeker & Gibbons, 2006).

Small area estimation

A more informative approach was suggested by Goldsmith et al. (2002) in which AE rates are stratified by demographic characteristics such as age, race, and sex within counties, and a mixed-effects Poisson regression model is used to analyze the data, treating the county as the unit of analysis. County population is used as an offset in the Poisson regression model. To evaluate drug–AE interactions, county-level prescription rates are added to the model to determine if changes in prescription rates are associated with changes in the AE rate. When longitudinal data are available, between-county effects and within-county effects can be uniquely estimated by expressing prescription rates as two variables, one for the mean over time (between) and the other for the yearly deviations from the mean (within). The methodology has been described in detail by Gibbons et al. (2005, 2006).

Illustrations

National rates

The recent decrease in suicide rate over time correlates with increased antidepressant use in Europe (Rihmer et al., 1998), Scandinavia (Isacsson, 2000), the USA (Olfson et al., 2003), and Australia (Hall et al., 2003). Doubling of prescriptions for SSRIs correlated with a 25% decrease in the suicide rate in Sweden (Isacsson, 2000). In an analysis of 27 countries, Ludwig and Marcotte (2005) showed that an increase of one pill per capita (a 13% increase over 1999 levels) was associated with a 2.5% reduction in suicide rates, a relationship that was more pronounced in adults than in children.

A curious anomaly is Japan, where a positive association between suicide rates and antidepressant prescriptions has been found (see Figure 9.2, Nakagawa et al., 2007). Figure 9.2 clearly shows an overall positive association between SSRI prescriptions and suicide rates; however, stratification by age illustrates that

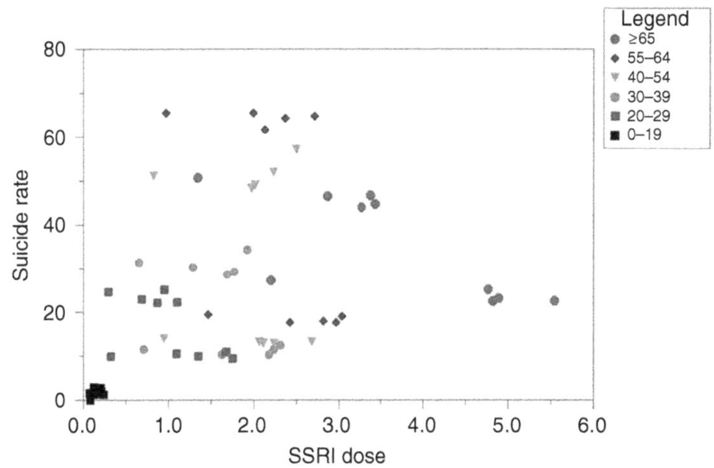

Figure 9.2. Suicide rate vs. SSRI dose in Japan, stratified by age. See plate section for color version.

within each age strata, an inverse association is observed. This is a classic illustration of Simpson's paradox. What it indicates is that in Japan, the elderly have the highest suicide rate and are also the largest users of antidepressants. However, even among the elderly, suicide rates are lowest in those years where SSRI prescriptions were the highest.

County-level analysis

Ecological modeling from large numbers of small areas can provide a stronger basis for understanding the association between antidepressant medication utilization and suicide completion. Gibbons et al. (2005) obtained US county-level data on suicide rates and antidepressant prescription rates for 1996–1998, and analyzed their relationship using mixed-effects Poisson regression adjusted for sex, race, age, income, and unobservable county-level effects. Results of the analysis revealed that increases in SSRI and SNRI prescriptions were associated with decreases in suicide rates both between counties and within counties over time. Conversely, counties with higher rates of TCA prescriptions were associated with higher suicide rates, which may be a function of their greater toxicity upon overdose and/or their increased use in areas with poorer access to quality mental health services.

Figure 9.3 (reprinted from Gibbons et al., 2005) provides an empirical Bayes map of county-level suicide rate multipliers that are adjusted for case-mix based on age, sex, and race. A rate multiplier of 2 indicates that the county-level suicide rate was twice the national suicide rate which at that time was 12/100 000 and a rate multiplier of 0.5 indicates that the county's suicide rate is half the national average. Subsequently, Gibbons and co-workers (2006) replicated these findings in children and young adolescents (aged 5–14 years).

Changes following the black box warning

Gibbons et al. (2007) showed that there were significant reductions in antidepressant prescriptions in children following the public health advisory in March of 2004 and record increases in youth suicide rates during the same time period. By contrast, in older adults aged 60 and over, the rate of antidepressant treatment continued to increase and the rate of suicide continued to decrease. Increases in youth suicide rates continued to be significantly above projected levels based on pre-2004 trends in 2005 as well (Bridge et al., 2009) (Figure 9.4).

Meta-analysis of RCTs

Prior to drug approval and/or release of a new drug, a series of RCTs are conducted that include information regarding AEs. While an individual study typically has insufficient power to detect a drug–AE relation, synthesis of data from several trials may provide a more powerful statistical inference. In many cases, the research synthesis is performed using meta-analysis. For example, the FDA black box warning of 2004 for suicide risk in children treated with antidepressants was based on a meta-analysis of 25 RCTs using suicidal thoughts and behavior as the primary endpoint. A second meta-analysis of 372 adult studies was used to extend the black box warning to young adults, ages 18–24.

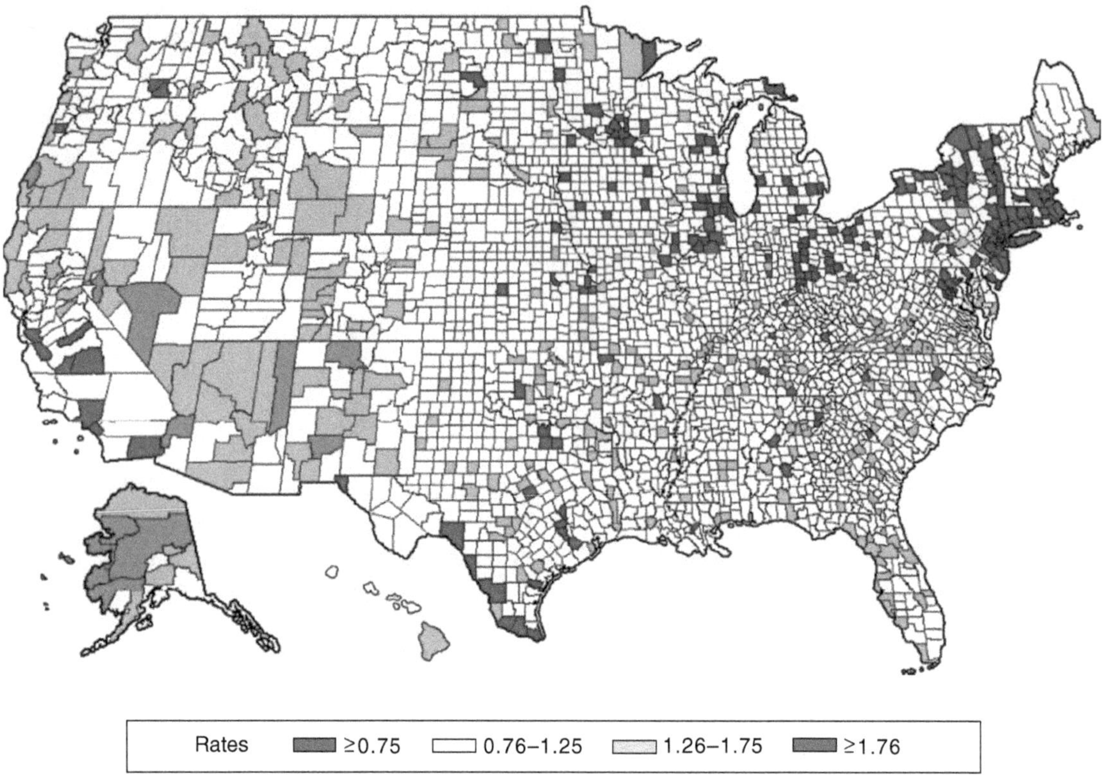

Figure 9.3. Statistical (empirical Bayes) estimates of county-specific adjusted annual suicide rates in the USA. A Bayes estimate of 1.0 indicates that the rate for the county was equal to the national rate of 12 per 100 000 population, a Bayes estimate of 2.0 represents a doubling of the national rate, and a Bayes estimate of 0.5 represents half the national rate. The estimates are based on all data from 1996 to 1998, adjusted for age, sex, and race. See plate section for color version.

Mantel–Haenszel method

The Mantel–Haenszel (MH) method is a moment-based fixed-effect estimator that combines studies using an inverse variance to determine the weight given to each study. It was originally developed to analyze odds ratios but it has been extended to include other measures. The basic idea for a fixed-effects model involves the calculation of a weighted average of the treatment effect across all of the eligible studies. The MH test assumes that the log odds ratio is equal across all studies.

DerSimonian and Laird (DL)

DerSimonian and Laird (1986) provide a moment-based random-effect estimate of the combined effect of multiple trials incorporating heterogeneity across studies. They assume a normal distribution for the treatment effects across studies with common mean θ and variance τ^2. This method provides a simple non-iterative way to compute the heterogeneity parameter τ^2 and adjusts the weight given to each study for the estimated heterogeneity across the studies. This method is more generalizable than the MH test that assumes a common effect across all studies. However, Malzahn, et al. (2000) and others have shown that the heterogeneity estimate has a large negative bias, leading to a biased estimate of the pooled treatment effect as well. In addition, the Q statistic that is used to test heterogeneity has low power to detect departure from homogeneity (Hardy & Thompson, 1998).

Mixed-effects logistic regression

Another approach to take heterogeneity into account while combining results across trials is mixed-effects logistic regression, which is a full likelihood random-effect estimator. The statistical properties of estimates of treatment effect and between study variance using

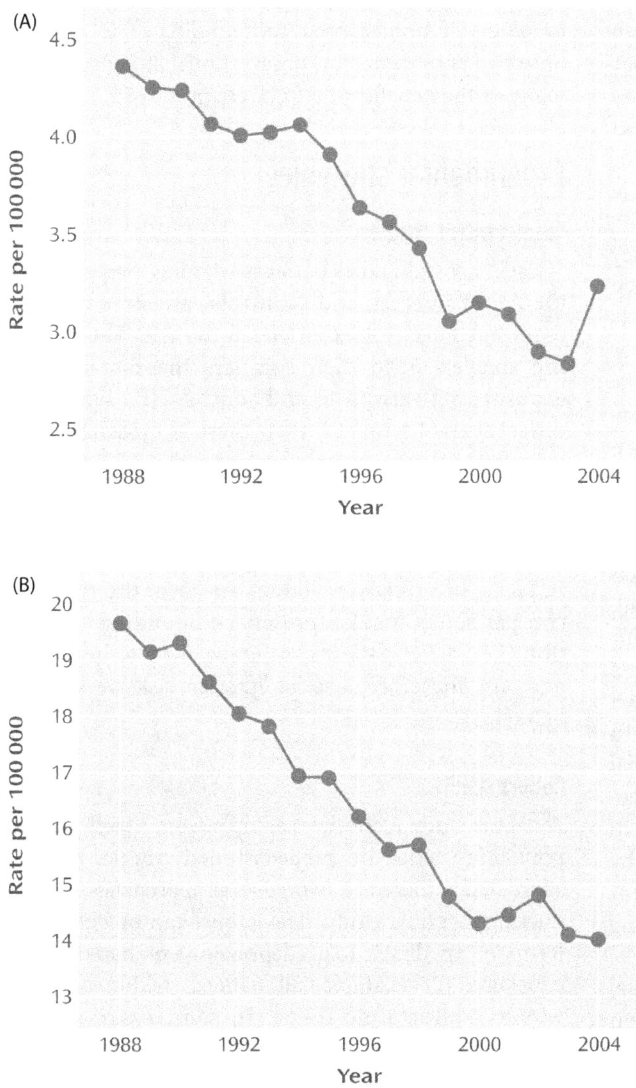

Figure 9.4. (**A**) Suicide rate in children and adolescents (ages 5–19 years) in USA, 1988–2004. (**B**) Suicide rate in older adults (age 60 years and over) in the USA, 1988–2004.

this method are well established (Hedeker & Gibbons, 2006). Unlike the previous two methods, studies with zero events can be included in the analysis and there is no need to add a continuity correction to studies that have a single arm with no events.

Comparison of statistical properties

Bhaumik et al. (2012) studied these moment-based estimators and found that the estimated treatment effect can be grossly overestimated when there is significant variability in the treatment effect across studies. The bias is smaller for the random-effect model than the fixed-effect model, but still appreciable. Likelihood-based alternatives do not suffer from bias due to treatment effect heterogeneity across studies and can incorporate variability in both the background rate and the treatment effect and permit them to be correlated.

Research synthesis

An even more general alternative to traditional meta-analysis of RCTs is research synthesis based on a reanalysis of a common longitudinal endpoint in a series of similarly designed RCTs. As an example, Gibbons and colleagues (Gibbons et al., 2012a, b) performed 3-level linear (efficacy) and non-linear (safety) mixed-effects regression analyses (Hedeker & Gibbons, 2006) of the data from a series of 41 RCTs on the efficacy and safety of antidepressants (all sponsor conducted placebo-controlled RCTs of fluoxetine and venlafaxine). Unlike meta-analysis which pools effect sizes (e.g., odds ratios), this approach to research synthesis involves a complete reanalysis of all available longitudinal data from all studies. In these analyses, the intercept and slope of the temporal trends in efficacy and safety measures are allowed to vary from individual to individual and the study means of these same effects are allowed to vary from study to study. With proper specification of the variance component structure, the overall pooled estimate of the treatment by time interaction tests the overall efficacy (or safety) of the medication of interest.

Results of these studies revealed that both drugs were efficacious, although the maximum benefit was observed for children and only marginal benefit was observed for the elderly following 6 weeks of treatment. With respect to suicidal thoughts and behavior, significant benefits of antidepressant treatment were observed in adults and the elderly, and these benefits were shown to be mediated by decreases in depressive severity. In children, no significant effect of treatment on suicidal thoughts and behavior were found, despite large benefits for depression. These results indicate that while in adults, suicidal thoughts and behavior are driven by depression; this does not appear to be the case for children. This finding is consistent with a recent finding by Nock and colleagues (2013) in which most suicidal adolescents (>80%) received some form of mental health treatment, but such treatment failed to prevent suicidal behavior from occurring.

Medical claims data

There are several advantages of the use of medical claims data for post-marketing drug surveillance. First, they represent person-level data, similar to RCTs, but unlike spontaneous reports, we know the population at risk. Second, several medical claims databases such as the VA or PharMetrics databases contain longitudinal information on AEs such as suicide attempts, concomitant medications, and comorbid diagnoses both before and after the drug exposure. Third, the populations that can be sampled are often large enough to study even the rarest of events. Their primary limitation is that they are observational, and any association identified may or may not represent a causal link between the drug and the AE of interest due to potential unmeasured confounding. The primary objective is to design an observational study such that many of the benefits of a RCT are preserved.

Experimental strategies

Case–control studies

"Cases" are defined as patients who have experienced the AE of interest, and "controls" are similar to the cases but have not experienced the AE. The goal of the analysis is to then compare the rate of drug exposure between cases and controls. If a significant difference is identified, then there is evidence of an association between the drug and the AE. A major limitation of case–control studies in drug surveillance is that the available potential confounders are often inadequate for matching the cases and controls in terms of severity of illness. As such, the resulting comparison may still represent confounding by selection (i.e., sicker patients are more likely to be treated and are therefore also at greater risk of suicidal behavior).

Cohort studies

A cohort study identifies a sample from a well-defined population based on predetermined criteria. In drug surveillance there are two general approaches to conducting a cohort study. The cohort can be defined in terms of an illness (e.g., depression) or based on an exposure; for example, all patients taking an SSRI within a given time frame. In some cases we may wish to identify "new cases" who have not been diagnosed or treated for some fixed period of time and have a minimum follow-up period. This strategy works well for databases with long-term enrollment patterns such as the VA, but may be less ideal for managed care databases where patients may not be continuously enrolled for long enough periods of time. In this case, the cohort study can be designed to have a fixed time window before and after the indication (either diagnostic date or first treatment date), for example a period of 1 year before and after the indication. The primary advantage of collecting data before and after diagnosis or drug exposure is that we can evaluate the suicide attempt rate both before and after the start of treatment. If the drug is producing the suicidal behavior, then rates should generally be higher following initiation of the drug compared with before it.

Within-subject designs

Within-subject designs are those in which the same patients are repeatedly measured over time, typically before and after initiating drug treatment. The basic idea is to compare the rate of a non-fatal AES before and after the exposure to the drug. The strength of the design is that it is restricted to only those patients who ultimately take the drug, thereby minimizing selection effects. A good example is a set of studies of lithium and suicide risk (Tondo et al., 2001). However, if patients with the disease are at higher risk of suicide or related events in general (e.g., depression and suicidality), then a limitation of the design is that the natural course of the disease (e.g., decrease in the severity of depressive symptomatology over time) can become confounded with the pre–post nature of the design.

Within-subject designs are also useful for understanding the effects of pattern or intensity of exposure on the AE rate. For example, breaking the surveillance time into discrete intervals (e.g., months), allows the analyst to explore the temporal association between drug exposure and the likelihood of suicidal behavior.

Between-subject designs

Between-subject designs involve comparison of patients who took the drug versus those that did not. Often it is most useful to compare monotherapy versus no therapy, at least with respect to the other drugs within the relevant class of drugs. Concomitant drug therapy with related classes of drugs can be included in the statistical model as covariates or as a separate comparison group. The importance of considering monotherapy is that patients using multiple drugs within the same class may be of greater initial severity and/or treatment-resistant and may in general have higher suicidal event rates. The primary limitation of between-subject designs is that they are subject to confounding by indication and/or severity of the indication. In general more severely ill patients will be treated with pharmacotherapy; therefore we would expect them to have a greater incidence of adverse effects in general that are related to the severity of illness. Various matching strategies, such as propensity score matching, to be described in the following section, are helpful for reducing bias; however, these techniques can only be done to the extent that the potential confounders are available and measurable.

Novel statistical strategies for studying suicide

Person-time logistic regression models

Person-time regression or discrete-time survival analysis (Efron, 1988) is an ingenious approach to fitting a time to event or survival analytic model in a parametric way using standard logistic regression software. The basic idea is to discretize time into a set of smaller intervals and to then record the number of subjects at risk in each interval, the number experiencing the event (e.g., suicide attempt), and the number censored. A similar approach can be taken using unstructured data in which each subject contributes n_i records either to the point in time in which the event was first experienced or to the end of the follow-up period. Advantages of the approach are that (a) time-varying predictors are easily accommodated, (b) random-effects such as the nesting of patients within hospitals or clinics, or counties can be easily included, (c) competing risks such as death by suicide or other causes of mortality can be examined, and (d) non-proportional hazard models can be estimated (Hedeker & Gibbons, 2006; Gibbons et al., 2003). The net result is that we can relax the assumption that once a subject is exposed they are always exposed and replace it with any exposure pattern (e.g., monthly) and produce a within-subject estimate of the effect of the exposure on the probability of experiencing the AE. Note that unlike a traditional mixed-effects logistic regression for a repeated binary event, these models are restricted to a single event per person and as such, the repeated observations within individuals are conditionally independent (Efron, 1988).

The general algorithm (Hedeker and Gibbons, 2006) as it relates to suicide attempts (SA) is as follows:

1. Create the following dataset.
   - Each subject has 2t months of observation, t months (or other unit of observation, e.g., weeks or days) before the index diagnosis (DX) and t after. There should be no DX during the first t (background) months. If a SA occurs before month t following treatment, the incomplete observation record should be retained in the analysis.
   - For the t months prior to index, if there was one or more SA, set prior SA (PSA) to 1 else PSA=0.
   - For each of the t months after the index DX determine if the patient took the drug and the day of the month they took it.

- If a SA occurred after the first day of medication then set the medication indicator to 1 otherwise 0.

2. From the data described in (1) create a new file in which each subject has the following number of records based on the post DX data only.
    - If there is no SA there are t records all with event=0.
    - If there is a SA then the number of records is equal to the month of the SA. Event=0 for all but the month of the SA, and the last record (i.e., month of the SA) has event=1.
    - If the SA occurred on the index date, it should be treated as a prior suicide attempt and the patient should be continued to be monitored for future attempts.
3. Fit a fixed-effects logistic regression model to the data using potential confounders such as age, sex, concomitant diagnoses, concomitant medications, and PSA as time-invariant covariates, and medication use and month as time-varying covariates (proportional hazards model).
4. Fit a second model that includes a month by medication interaction (non-proportional hazards model).

The proportional hazards model assumes that the effect of the medication is constant over time, whereas the non-proportional hazards model allows the effect of the medication on the SA to vary over time. Note that since each subject can have no more than one SA, the records are conditionally independent (Efron, 1988).

Illustration

Gibbons et al. (2010), re-analyzed data for a sample of 226 000 veterans with new episodes of major depressive disorder. Comparison of the suicide attempt rate was restricted to patients with SSRI treatment (monotherapy) and patients with no medication treatment, and covariates included sex, age, race, and previous suicide attempt (prior to diagnosis). The person–time analysis revealed a significant decrease in suicide attempt rate for patients with SSRI monotherapy treatment (hazard ratio (HR)=0.17, CI=0.10–0.28, $p<0.0001$). This compares favorably with the observed data, for which there were a total of 1 134 173 observations (i.e., number of months). Of these, 805 525 months were without medication and 328 648 months with medication. The corresponding number of suicide attempts were 207 (0.026%) and 17 (0.005%), respectively, yielding an observed HR=0.19 (estimated HR=0.17).

Figure 9.5 provides the estimated hazard functions for the non-proportional hazards model. A significant interaction was found indicating that the magnitude of the difference between SSRI monotherapy and no antidepressant treatment groups decreased over time ($p<0.0001$). The difference in hazard rates is largest early in treatment (HR=0.08), but decreases by

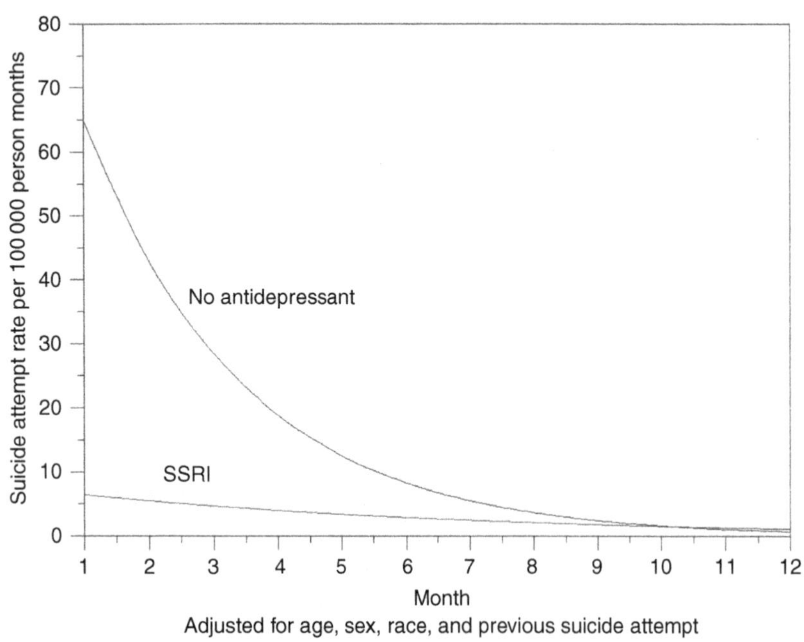

Figure 9.5. Non-proportional hazards model for suicide attempts over time: comparison of SSRI monotherapy versus no antidepressant.

approximately 30% per month (HR=1.29 for the drug by month interaction), such that the monthly hazard rates are essentially equivalent by approximately 9 months following the index episode. These data do not support the conclusion that antidepressants increase suicide attempts in adults, and if anything, the effects are protective, particularly early in the course of treatment when suicide attempt rates are highest.

Drawing causal inferences from observational data

Since suicidal events are rare, research in this area often is based on large-scale pharmacoepidemiologic studies. In the following, I discuss several approaches for minimizing bias in such studies produced by the non-random assignment of patients to treatments.

Propensity score matching

Propensity score matching (Rosenbaum & Rubin, 1983) provides a way to balance cases (treated) and controls when there are numerous potential confounders that are measured. The first step is to develop a model for the probability of being treated with a certain drug (i.e., the propensity score) based on all measured confounders. Then matching on the propensity score rather than each confounder can provide balance between the groups leading to between-group comparisons with greatly reduced bias. Equally important, matching on the propensity score can also identify the presence of bias that is inherent in the particular between-group comparison of interest that cannot be controlled through simple adjustment. For example, in the now classic example of relationship between smoking and mortality (Cochran, 1968), pipe smoking is seen to have the highest risk of mortality not cigarette smoking. However, pipe smokers were on average older than cigarette smokers, so the actual comparison was potentially between a 30-year-old cigarette smoker and a 70-year-old pipe smoker. Stratification on age produced an unbiased comparison (at least with respect to observed covariates) that showed a clear effect of cigarette smoking on mortality, above that for both cigar and pipe smoking throughout the life cycle. Propensity score matching is therefore a multivariate extension of the single univariate stratification procedure described by Cochran (Cochran, 1968).

The general idea involves fitting a logistic regression to model the association between the potential confounders (age, sex, concomitant treatments, comorbid diagnoses, prior attempts) and the likelihood of receiving treatment (e.g., an antidepressant). By matching patients who did or did not receive the treatment on the log odds of receiving the treatment based on the confounders alone, we have in essence matched patients and controls in terms of all observed potential confounders, at least in probability. There are several different ways of matching which include 1:1, 1:n, stratification, and use of the propensity score as a covariate in a subsequent regression which relates treatment to the probability of the AE of interest. There are strengths and weaknesses to all of the procedures; however, stratification into quintiles is often the most informative (in that it reveals hidden bias produced by lack of overlap in covariate distributions), and use of the propensity score as a covariate in a subsequent regression model is the weakest, because it is based on a strong linearity assumption. The fundamental idea is to carve a RCT out of an observational study, without eliminating so much of the data that the "RCT" is no longer generalizable.

A limitation of using propensity score matching in drug surveillance studies is that medical claims data often have limited information regarding potential confounders. Good choices include demographic variables, diagnostic variables, and concomitant medications, as well as comorbidities. In some cases, longitudinal medical records can be used to identify whether there is a history of related AEs prior to exposure to the drug of interest. The key here is to adjust for the severity of illness which may be related to both the use of the drug and the AE.

Differential effects

Consider two different pharmacologic treatments given for the same or similar clinical indications. While the observed response of each treatment relative to no treatment may be subject to confounding by indication, the relative effect of these two treatments may be less biased by unmeasured prognostic factors (called generic biases) that promote the use of either treatments (Rosenbaum, 2006).

To study suicidal events and antidepressant treatment using differential effects, we can contrast the frequency of suicide attempts in depressed patients who received either an SSRI or an older TCA, but not both, adjusting for known prescribing predictors such as age. In parallel, the frequency of suicide attempts are then also contrasted for patients who received SSRIs + psychotherapy or TCAs + psychotherapy but not both. If SSRIs are stimulating suicide attempts, we would expect to see an excess of suicide attempts in many if not most comparisons of SSRIs with other treatments for depression, otherwise, this pattern is compatible with confounding by indication. Rosenbaum (2006) describes sensitivity analyses and adjustment for additional covariates using differential propensity score adjustment.

Coherence

The term coherence is used both informally and formally, and both are relevant in the current context. Informally, we may predict that a treatment will produce several observable associations, and there is coherence if each prediction is checked and confirmed. Formally, we may devise a measure of how much the outcomes of a patient resemble those predicted for the treatment in question, and use that measure of coherence as an outcome in the analysis (Rosenbaum, 2004). In drug surveillance, examples of relevant predicted associations are the following:

1. Suspected drugs should be associated with higher frequency of AEs compared to rates for other treatments.
2. The increase in frequency should occur after, not before, the start of treatment.
3. There should be no corresponding increase in frequency after the start of other pharmacological or non-pharmacologic (e.g., psychotherapy) treatments that are not directly related to the AE of interest.
4. An AE (e.g., suicide attempt) shortly after the start of treatment is stronger evidence of an effect than an event years later, and an AE shortly before treatment is stronger evidence of confounding by indication than an AE many years earlier.

Rosenbaum (2004) has suggested methods for creating a coherence score that measures the degree to which these predictions hold, and how it can be used as an outcome to study its sensitivity to unobserved biases.

Marginal structural models

While propensity score matching is useful conceptually, drug exposures are typically dynamic and the exposure status takes on different values over time. Traditional propensity score matching assumes that treatment status does not change over time. While some work has been done in the area of dynamic propensity score matching (Leon et al., 2011), an equally if not more promising approach for dynamic treatment exposures is based on the idea of marginal structural models (MSM – Robins et al., 2000). The basic idea of MSM is that we compute the probability of treatment at each of T time-points and the likelihood of treatment at time-point t is the product of the individual occasion probabilities to that point in time. These probabilities are then standardized and used as weights in a second stage regression that models the dynamic effects of treatment on the AE of interest (e.g., suicide attempt) weighted by the likelihood to receive treatment at any particular point in time. While the traditional approach described by Robins and co-workers rests strongly on the assumption that all of the important confounders have been measured and are available for the analysis, the analysis may be further expanded to include the effects of unmeasured confounders by adding one or more random-effects to the treatment selection model as described by Leon and Hedeker (2007) in the context of computing dynamic propensity score adjustments.

Discussion

The statistics of suicide provides a fruitful area for both statistical research and practice. Contributions to this area are useful in the area of drug safety in general, and in fact, suicide and related events are among the most difficult safety endpoints to study. Not only may pharmaceuticals increase the risk of suicide and related behaviors, suicidal thoughts and behavior increase the likelihood of treatment, resulting in serious problems of confounding that can only be dealt with properly using advanced statistical methods. The statistical issues are further complicated by the rarity of suicidal events, where randomized studies are often not possible. This review should encourage practitioners to improve the quality of their measures and statisticians to further add to the arsenal of methods to deal with the myriad of issues related to experimental design and analytic work in this fundamentally important area.

References

Bhaumik, D. K., Amatya, A., Normand, S. L., et al. (2012). Meta-analysis of rare binary adverse event data. *Journal of the American Statistical Association*, **107**, 555–567.

Bridge, J. A., Greenhouse, J. B., Weldon, A. H., Campo, J. V., & Kelleher, K. J. (2009). Suicide trends among youths aged 10 to 19 years in the United States, 1996–2005. *JAMA*. **300**, 1025–1026.

Cochran, W. G. (1968). The effectiveness of adjustment by subclassification in removing bias in observational studies. *Biometric*, **24**, 295–313.

DerSimonian, R., & Laird, N. (1986). Meta-analysis in clinical trials. *Controlled Clinical Trials*, **7**, 177–188.

DuMouchel, W. (1999). Bayesian data mining in large frequency tables, with an application to the FDA Spontaneous Reporting System. *The American Statistician*, **53**, 177–190.

Efron, B. (1988). Logistic regression, survival analysis, and the Kaplan Meier curve. *JASA*, **83**, 414–425.

Evans, S. J. W., Waller, P. C., & Davis, S. (2001). Use of proportional reporting ratios (PRR) for signal generation from spontaneous adverse drug reaction reports. *Pharmacoepidemiology and Drug Safety*, **10**, 483–486.

FDA (2012). Guidance for industry: Suicidal ideation and behavior: Prospective assessment of occurrence in clinical trials. www.fda.gov/Drugs/GuidanceCompliance RegulatoryInformation/Guidances/ucm315156.htm (accessed January 14, 2013).

Gibbons, R. D., & Mann, J. J. (2011). Strategies for quantifying the relationship between medications and suicidal behavior: what has been learned? *Drug Safety*, **34**, 375–395.

Gibbons, R. D., Duan, N., Meltzer, D., et al. (2003). Waiting for organ transplantation: results of an analysis by Institute of Medicine Committee. *Biostatistics*, **4**, 207–222.

Gibbons, R. D., Hur, K., Bhaumik, D. K., & Mann, J. J. (2005). The relationship between antidepressant medication use and rate of suicide. *Archives of General Psychiatry*, **62**, 165–172.

Gibbons, R. D., Hur, K., Bhaumik, D. K., & Mann, J. J. (2006). The relationship between antidepressant prescription rates and rates of early adolescent suicide. *American Journal of Psychiatry*, **163**, 1898–1904.

Gibbons, R. D., Brown, C. H., Hur, K., et al. (2007). Early evidence on the effects of the FDA black box warning on SSRI prescriptions and suicide in children and adolescents. *American Journal of Psychiatry*, **164**, 1356–1363.

Gibbons, R. D., Segawa, E., Karabatsos, G., et al. (2008). Mixed-effects Poisson regression analysis of adverse event reports: The relationship between antidepressants and suicide. *Statistics in Medicine*, **27**, 1814–1833.

Gibbons, R. D., Amatya, A. K., Brown, C. H., et al. (2010). Post-approval drug safety surveillance. *Annual Review of Public Health*, **31**, 419–437.

Gibbons, R. D., Hur, K., Brown, C. H., Davis, J. M., & Mann, J. J. (2012a). Benefits from antidepressants: Synthesis of 6-week patient-level outcomes from double-blind placebo controlled randomized trials of fluoxetine and venlafaxine. *Archives of General Psychiatry*, **69**, 572–579.

Gibbons, R. D., Brown, C. H., Hur, K., Davis, J. M., & Mann, J. J. (2012b). Suicidal thoughts and behavior with antidepressants treatment: re-analysis of the randomized placebo controlled studies of fluoxetine and venlafaxine. *Archives of General Psychiatry*, **69**, 580–587.

Goldsmith, S. K., Pellmar, T. C., Kleinman, A. M., et al. (2002). *Reducing Suicide: A National Imperative.* Washington, DC: National Academy Press.

Hall, W. D., Mant, A., Mitchell, P. B., et al. (2003). Association between antidepressant prescribing and suicide in Australia, 1991–2000: trend analysis. *BMJ*, **326**, 1008.

Hardy, R. J., & Thompson, S. G. (1998). Detecting and describing heterogeneity in meta-analysis. *Statistics in Medicine*, **17**, 841–856.

Hauben, M., Riech, L., DeMicco, J., & Kim, K. (2007). 'Extreme duplication' in the US FDA adverse events reporting system database. *Drug Safety*, **30**, 551–554.

Hedeker, D., & Gibbons, R. D. (2006). *Longitudinal Data Analysis.* New York:Wiley.

Huber, P. J. (1967). The behavior of maximum likelihood estimates under nonstandard conditions. In *Proceedings of the Fifth Berkeley Symposium on Mathematical Statistics and Probability*, Vol **1** (pp. 221–233). Berkeley, CA: University of California Press.

Isacsson, G. (2000). Suicide prevention: a medical breakthrough? *Acta Psychiatrica Scandinavica*, **102**, 113–117.

Leon, A. C., & Hedeker, D. (2007). Quantile stratification based on a misspecified propensity score in longitudinal treatment effectiveness analyses of ordinal doses. *Computational Statistics and Data Analysis*, **51**, 6114–6122.

Leon, A. C., Solomon, D. A., Li, C., et al. (2011). Antidepressants and risks of suicide attempts: a 27-year observational study. *Journal of Clinical Psychiatry*, **72**, 580–586.

Ludwig, J., & Marcotte, D. (2005). Anti-depressants, suicide and drug regulation. *Journal of Policy Analysis and Management*, **2**, 249–272.

Malzahn, U., Bohning, D., & Holling, H. (2000). Nonparametric estimation of heterogeneity variance for the standardized difference used in meta-analysis. *Biometrika*, **87**, 619–632.

Nakagawa, A., Grunebaum, M. F., Ellis, S. P., et al. (2007). Suicide and antidepressant prescription rates in Japan, 1999–2003. *Journal of Clinical Psychiatry*, **68**, 908–916.

Nock, M. K., Green, J. G., Hwang, I., et al. (2013). Prevalence, correlates, and treatment of lifetime suicidal behavior among adolescents: Results from the national comorbidity survey replication adolescent supplement. *JAMA Psychiatry*, **70**(3), 300–310.

Olfson, M., Shaffer, D., Marcus, S. C., & Greenberg, T. (2003). Relationship between antidepressant medication treatment and suicide in adolescents. *Archives of General Psychiatry*, **60**, 978–82.

Rihmer, Z., Rutz, W., Pihlgren, H., & Pestality, P. (1998). Decreasing tendency of seasonality in suicide may indicate lowering rate of depressive suicides in the population. *Psychiatry Research*, **81**, 233–240.

Robins, J. M., Hernán, M. A., & Brumback, B. (2000). Marginal structural models and causal inference in epidemiology. *Epidemiology*, **11**, 550–560.

Rosenbaum, P. R. (2004). Design sensitivity in observational studies. *Biometrika*, **91**, 153–164.

Rosenbaum, P. R. (2006). Differential effects and generic biases in observational studies. *Biometrika*, **93**, 573–586.

Rosenbaum, P., & Rubin, D. B. (1983). The central role of the propensity score in observational studies for causal effects. *Biometrika*, **70**, 41–50.

Sonesson, C., & Bock, D. (2003). A review and discussion of prospective statistical surveillance in public health. *Journal of Royal Statistical Society A*, **166**, 5–21.

Tondo, L., Hennen, J., & Baldessarini, R. J. (2001). Lower suicide risk with long-term lithium treatment in major affective illness: a meta-analysis. *Acta Psychiatrica Scandinavica*, **104**, 163–172.

Chapter 10

Current and chronic signs and symptoms

Jan Fawcett

The most difficult diagnostic determination that clinicians must make is whether their patient is on the verge of suicide. This is because it is not possible to accurately predict if and when an individual is going to commit suicide. It is not the standard of care that a clinician prevents a suicide. It is the standard of care that a clinician makes a competent risk assessment and does whatever a reasonable clinician would do to prevent a suicide. This means that the clinician is expected to assess the risk of suicide in each patient at any time when a person of similar clinical training would find it prudent to do so.

Because a clinician can be held legally responsible for dereliction of duty leading directly to damages, and the death of a loved one is an obvious example of major damage, a suicide is a common basis for a lawsuit against psychiatrists. Although the clinician has not fallen below the standard of care for failing to prevent a suicide, the question that usually arises is whether the clinician met the standard of doing a competent assessment of suicide risk and whatever is deemed appropriate to prevent a suicide. This means that the clinician is expected to not only make a competent risk assessment at the appropriate time in the patient's course of treatment, but also to adequately document that this was done in the patient's clinical record.

Various studies have shown that from 70% to 33% of patients commit suicide while receiving psychiatric or mental health treatment (Baraclough et al., 1974; Robins, 1981; Luoma et al., 2002). Forty-five percent of patients who commit suicide have been found to have seen a primary care physician within a month before their suicide (Luoma et al., 2002). Khan et al.'s analysis of FDA treatment studies show that neither SSRI and TCA antidepressants or antipsychotic medications over 8–12 weeks result in lower suicide rates than placebo treatment (Khan et al., 2003).

On the other hand studies by Angst et al. and Leon et al. show that antidepressant, lithium, or antipsychotic treatments alone or especially in combination maintained for at least 6 months, or antidepressant medications taken with a high propensity over a 16- to 20-year follow-up, significantly reduce suicide rates (Angst et al., 2005; Leon et al., 2011)

There are two major issues that need emphasis in the assessment of suicide risk and treatment planning for the management of patients at high risk. One important issue is the question of whether a patient is at high acute or high chronic risk of suicide. The other issue is when in the patient's course a full suicide risk assessment should be performed by a treating clinician. This chapter will focus on these two important issues.

With regard to assessing the presence of acute or chronic suicide risk, it is known that a patient may be at high chronic risk for suicide, but a careful clinical assessment may conclude that a patient at high chronic risk for suicide is actually at low acute risk for suicide. This is a crucial issue for the determination of the treatment plan at any given point.

For example, consider a patient who has a history of barely surviving an attempt at hanging, having been found hanging from a rafter in his garage early in the attempt by his wife and being cut down, falling between the cars. The patient, who suffered from a bipolar mixed state, had started drinking, become increasingly agitated over a period of 24 hours, and hanged himself with his leather belt. The patient suffered only superficial neck injuries and a minor back injury from hitting the garage floor. He was mood stabilized and treated successfully for depression. He has been followed for 3 years since this attempt: he has remained stable, is able to work part-time, and enjoys visiting his grown-up children on vacation with his wife.

A Concise Guide to Understanding Suicide, ed. Stephen H. Koslow, Pedro Ruiz, and Charles B. Nemeroff. Published by Cambridge University Press.

In the time just before his suicide attempt he moved from a state of depression, for which he was treated with mood stabilizers and antidepressant medication, into a mixed state, with severe anxiety and agitation within 2 days. He relapsed into his alcohol substance use disorder, drinking two six-packs, expressing suicidal ideation, and making the attempt at hanging before his wife could see and react to the danger and call his psychiatrist as she had been instructed to do.

He had multiple acute risk factors for imminent suicide, including severe depressed mood, worthlessness, hopelessness, suicidal threats, severe anxiety and agitation, increased alcohol abuse, increased impulsiveness, and severe insomnia. He made a potentially lethal suicide attempt within hours of his clinical deterioration. Prior to his suicide he clearly manifested signs of high acute suicide risk, but his condition progressed too rapidly for his wife to call for help.

Over the past 3 years, the patient has been a high chronic suicide risk on the basis of this lethal attempt, but has not met criteria for acute high risk for suicide during this time. His chronic high-risk factors include a bipolar diagnosis, history of alcohol abuse, binge-drinking type with increased aggressive impulsivity, severe anxiety and agitation, and a prior highly lethal suicide attempt. Despite being a chronic high risk for suicide, he has returned to work, maintained a loving relationship with his wife, and the couple has enjoyed two vacations.

Though it can be anticipated that a relapse of depressive or mixed symptoms could rapidly revert to an acute risk state, thus far the patient has remained stable and in remission. At this point, the patient does not require full suicide assessments. If the patient begins to show signs of relapse of mood symptoms, anxiety symptoms, or experiences a severe loss or stress (e.g., loss of pension benefits, a severe conflict with his wife, who he is quite dependent on, or the onset of a painful or adverse medical condition, e.g., a diagnosis of prostate cancer) a careful and ongoing suicide risk assessment would be indicated. For the present, this patient is in remission and doing well, despite being a high chronic risk for suicide.

This case illustrates the dramatic difference of a patient being at high chronic risk for suicide contrasting with a sudden onset of acute high-risk factors leading to a near lethal suicide attempt.

Problems in assessing suicide risk

In considering the state of the suicide assessment, it is clear that the long-term risk factor of a prior suicide attempt in study after study (Hoyer et al., 2009; Hawton et al., 2013), or "suicidal tendencies" (Coryell & Young, 2005) which includes "preparations for suicide" or rehearsal behavior and increases predictability over that of only a history of a prior attempt, is the most potent factor predicting subsequent suicidal behavior (Coryell & Young, 2005). Unfortunately, a history of a prior attempt does not predict when a suicide might occur – it is more of an actuarial predictor. Since a clinician must try to assess suicide risk in terms of immediate or acute risk over the next hours, days, or weeks, and since it is not uncommon to be treating patients with a history of recurrent illness who may have a history of a suicide attempt, this history may be additive to a clinician's judgment, but it is not of great help in estimating what is likely to transpire in the near future. That is, it is not as crucial as a clinician's estimate of recent or current risk factors. Also Isometsa's data that 62% of males and 38% of females kill themselves by their first suicide attempt tempers the value of the patient denying prior suicide attempts (Isometsa & Lonnqvist, 1998).

Another problem is the validity of a patient's denial of suicide thoughts or intent. It is clear that if a patient makes a statement indicating that they have planned a suicide or intend to end their lives, that this statement deserves full clinical attention.

The evidence is overwhelming that the reverse is not clinically valid. Study after study has shown that denial of suicidal ideation, denial of suicidal intent, and even the patient's willingness to "contract" that they will talk to a therapist or nursing staff before initiating any self-harmful or suicidal behavior cannot be taken at face value (Isometsa et al., 1995; Busch et al., 2003).

It may be the human brain's tendency to accept that if an affirmative statement implies danger, that a negative statement or denial automatically implies safety, or simply the wish for and eagerness to accept reassurance around an anxiety-provoking situation such as the possibility of a suicide that leads a clinician to readily accept denials of suicidal intent uncritically from a patient, without taking into account the entire clinical situation at that moment in time. Can a highly impulsive patient who is depressed and severely anxious really be trusted to keep a no-harm contract?

If a patient is truly hopeless and has made a plan to commit suicide, is he likely to admit to a suicide plan to someone he knows is dedicated to preventing his suicide? Should we accept denial of suicide intent from a patient who after awaking from a failed suicide attempt stated, "I should have used a gun"?

The fact is that the frequent chart notation "no HI, SI" is not even evidence that a suicide assessment was done. Asking a patient if they have suicidal ideation or plan is not really a suicide assessment, yet this notation is all that is noted to indicate a suicide assessment. If the clinician does not make an adequate note, in the unfortunate case of a suicide, how can an expert base a defense on the fact that a full suicide assessment was done and the standard of care was met? Of course clinicians cannot be expected to record everything that transpired in a clinical evaluation. Perhaps a note concluding, "chronic high-risk factors present but no acute suicide risk factors found," implying that the assessment involved more than a denial of suicidal ideation or plan would be more informative. This is more of a clinician's conclusion implying that an assessment was done, which if questioned, allows the clinician to state what was included in the assessment.

When should full suicide risk assessments be done?

A full suicide risk assessment takes time to perform. The clinician has many other tasks to address in a clinical encounter. A suicide risk assessment is not necessary if the patient is not found to be in a situation that suggests increased risks. If the patient's therapy is progressing and their condition is improving a full risk assessment is not necessary. What are the conditions that call for suicide risk assessments?

Certainly the patient's initial or a repeated full clinical assessment requires a full suicide risk assessment. If the patient suffers a relapse of symptoms, or encounters a major loss or stress, a full assessment is important.

Another time when suicide risk is known to be increased is the period immediately after discharge from hospital. This risk is greatest the week after discharge, but remains elevated over the year following the discharge. Repeated suicide risk assessments are indicated in this time frame – especially in the early period, but depending on the patient's clinical course. Bostwick and Pancratz re-analyzed long-term suicide risk data and reported that the lifetime risk for suicide was 8.2% for patients admitted to the hospital for suicide risk and 4.0% for patients admitted without an indication of suicide risk. Depressive outpatients were found to have a suicide risk of 2.2% (Bostwick & Pancratz, 2000).

Current risk factors

These factors are the most important to assess, but also the most difficult. Some acute risk factors may be present in patients who are denying suicidal ideations. It is important to determine the presence of these factors because a mounting amount of data has shown them to be associated with an elevated risk of suicide and they may be modifiable by treatment.

The most important current risk factor is the occurrence of a major loss, anticipated loss, or severe life stress from the patient's point of view.

Patients often minimize or dismiss or even suppress mention of these events, so it is very important for the clinician to be sensitive and question the impact of these events as well as assessing the patient's ability to cope with actual or anticipated stress, perhaps using a statement such as "This would be devastating for many people, how are you going to handle it?" This clinician has found this the most difficult area in assessing suicide risk.

A resident sought help in dealing with the clinical deterioration and increased suicidal ideation and distress of his patient. The patient was hospitalized for suicidal ideation and threats. After discharge she reverted to the same state of agitation with suicidal ideation. The patient's agitation was treated successfully with olanzapine. On the fourth visit the patient admitted that she had been raped in a parking lot and this precipitated her suicidal crisis. The patient was too guilty and embarrassed to admit the rape to her male physician–therapist, and her admission about the event did not occur until her agitated state had been successfully treated.

The occurrence of a medical condition, especially a cancer diagnosis, and in particular after the diagnosis of prostate cancer in men (before any evidence of progression) (Feng et al., 2010) or the development of a medical condition causing chronic pain, increases the risk for suicide and mandates a suicidal assessment (Igen et al., 2010)

One of few prospective studies of suicide has produced indications of the importance of acute risk factors, which has been supported by subsequent studies (Fawcett et al., 1990). It is difficult to recognize time-related suicide risk factors without a prospective study design and a sufficiently large sample of high suicide risk patients. This study consisted of 954 patients with major affective disorder who were followed for at least 10 years. Over 80% of the patients were hospitalized when entered into the study, meaning that they were followed at a period of known increased suicide risk.

The initial data analysis showed no significant differences in the presence of the classic risk factors including severity of suicidal ideation, prior suicide attempts (past or recent), or hopelessness between patients who suicided and survivors.

When the analysis separated the analyses to look at suicides occurring over the first year of follow-up and the subsequent 9 years of follow-up, the above classic risk factors were significantly higher for suicides at the 10-year follow-up point (N = 34 suicides), but the suicide risk factors emerging significantly at year 1 (N = 13 suicides) were severity of psychic anxiety, panic attacks, severe insomnia, agitation, severe hopelessness, and recent increased alcohol abuse (Fawcett et al., 1990).

A subsequent study of 100 suicide attempts requiring hospitalization (Hall et al., 1999) found from interviews using similar measures to the former study that 90% of patients endorsed severe psychic anxiety over the month prior to the suicide attempt, as well as increased panic attacks. Over 80% of the patients had made no-suicide commitments to their therapists.

A study of 76 inpatient suicides had reviewed the patients' hospital records finding that 75% of the patients had either episodes of severe anxiety or agitation within the week of their suicide. No-suicide contracts were recorded in 28% of the suicides and 76% of the patients had denied suicidal ideation to a nurse as their last communication prior to their suicide. Forty percent of these patients were followed on q15 minute checks (Fawcett et al., 1990).

A study by Stordal et al. collected monthly (except for July) Hospital Anxiety and Depression Scale ratings of over 60 000 subjects from 1996 to 2004 (Stordal et al., 2008). The sample contained over 6000 males and 3000 females who committed suicide during the study period. It was found that suicide occurred in months when anxiety symptoms and depressive symptoms were at their maximum severity ($r = 0.72$, $p < 0.05$) with peaks in the months of May and June, as well as October.

A study by Pfeiffer et al., (2009) of 887 000 depressed veterans found a significantly increased rate of comorbid generalized anxiety disorder (GAD), Anx NOS, and panic disorder associated with suicide. Patients receiving benzodiazepines, buspirone showed a significantly elevated odds ratio for suicide and those with high dose anxiolytic medications had a higher odds ratio (2.4) for suicide, suggesting a relationship between severity of anxiety and suicide (Stordal et al., 2008).

An epidemiologic study of suicide attempts by Nock et al. in 2009 in 121 000 subjects across 21 countries, both developed and developing, found that suicidal ideation did not alone predict suicide attempts, but suicide ideation plus anxiety or impulsivity predicted suicidal behavior (Nock et al., 2009). Taylor et al. found a significant relationship between levels of impulsivity and anxiety in a clinical sample (Taylor et al., 2008).

The concept of suicidal ideation plus anxiety/high impulsivity leading to suicidal behavior seems a useful one for anticipating increased suicide risk. This suggests that a combination of factors may more usefully be predictive of suicidal behavior.

There is no evidence that any given treatment over a 2- to 3-month period of time will reduce suicide. There is evidence that medications such as quetiapine will rapidly reduce anxiety and agitation, while olanzapine has been shown to reduce suicidal ideation in patients suffering from bipolar mixed state, while reducing agitation (Khan et al., 2003; Houston et al., 2006; Hirschfeld et al., 2006).

Not all patients manifest severe anxiety as a suicide risk factor although 90% of outpatients did so in the Hall study and 79% of inpatients manifested anxiety/agitation in the Busch study. Other current risk factors – a statement of suicidal plan or intent, and particularly some loss or stressful event, actual or anticipated – can precipitate a suicide, particularly in a patient struggling with depression or psychosis.

We need to know more about how to obtain information on current risk factors in order to be more effective at evaluating patients for current suicide risk, and we need more effective treatments to minimize this risk.

Research challenges

We need more research to improve the accuracy of our suicide risk assessments as well as more effective preventive treatments. To improve our knowledge of risk factors, a fine-grained study of patients at high risk for suicide would help reveal more about risk factors. A follow-up study of patients admitted to the hospital for suicide risk over a 2- to 5-year period would be revealing.

The Collaborative Study of Depression (CDS) was not designed to study suicide, but was able to reveal the distinction between acute and chronic risk factors as well as the role of severe psychic anxiety in suicide over a follow-up period of a year. The CDS studied a high-risk group, based on studying the course of major affective disorder patients, over a high-risk period, in that over 80% of the patients followed had been enrolled in the study while inpatients and were followed for over a year after hospital discharge, a known high-risk period for suicide. In this study, treatment participation was recorded, but not provided by the study. In a sample of 954 patients followed at five university medical centers, 13 suicides had occurred within 1 year, 25 suicides had occurred within 5 years, and 34 suicides had occurred within 10 years, showing the increased risk for suicide in the year following hospital discharge (Nock et al., 2009).

A similarly designed follow-up study of patients hospitalized for a documented suicide attempt would probably result in more suicides at year 1, with a higher long-term rate. Such a study could build in treatments showing promise of reducing suicides, which could then be tested for effectiveness. A separate follow-up study of military personnel and/or veterans could be designed, since this group may produce different information on risk factors. A recent retrospective study of a large group of veterans mentioned above produced useful information about the role of anxiety disorders and anxiety severity and suicide in depressed patients (Pfeiffer et al., 2009).

Newly developed and developing assessment methods which do not depend on the patient's manifest response to questions about suicide risk, such as implicit responses (Nock et al., 2010), biomarkers in response to suicide assessment interviews, and perhaps physiological responses could be tested in such studies of high-risk patients. Both developed (cognitive behavioral and dialectic behavioral therapy) and novel treatments could be tested for their effectiveness (e.g., using acupuncture to elicit emotional responses and engage military personnel in therapy (Koffman & Helms, 2013)), in order to find candidate treatments for focused treatment effectiveness studies.

To date prospective studies of suicide and the application of new techniques for gathering clinically relevant data have been missing from suicide research. To study these issues, large samples of high-risk patients during periods of increased risk are needed to yield sufficient numbers of suicides. Suicide is at its highest rate for 20 years (American Foundation for Suicide Prevention, 2012). We should be learning from these personal tragedies how to detect the possibility of suicide in advance and how to deploy effective treatments to prevent these outcomes.

Suicide is a growing national and worldwide problem; in 2010 it was the 10th leading cause of death and the 4th leading cause of death in the 18 to 65 age group (American Foundation for Suicide Prevention, 2012). We know that diagnosis matters by comparing the ratios of suicide attempts to suicide deaths. The ratio was 25 suicide attempts for every suicide in 2010. Baldessarini et al. found that the ratio in bipolar patients was 3 attempts for every suicide (Baldessarini et al., 2006). Further studies are needed in this area with the aim of reducing levels of suicide. Studying convenient clinical and epidemiological samples alone will not inform us adequately in the prevention of suicide. We must learn to separate "suicidality" from high suicide risk, and find preventive treatments.

References

American Foundation for Suicide Prevention. (2012). www.asfg.org.

Angst, J., Angst, F., Gerber-Werder, R., & Gamma, A. (2005). Suicide in 406 mood-disorder patients with and without long term medication: a 40 to 44 years follow-up. *Archives of Suicide Research*, **9**, 279–300.

Baldessarini, R. J., Pompili, M., & Tondo, L. (2006). Suicide in bipolar disorder: risks and management. *CNS Spectrums*, **11**(6), 466–471.

Baraclough, B., Bunch, J., Nelson, B., & Sainsbury, P. (1974). A hundred cases of suicide: Clinical aspects. *British Journal of Psychiatry*, **125**, 355–373.

Bostwick, J. M., & Pancratz, V. S. (2000). Affective disorders and suicide risk: a reexamination. *American Journal of Psychiatry*, **157**(12), 1925–1932.

Busch, K. A., Fawcett, J., & Jacobs, D. (2003). Clinical correlates of inpatient suicide. *Journal of Clinical Psychiatry*, **64**, 14–19.

Coryell, W., & Young, E. A. (2005). Clinical predictors of suicide in primary major depressive disorder. *Journal of Clinical Psychiatry*, **66**, 412–417.

Fawcett, J., Scheftner, W. A., Fogg, L. et al. (1990). Time-related predictors of suicide in major affective disorder. *American Journal of Psychiatry*, **147**(9), 1189–1194.

Feng, F., Keating, N. L., Mucel, I. A., et al. (2010). Immediate risk of suicide and cardiovascular death after a prostate cancer diagnosis: cohort study in the United States. *Journal of the National Cancer Institute*, **103**, 307–314.

Hall, R. C., Platt, D. E., & Hall, R. C. (1999). Suicide risk assessment: a review of risk factors for suicide in 100 outpatients who make severe suicide attempts. *Psychosomatics*, **40**(1), 18–27.

Hawton, K., Casanas, C., Haw, C., & Saunders, K. (2013). Risk factors for suicide in individuals with depression. *Journal of Affective Disorders*, **147**, 17–28.

Hirschfeld, R. M., Weisler, R. H., Raines, S. R. et al. (2006). Quetiapine in the treatment of anxiety in patients with bipolar I or II depression: a secondary analysis from a randomized, double-blind, placebo-controlled study. *Journal of Clinical Psychiatry*, **67**(3), 355–362.

Houston, J. P., Ahl, J., Meyers, A. L., et al. (2006). Reduced suicide ideation in bipolar I mixed episode in a placebo-controlled trial of Olanzapine combined with lithium or divalproex. *Journal of Clinical Psychiatry*, **67**(8), 1246–1252.

Hoyer, E. H., Licht, R. W., & Mortensen, P. B. (2009). Risk factors of suicide in inpatients and recently discharged patients with affective disorders: A case-control study. *European Psychiatry*, **24**(5), 317–321.

Igen, M. A., Zivin, M. K., Austin, K. L., et al. (2010). Severe pain predicts greater likelihood of subsequent suicide. *Suicide and Life-Threatening Behavior*, **40**(6), 597–608.

Isometsa, E. T., & Lonnqvist, J. K. (1998). Suicide attempts preceding completed suicide. *British Journal of Psychiatry*, **173**, 531–535.

Isometsa, E. T., Heikkinen, M. E., Martunen, M. J., et al. (1995). The last appointment before suicide: is suicide intent communicated? *American Journal of Psychiatry*, **152**, 919–922.

Khan, A., Khan, S., Kolts, R., & Brown, W. A. (2003). Suicide rates in clinical trials of SSRIs, other antidepressants, and placebo: analysis of FDA reports. *American Journal of Psychiatry*, **160**(40), 790–792.

Koffman, R. L., & Helms, J. M. (2013). Come for the needles, stay for the therapy. *Psychiatric Annals*, **43**(5), 226–339.

Leon, A. C., Solomon, D. A., Li, C., et al. (2011). Antidepressants and risk of suicide and suicide attempts: a 27-year observational study. *Journal of Clinical Psychiaty*, **72**(5), 580–586.

Luoma, J. B., Martin, C. E., & Oearson, J. L. (2002). Contact with mental health and primary care providers before suicide. *American Journal of Psychiatry*, **159**, 908–916.

Nock, M. K., Hwang, I., Sampson, N., et al. (2009). Cross-national analysis of the associations among mental disorders and suicidal behavior: findings from the WHO World Mental Health Surveys. *PLoS Medicine*, **6**(8), 1–17.

Nock, M. K., Park, J. M., Finn, C. T., et al. (2010). Measuring the suicidal mind: implicit cognition predicts suicidal behavior. *Psychological Science*, **21**(4), 511–517.

Pfeiffer, P. N., Ganoczy, D., Ilgen, M. et al. (2009). Comorbid anxiety as a suicide risk factor among depressed veterans. *Depression and Anxiety*, **26**(8), 166–170.

Robins, E. (1981). *The Final Months* (p 47). Oxford UK: Oxford University Press.

Stordal, E., Morken, G., Mykietun, A., et al. (2008). A monthly variation in prevalence rates of comorbid depression and anxiety in the general population at 63–65 degrees North: the HUNT study. *Journal of Affective Disorders*, **106**(3), 273–278.

Taylor, C. T., Hirshfeld-Becker, D. R., Ostracher, M. J., et al. (2008). Anxiety is associated with impulsivity in bipolar disorder. *Journal of Anxiety Disorder*, **22**(5), 868–875.

Chapter 11

Anxiety, depression, and suicide: epidemiology, pathophysiology, and prevention

Giampaolo Perna and Alan F. Schatzberg

Introduction

The association between depression/mood disorders and suicide attempts or ideation is well known with suicidal ideation and behavior frequently present during depressive episodes. In contrast, the association of suicidal activity with anxiety disorders is less intuitive. Epidemiology studies clearly underline the link between depression and suicide risk; however, the rubric of major depression contains heterogeneous subtypes that do not share the same risk of suicide. Fulfilling DSM criteria for major depression by itself often does not allow for distinguishing between a more severe, melancholic, or "true" depressive episode related to a recurrent mood "disorder" from a milder, less endogenous-like depressive syndrome that is a secondary consequence of environmental, relational difficulties or even other disorders. The role of anxiety disorders in increasing suicidal risk is still a matter of debate although it is well recognized that the association between depression and anxiety disorders has a synergistic role in increasing the risk. Possible pathophysiological factors that link depression or anxiety to suicidal risk are not yet fully understood; however, genetics, the hypothalamic–pituitary–adrenal (HPA) axis and serotonergic systems seem to play relevant roles. Finally prevention of suicide, one of the main goals in psychiatry, is a complex process that starts with the identification of risk factors and moves on to finding the most effective treatment resources for the condition that has created the background for such dangerous activity. In the present chapter, we try to disentangle the many factors related to suicide in anxiety and depression and attempt to give useful suggestions for effectively managing this risk.

Epidemiology

Keith Hawton and Kees van Heeringen, in a recent paper in the *Lancet* (Hawton & van Heeringen, 2009) on the impact of suicide estimated global burden of suicide to be a million deaths per year and WHO estimated that one suicide death occurs every 40 seconds (WHO, 2002). The burden is higher in developing countries and although suicide rates in elderly people have fallen in many countries, those of young people have risen, peaking in the spring – particularly in women born in the spring and early summer. Psychiatric disorders are present in 90% of people who commit suicide and affective disorders are the most common disorders present: more than half of all people who lost their lives by suicide met the criteria for a current depressive disorder. Moreover, emerging evidence from the WHO that in the next few years depression will become the most important cause of disability in developing countries together with data showing that 4% of depressed patients die by suicide (Coryell & Young, 2005) clearly point out the importance of mood disorders in suicide. Moreover, 10–15% of patients with bipolar disorder die by suicide, particularly during the early phases of the disorder.

Although the co-occurrence of anxiety and depressive disorders is firmly established, there is a lack of empirical studies on the relationships between anxiety disorders and suicide. Data reported are limited and somewhat inconclusive; however, a recent systematic review and meta-analysis (Kanwar et al., 2013) concluded that patients with anxiety disorders, except obsessive-compulsive disorder, are more likely to have completed suicides, and to experience suicide attempts, suicidal ideation, and any

A Concise Guide to Understanding Suicide, ed. Stephen H. Koslow, Pedro Ruiz, and Charles B. Nemeroff. Published by Cambridge University Press.

other type of suicidal behaviors. Of the 42 studies included in the meta-analysis, 31 studies reported a significant association while 11 did not. The latter, however, suffered from several limitations: small samples, limited length of follow-up, uncertain ascertainment of diagnosis, variability in the outcome, no differentiation between separate anxiety disorders, etc. In a previous assessment of the relationships between anxiety disorders and suicide in the National Comorbidity Survey-Replication (Cougle et al., 2009), data suggested that generalized anxiety, post-traumatic stress, social anxiety, and panic disorders are uniquely predictive of suicidal ideation while only the first three were associated with suicide attempts. The results were obtained after controlling for a range of covariates, including personality disorders, substance abuse, and depression. Among the different anxiety disorders the most studied and controversial is panic disorder. If there is an agreement on a higher risk of suicidal ideation and suicide attempts, many studies, but not all, indicate that the risk is not related to panic disorder itself but explained by comorbid mood, substance abuse, and personality disorders (Hornig & McNally, 1995; Vickers & McNally, 2004; Goodwin & Roy-Byrne, 2006) and a study on panic disorder in completed suicide reported that this diagnosis in its non-complicated form was rarely found in completed suicide (Henriksson et al., 1996). Finally, Jonson and co-workers (Jonson et al., 2012; Boyce, 2010) investigated 560 subjects aged 70 years or older and reported an association between anxiety symptoms and suicidal feelings underlying the importance of assessing and treating anxiety in the elderly.

One of the most interesting pieces of data from the epidemiological studies is the effect of anxiety symptoms and disorders on the risk of suicidal behaviors in patients with mood disorders. A recent review (Goldberg & Fawcett, 2012) investigating the importance of anxiety in both major depression and bipolar disorder pointed out that there is a substantially increased rate of suicide in patients when major depression is accompanied by anxiety symptoms, and a recent 10-year longitudinal study (May et al., 2012) confirmed that anxiety disorders were among the predictors of suicide attempts among depressed suicide ideators; however, there was a suggestion that this relationship was mediated by the presence of cluster B personality disorder. Simon and co-workers (Simon et al., 2007) reported in bipolar patients that lifetime anxiety disorder more than doubled the odds of past suicide attempts and that current comorbid anxiety increased the risk of suicidal ideation. This association was confirmed in a large meta-analysis (Tondo et al., 2003), although not all the studies are in line with this finding (Gonda et al., 2012).

Katz and co-workers (2011) analyzed data from the National Epidemiological Survey on Alcohol and Related Conditions and reported two primary findings. First, past history of panic attacks was significantly associated with suicidal behaviors in patients with depression but panic seemed to be related more to suicide attempts than to suicidal ideation, representing a factor mediating the transition from ideation to action. Second, focusing on panic attack symptoms, catastrophic cognitions (fears of dying, losing control, or going insane) had a stronger association with suicide attempts while dissociation, chocking, and chest pain were more closely associated with suicide ideation. The same group of researchers (Yaseen et al., 2013) reported that fear of dying during panic attacks is an independent risk factor for subsequent suicide attempts among individuals with depressive disorders.

Risk factors

Given the high association of depressive (and anxiety) disorders with suicide, it is crucial to investigate suicidal thoughts and/or behaviors in every patient with a depressive episode (Nemeroff et al., 2001). Risk factors are important, although we should keep in mind that it is not possible to predict accurately whether or when a particular individual with a depressive episode will attempt suicide.

Genetic loading, personality disorders, early traumatic events, and possibly abnormal function in serotonergic and hypothalamic pituitary axis play roles in conferring distal risks for suicide. Psychiatric and physical disorders together with psychosocial crises, availability of means, and exposure to "role models" are proximal risk factors (Hawton & van Heeringen, 2009). Taken together, the literature leads to a number of conclusions regarding risk factors for suicide in mood and anxiety disorders.

In patients with major depressive disorder, risk factors can be further divided into those that affect the threshold for suicidal behavior and those that serve as triggers. Among the former are: male gender, personal history of attempted suicide, positive family history of suicide, early onset and first episode of depression, comorbid substance use disorders, comorbid cluster B personality disorders, impulsive aggressive personality traits, chronic physical illness, marital isolation, parental loss through death before the age of 11, childhood history of physical or sexual abuse, corporal punishment in adolescence, presence of hopelessness, and low self-esteem. Risk factors that may serve as triggers include: severity of depressive episode, symptoms of anxiety, bipolar disorder, presence of psychosis, acute substance intoxication, social, financial, or family crisis or loss, and contagion or recent exposure to suicide. We cannot forget that some factors might be protective, including religious or moral constraints, concern about social disapproval, better coping skills, feelings of responsibility toward family, living with children under the age of 18, and supportive relationships (Oquendo et al., 1997; Hawton et al., 2013). To this list we should also add as risk factors: inadequate treatment of the depressive episode and heightened risk during the first weeks after discharge from inpatient care.

In patients with bipolar disorder, previous self-harm, positive family history of suicide, early onset, depressive symptoms, mixed affective states, rapid cycling, comorbid psychiatric disorders, and alcohol and drug abuse increase the risk of committing suicide (Gonda et al., 2012).

Pathophysiology

Suicide is a complex behavior that ranges from suicidal ideation to suicide attempts to completion. This complex phenomenon is not due to a simple etiology but rather is the result of the complex interaction of genetic vulnerability, stress factors, underlying psychopathology, and social aspects. The precise pathophysiological mechanisms underlying this behavior are not yet fully understood. However, there have been a great many studies on possible causes with some variables being consistently associated with suicidal behaviors and often with mood and anxiety disorders as well. These include:

a. Genetic vulnerability
b. HPA axis
c. Serotonergic system
d. Neuroplasticity and brain-derived neurotrophic factor (BDNF)
e. Neuropsychological functions
f. Epigenetics
g. Cholesterol

This list is not complete and several of these interact with one another; however, each of these neurobiological aspects appears to be relevant to suicidal behaviors.

a. *Genetic vulnerability*. Family history of suicide increases the risk at least two-fold and the concordance among monozygotic twins is higher than among dizygotic twins. Genetic factors account for 45% of the variance. There is an association between family history of suicide and mood disorders (Lopez de Lara et al., 2006; Nierenberg et al., 2008; Serretti et al., 2013) that confirms a genetic relationship between depression and suicide. An intron 2 (STin2) variant of 5-HTT promoter region (5HTTLPR) is a significant predictor of suicide in major depression when jointly considered with a family history of suicide (Lopez de Lara et al., 2006) suggesting a genetic link between serotonergic abnormalities and suicide.

b. *HPA axis*. HPA axis dysfunction predicts suicide in patients with depression (Coryell & Schlesser, 2001). The relationships between suicide and depression were originally observed more than 40 years ago (Bunney & Fawcett, 1965) and since then multiple studies have confirmed this association (Pompili et al., 2010). The main findings in suicidal subjects are HPA axis hyperactivity, as expressed by elevated 24-hour urinary cortisol levels, a non-suppression of cortisol on the dexamethasone suppression test, increased levels of corticotropin-releasing hormone (CRH) in the hypothalamus, and pituitary abnormalities. Reduced CRH binding sites in the frontal cortex have been observed in suicide victims (Nemeroff et al., 1988). Chronic abnormalities in the stress system could lead to abnormalities in activity of brain areas related to memory and decision-making, abnormalities that have been reported to be associated with suicide in depressed patients (Jollant et al., 2011). An increasing number of studies are examining the association between variation in expression of genes related to HPA axis in brain areas and suicide in depressed patients, for example, corticotropin-releasing hormone receptor 1 gene (Wasserman et al., 2010) and metallothionein subfamilies 1 and 2 genes (Sequeira et al., 2012), with promising results. A recent study indicated decreased expression for both glucocorticoid receptor and the FKBP-5 co-chaperone for the glucocorticoid receptor in the amygdala of suicide victims (Perez-Ortiz et al., 2013). Childhood maltreatment is one of the main sources of disruption of HPA axis function and its effects have been related to the development of depression in adulthood, particularly in those with specific FKBP5 variation, as well as to suicidal behaviors in both childhood and adulthood. A gene–environment interaction of childhood maltreatment and HPA axis genetic variation seems to play a relevant role in suicidal behaviors (Roy et al., 2012; Braquehais et al., 2012; Guillaume et al., 2013).

c. *Serotonergic system.* There is clear evidence that suicide is associated with abnormal function of the serotonergic system (Nemeroff et al., 2001; Purselle & Nemeroff, 2003). The first evidence of this link is dated more than 35 years ago: Asberg and co-workers (1976) reported that patients with major depression who attempted suicide have lower levels of 5-hydroxyindoleacetic acid (5-HIAA) in the cerebrospinal fluid and this reduction is correlated with lethality and medical consequences. Most studies, but not all (Secunda et al., 1986), confirmed this relationship to low metabolite levels that has also been associated with impulsivity and aggressive and violent behavior. As mentioned there is evidence of a genetic link between serotonin and suicide, although results on the association between 5HTTLPR variants and suicide are conflicting. There are some positive studies on an association between the short (s) form of the 5HTTLPR and the use of violent or highly lethal means of suicide; however, a recent meta-analysis of over 100 studies indicates the increased risk appears to be associated primarily with suicide attempts. In addition, this recent meta-analysis indicated that an association of a variation for the tryptophan hydroxylase (TPH) gene with suicide was also seen in attempters (Clayden et al., 2012). A decrease in 5-HT2A receptor gene expressions in the dorsolateral prefrontal cortex has been reported in mood disorder subjects who committed suicide versus non-suicide mood disorder subjects (Sequeira et al., 2012).

d. *Neuroplasticity and brain-derived neurotrophic factor (BDNF).* Neuroplasticity and neuroprotection are two aspects traditionally related to adaptation to stress. Neurotrophins in the brain may promote neuroplasticity and have a protective role on brain function. The BDNF gene and its high affinity receptor, tyrosine receptor kinase B (TRKB), have been studied in relation to suicide and both were shown to be altered in suicide. This alteration might increase the vulnerability to chronic stress and early life adverse experiences. Metallothioneins, small single chain proteins, play an important role in neuroprotection, and are reduced in mood disorder suicides compared to non-suicides.

e. *Neuropsychological functions.* Neuropsychological functions also are altered in suicide attempters (Jollant et al., 2011). In particular, data suggest a higher attention to specific emotional stimuli, impaired decision-making, lower problem solving ability, reduced verbal fluency, cognitive inflexibility, and a cognitive inhibition deficit (Richard-Devantoy et al., 2012), the latter specifically observed in patients with mood disorders. Impaired decision-making, cognitive inflexibility (Miranda et al., 2012), and attention to specific negative stimuli could be a neuropsychological style that predisposes to suicidal behaviors.

f. *Epigenetics.* Epigenetic modifications are reversible, mitotically heritable alterations in genomic expression that occur independent of changes in gene sequence. Several studies focused on the epigenetic mechanism related to suicide. Methylation of genes related to BDNF and its receptor tropomyosin-related kinase B, 5-HT2A receptor gene, neuron-specific glucocorticoid receptor (NR3C1), and oligodendrocyte-specific RNA binding protein (QK1) has been assessed in suicide attempters and completers with some evidence of genetic modifications in contrast to non-suicidal subjects. These alterations are thought to be induced by stress-related events, for example childhood maltreatment, and they can lead to behavioral consequences that could predispose to suicidal behaviors.

g. *Cholesterol.* Several, but not all, studies have reported a link between lower total cholesterol levels and suicide (De Berardis et al., 2012). There are several possible explanations: low cholesterol levels have been related to decreased serotonin activity possibly via reduced lipid viscosity of neuronal cell membranes; alternatively low cholesterol could result in a reduced synaptic plasticity.

The neurobiological vulnerability to suicide is possibly linked to genetic predisposition and physiologic abnormalities, mainly involving stress biology – the HPA axis as well as the serotonergic system. Abnormal functions of both these two systems relate to genetic variation and/or psychosocial factors. For example, negative childhood experiences could lead to epigenetic modifications in HPA axis genes such as FKBP-5 co-chaperone for the glucocorticoid receptor and greater stress responsiveness. Abnormal brain functions that are related to neuropsychological aspects, aggressive behaviors, impulsivity, and neuroticisms could create the background for mood or anxiety disorders leading to suicidal behaviors.

Finally we can make a tentative explanation of the potentiating effect of panic attacks on suicidal behaviors in depressed patients referring to "positive feedback model of suicide" (Katz et al., 2011). In this model autonomic arousal and the catastrophic thinking in panic attacks are mutually reinforcing. Depression is accompanied by negative cognitions that are amplified during panic attacks. The physical discomfort related to panic attacks escalates catastrophic cognition thus increasing suicidal ideation. In the last step, autonomic-limbic activation seen with suicidal ideation can transform behavior into action, i.e., the suicide attempt.

Prevention

Prevention of suicide relies first of all on the identification of "false" suicide attempts or ideation related often to a histrionic personality disorder where the act is an attempt to obtain attention rather than a true intention to put an end to one's life. Depressed and anxious patients often have comorbid personality disorders that may help to explain frequently observed suicidal declarations or multiple "false" or attention seeking suicidal attempts.

In the presence of a major suicide risk with depression, it is important to evaluate carefully the presence of severe anxiety, panic attacks, agitation, and severe insomnia since these are considered acute risk factors for suicide that might precede suicide attempts within hours, days or weeks (Fawcett et al., 1990; Hall et al., 1999).

The careful use of benzodiazepines or mood stabilizers together with cognitive behavioral psychotherapy can help to control these symptoms. The use of antidepressants, although effective in the treatment of anxiety disorders and panic attacks, should be evaluated carefully, given the possible increase in suicidal ideation during the first 2 weeks of treatment.

When a patient is depressed the presence of suicidal ideation is understandable and the most logical way to prevent suicide attempts and behaviors is to treat the depressive episode with antidepressant medications. To date there is still a debate on the relationships between use of antidepressants and risk of suicide. In 2004 the US FDA issued a black box warning for antidepressants and risk of suicide in children and adolescents, mainly based on reported increase of suicidal ideation and attempts in clinical settings although no actual suicides had been reported in trials. In 2006 the warning was extended also to young adults between 18 to 25 years based on analysis of data that approached significance in this age range obtained from a larger data set of 100 000 subjects who participated in all registered clinical trials. In contrast, no increased risk was seen in adults aged 25 to 64 and in the elderly a significant decrease was observed. The debate is still open (Pompili et al., 2008) although a recent well done reanalysis of randomized placebo-controlled studies on fluoxetine and venlafaxine reported that there was no increase of suicide risk among youths and confirmed the protective effect in adult and geriatric depressed patients in parallel with an improvement in depressive symptoms. Of particular importance is that the warning in children did lead to a decrease in prescription of antidepressants in the USA – primarily by pediatricians (Nemeroff et al., 2007) – and in one study to an increase in suicides in youths in the Netherlands where a similar warning had been instituted (Gibbons et al., 2007).

Although recent studies in adults suggest that antidepressant use is relatively safe, there are some specific circumstances that make their use risky. Administration of antidepressants in bipolar patients could increase impulsivity and irritability and thus the risk of suicidal behaviors. In mixed states, mood stabilizers should be preferred to antidepressants. Lithium has been proven to reduce suicide risk in a significant way (Guzzetta et al., 2007). A relevant risk factor for suicidal behaviors in mood disorder patients is impulsivity and some data suggest that mood stabilizers could be a protective factor against suicide risk (Pompili et al., 2008).

Looking at non-pharmacological prevention strategies, a systematic review published in 2005 in *JAMA* (Mann et al., 2005) reported that only educating physicians in depression recognition and treatment and restricting access to lethal methods reduce suicide rates. Other methods could help but are not sufficiently supported by evidence.

Final remarks

Suicide is a major public health problem that should not be ignored. Pathophysiologic studies are making progress in the understanding of the biological and genetic roots of suicidal behaviors – mainly focusing on the HPA axis, the serotonergic system, and neuropsychological dysfunction with the promise/hope of finding neurobiological markers useful in clinical practice. However, to date the evaluation of suicide risk is still based mainly on clinical interview.

When we see patients who report suicidal ideation and attempts, it is crucial to make a careful psychopathological assessment. True suicide risk should not be confused with declaration of suicidal ideation or even the reporting of suicidal behavior. Often in patients with mood and anxiety disorders, in particular when comorbid with personality disorders, suicidal behavior is mainly the consequence of a cry-for-help rather than the expression of true suicidal intention. This difference often is not taken into account in epidemiological studies. When seeing patients who declare current suicidal behavior, we should carefully investigate the nature of this declaration. What clearly emerges from the literature is the expectedly high suicide risk related to mood disorder, and most interestingly, the amplification of this risk in the presence of comorbid anxiety disorders, in particular panic attacks and panic disorder. Anxiety phenomena might be considered triggers of action in those who experience suicidal ideation. This underlines the importance of treating anxiety in depressed patients to reduce the risk of suicidal behaviors. The best prevention strategies involve early recognition and treatment of anxiety and mood disorders by appropriate pharmacological and psychotherapeutic therapies, physician education of patients, recognizing their symptoms and restricting their access to lethal methods (Yip et al., 2012). Some recent papers also suggest the usefulness of modern technologies, including online courses, websites, and social networking; however, to date these methods have not been systematically evaluated. Finally, the impact of publicity concerning the waves of suicide seen at times in cohorts of teenagers as well as that concerning the phantom increased risk of suicide in adults caused by antidepressants needs to be countered by evidence-based and appropriate reporting.

References

Asberg, M., Traskman, L., & Thoren, P. (1976). 5-HIAA in the cerebrospinal fluid. A biochemical suicide predictor? *Archives of General Psychiatry*, **33**(10), 1193–1197.

Boyce, N. (2010). Pilots of the future: suicide prevention and the internet. *Lancet*, **376**(9756), 1889–1890.

Braquehais, M. D., Picouto, M. D., Casas, M., & Sher, L. (2012). Hypothalamic-pituitary-adrenal axis dysfunction as a neurobiological correlate of emotion dysregulation in adolescent suicide. *World Journal of Pediatrics*, **8**(3), 197–206.

Bunney, W. E., Jr., & Fawcett, J. A. (1965). Possibility of a biochemical test for suicidal potential: an analysis of endocrine findings prior to three suicides. *Archives of General Psychiatry*, **13**, 232–239.

Clayden, R. C., Zaruk, A., Meyre, D., Thabane, L., & Samaan, Z. (2012). The association of attempted suicide with genetic variants in the SLC6A4 and TPH genes depends on the definition of suicidal behavior:a systematic review and meta-analysis. *Translational Psychiatry*, **2**, e166.

Coryell, W., & Schlesser, M. (2001). The dexamethasone suppression test and suicide prediction. *The American Journal of Psychiatry*, **158**(5), 748–753.

Coryell, W., & Young, E. A. (2005). Clinical predictors of suicide in primary major depressive disorder. *The Journal of Clinical Psychiatry*, **66**(4), 412–417.

Cougle, J. R., Keough, M. E., Riccardi, C. J., & Sachs-Ericsson, N. (2009). Anxiety disorders and suicidality in the National Comorbidity Survey-Replication. *Journal of Psychiatric Research*, **43**(9), 825–829.

De Berardis, D., Marini, S., Piersanti, M., et al. (2012). The relationships between cholesterol and suicide: an update. *ISNR Psychiatry*, **6**.

Fawcett, J., Scheftner, W. A., Fogg, L., et al. (1990). Time-related predictors of suicide in major affective disorder. *The American Journal of Psychiatry*, **147**(9), 1189–1194.

Gibbons, R. D., Brown, C. H., Hur, K., et al. (2007). Early evidence on the effects of regulators' suicidality warnings on SSRI prescriptions and suicide in children and adolescents. *The American Journal of Psychiatry*, **164**(9), 1356–1363.

Goldberg, D., & Fawcett, J. (2012). The importance of anxiety in both major depression and bipolar disorder. *Depression and Anxiety*, **29**(6), 471–478.

Gonda, X., Pompili, M., Serafini, G., et al. (2012). Suicidal behavior in bipolar disorder: epidemiology, characteristics and major risk factors. *Journal of Affective Disorders*, **143**(1–3), 16–26.

Goodwin, R. D., & Roy-Byrne, P. (2006). Panic and suicidal ideation and suicide attempts: results from the National Comorbidity Survey. *Depression and Anxiety*, **23**(3), 124–132.

Guillaume, S., Perroud, N., Jollant, F., et al. (2013). HPA axis genes may modulate the effect of childhood adversities on decision-making in suicide attempters. *Journal of Psychiatric Research*, **47**(2), 259–265.

Guzzetta, F., Tondo, L., Centorrino, F., & Baldessarini, R. J. (2007). Lithium treatment reduces suicide risk in recurrent major depressive disorder. *The Journal of Clinical Psychiatry*, **68**(3), 380–383.

Hall, R. C., Platt, D. E., & Hall, R. C. (1999). Suicide risk assessment: a review of risk factors for suicide in 100 patients who made severe suicide attempts. Evaluation of suicide risk in a time of managed care. *Psychosomatics*, **40**(1), 18–27.

Hawton, K., & van Heeringen, K. (2009). Suicide. *Lancet*, **373**(9672), 1372–1381.

Hawton, K., Casanas, I. C. C., Haw, C., & Saunders, K. (2013). Risk factors for suicide in individuals with depression: A systematic review. *Journal of Affective Disorders*, **147**(1–3), 17–28.

Henriksson, M. M., Isometsa, E. T., Kuoppasalmi, K. I., et al. (1996). Panic disorder in completed suicide. *The Journal of Clinical Psychiatry*, **57**(7), 275–281.

Hornig, C. D., & McNally, R. J. (1995). Panic disorder and suicide attempt. A reanalysis of data from the Epidemiologic Catchment Area study. *The British Journal of Psychiatry*, **167**(1), 76–79.

Jollant, F., Lawrence, N. L., Olie, E., Guillaume, S., & Courtet, P. (2011). The suicidal mind and brain: a review of neuropsychological and neuroimaging studies. *The World Journal of Biological Psychiatry*, **12**(5), 319–339.

Jonson, M., Skoog, I., Marlow, T., Mellqvist Fassberg, M., & Waern, M. (2012). Anxiety symptoms and suicidal feelings in a population sample of 70-year-olds without dementia. *International Psychogeriatrics*, **24**(11), 1865–1871.

Kanwar, A., Malik, S., Prokop, L. J., et al. (2013). The association between anxiety disorders and suicidal behaviors: a systematic review and meta-analysis. *Depression and Anxiety*, **30**(10), 917–929.

Katz, C., Yaseen, Z. S., Mojtabai, R., Cohen, L. J., & Galynker, I. I. (2011). Panic as an independent risk factor for suicide attempt in depressive illness: findings from the National Epidemiological Survey on Alcohol and Related Conditions (NESARC). *The Journal of Clinical Psychiatry*, **72**(12), 1628–1635.

Lopez de Lara, C., Dumais, A., Rouleau, G., et al. (2006). STin2 variant and family history of suicide as significant predictors of suicide completion in major depression. *Biological Psychiatry*, **59**(2), 114–120.

Mann, J. J., Apter, A., Bertolote, J., et al. (2005). Suicide prevention strategies: a systematic review. *JAMA*, **294** (16), 2064–2074.

May, A. M., Klonsky, E. D., & Klein, D. N. (2012). Predicting future suicide attempts among depressed suicide ideators: a 10-year longitudinal study. *Journal of Psychiatric Research*, **46**(7), 946–952.

Miranda, R., Gallagher, M., Bauchner, B., Vaysman, R., & Marroquin, B. (2012). Cognitive inflexibility as a prospective predictor of suicidal ideation among young adults with a suicide attempt history. *Depression and Anxiety*, **29**(3), 180–186.

Nemeroff, C. B., Owens, M. J., Bissette, G., Andorn, A. C., & Stanley, M. (1988). Reduced corticotropin releasing factor binding sites in the frontal cortex of suicide victims. *Archives of General Psychiatry*, **45**(6), 577–579.

Nemeroff, C. B., Compton, M. T., & Berger, J. (2001). The depressed suicidal patient. Assessment and treatment. *Annals of the New York Academy of Sciences*, **932**, 1–23.

Nemeroff, C. B., Kalali, A., Keller, M. B., et al. (2007). Impact of publicity concerning pediatric suicidality data on physician practice patterns in the United States. *Archives of General Psychiatry*, **64**(4), 466–472.

Nierenberg, A. A., Alpert, J. E., Gaynes, B. N., et al. (2008). Family history of completed suicide and characteristics of major depressive disorder: a STAR*D (sequenced treatment alternatives to relieve depression) study. *Journal of Affective Disorders*, **108**(1–2), 129–134.

Oquendo, M. A., Malone, K. M., & Mann, J. J. (1997). Suicide: risk factors and prevention in refractory major depression. *Depression and Anxiety*, **5**(4), 202–211.

Perez-Ortiz, J. M., Garcia-Gutierrez, M. S., Navarrete, F., Giner, S., & Manzanares, J. (2013). Gene and protein alterations of FKBP5 and glucocorticoid receptor in the amygdala of suicide victims. *Psychoneuroendocrinology*, **30**(10), 917–929.

Pompili, M., Innamorati, M., Raja, M., et al. (2008). Suicide risk in depression and bipolar disorder: Do impulsiveness-aggressiveness and pharmacotherapy predict suicidal intent? *Neuropsychiatric Disease and Treatment*, **4**(1), 247–255.

Pompili, M., Serafini, G., Innamorati, M., et al. (2010). The hypothalamic-pituitary-adrenal axis and serotonin abnormalities: a selective overview for the implications of suicide prevention. *European Archives of Psychiatry and Clinical Neuroscience*, **260**(8), 583–600.

Purselle, D. C., & Nemeroff, C. B. (2003). Serotonin transporter: a potential substrate in the biology of suicide. *Neuropsychopharmacology*, **28**(4), 613–619.

Richard-Devantoy, S., Gorwood, P., Annweiler, C., et al. (2012). Suicidal behaviours in affective disorders: a deficit of cognitive inhibition? *Canadian Journal of Psychiatry*, **57**(4), 254–262.

Roy, A., Hodgkinson, C. A., Deluca, V., Goldman, D., & Enoch, M. A. (2012). Two HPA axis genes, CRHBP and FKBP5, interact with childhood trauma to increase the risk for suicidal behavior. *Journal of Psychiatric Research*, **46**(1), 72–79.

Secunda, S. K., Cross, C. K., Koslow, S., et al. (1986). Biochemistry and suicidal behavior in depressed patients. *Biological Psychiatry*, **21**(8–9), 756–767.

Sequeira, A., Morgan, L., Walsh, D. M., et al. (2012). Gene expression changes in the prefrontal cortex, anterior cingulate cortex and nucleus accumbens of mood disorders subjects that committed suicide. *PloS one*, **7**(4), e35367.

Serretti, A., Chiesa, A., Calati, R., et al. (2013). Influence of family history of major depression, bipolar disorder, and suicide on clinical features in patients with major depression and bipolar disorder. *European Archives of Psychiatry and Clinical Neuroscience*, **263**(2), 93–103.

Simon, N. M., Zalta, A. K., Otto, M. W., et al. (2007). The association of comorbid anxiety disorders with suicide attempts and suicidal ideation in outpatients with bipolar disorder. *Journal of Psychiatric Research*, **41**(3–4), 255–264.

Tondo, L., Isacsson, G., & Baldessarini, R. (2003). Suicidal behaviour in bipolar disorder: risk and prevention. *CNS Drugs*, **17**(7), 491–511.

Vickers, K., & McNally, R. J. (2004). Panic disorder and suicide attempt in the National Comorbidity Survey. *Journal of Abnormal Psychology*, **113**(4), 582–591.

Wasserman, D., Wasserman, J., & Sokolowski, M. (2010). Genetics of HPA-axis, depression and suicidality. *European Psychiatry*, **25**(5), 278–280.

WHO. (2002). *World Report on Violence and Health.* Geneva: World Health Organization.

Yaseen, Z. S., Chartrand, H., Mojtabai, R., Bolton, J., & Galynker, I. I. (2013). Fear of dying in panic attacks predicts suicide attempt in comorbid depressive illness: prospective evidence from the National Epidemiological Survey on Alcohol and Related Conditions. *Depression and Anxiety*, **30**(10), 930–939.

Yip, P. S., Caine, E., Yousuf, S., et al. (2012). Means restriction for suicide prevention. *Lancet*, **379**(9834), 2393–2399.

Chapter 12

Suicide in schizophrenia

Philip D. Harvey and Stacey Espaillat

Suicide is a leading cause of death in schizophrenia and the primary cause of death before age 40 in the illness (Harris & Barraclough, 1997). Like all severe mental illnesses, there is an increase in suicidality compared to the general population and death by suicide is even more common in certain patient subgroups. In this chapter, we address several critical features of suicide in schizophrenia with a focus on detection and treatments. There is less literature on many aspects of suicide in schizophrenia than would be expected and we will consider why. Further, there is a popular press preoccupation with risk of dangerous and even homicidal behavior on the part of people with psychosis. We will address relative risks of suicide, homicide, and murder-suicide in this population.

We will review the demographics of suicide (age and gender), the prediction of suicide risk, and treatments. Differentiating between suicide attempts, actual suicides, and non-suicidal self-injurious acts, we will evaluate the level of seriousness on the part of suicidal people with schizophrenia. We will also examine the correlations between suicide risk and psychotic symptoms and the association between suicide and other symptoms of the illness, such as disorganized behavior. The literature on the association between awareness of illness (i.e., insight), cognitive impairment, substance abuse, and medical comorbidities will also be considered. Finally, after full consideration of the risk factors for suicide, we will consider treatments. Remarkably, there is a pharmacological treatment approved for suicide in schizophrenia, clozapine, which is rarely used. We will consider reasons for this low rate of use and examine non-pharmacological interventions for schizophrenia.

Demographic predictors of risk for suicide

Schizophrenia is associated with increased all-cause mortality, and suicide is a major contributor to early death of people with schizophrenia. At least 90% of individuals who die by suicide have a mental disorder at the time of death, with 10% of all people successfully completing suicide suffering from schizophrenia (Mann, 2002). More than 50% of all people with schizophrenia attempt suicide at some point in their life and some estimates are as high as 75% (Caldwell & Gottesman, 1990). Rates of suicidal ideation are considerably higher than the rates of suicide attempts. As a result, it is a reasonable conclusion that suicidality, in some level of severity and intention, is ubiquitous in schizophrenia and should be assessed in every patient at every clinical contact.

The most commonly cited suicide rate for people with schizophrenia is 10%, based on a review by Miles (1977). More recent evidence, however, supports a somewhat lower lifetime completed suicide rate of approximately 5% (Palmer et al., 2005; Hor & Taylor, 2010). Approximately 50% of suicides and homicides perpetrated by individuals with schizophrenia occur during or shortly after the first episode of psychosis, sometimes prior to the initiation of treatment (Nielssen et al., 2012). These young patients at highest risk are typically men, with some evidence of higher level of education, which may increase their awareness of the negative impact their disease will confer on their futures (we return to this discussion below). Another major time period for increased suicide risk is after partial recovery from the first episode of illness (Bakst et al., 2009). Thus, one of the critical early interventions required, in addition to reduction of psychosis

A Concise Guide to Understanding Suicide, ed. Stephen H. Koslow, Pedro Ruiz, and Charles B. Nemeroff. Published by Cambridge University Press.

Table 12.1. Suicide risk factors in people with schizophrenia

History of previous attempts	++++
Younger age	+++
Male gender	+++
Command hallucinations	+++
Depression	+++
Hopelessness	+++
Substance abuse	+++
Poor premorbid functioning	+
Social isolation	++
Higher educational attainment	+
Disability compensation	–

++++, Highest risk; +++, high consistent risk; ++, high-risk; +, mixed evidence; –, protective factor.

and promotion of functional recovery, is reduction of suicide risk in this particularly high-risk group.

Prediction/suicide risk assessment

There is no single indicator of suicide risk (Table 12.1). Thus, psychiatrists and other mental health professionals must focus on assessing patients for the presence and severity of multiple risk factors and then providing appropriate interventions to reduce the patient's risk. Many of the risk factors are common among all people, including those with schizophrenia. The clinician must consider demographic risk factors (age, gender, education), familial and genetic risk factors (family history of suicide), illness-related factors (mood or psychotic disorder, substance abuse, presence of suicidal ideation, history and severity of suicide attempts, impulsivity, insomnia, and hopelessness), and the presence of psychosocial stressors such as poverty and social isolation.

As noted above, in patients with schizophrenia, the most substantial demographic risk factors are age and male gender (De Hert et al., 2001). The strongest illness-related risk factors are the number of prior attempts, the presence of depressive symptoms, substance abuse, and certain active hallucinations as described below (Fenton, 2000). While insight has been proposed to be a strong risk factor, because patients with high levels of awareness may be more realistic about their prognosis, a recent meta-analysis could not find evidence to support this hypothesis (López-Moríñigo et al., 2012). Instead of insight as a risk factor, the meta-analysis of the data in the previous studies implicated depression and, even more strongly, hopelessness (Kim et al., 2003), as risk factors for suicide in the early stages of the illness. We will return to other factors that may be as important as insight later.

Assessment of depression and hopelessness is critically important. Just because depression is considered as an exclusionary factor for the diagnosis of schizophrenia in the DSM, this does not mean that depression is not a major factor in schizophrenia. In fact, 50% of people with schizophrenia experience at least one episode of major depression over the course of their illness and their risk for suicide during these episodes is increased (Hawton et al., 2005). Hopelessness is a consistent risk factor for suicide across neuropsychiatric conditions and its influence in schizophrenia is similar to that in other conditions (Kim et al., 2003). Assessment of major depression and hopelessness is easy to accomplish with simple self-report measures or a couple of interview questions.

A major risk factor for suicide in schizophrenia is a symptom that is quite unique to psychotic conditions: command hallucinations. Both depressed and schizophrenic patients can experience these symptoms, which consist of a voice speaking directly to the patient. These voices can either tell the patient to hurt or kill themselves or they may simply be so abusive or derogatory that the patient considers killing themselves to escape them. As a result, in patients who have a history of command hallucinations combined with positive medication response, medication adherence becomes a major clinical goal in order to prevent the recurrence of these symptoms. Interestingly, command hallucinations have been reported to be associated with suicide attempts only in previous attempters (Harkavy-Friedman et al., 2003). The combination of paranoid delusions and command hallucinations has also been proposed to augment suicide risk considerably, but it is not clear if command hallucinations alone account for all of the increased risk. The presence of command hallucinations is also associated with acts that injure others as well, suggesting that command hallucinations need to be taken seriously in all cases.

Other strong risk factors include family history of suicide and comorbid substance abuse, especially alcohol abuse (Hor & Taylor, 2010). Family history of suicide has been investigated across neuropsychiatric conditions, with the question being whether the familiality of suicidality is based on genetics or environmental factors. Being exposed to the suicide of a parent or sibling could be argued to have multiple learning effects, both increasing (through modeling of suicide as an acceptable problem solving strategy), or reducing (through exposure to the adverse impact on others) risk. As suicide in family members clearly increases risk, the deterrent effects of suicide appear not to exert a major influence.

Both suicidal and self-injurious acts are increased in prevalence during periods of intoxication. Intoxication and substance abuse are risk factors for suicide in the general population and their risk is approximately equivalent in people with schizophrenia. As the prevalence of substance abuse in schizophrenia may be increasing, the suicide risk associated with substance abuse may be increasing as well. Further, as some research suggests that homicidal behavior may also be associated with substance abuse, these risks may be increased as well (Swinson et al., 2011). Substance abuse in schizophrenia presently occurs in as many as 50% of cases with the illness. However, only about a third of psychiatrists indicate that they regularly assess their patients for substance abuse (West et al., 2005). As a result, assessment and treatment of substance abuse is an area where treatment could possibly reduce suicide risk.

One perspective on suicide in schizophrenia that has not received substantial attention is the role of early life stress (ELS) on suicidality in schizophrenia. In major depression, ELS has been found to be the predominant environmental factor associated with increased suicide risk as noted in other chapters in this volume. As ELS has recently been identified as a potential risk factor for the development of the illness, this may also be an important factor for increasing suicide risk in schizophrenia. In contrast to the research on ELS and suicide in depression, a literature search on this topic in schizophrenia yields a single hit. In this study, ELS was associated with increases in both suicidality and several of its correlates (Rosenberg et al., 2007). In contrast, the effect of ELS on cognition and functional outcomes has been studied in considerably more detail. As a result, these discrepancies in research coverage of this suggest that much more effort is needed. In the absence of information to the contrary, an assessment of childhood trauma would seem to be indicated in schizophrenia. Whether the results of the assessment lead in the direction of cognitive remediation or suicide prevention, a self-report assessment of childhood trauma is a very valuable source of information that requires little burden to collect.

An important additional correlate of ELS in schizophrenia is the finding that ELS has several additional adverse impacts on functioning in people with schizophrenia (McCabe et al., 2012). ELS correlates with increased depression, impulsivity, and substance abuse. As noted above, all of these factors also increase risk for suicide independently. As a result, childhood trauma of various forms is a substantial risk factor for adverse suicide outcomes in schizophrenia and should be part of the initial assessment of all patients.

Methods of suicide attempts

It is believed that people with schizophrenia are more likely to attempt suicide using means with higher potential lethality than other suicidal individuals. However, there is a lack of objective evidence to support this conclusion as evidenced by very limited empirical evidence regarding methods. One small-scale study reported no differences between patients with schizophrenia and adjustment disorders in terms of the violence of their self-injurious acts (Symonds et al., 2006). Further study is needed to understand this situation, as it may be influenced by well-established demographic differences, such as the increased risk of suicide attempts in males with schizophrenia and the tendency for males to use higher lethality methods in suicide attempts.

It is important to consider that not all self-injurious behaviors are suicidal in nature. A suicide attempt is a self-injurious behavior in which the person intends to die and utilizes a method that they believe (correctly or not) to be potentially lethal. This is differentiated from non-suicidal self-injurious behaviors, or parasuicide, in which the person injures themself without the intention of causing death while using methods that they believe will not be lethal. Non-suicidal self-injurious behaviors are more common in people with adjustment and personality disorders.

Cognition, education, and suicide

Cognitive impairments are central in schizophrenia and present in nearly all cases. Higher levels of cognitive impairments are associated with greater disability in everyday functioning, poorer premorbid functioning, and more severe negative symptoms. Interestingly, the theory that greater insight and awareness of illness increases suicide risk would suggest that higher levels of cognitive functioning might confer greater risk for suicide. Research on this question is somewhat divided in its results. Some studies (e.g., Delaney et al., 2012) have found that better cognitive functioning was associated with increased risk for suicide and other studies have found no differences (e.g., Barrett et al., 2011). No studies to date have found that poorer cognitive functioning was associated with increased suicide risk. As a result, cognitive impairment on formal neuropsychological assessment does not provide much reliable information for the prediction of suicide risk.

Another way to index cognitive abilities is to examine the levels of educational attainment on the part of people with schizophrenia. Many people with schizophrenia have reduced attainment compared to their relatives. At the same time, some individuals with schizophrenia complete college and even graduate education, so the illness in no way precludes high levels of achievement in all cases. One of the possible risks associated with high levels of educational attainment is that individuals with this level of attainment are likely to have higher levels of awareness of the implications of their illness and have had exposure to high functioning both on the part of others and themselves. Thus, higher levels of education are likely a moderate risk factor for suicide in people with schizophrenia (Bakst et al., 2009).

A related construct is that of premorbid functioning. Partially overlapping with education, premorbid functioning is indexed in terms of social, educational, and behavioral adjustment prior to the onset of illness. Poorer premorbid functioning is associated with poorer outcome after the onset of illness and is also associated with earlier age of onset. There have been reports suggesting that poorer premorbid functioning is associated with increased risk of suicide (Stephens et al., 1999). This finding seems somewhat paradoxical in the context of reports of higher educational attainment predicting increased suicide risk and requires some closer analysis.

In a large sample of early course patients selected from a national registry of first episode patients followed up about 5 years later, some of these paradoxical questions were partially answered (Bakst et al., 2010). In this sample, the largest single risk factor for a suicide attempt after a first admission to psychiatric care was a previous suicide attempt during or prior to the current episode. However, there were other combinations of risk factors that predicted increased risk. Particularly low levels of educational attainment (failing to complete high school) were associated with a greater suicide risk in females than higher levels of attainment, while quite high levels of educational attainment (greater than college education) were also associated with increased suicide risk (in both genders). Interestingly, in both males and females, high levels of education were associated with increased suicide risk only in the context of some evidence of social dysfunction (never having been married or experiencing an equivalent social relationship). Thus, better intellectual functioning in the context of other functional limitations may interact to increase risk.

There has been considerable recent research on two previously under-researched aspects of schizophrenia: disability and its determinants, including cognitive deficits, and the medical complications of schizophrenia and its treatment, with a specific focus on metabolic syndrome. Disability after diagnosis is the norm in people with schizophrenia, with the majority of cases failing to consistently achieve functional milestones in social, vocational, or residential domains. As disability is often a consequence of cognitive impairments, lower educational attainment, and other aspects of poor premorbid functioning, it might be the case that disability can increase suicide risk through increasing psychosocial stress and isolation.

While this premise seems reasonable in terms of the cascade of risk factors (isolation, stress, poor premorbid functioning), the evidence does not suggest that disability by itself increases suicide risk. Interestingly, receipt of a pension or other disability compensation is associated with reduced suicidality relative to people with schizophrenia in general (Kiviniemi et al., 2011). Thus, reduced financial stress, which also helps to prevent homelessness and other complications of disability, may reduce desperation and lead to reduced suicide risk. As a result, simply failing to achieve functional milestones does not appear to lead to increased suicide risk and receiving compensation is associated with reductions in risk.

Metabolic syndrome, obesity, and suicide

Metabolic syndrome and associated weight changes are common in schizophrenia and are associated with the substantial morbidity and mortality in the illness. In fact, the shortened life expectancy in patients with schizophrenia after the first episode is largely associated with metabolic syndrome and associated cardiac risk (Newcomer & Hennekens, 2007). A number of psychotropic medications used for schizophrenia cause weight gain, and associated complications such as diabetes.

What is less well known is whether obesity and metabolic complications have indirect influences on mortality through increasing suicide risk.

There have been several large epidemiological studies demonstrating an association between obesity and reduced rates of suicide completion in the general population, despite an increased rate of depression among obese individuals (see Magnusson et al., 2006, for a study with more than a million participants). The mechanism of this relationship is not particularly clear, but the consistent replications underscore the validity of these findings. At this time, there is minimal information available to address the issue of whether this same relationship is present in people with schizophrenia, as evidenced by no current publications in the English language psychiatric literature. Further study is needed to understand if these findings extend to the subpopulation of people with schizophrenia. Given the increasing rate of obesity in people with schizophrenia, this would be an easy research question to address.

Protective factors are also important and in the general population may include factors such as duty to family, religious beliefs, fear of dying, or evidence of future planning. These factors may be operative in schizophrenia as well. However, these domains of everyday functioning are areas where people with schizophrenia appear to be additionally disadvantaged. Family relationships are more likely to be strained or fractured than in the general population. Future planning and the ability to anticipate future outcomes, including adverse illness outcomes, are impaired in people with schizophrenia. Thus, typically protective factors in the general population require skills that are impaired in schizophrenia and may be reduced in their potential to truly protect people with schizophrenia. As cognitive impairment appears not be associated with increased suicide risk, it is presently unclear as to whether these deficits in planning and anticipating the future shape suicide risk in people with schizophrenia.

While these risk factors have all been examined in different studies, there was one prospective, randomized study of treatment for suicide in schizophrenia, the International Suicide Prevention Trial (InterSePT). We will describe the results of the intervention study below, but the predictive results of the study are also quite informative (Potkin et al., 2003). Patients (N = 980) were selected for this study on the basis of a history of suicide attempts or persistent suicidal ideation. Historical predictors of increased risk for suicide attempts in a 24-month period were a diagnosis of schizoaffective disorder (as compared to schizophrenia), history or current use at baseline of alcohol or substance abuse, cigarette smoking, the total number of lifetime suicide attempts, and the number of hospitalizations to prevent suicide in the previous 36 months. Predictive clinical features included greater baseline scores on the InterSePT scale for suicidal thinking, the Covi Anxiety Scale, the Calgary Depression Scale (CDS), and severity of parkinsonism. Subsequent multivariate analysis revealed the number of hospitalizations in the previous 36 months, baseline CDS, severity of Parkinson's, history of substance abuse, and lifetime suicide attempts were the best predictors of attempting suicide in the next 24 months. These data are important, because they represent a study of individuals who have survived the early course of their illness despite persistent suicidality. Although older patients with schizophrenia have a slightly reduced risk for suicide compared to first episode patients, the risk for suicide does not go away with time and persistently suicidal patients are still at high risk for completion of suicide.

Pharmacological treatment for suicidality: clozapine in the InterSePT Study

Remarkably, there is a pharmacological treatment approved for suicidality in schizophrenia, clozapine, which is rarely used for this indication and others as well. We will consider reasons for this low rate of use and examine non-pharmacological interventions for schizophrenia. The most effective empirically validated method employed for the reduction of suicide risk in schizophrenia is the successful treatment of psychosis, particularly hallucinations, with antipsychotic medications. There is evidence that treatment of psychosis and other comorbidities in general reduces suicide risk (Hor and Taylor, 2010). In particular, clozapine was approved in 2002 to reduce the risk of recurrent suicidal behaviors in patients with schizophrenia or schizoaffective disorder, based on results of the InterSePT trial. Clozapine has several other well-established benefits, including superiority for positive symptoms (hallucinations and delusions) in treatment-resistant patients, lower risk for tardive dyskinesia and suppression of established tardive dyskinesia, higher quality of life and longer time to discontinuation, and decreased relapse.

The InterSePT trial (Meltzer et al., 2003) was a remarkable achievement and still remains the high water mark for a collaborative study involving the pharmaceutical industry and academia in schizophrenia. In this trial, patients with high suicide risk, including recent hospitalizations for suicide attempts and suicidal ideation, were identified and randomized to treatment with two antipsychotic medications with clear evidence of efficacy for the treatment of psychosis. Patients were randomized to treatment with one of the two treatments and their 2-year course of suicidality was examined. Even with a 5–10% lifetime risk of suicide and 50% suicide attempts, the trial would have been underpowered for the detection of treatment effects on these outcomes. As a result, significant suicidal ideation, judged by a board composed of experienced clinicians, was the outcome measure, along with the other more major outcomes including suicide attempts and suicides.

Patients randomized to clozapine had significantly less suicidal behavior versus olanzapine (hazard ratio, 0.76; 95% confidence interval, 0.58–0.97; P = 0.03). Fewer clozapine-treated patients attempted suicide (34 vs. 55; P = 0.03), and fewer required hospitalizations (82 vs. 107; P = 0.05) or rescue interventions (118 vs. 155; P = 0.01) to prevent suicide. In addition, there was a reduction in concomitant treatment with antidepressants (221 vs. 258; P = 0.01). The US Food and Drug Administration approved clozapine for the treatment of suicidality in schizophrenia, the only such indication ever approved.

Unfortunately, there has been no change in the use of clozapine since the InterSePT study, despite the FDA indication, and the use of this medication is markedly less than would be expected compared to the number of patients who could benefit. Clozapine carries several serious risks which apparently limit its use in clinical practice. There is a 0.7–1% risk of developing agranulocytosis (Honigfeld et al., 1998), a condition in which the number of infection-fighting white blood cells decreases. This condition is generally reversible if identified early and occurs most frequently during the first 6 months of treatment, and thus a mandatory, nationwide system for monitoring has been enacted in the USA. In order to prescribe clozapine, a physician must register with the national clozapine registry. White blood cell counts must be reported to the registry and pharmacy weekly for the first 6 months of treatment, every other week for the second 6 months of treatment, and then monthly for the duration of treatment. While this system allows early detection of changes in white blood cell counts, in practice it creates a significant perceived barrier to treatment. Clozapine carries a risk of metabolic side effects similar to olanzapine and greater than other second-generation antipsychotics. This includes risks of weight gain, hyperlipidemia, and elevations in blood glucose that can lead to diabetes mellitus.

Due to these concerns about safety in addition to the logistical challenges they create, Clozaril is significantly underutilized in clinical practice. In fact, 35–40% of patients with schizophrenia are candidates for Clozaril treatment due to treatment resistance or suicide attempts, yet clozapine has only 4.4% of the market share (Meltzer, 2012). Despite its risks, multiple studies have demonstrated significantly decreased all-cause mortality in patients treated with clozapine, and it is estimated that one-third of the approximately 5000 annual suicide deaths in persons with schizophrenia and schizoaffective disorder could be prevented with the use of clozapine (Meltzer, 2012). When the relative risks of clozapine and suicide are compared to each other, the balance is clearly in support of the use of clozapine. Patient acceptance of clozapine is not the barrier to its use, as previous studies have shown that adherence to clozapine is not lower than for other medications. This underutilization seems more a result of practitioner choices rather than objective evidence regarding the relative cost–benefit of this medication.

Psychotherapy for suicide

Cognitive behavioral therapy (CBT) interventions have shown promise for the treatment of persistent or residual psychotic symptoms in people with schizophrenia. As suicidal ideation is a domain of thinking that is quite relevant to the targets of CBT interventions (persistent, intrusive, troubling), CBT interventions have been tried for suicidal ideation. In a study of 90 chronic patients, CBT was found to reduce suicidal ideation, both immediately and over follow-ups (Bateman et al., 2007). However, in an 18-month study of first episode patients, there was no benefit of CBT on suicidal ideation or attempts (Tarrier et al., 2006). Thus, the evidence for CBT treatments is decidedly mixed and it should certainly not be considered as an effective stand-alone therapy.

Conclusions

Suicidal behavior is a major public health problem and schizophrenia is markedly affected by suicide. Early and continuous monitoring of suicidality is important and high-risk groups are easily identified. Suicide risk is treated in the same way that other symptoms are treated, with antipsychotic medications. Use of clozapine is surprisingly low and the risks of clozapine are less than the risks of suicide. More serious consideration for greater use of clozapine seems to be a consistent suggestion across multiple different sources and despite the fact that suicide risk peaks early, it never completely goes away.

References

Bakst, S., Rabinowitz, J., & Bromet, E. J. (2009). Antecedents and patterns of suicide in first admission psychosis. *Schizophrenia Bulletin*, **36**, 880–889.

Bakst, S., Rabinowitz, J., & Bromet, E. J. (2010). Is poor premorbid functioning a risk factor for suicide attempts in first-admission psychosis? *Schizophrenia Research*, **116**, 210–216.

Barrett, E. A., Sundet, K., Simonsen, C., et al. (2011). Neurocognitive functioning and suicidality in schizophrenia spectrum disorders. *Comprehensive Psychiatry*, **52**, 156–163.

Bateman, K., Hansen, L., Turkington, D., & Kingdon, D. (2007). Cognitive behavioral therapy reduces suicidal ideation in schizophrenia: results from a randomized controlled trial. *Suicide and Life Threatening Behavior*, **37**, 284–290.

Caldwell, C. B., & Gottesman, I. I. (1990). Schizophrenics kill themselves too: a review of risk factors for suicide. *Schizophrenia Bulletin*, **16**, 571–589.

De Hert, M., McKenzie, K., & Peuskens, J. (2001). Risk factors for suicide in young people suffering from schizophrenia: a long-term follow-up study. *Schizophrenia Research*, **47**, 127–134.

Delaney, C., McGrane, J., Cummings, E., et al. (2012). Preserved cognitive function is associated with suicidal ideation and single suicide attempts in schizophrenia. *Schizophrenia Research*, **140**, 232–236.

Fenton, W. S. (2000). Depression, suicide, and suicide prevention in schizophrenia. *Suicide and Life Threatening Behavior*, **30**, 34–49.

Harkavy-Friedman, J. M., Kimhy, D., Nelson, E. A. et al., (2003). Suicide attempts in schizophrenia: the role of command auditory hallucinations for suicide. *Journal of Clinical Psychiatry*, **64**, 871–874.

Harris, E. C., & Barraclough, B. (1997). Suicide as an outcome for mental disorders. A meta-analysis. *British Journal of Psychiatry*, **170**, 205–228.

Hawton, K., Sutton, L., Haw, C., et al. (2005). Schizophrenia and suicide: systematic review of risk factors. *British Journal of Psychiatry*, **187**, 9–20.

Honigfeld, G., Arellano, F., Sethi, J. et al. (1998). Reducing clozapine related morbidity and mortality: 5 years of experience with the Clozaril National Registry. *Journal of Clinical Psychiatry*, **59**(Suppl 3), 3–7.

Hor, K. & Taylor, M. (2010). Suicide and schizophrenia: a systematic review of rates and risk factors. *Journal of Psychopharmacology*, **24** (Supp 4), 81–90.

Kim, C. H., Jayathilake, K., & Meltzer, H. Y. (2003). Hopelessness, neurocognitive function, and insight in schizophrenia: relationship to suicidal behavior. *Schizophrenia Research*, **60**, 71–80.

Kiviniemi, M., Suvisaari, J., Pirkola, S., et al. (2011). Five-year follow-up study of disability pension rates in first-onset schizophrenia with special focus on regional differences and mortality. *General Hospital Psychiatry*, **33**, 509–517.

López-Moríñigo, J. D., Ramos-Ríos, R., David, A. S., et al. (2012). Insight in schizophrenia and risk of suicide: a systematic update. *Comprehensive Psychiatry*, **53**, 313–322.

Magnusson, P. K., Rasmussen, F., Lawlor, D. A., et al. (2006). Association of body mass index with suicide mortality: a prospective cohort study of more than one million men. *American Journal of Epidemiology*, **163**, 1–8.

Mann, J. J. (2002). A current perspective of suicide and attempted suicide. *Annals of Internal Medicine*, **136**, 302–311.

McCabe, K. L., Maloney, E. A., Stain, H. J., et al. (2012). Relationship between childhood adversity and clinical and cognitive features in schizophrenia. *Journal of Psychiatric Research*, **46**, 600–607.

Meltzer, H. Y. (2012). Clozapine: Balancing safety with superior antipsychotic efficacy. *Clinical Schizophrenia & Related Psychoses*, **6**, 134–144.

Meltzer, H. Y., Alphs, L., Green, A. I., et al. (2003). Clozapine treatment for suicidality in schizophrenia: International Suicide Prevention Trial (InterSePT). *Archives of General Psychiatry*, **60**, 82–91.

Miles, C. (1977). Conditions predisposing to suicide: a review. *Journal of Nervous and Mental Disease*, **164**, 231–246.

Newcomer, J., & Hennekens, C. H. (2007). Severe mental illness and risk of cardiovascular disease. *Journal of the American Medical Association*, **298**, 1794–1796.

Nielssen, O., Malhi, G., McGorry, P., et al. (2012). Overview of violence to self and others during the first episode of psychosis. *Journal of Clinical Psychiatry*, **73**, e580–e587.

Palmer, B., Pankratz, V., & Bostwick, J. (2005). The lifetime risk of suicide in schizophrenia: a reexamination. *Archives of General Psychiatry*, **62**, 247–253.

Potkin, S. G., Alphs, L., Hsu, C., et al. (2003). Predicting suicidal risk in schizophrenic and schizoaffective patients in a prospective two-year trial. *Biological Psychiatry*, **54**, 444–452.

Rosenberg, S. D., Lu, W., Mueser, K. T., et al. (2007). Correlates of adverse childhood events among adults with schizophrenia spectrum disorders. *Psychiatric Services*, **58**, 245–253.

Stephens, J. H., Richard, P., & McHugh, P. R. (1999). Suicide in patients hospitalized for schizophrenia: 1913–1940. *Journal of Nervous and Mental Disease*, **187**, 10–14.

Swinson, N., Flynn, S. M., While, D., et al. (2011). Trends in rates of mental illness in homicide perpetrators. *British Journal of Psychiatry*, **198**, 485–489.

Symonds, C. S., Taylor, S., Tippins, V., et al. (2006). Violent self-harm in schizophrenia. *Suicide and Life Threatening Behavior*, **36**, 44–49.

Tarrier, N., Haddock, G., Lewis, S., et al. (2006). Suicide behaviour over 18 months in recent onset schizophrenic patients: the effects of CBT. *Schizophrenia Research*, **83**, 15–27.

West, J. C., Wilk, J. E., Olfson, M., et al. (2005). Patterns and quality of treatment for patients with schizophrenia in routine psychiatric practice. *Psychiatric Services*, **56**, 283–291.

Chapter 13

Personality disorders and suicide

Katharine J. Nelson, Michael J. Miller, Alexandra Zagoloff, Melinda K. Westlund, and S. Charles Schulz

Introduction

Perhaps the most relevant and overlooked consideration in the worldwide effort to end suicide is the role of maladaptive personality or the presence of dysfunctional personality traits. Personality disorders have previously been classified under *Axis II* of the multi-axial diagnostic system as defined by *Diagnostic and Statistical Manual-IV-Text Revision (DSM-IV-TR)* as disorders characterized by an "enduring pattern of inner experience and behavior that deviates markedly from the expectations of the individual's culture, is pervasive and inflexible, has an onset in adolescence or early adulthood, is stable over time, and leads to distress or impairment" (American Psychiatric Association, 2000). In the *Diagnostic and Statistical Manual 5 (DSM5)*, the criteria for personality disorders remained unchanged, although there is no longer a multi-axial system on which to organize diagnoses (American Psychiatric Association, 2013). The discontinuation of Axis II is considered a positive step in the direction of personality disorders treatment, as Axis II was meant to designate conditions that were classically considered untreatable. The consequences of classifying disorders on Axis II included undue stigmatization of patients with these disorders and access to treatment difficulties related to reimbursement and compensation of care.

Personality disorders have long been studied to determine their role in suicidal behavior. A large-scale epidemiologic study examining over 40 000 community participants noted those who received a personality disorder diagnosis using strict criteria were 9.66 times more likely to report history of a suicide attempt (Trull et al., 2010). Additionally, "psychological autopsies" have sought to identify factors that might have contributed to an individual's suicide postmortem. This method consists of retrospective interviews and review of medical records (Arsenault-Lapierre et al., 2004). A meta-analysis of such research included 27 studies for a total of 3275 suicides. Studies included in the meta-analysis were conducted in Europe, North America, Australia, and Asia. Only 14 studies included diagnostic information for both personality and other psychiatric disorders. Of those that included information on personality disorders, 16.2% of the individuals who completed suicide had received a personality disorder diagnosis based on psychological autopsy. There were no differences in rates of personality disorder diagnosis by geographic region. Based on these results, it appears that the role of personality disorders in suicide risk appears consistent worldwide.

The field of study of personality disorders has been faced with controversy over the past decade. In the development of the DSM5, the Personality Disorders workgroup questioned the validity and usefulness of the DSM-IV-TR conceptualization and categorization of personality disorders and proposed a new dimensional analysis of specific personality traits and facets. A description of this proposal is contained within Section III of the DSM5, the section reserved for emerging measures and models (American Psychiatric Association, 2013). No method has been described for translating the existing body of literature which has relied on the current criteria to the new proposed model. Other challenges in the interpretation of personality disorder literature lie in the high rates of comorbidity of personality disorders and other psychiatric diagnoses, which tend to confound available data and are difficult to control in large-scale studies. Additionally, emerging evidence challenges the idea that dysfunctional personality traits or criteria are stable over time or untreatable as once assumed. Nonetheless, this chapter will provide a review of the literature examining the relationship between personality disorders and suicide as currently described in the DSM5 with

A Concise Guide to Understanding Suicide, ed. Stephen H. Koslow, Pedro Ruiz, and Charles B. Nemeroff. Published by Cambridge University Press.

an additional discussion describing the role of specific personality traits as may pertain to proposed changes to personality categorization in future editions.

Cluster B personality disorders

The DSM5 divides personality disorders into three "clusters" based on their similar features. Historically the most relevant and studied group related to suicide has been cluster B, with shared traits described as individuals often appearing "dramatic, emotional, or erratic" and include Borderline Personality Disorder (BPD), Narcissistic Personality Disorder (NPD), Antisocial Personality Disorder (ASPD), and Histrionic Personality Disorder (HPD) (APA, 2013). A 10-year longitudinal study of 49 participants with major depressive disorder (MDD) and suicidal ideation assessed several demographic, psychological, personality, and psychosocial risk factors with the goal of identifying prospective predictors of suicide attempts and found the only unique predictor to be the presence of a comorbid cluster B personality disorder (May et al., 2012). Further inquiry has attempted to identify specific disorders and characteristics within cluster B associated with increased risk for suicide.

Borderline personality disorder

The personality disorder most commonly associated with suicidality is BPD, a heterogeneously presenting disorder commonly characterized by non-suicidal self-injury and suicidality. Other associated features include affective and interpersonal instability, lack of self-identity and cognitive perceptual symptoms including stress-related paranoid ideation (APA, 2013). The prevalence of BPD in the population based on a large-scale epidemiologic study of 34 653 adults is estimated to be around 2.7–5.9% (depending on strictness of criteria applied to the calculation) with equal distribution between men and women. Women are more likely to present for mental health care and appear to be more disabled by the disorder (Trull et al., 2010). Longitudinal studies indicate the disorder is treatable and remitting with low rates of relapse; however social and occupational functioning remain impaired (Zanarini et al., 2012). Based on this evidence, BPD is now being conceptualized as having a better prognosis than previously believed. Despite this evolving optimism, 75% of patients with BPD attempt suicide (Soloff et al., 1994) and 10% of patients with BPD complete suicide; a tragic outcome highlighting the critical need for early identification and treatment (Paris & Zweig-Frank, 2001).

Common comorbidities

Several studies have attempted to examine the relationship between Axis I disorders, mainly major depression, and BPD to explore defining aspects of these disorders related to suicide. A 10-year prospective study examining individuals diagnosed with personality disorders and/or major depression with single versus multiple suicide attempts found a distinguishing feature of participants with multiple suicide attempts to be the presence of BPD and higher impulsivity scores (Boisseau et al., 2013). A study of 81 psychiatric inpatients with BPD, major depression, or both examined suicidal behavior in these three groups and found patients with both major depression and BPD had the greatest number of suicide attempts and objective planning (Soloff et al., 2000). This finding highlights the need to screen for the presence of BPD among depressed patients and provide appropriate treatment which takes into account this important comorbidity.

BPD characteristic associated with suicide

Owing to the high rates of suicide attempts and high lethality associated with BPD, a related field of inquiry has sought to identify particular characteristics of BPD most highly correlated with suicide. The largest and longest running study of longitudinal outcomes for patients with BPD is the McLean Study of Adult Development (MSAD). This study has followed a series of prospective predictors of suicide attempts over 16 years in a sample of 290 patients meeting criteria for BPD using both *Diagnostic and Statistical Manual-III-Revised* and *Revised Diagnostic Interview for Borderlines* (DIB-R) criteria. The participants were assessed every 2 years. Sadly, at the 16-year follow-up point, 13 participants had completed suicide and 13 died of other causes. Variables which emerged as significant in multivariate analyses included a comorbid diagnosis of major depression, substance use, PTSD, non-suicidal self-injury (NSSI), adult sexual assault, caretaker suicide, affective instability, and more severe dissociation. The authors interpreted the results of this study to suggest that the practice of predicting suicide attempts among patients with BPD is difficult and complex. Relevant factors include the presence of comorbidities, co-occurring symptoms of BPD, adversity and a family history of completed suicide (Wedig et al., 2012). This patient sample has also produced data demonstrating high rates of BPD remission and relatively low rates of relapse over the course of the study period (Zanarini et al., 2012).

Non-suicidal self-injury

NSSI and suicidality are both core features of BPD accomplishing different behavioral functions, although, distinguishing these two behaviors can be difficult due to frequent comorbidity. NSSI appears to double the risk of suicide and may be potentially life-threatening, even in the absence of motivation to die. NSSI may take the form of cutting, head-banging, scratching, burning, or ingestion and generally occurs in the context of emotional crisis. Consequences of NSSI include disfigurement, injury, disability, or accidental death (i.e., cutting too deeply and severing an artery) (Black et al., 2004). In a study examining self-reported reasons for suicide attempts versus NSSI in patients with BPD, Brown et al. (2002) identified a significant association with the report of suicide attempters wanting to "make others better off." NSSI was associated with reports of wanting to "express anger, punish oneself, generate normal feelings, and distract oneself." These studies highlight the importance of differentiating the motivation and psychopathology underlying NSSI and behaviors with suicidal intent to identify treatment targets to decrease the risk of both of these serious behavioral symptoms of BPD.

Biological underpinnings

In addition to studies examining characteristics and correlates of suicidal behavior in BPD, several studies have sought to determine the neurobiological underpinnings of this disorder. New and colleagues (New et al., 2012) conducted a review of current structural and functional neuroimaging, neurochemical markers, and genetic studies relevant to BPD symptomatology. Although, like many other psychiatric disorders, there is no clear pathophysiological pattern, some consistent findings may serve as an early foundation to better understanding this disorder. BPD is proposed to arise from the lack of medial prefrontal control of overactive limbic structures. This results in an unmodulated fear response, primarily in response to interpersonal prompts. Specific findings relative to suicide include one study in adolescents that identified a negative correlation with anterior cingulate gyrus (ACG) volume with the number of suicide attempts and BPD symptoms severity. This correlation was not shown with depressive symptoms. This study suggests ACG volume reduction is present early and specific to BPD. Soloff et al. (2012) examined adults with BPD versus healthy controls and found structural abnormalities in the brain which discriminated participants with BPD and a history of suicide attempts from those without prior suicide attempts. Abnormalities were also present which separated high from low lethality attempters. New et al. (2012) also reviewed studies examining cerebrospinal fluid metabolite abnormalities in serotonin levels and noted this finding was more consistent generally in individuals with a history of suicide attempts or impulsive aggressive behavior. Other studies have examined the role of endogenous opioids and propose that patients with BPD have an intrinsic opioid deficit which explains the symptoms of NSSI which may prompt endogenous opioid release during self-injury behaviors.

Adolescents and BPD

Despite the fact that DSM5 allows for the diagnosis of BPD when the adolescent meets criteria for more than a year (APA, 2013), BPD, like other personality disorders, is not considered a viable diagnosis for adolescents by many psychiatric providers. Instead, providers frequently write "deferred" or "borderline features" when considering a personality disorder diagnosis. This leads to BPD being underdiagnosed in adolescents leading to a lack of accurate study of the early end of the longitudinal course of the disorder. More distressing is the lack of treatment that these individuals receive due to the inaccurate diagnosis leading to years of suffering with maladaptive and self-destructive behaviors (Aguirre, 2012).

Evidence from Miller et al. (2008) clearly shows that BPD can reliably be diagnosed in adolescence. Crick et al. (2005) showed that the symptoms of adolescent girls are similar to that of adults with BPD, while adolescent males meeting BPD criteria are more aggressive, disruptive, and antisocial. At the same time, other studies show that the diagnosis is not necessarily reliable over time. In a 2-year follow-up study in Australia a prospective study found that only 40% of adolescents aged 15–18 with BPD met criteria at the follow-up point (Chanen et al., 2004). Similar to the adult data indicating the natural course of this disorder in remission, a community sample looked at symptoms at 2- and 3-year intervals from age 14 to 24 in adolescent twins with BPD. The results showed that there was a steady decrease in the symptoms at each study interval in the 10-year follow-up (Bornovalova et al., 2009).

The neuropsychological findings of executive functioning impairments suggestive of decreased frontal processing in adult BPD patients (LeGris & van Reekum, 2006) have never been systematically examined in adolescents. These deficits are consistent with the behavioral pattern of BPD that includes poor planning abilities, impulsivity, and increased difficulty in emotion regulation. Adolescents have developmentally determined deficits in areas of executive functioning, putting adolescents with BPD at greater risk of impulsive behavior. These deficits lead to behaviors such as substance abuse, impulsive aggression, and other maladaptive coping strategies to deal with the emotional imbalance. All of these data suggest that although BPD is a controversial diagnosis in adolescence, it still is consistent with the adult population and earlier intervention is warranted.

Treatment

Historically, patients with BPD have faced tremendous stigma due to the perception that this disorder was treatment non-responsive and individuals with BPD were viewed as being problematic by nature. More recent work in developing effective and evidence-based therapies for BPD has started to shift perceptions and improve the prognosis. The most widely studied psychotherapeutic treatment for BPD is dialectical behavioral therapy (DBT). DBT was developed by Marsha Linehan, PhD, originally as a cognitive behavioral treatment for patients with "parasuicidal" behavior. DBT has been shown to significantly reduce rates of suicidality and NSSI for both adult and adolescent patients with BPD. Other therapies demonstrating positive outcomes for the treatment of BPD include mentalization-based therapy, systems training for emotional predictability and problem solving, and schema-focused therapy. Early evidence for pharmacotherapeutic strategies for symptom-domain targeted treatment has also been described (Nelson & Schulz, 2012).

Histrionic personality disorder

Histrionic personality disorder (HPD) falls into Cluster B and is described as a pattern of "pervasive and excessive emotionality and attention seeking" (APA, 2013). Prevalence estimates of this disorder in the general population range from 0.3 to 1.8%, HPD is more likely to be diagnosed in women, and is associated with high rates of comorbidity with alcohol and drug dependence (Trull et al., 2010). HPD is relatively understudied compared to BPD and even less is known about the risk of suicide in this population.

Narcissistic personality disorder

NPD falls into Cluster B and is described as a pattern of "grandiosity, need for admiration, and lack of empathy" (APA, 2013). Prevalence estimates of this disorder in the general population range from 1 to 6.2% with more frequent diagnosis in men (Trull et al., 2010). Narcissism as a trait predates the current medical classifications. It is based on the Greek myth of Narcissus who loved his own reflection in a lake to the degree that he eventually died because he could not remove himself from viewing his own image. In psychiatry, the term has been used to focus on a group of individuals who experience a cluster of symptoms including excessive vanity and self-centeredness. Otto Kernberg introduced the concept of the "narcissistic personality structure" in 1967; and the personality disorder was proposed by Heinz Kohut in 1968 to define this group of patients.

Researchers agree that while suicide is a clinically significant issue for individuals with NPD, there currently are no reliable data on the actual number of individuals with narcissistic personality disorder who commit suicide. The only current research on the topic is by Blasco-Fontecilla et al. (2009) that looked at the impulsivity of NPD individuals and whether they differed in their profile from both controls and other personality disorders. They found that individuals with NPD are not more impulsive than those with other personality disorders, but they are more lethal than other suicide attempters in this population. This may be an artifact of the preponderance of males with NPD, being anywhere from 50% to 75% of the total number of diagnoses, and that males have been shown to be more lethal in their suicide attempts.

Antisocial personality disorder

ASPD falls into cluster B and is described as a pattern of "disregard for, and violation of, the rights of others" (APA, 2013). Prevalence of this disorder in the general population is estimated to be around 3.8% of the population with more frequent diagnosis in men (Trull et al., 2010). Verona et al. (2001) investigated the relationship between suicide attempts and antisocial tendencies among incarcerated male offenders. Offenders diagnosed with ASPD were significantly more likely to have a history of suicidal behaviors than those without the diagnosis. Results indicated that impulsive/antisocial behavior, but not affective/interpersonal symptoms, was a significant predictor of suicide attempt. The authors noted that they did not gather detailed information of suicide history which made it impossible to determine what percentage of attempts were "manipulative" versus "genuine" and that such a distinction may be important when studying the relationship between suicide and psychopathy. The relationships among antisocial behavior, negative emotionality (anxiousness, neuroticism, alienation, hostility), constraint (impulsivity, sensation seeking, socialization, psychoticism), and suicide suggest the presence of a basic predisposition toward destructive, self-damaging interests. The authors suggest future studies are needed to compare the suicidal acts of individuals diagnosed with ASPD versus major depression with respect to mood state, method, and degree of planning to evaluate the roles of impulsivity and negative affect.

Cluster A personality disorders

Cluster A is characterized by the DSM5 (APA, 2013) as having shared traits described as individuals often appearing "odd or eccentric" and include schizotypal personality disorder (StPD) (0.6–3.9% prevalence), schizoid personality disorder (SPD) (0.6–3.1% prevalence), and paranoid personality disorder (PPD) (1.9–4.4% prevalence) (Trull et al., 2010). These disorders are relatively understudied compared to Cluster B. Lentz et al. (2010) analyzed data from a large epidemiological survey with particular attention to StPD. After controlling for demographic variables and other psychiatric and personality disorder diagnoses, individuals with StPD were 1.5 times more likely than those without the diagnosis to attempt suicide. While men with StPD were significantly more likely to attempt suicide than men without this diagnosis, this difference was non-significant for women. After controlling for childhood adversity (abuse, violence, neglect, assault), the relationship between StPD and suicide attempts was reduced but remained significant. Taken together, these results indicate that clinicians working with individuals with a diagnosis of StPD should remain vigilant to factors associated with suicide risk.

Cluster C personality disorders

Cluster C is characterized by the DSM5 (APA, 2013) as having shared traits described as individuals often appearing "anxious or fearful" and include avoidant personality disorder (APD) (1.2–2.4% prevalence), obsessive-compulsive personality disorder (OCPD) (1.9–7.9% prevalence), and paranoid personality disorder (PPD) (1.9–4.4% prevalence) (Trull et al., 2010). While the majority of the literature investigating suicidal behavior and personality disorders focuses on cluster B, the rigidity and lack of coping mechanisms associated with cluster C may present significant risk factors (Diaconu & Turecki, 2009). These authors note that cluster C comorbidity is a poor prognostic indicator for recovery from a major depressive episode and they focused their study on OCPD since it is the most prevalent cluster C diagnosis. Among the 311 outpatients included, 31 received comorbid diagnoses of OCPD and a depressive disorder. They were compared with depressed individuals without a personality disorder diagnosis and outpatients without depressive or personality disorder diagnoses. While only 46% of the latter two groups reported significant current or lifetime suicidal ideation, 77% of the OCPD group endorsed suicidality. Fifty-two percent of the OCPD group had attempted suicide, which was higher than the depressed and non-depressed groups (38% and 24%, respectively). The rate of multiple suicide attempts for the OCPD group was three times higher than that of the non-depressed group. The OCPD group, compared with the non-depressed group, had significantly fewer reasons for living, ruminated more about death and dying, paid less attention to external disapproval and fear of suicide, and had fewer coping beliefs and a lower moral objection to suicide. The results of this study indicate that suicide risk is affected by cluster C traits in addition to those of cluster B. Additionally, anxiety is often conceptualized as protective against suicide risk, but these results suggest that the anxious traits associated with OCPD are risk factors. In contrast to cluster B disorders which wax and wane, cluster C disorders are relatively stable which might suggest a need to investigate these conditions among geriatric populations. Finally, this research was conducted with individuals who *attempted* suicide, and the role of cluster C traits in *completed* suicides requires additional attention.

Longitudinal findings

The Collaborative Longitudinal Personality Disorders Study (CLPS; Skodol et al., 2005) gathered a wealth of information related to the comorbidities, antecedents, course, and impact of personality disorders. Study participants included individuals diagnosed with StPD, BPD, APD, and OCPD. These disorders were selected based upon psychobiology, prevalence rates, and theoretical frameworks. Individuals diagnosed with MDD were chosen as the comparison group based on its episodic course, prevalence, and available data regarding its phenomenology and course. The total sample size was composed as follows: StPD = 13%, BPD = 26%, APD = 24%, OCPD = 23%, MDD = 14%. Nine percent of participants reported at least one suicide attempt within the first 2 years of follow-up and 44% of these reported multiple suicidal behaviors. After controlling for baseline BPD diagnosis, suicide attempts were significantly predicted by worsening of MDD and substance use disorders (SUDs). After excluding self-injury, the BPD criteria of affective instability, identity disturbance, and impulsivity were significant predictors of suicidal behaviors. Suicide attempts (behavior with intent to die) were significantly associated with affective instability and childhood sexual abuse. At the 3-year follow-up, 12% of the personality disorder participants had attempted suicide. Negative life events, especially those related to love/marriage and legal matters, were significant predictors of attempts after controlling for childhood sexual abuse and baseline diagnoses of BPD, MDD, and SUDs.

DSM5 emerging models of personality traits

Proposed changes to the classification and diagnosis of personality disorders have been included in Section III of the DSM5. The proposed new model suggests personality disorder diagnosis be based on significant impairment in both self- and interpersonal functioning. Impairment in self-functioning would include difficulties in self-identification, whereas impairment in interpersonal functioning would involve deficits in forming close relationships and taking the perspective of another. An individual also must have personality traits within one of five areas that are deemed pathological. These traits include disinhibition, antagonism, negative affectivity, detachment, and psychoticism and are further broken down into several sub-traits (APA, 2013). Given the current literature, this proposition may be of relevance to the understanding of psychopathology and suicidal behaviors. In order to incorporate this perspective, the involvement of specific personality traits in suicidal behavior is reviewed.

Research has associated certain specific personality *traits* with suicidality, NSSI, suicidal ideation, suicide attempts, and completed suicide. In a comprehensive review by Brezo et al., (2006), personality traits are examined in the context of suicidal ideation, attempts, and completions. Regarding suicidal ideation, hopelessness appears to have a predominant association along with neuroticism, psychoticism, aggression, and introversion. Introversion is also higher among those who attempt suicide, which has been found across age and diagnosis. Furthermore, impulsivity and hostility appear to be present among suicide *attempters*, whereas traits associated with *completed* suicide include hopelessness, impulsivity, and neuroticism. These findings presented by Brezo and colleagues were further corroborated by a more recent review by Courtet et al. (2011) which described the traits of impulsivity and aggression as being endophenotypes of suicidal behaviors. These traits have also been linked with serotonin dysfunction, which is also related to disadvantageous decision-making. The information presented by Courtet and colleagues highlights the importance of recognizing that suicidal behaviors, which are linked with certain personality traits, may have a heritable neurobiological component that is worth examining in the context of intervention and prevention.

Research has also examined the association between personality traits and suicide among more focused populations such as those with personality disorders. In a longitudinal study involving individuals with personality disorders, Yen et al. (2009) examined suicide attempts and the possible influence of negative affectivity and disinhibition, which are two of the five personality traits proposed by the DSM-5 workforce (Skodol, 2012). Compared to disinhibition and the multiple facets of impulsivity, negative affectivity was found to be a more robust predictor of suicide attempts. Lack of premeditation was the only facet of impulsivity found to be significant in the prediction of suicide attempts.

Although Yen and colleagues (2009) did not find a large amount of evidence regarding the role of impulsivity in suicidal behaviors, other studies have found a more promising link between this trait and suicide. Lynam et al. (2011) examined the relationship between suicidal behaviors and four traits related to impulsivity – lack of perseverance, lack of premeditation, negative urgency and sensation seeking – among patients with both borderline personality and substance use disorders. The impulsivity-related traits, with the exception of sensation seeking, were found to be related to both suicidal injury and NSSI. The largest effect sizes were found with the lack of premeditation and negative urgency and individuals possessing high levels of both of these traits were at an even greater risk of suicidal behaviors. The finding by Lynam and colleagues regarding lack of premeditation are well aligned with that by Yen et al., and also demonstrates the importance of conceptualizing broader traits as being multi-faceted and consisting of several sub-traits.

The personality trait of impulsivity is perhaps the most well studied in terms of its influence on suicidal behavior in both the general and BPD population. However, further research should examine this trait, as well as others such as aggression and negative affectivity, within other personality disorder diagnoses. Additionally, caution must be exercised regarding the generalization of findings between men and women as risk and protective traits may be different between genders.

Understanding the presence and influence of personality disorders and pathological personality traits is essential for the identification of patients who are at high risk for suicidal behavior and may also be helpful in the development of individualized treatment strategies.

References

Aguirre, B. (2012). Borderline personality disorder in adolescents. *Psychiatric Times*, **29**(5), 22–24.

American Psychiatric Association (APA). (Ed.). (2000). *Diagnostic and Statistical Manual of Mental Disorders*, 4th edn, Text Revision. Washington, DC: American Psychiatric Association.

American Psychiatric Association (APA). (2013). *Diagnostic and Statistical Manual of Mental Disorders*, 5th edn. Washington, DC: American Psychiatric Publishing.

Arsenault-Lapierre, G., Kim, C., & Turecki, G. (2004). Psychiatric diagnoses in 3275 suicides: A meta-analysis. *BMC Psychiatry*, **4**(37), 1–11.

Black, D. W., Blum, N., Pfohl, B., & Hale, N. (2004). Suicidal behavior in borderline personality disorder: prevalence, risk factors, prediction, and prevention. *Journal of Personality Disorders*, **18**(3), 226–239.

Blasco-Fontecilla, H., Baca-Garcia, E., Dervic, K., et al. (2009). Specific features of suicidal behavior in patients with narcissistic personality disorder. *The Journal of Clinical Psychiatry*, **70**(11), 1583–1587.

Boisseau, C. L., Yen, S., Markowitz, J. C., et al. (2013). Individuals with single versus multiple suicide attempts over 10 years of prospective follow-up. *Comprehensive Psychiatry*, **54**(3), 238–242.

Bornovalova, M. A., Hicks, B. M., Iacono, W. G., & McGue, M. (2009). Stability, change, and heritability of borderline personality disorder traits from adolescence to adulthood: a longitudinal twin study. *Developmental Psychopathology*, **21**, 1335–1353.

Brezo, J., Paris, J., and Turecki, G. (2006). Personality traits as correlates of suicidal ideation, suicide attempts, and suicide completions: A systematic review. *Acta Psychiatrica Scandinavica*, **113**, 180–206.

Brown, M. Z., Comtois, K. A., & Linehan, M. M. (2002). Reasons for suicide attempts and nonsuicidal self-injury in women with borderline personality disorder. *Journal of Abnormal Psychology*, **111**(1), 198–202.

Chanen, A. M., Jackson, H. J., McGorry, P. D., et al. (2004). Two-year stability of personality disorder in older adolescent outpatients. *Journal of Personality Disorders*, **18**, 526–541.

Courtet, P., Gottesman, I. I., Jollant, F., & Gould, T. D. (2011). The neuroscience of suicidal behaviors: What can we expect from endophenotype strategies? *Translational Psychiatry*, 1.

Crick, N. R., Murray-Close, D., & Woods, K. (2005). Borderline personality features in childhood: A short-term longitudinal study. *Developmental Psychopathology*, **17**(1), 551–570.

Diaconu, G., & Turecki, G. (2009). Obsessive-compulsive personality disorder and suicidal behavior: Evidence for a positive association in a sample of depressed patients. *Journal of Clinical Psychiatry*, **70**(11), 1551–1556.

LeGris, J., & van Reekum, R. (2006). The neuropsychological correlates of borderline personality disorder and suicidal behaviour. *Canadian Journal of Psychiatry*, **51**, 131–142.

Lentz, V., Robinson, J., & Bolton, J. M. (2010). Childhood adversity, mental disorder comorbidity, and suicidal behavior in schizotypal personality disorder. *Journal of Nervous and Mental Disorders*, **198**, 795–801.

Lynam, D. R., Miller, J. D., Miller, D. J., Bornovalova, M. A., & Lejuez, C. W. (2011). Testing the relations between impulsivity-related traits, suicidality, and nonsuicidal self-injury: A test of the incremental validity of the UPPS model. *Personality Disorders: Theory, Research, and Treatment*, **2**, 151–160.

May, A. M., Klonsky, E. D., & Klein, D. N. (2012). Predicting future suicide attempts among depressed suicide ideators:

a 10-year longitudinal study. *Journal of Psychiatric Research*, **46**(7), 946–952.

Miller, A. L., Muehlenkamp, J. J., & Jacobson, C. M. (2008). Fact or fiction: Diagnosing borderline personality disorder in adolescents. *Clinical Psychology Review*, **28**, 969–981.

Nelson, K. J., & Schulz, S. C. (2012). Treatment advances in borderline personality disorder. *Psychiatric Annals*, **42**(2), 59–64.

New, A. S., Perez-Rodriguez, M., & Ripoll, L. H. (2012). Neuroimaging and borderline personality disorder. *Psychiatric Annals*, **42**(2), 65–71.

Paris, J., & Zweig-Frank, H. (2001). A 27-year follow-up of patients with borderline personality disorder. *Comprehensive Psychiatry*, **42**(6), 482–487.

Skodol, A. E. (2012). Personality disorders in DSM-5. *Annual Review of Clinical Psychology*, **8**, 317–344.

Skodol, A. E., Gunderson, J. G., Shea, M. T., et al. (2005). The Collaborative Longitudinal Personality Disorders Study (CLPS): Overview and implications. *Journal of Personality Disorders*, **19**(5), 487–504.

Soloff, P. H., Lis, J. A., Kelly, T., Cornelius, J., & Ulrich, R. (1994). Risk factors for suicidal behavior in borderline personality disorder. *American Journal of Psychiatry*, **151**(9), 1316–1323.

Soloff, P. H., Lynch, K. G., Kelly, T. M., Malone, K. M., & Mann, J. J. (2000). Characteristics of suicide attempts of patients with major depressive episode and borderline personality disorder: A comparative study. *American Journal of Psychiatry*, **157**, 601–608.

Soloff, P. H., Pruitt, P., Sharma, M., et al. (2012). Structural brain abnormalities and suicidal behavior in borderline personality disorder. *Journal of Psychiatric Research*, **46**(4), 516–525.

Trull, T. J., Jahng, S., Tomko, R. L., Wood, P. K., & Sher, K. J. (2010). Revised NESARC personality disorder diagnoses: gender, prevalence, and comorbidity with substance dependence disorders. *Journal of Personality Disorders*, **24**(4), 412–426.

Verona, E., Patrick, C. J., & Joiner, T. E. (2001). Psychopathy, antisocial personality, and suicide risk. *Journal of Abnormal Psychology*, **110**(3), 462–470.

Wedig, M. M., Silverman, M. H., Frankenburg, F. R., et al. (2012). Predictors of suicide attempts in patients with borderline personality disorder over 16 years of prospective follow-up. *Psychological Medicine*, **42**(11), 2395–2404.

Yen, S., Shea, M. T., Sanislow, C. A., et al. (2009). Personality traits as prospective predictors of suicide attempts. *Acta Psychiatrica Scandinavica*, **120**, 222–229.

Zanarini, M. C., Frankenburg, F. R., Reich, D. B., & Fitzmaurice, G. (2012). Attainment and stability of sustained symptomatic remission and recovery among patients with borderline personality disorder and Axis II comparison subjects: A 16-year prospective follow-up study. *American Journal of Psychiatry*, **169**, 476–483.

Chapter 14

Suicide and substance use disorders

Timothy W. Lineberry and Kathleen T. Brady

Overview

Suicide is a worldwide public health problem with far-reaching consequences. In the USA, conservative estimates are that over one million individuals per year attempt suicide and nearly 40 000 individuals died by suicide in 2010 (NSDUH, 2012). The causes of suicide are multi-factorial with genetic, biological, personality, diagnostic, and cultural factors involved in suicidal behavior and death by suicide.

At the individual level, the relationship between substance use disorders (SUDs), suicidal thoughts, and suicidal behavior is an important one. SUDs have long been recognized as an important risk factor for suicidal behaviors (Cornelius et al., 1996; Mino et al., 1999; Sher et al., 2005). It is likely that there are common predisposing factors for suicidality and SUDs (e.g., trauma and victimization), neurobiologic connections between the two, and both short- and long-term psychosocial consequences of SUDs are associated with increased rates of suicidal behavior and suicide. SUDs have varying effects over the lifespan based on associated developmental tasks, biological changes, and the natural history of addictive disorders. Even in individuals who do not have an established substance use diagnosis, acute intoxication with substances can be associated with impulsivity and impaired judgment facilitating suicidal behavior and completed suicide in at risk individuals. At a societal level, substance use patterns may impact suicide rates, as seen in Russia where increases in alcohol availability and consumption in the 1980s and 1990s was associated with an increase in completed suicides (Nemtsov, 2003).

Prevalence

In general, individuals with SUDs are 10 times more likely to die by suicide (Wilcox et al., 2004). In a large population-based study using the Danish Psychiatric Case Register from 1973 to 1993, the highest relative risks for unnatural causes of death were associated with drug use disorders (Hiroeh et al., 2001). Those with drug use disorders alone were at the highest risk for suicide death while those with drug or alcohol use disorders were at highest risk for accidental death. The 2010 United States National Household Survey found that adults (18 or older) with a SUD were four times more likely to have had serious thoughts of suicide and to have made a suicide attempt in the past year compared to those without a SUD (NSDUH, 2012) (see Table 14.1). As shown in Table 14.1, suicidal ideation, planning, attempts, and completed suicides are seen at much higher rates in those with an SUD. This association has been found in studies focused on the general population, outpatient and inpatient treatment samples, and across all substances of abuse.

Explanatory models and substance use – suicide connection

The combination of an affective disorder and/or a SUD is particularly concerning for suicidal behavior and suicide at population levels (Harris & Barraclough, 1997; Inskip et al., 1998; Hiroeh et al., 2001). Both affective disorders and SUDs are independently associated with suicidal thoughts, plans, and completed suicide (Nock et al., 2009a).

From an individual perspective, suicide risk fluctuates over time and is dependent on psychosocial stressors, loss and shame, and illness course. Worsening symptoms of an affective disorder, relapse to substance use, and severity of illness are all factors potentially associated with development of/or exacerbation of suicidal thoughts and behaviors. Treatment setting also appears to denote different levels of risk, particularly for those who have required hospital-level care (Bostwick & Pankratz, 2000).

A Concise Guide to Understanding Suicide, ed. Stephen H. Koslow, Pedro Ruiz, and Charles B. Nemeroff. Published by Cambridge University Press.

Table 14.1.

	Ideation	Planning	Attempt	Suicide
Adults 18 or older Substance Dependence or Abuse Past Year (NSDUH) (SAMHSA, 2012)	SUD 12.2% No SUD 3.0% *(serious thoughts)	SUD 3.1% No SUD 0.9%	SUD 1.7% No SUD 0.4% (past year)	
Adolescents (15–19 years) with substance dependence receiving residential addiction treatment (Deykin & Buka, 1994)	Females: 75% Males: 40.3% (lifetime)		Females: 60.5% Males: 28.1% (lifetime)	
Meta-analysis of suicide autopsy data by individual diagnosis present (Bertolote et al., 2004)				18% of total deaths had substance use disorder
Community study of alcohol dependence			24% lifetime attempts vs. 5% with other psychiatric disorders	
Depressed with alcohol dependence (hospitalized) (Cornelius et al., 1997)			40% attempted in the week prior 70% lifetime	
Current or historic methadone maintenance vs.controls (Frederick et al., 1973)			16–18 times more likely to have attempted suicide	
Heroin dependence			14 times more likely to have attempted suicide	
Methamphetamine dependence in treatment			Females: 28% Males: 13% (lifetime)	

In individuals with SUDs alone or a comorbid SUD/psychiatric disorder, acute effects of intoxication may facilitate suicidal thoughts and behavior or chronic effects of substance use, which may promote impulsivity and decreased executive function (Scott et al., 2007). Epidemiologic data show that the transition from thoughts of suicide in affective disorders to actual planning and subsequent impulsive or planned suicide attempts is mediated by anxiety and impulse control disorders, including SUDs (Nock et al., 2009b). Clinically, intoxication or the anxiety and agitation associated with craving and early recovery may be critical factors associated with transitions to active suicidal behavior.

An active SUD may exacerbate symptom severity and lead to medication non-compliance or other behaviors that are associated with poor symptom management of a comorbid disorder (e.g., affective and psychotic disorders) associated with suicide. Finally, the hopelessness associated with psychosocial losses that often accompany SUDs, including occupational problems and lost relationships, can be a critical suicide risk factor.

A developmental approach can be helpful in integrating substance use-related issues over the lifespan. Recent research findings have reinforced the clinical wisdom that suicide attempts in adolescents are much less likely to be planned (Nock et al., 2013). The effect of intoxication on decreasing impulse control in adolescents who are at risk for impulsive suicide attempts is concerning. With onset of affective disorders and psychosis in adolescents and young adults, the convergence of the risk for suicide associated with the comorbid psychiatric illness and the use of disinhibiting substances may be more pronounced and dangerous. Later in life, the cumulative consequences of many years of damaging substance use, including occupational, financial and relationship failures, can lead to hopelessness about recovery and increased suicidal thoughts and behavior. In an interesting study of age-related patterns associated with completed suicide in alcohol-dependent men, younger victims had early onset alcohol dependence, unemployment, and recent separation from a domestic partner while older victims were more likely to have a mood disorder and serious medical illness (Conner et al., 1999).

Neurobiologic connections

A growing body of evidence from basic science and translational studies implicates common neurobiological pathways and abnormalities involved in SUDs and a number of psychiatric disorders that are associated with suicidal behavior. Within a neurobiological framework, it is possible that SUDs and suicidal behavior disorders are different symptomatic expressions of similar pre-existing neurobiological abnormalities and/or that repeated drug administration, through neuroadaptation, leads to biological changes that may predispose to suicidal behavior. For example, multiple lines of evidence suggest an association between low serotonin, impulsive and aggressive behavior, alcohol dependence, and suicidal behavior. Acute alcohol consumption can increase serotonin release, but chronic consumption is associated with serotonin deficits. Alcohol-dependent individuals have lower levels of serotonin metabolites (5-HIAA) in the cerebrospinal fluid (CSF) compared to controls (Ratsma et al., 2002) and the 5-HIAA levels are lower in high lethality, depressed, alcohol-dependent suicide attempters as compared to low-lethality attempters (Sher et al., 2007). In other studies, an inverse relationship between impulsive, aggressive behavior and CSF 5-HIAA in violent offenders has been demonstrated leading to a postulated "low serotonin syndrome" in which acute alcohol consumption may provide some relief of dysphoria related to low serotonin levels, but with chronic consumption there is a combination of enhanced dysphoria and disinhibition and an associated increased risk for impulsive aggression (Linnoila & Virkkunen, 1992). Abnormalities of the dopaminergic system are also associated with both SUDs and pathologic aggression (Chen et al., 2005). It has been demonstrated that CSF levels of dopaminergic metabolites are decreased in individuals with a suicide attempt compared to controls (Engstrom et al., 1999; Sher et al., 2006). Therefore, dopaminergic and/or serotonergic dysfunction may predispose to impulsive, aggressive behavior. In addition, alcohol and drug dependence can cause abnormalities in these systems that can exacerbate suicidal, impulsive, and aggressive behavior leading to a cycle, which can escalate both the substance use and the suicidal behavior.

Clinical characteristics

A number of investigations have focused on risk factors for suicidal thoughts and behavior in the general population. Depression, a history of sexual/physical victimization, family dysfunction, serious medical illness, and social isolation/dysfunction are all associated with suicidal behavior in the general population. A number of studies have identified these same risk factors for suicidal behavior in individuals with SUDs (Conner et al., 1999; Rossow, 2000; Darke & Ross, 2002; Roy, 2003; Glasner-Edwards et al., 2010). Of importance, however, is the fact that studies have also demonstrated the extremely high prevalence of these risk factors in individuals with SUDs. A number of epidemiologic studies have demonstrated that individuals with SUDs are more likely to have an affective disorder as compared to the general population (Kessler et al., 1994; Grant et al., 2004). Childhood sexual and physical victimization are much more common in individuals with SUDs as compared to the general population (Kilpatrick et al., 1998; Kendler et al., 2000). Family discord, job loss, and social isolation are also common in the lives of individuals with SUDs. Of interest, studies have found that among substance users, polysubstance use and severity of addiction are associated with suicidal behavior (Darke & Ross, 2002). A recent study of individuals entering addiction treatment (N = 5892) found that those who endorsed a suicide attempt were more likely to have depression and a history of sexual or physical abuse as compared to those who had an unintentional, non-fatal overdose (Bohnert et al., 2011).

In conclusion, while the risk factors for suicide do not fundamentally differ for individuals with SUDs, the fact that these risk factors are so commonly found in individuals with SUDs makes screening for suicidality in this population critical.

Assessment

Because of the known associations between SUDs and suicidal behavior, individuals with SUDs, whether presenting in the emergency room, primary care, SUD or psychiatric treatment setting, must be carefully screened for suicidal thoughts and behaviors. Assessment of suicide risk should be incorporated within all clinical interviews with a careful initial assessment of past suicidal behavior, family history of suicide and suicidal ideation, plans, and intent. Past suicide attempts are one of the strongest predictors of a future suicide attempt (Oquendo et al., 2002; Joiner, 2005). Sleep problems and alcohol misuse, often ubiquitous in presentations in this clinical group, have been shown prospectively to be associated with completed suicide. Standardizing assessment with brief evidence-based self-report scales enhances assessment. Use standardized depression rating scales such as the PHQ-9 (Wittkampf et al., 2007) and BDI-II (Dum et al., 2008) at initial assessment and to monitor response. The Suicide Status Form-II (Jobes et al., 1997; Conrad et al., 2009) is a helpful assessment tool incorporating qualitative and quantitative assessment of factors associated with suicide including hopelessness, self-hate, psychological pain, and the patient's own rating of their risk of suicide. Patients should be asked about access to lethal means and specifically, about access to firearms along with providing recommendations about safe storage or removal.

Treatment/prevention

Individuals with SUDs who commit suicide often see a physician or other treatment care provider in the months prior to their death (Sher et al., 2001, 2006). Clinicians in primary care settings are more likely to see individuals at risk for suicide at their last contact versus mental health professionals. Clinically, if patients have exacerbation or recurrence of symptoms of depression, anxiety disorders or SUDs, or pronounced psychosocial stressors, suicide risk should be reassessed and monitored until resolve of symptoms. Particularly concerning periods of risk include change in physicians and discharge from inpatient treatment to outpatient care.

The use of crisis safety planning intervention may be particularly helpful in formalizing and developing coping tactics for patients in suicidal crises (Stanley & Brown, 2012). As opposed to "contracting for safety," a written agreement in which a patient "agrees" to not hurt themselves and is not evidence based nor recommended, crisis safety planning intervention outlines a response in the event of suicidal crisis. Starting first with interventions the patient can make, the plan also includes patient-derived contact points for support and plans to restrict access to means for suicide. If the clinician does not feel comfortable with the patient's level of risk, the patient should be referred to an appropriate service. Patients can be at higher risk of attempting suicide when intoxicated, so a suicidal, intoxicated individual should be kept under observation. Often, the suicidality is transient and will pass when the individual is no longer intoxicated. Observation facilities associated with emergency rooms can be useful and less costly than hospitalization, but holding suicidal individuals in a busy emergency room can be dangerous and challenging for staff. This is a difficult and unresolved issue for many mental health care providers in emergency room settings as well as emergency room personnel.

For individuals with suicidal thoughts who are not an imminent threat for suicide, close follow-up with continuous assessment of risk factors should be arranged. Firearms should be removed from the homes and medications should be prescribed with caution and carefully monitored. Treatment addressing the SUD, psychiatric disorder as needed, and social stabilization should be implemented. Caplehorn and colleagues (1996) found that mortality related to overdose in out-of-treatment drug users was four times as high as in those on methadone maintenance. In a study of suicide rates in Estonia during a major government anti-alcohol campaign, average per capita alcohol consumption fell by 40% and alcohol-positive suicides decreased by 39% for males and 41% for females suggesting that public health interventions can be useful in decreasing SUD-related suicide (Caplehorn et al., 1996).

Conclusions: research recommendations

In conclusion, there is a robust relationship between both acute intoxication and chronic use of substances and suicidal behavior. The relationship is complex and includes neurobiologic commonalities, common predisposing factors (physical and sexual victimization) as well as the fact that substance use can aggravate known risk factors for suicide (family dysfunction, social isolation), and acute intoxication can disinhibit and impair judgment such that an ambivalently conceived suicide attempt is more likely to be successful.

Further exploration of the relationship between suicide and SUDs is needed to inform prevention and treatment strategies. Specifically, more information about neural connections between SUDs, mood disorders, aggression, and impulsivity may lead to the development of targeted pharmacological and cognitive behavioral treatments to decrease risk for suicidal behavior. In addition, exploration of the best strategies for the assessment and management of suicidal behavior in individuals with SUDs in primary care, emergency room, and mental health settings is needed. On a public health level, exploration of the impact of policies related to substance use on suicide rates will be critical to the development of informed prevention strategies.

References

Bertolote, J. M., Fleischmann, A., De Leo, D., & Wasserman, D. (2004). Psychiatric diagnoses and suicide: revisiting the evidence. *Crisis*, **25**(4), 147–155.

Bohnert, A. S., Roeder, K. M., & Ilgen, M. A. (2011). Suicide attempts and overdoses among adults entering addictions treatment: comparing correlates in a U.S. National Study. *Drug and Alcohol Dependence*, **119**(1–2), 106–112.

Bostwick, J. M., & Pankratz, V. S. (2000). Affective disorders and suicide risk: a reexamination. *American Journal of Psychiatry*, **157**(12), 1925–1932.

Caplehorn, J. R., Dalton, M. S., Haldar, F., Petrenas, A. M., & Nisbet, J. G. (1996). Methadone maintenance and addicts' risk of fatal heroin overdose. *Substance Use and Misuse*, **31**(2), 177–196.

Chen, T. J., Blum, K., Mathews, D., et al. (2005). Are dopaminergic genes involved in a predisposition to pathological aggression? Hypothesizing the importance of "super normal controls" in psychiatric genetic research of complex behavioral disorders. *Medical Hypotheses*, **65**(4), 703–707.

Conner, K. R., Duberstein, P. R., & Conwell, Y. (1999). Age-related patterns of factors associated with completed suicide in men with alcohol dependence. *American Journal of Addiction*, **8**(4), 312–318.

Conrad, A. K., Jacoby, A. M., Jobes, D. A., et al. (2009). A psychometric investigation of the Suicide Status Form II with a psychiatric inpatient sample. *Suicide and Life-Threatening Behavior*, **39**(3), 307–320.

Cornelius, J. R., Salloum, I. M., Day, N. L., Thase, M. E., & Mann, J. J. (1996). Patterns of suicidality and alcohol use in alcoholics with major depression. *Alcoholism, Clinical and Experimental Research*, **20**(8), 1451–1455.

Cornelius, J. R., Salloum, I. M., Ehler, J. G., et al. (1997). Fluoxetine in depressed alcoholics: A double-blind, placebo-controlled trial. *Archives of General Psychiatry*, **54**(8), 700–705.

Darke, S., & Ross, J. (2002). Suicide among heroin users: rates, risk factors and methods. *Addiction*, **97**(11), 1383–1394.

Deykin, E. Y., & Buka, S. L. (1994). Suicidal ideation and attempts among chemically dependent adolescents. *American Journal of Public Health*, **84**(4), 634–639.

Dum, M., Pickren, J., Sobell, L. C., & Sobell, M. B. (2008). Comparing the BDI-II and the PHQ-9 with outpatient substance abusers. *Addictive Behaviors*, **33**(2), 381–387.

Engstrom, G., Alling, C., Blennow, K., Regnell, G., & Traskman-Bendz, L. (1999). Reduced cerebrospinal HVA concentrations and HVA/5-HIAA ratios in suicide attempters: Monoamine metabolites in 120 suicide attempters and 47 controls. *European Neuropsychopharmacology*, **9**(5), 399–405.

Frederick, C. J., Resnik, H. L., & Wittlin, B. J. (1973). Self-destructive aspects of hard core addiction. *Archives of General Psychiatry*, **28**(4), 579–585.

Glasner-Edwards, S., Mooney, L. J., Marinelli-Casey, P., et al. (2010). Anxiety disorders among methamphetamine dependent adults: association with post-treatment functioning. *American Journal of Addiction*, **19**(5), 385–390.

Grant, B. F., Stinson, F. S., Dawson, D. A., et al. (2004). Prevalence and co-occurrence of substance use disorders and independent mood and anxiety disorders: results from the National Epidemiologic Survey on Alcohol and Related Conditions. *Archives of General Psychiatry*, **61**(8), 807–816.

Harris, E. C., & Barraclough, B. (1997). Suicide as an outcome for mental disorders; A meta-analysis. *British Journal of Psychiatry*, **170**, 205–228.

Hiroeh, U., Appleby, L., Mortensen, P. B., & Dunn, G. (2001). Death by homicide, suicide, and other unnatural causes in people with mental illness: a population-based study. *Lancet*, **358**(9299), 2110–2112.

Inskip, H. M., Harris, E. C., & Barraclough, B. (1998). Lifetime risk of suicide for affective disorder, alcoholism and schizophrenia. *British Journal of Psychiatry*, **172**, 35–37.

Jobes, D. A., Jacoby, A. M., Cimbolic, P., & Hustead, L. A. T. (1997). Assessment and treatment of suicidal clients in a university counseling center: Research in counseling centers. *Journal of Counseling Psychology*, **44**(4), 368–377.

Joiner, T. E., Jr., Conwell, Y., Fitzpatrick, K. K., et al. (2005). Four studies on how past and current suicidality relate even when "everything but the kitchen sink" is covaried. *Journal of Abnormal Psychology*, **114**(2), 291–303.

Kendler, K. S., Bulik, C. M., Silberg, J., et al. (2000). Childhood sexual abuse and adult psychiatric and substance use disorders in women: an epidemiological and cotwin control analysis. *Archives of General Psychiatry*, **57**(10), 953–959.

Kessler, R. C., McGonagle, K. A., Zhao, S., et al. (1994). Lifetime and 12-month prevalence of DSM-III-R psychiatric disorders in the United States: Results from the National Comorbidity Survey. *Archives of General Psychiatry*, **51**(1), 8–19.

Kilpatrick, D. G., Resnick, H. S., Saunders, B. E., & Best, C. L. (1998). Victimization, post-traumatic stress disorder, and substance use and abuse among women. In C. L. Wetherington & A. B. Roman (Eds.) *Drug Addiction Research and the Health of Women*. NIH Publication No. 98–4290 (pp. 285–307). Rockville, MD: US Department of Health and Human Services.

Linnoila, V. M., & Virkkunen, M. (1992). Aggression, suicidality, and serotonin. *Journal of Clinical Psychiatry*, **53** (Suppl), 46–51.

Mino, A., Bousquet, A., & Broers, B. (1999). Substance abuse and drug-related death, suicidal ideation, and suicide: a review. *Crisis*, **20**(1), 28–35.

National Survey on Drug Use and Health (NSDUH) (2012). https://nsduhweb.rti.org.

Nemtsov, A. (2003). Suicides and alcohol consumption in Russia, 1965–1999. *Drug and Alcohol Dependence*, **71**(2), 161–168.

Nock, M. K., Hwang, I., Sampson, N., et al. (2009a). Cross-national analysis of the associations among mental disorders and suicidal behavior: findings from the WHO World Mental Health Surveys. *PLoS Med*, **6**(8), e1000123.

Nock, M. K., Prinstein, M. J., & Sterba, S. K. (2009b). Revealing the form and function of self-injurious thoughts and behaviors: A real-time ecological assessment study among adolescents and young adults. *Journal of Abnormal Psychology*, **118**(4), 816–827.

Nock, M. K., Green, J. G., Hwang, I., et al. (2013). Prevalence, correlates, and treatment of lifetime suicidal behavior among adolescents: results from the National Comorbidity Survey Replication Adolescent Supplement. *JAMA Psychiatry*, 1–11.

Oquendo, M. A., Kamali, M., Ellis, S. P., et al. (2002). Adequacy of antidepressant treatment after discharge and the occurrence of suicidal acts in major depression: a prospective study. *American Journal of Psychiatry*, **159**(10), 1746–1751.

Ratsma, J. E., Van Der Stelt, O., & Gunning, W. B. (2002). Neurochemical markers of alcoholism vulnerability in humans. *Alcohol Alcohol*, **37**(6), 522–533.

Rossow, I. (2000). Successful drinking – or drinking among the successful? *Addiction*, **95**(10), 1584.

Roy, A. (2003). Characteristics of drug addicts who attempt suicide. *Psychiatry Research*, **121**(1), 99–103.

Scott, J. C., Woods, S. P., Matt, G. E., et al. (2007). Neurocognitive effects of methamphetamine: a critical review and meta-analysis. *Neuropsychology Review*, **17**(3), 275–297.

Sher, L., Oquendo, M. A., & Mann, J. J. (2001). Risk of suicide in mood disorders. *Clinical Neuroscience Research*, **1**, 337–344.

Sher, L., Oquendo, M. A., Conason, A. H., et al. (2005). Clinical features of depressed patients with or without a family history of alcoholism. *Acta Psychiatrica Scandinavica*, **112**(4), 266–271.

Sher, L., Mann, J. J., Traskman-Bendz, L., et al. (2006). Lower cerebrospinal fluid homovanillic acid levels in depressed suicide attempters. *Journal of Affective Disorders*, **90**(1), 83–89.

Sher, L., Oquendo, M. A., Grunebaum, M. F., et al. (2007). CSF monoamine metabolites and lethality of suicide attempts in depressed patients with alcohol dependence. *European Neuropsychopharmacology*, **17**(1), 12–15.

Stanley, B., & Brown, G. K. (2012). Safety planning intervention: A brief intervention to mitigate suicide risk. *Cognitive and Behavioral Practice*, **19**, 256–264.

Substance Abuse and Mental Health Services Administration (SAMHSA). (2012). Results from the 2010 National Survey on Drug Use and Health: Mental Health Findings, NSDUH Series H-42, HHS Publication No. (SMA) 11–4667. Rockville, MD: Substance Abuse and Mental Health Services Administration.

Wilcox, H. C., Conner, K. R., & Caine, E. D. (2004). Association of alcohol and drug use disorders and completed suicide: an empirical review of cohort studies. *Drug and Alcohol Dependence*, **76** (Suppl), S11–19.

Wittkampf, K. A., Naeije, L., Schene, A. H., Huyser, J., & van Weert, H. C. (2007). Diagnostic accuracy of the mood module of the Patient Health Questionnaire: a systematic review. *General Hospital Psychiatry*, **29**(5), 388–395.

Chapter 15

Eating disorders and suicide

April R. Smith, Tracy K. Witte, and Scott J. Crow

Anorexia nervosa (AN) is characterized by extreme caloric restriction that results in a body weight below what is considered normal for an individual's height and age. AN has a lifetime prevalence of 0.3% in men and 0.9% in women (Hudson et al., 2007). There are two AN subtypes: the restricting subtype (RAN) and the binge-eating/purging subtype (BPAN). Bulimia nervosa (BN) is characterized by a pattern of binge eating and inappropriate compensatory behaviors, which may include self-induced vomiting, use of laxatives/diuretics, excessive exercise, and/or fasting. BN has lifetime prevalence rates of 0.5% in men and 1.5% in women (Hudson et al., 2007). Longitudinal research suggests that diagnostic crossover between AN and BN is common (Eddy et al., 2008). This introduces complexity when determining each disorder's relationship with suicidal behavior, particularly when considered over the course of an individual's lifetime.

Binge eating disorder (BED) is characterized by recurrent episodes of binge eating accompanied by perceived lack of control over eating; however, unlike BN, individuals with BED do not engage in compensatory behaviors. The lifetime prevalence for BED is 3.5% in women and 2% in men (Hudson et al., 2007). In DSM IV TR 'eating disorder not otherwise specified' (EDNOS) was a catch-all category reserved for individuals who did not meet criteria for AN or BN, but exhibited clinically significant eating disorder symptoms. EDNOS has been renamed 'other specified feeding or eating disorder' (OSFED) in DSM5 (APA, 2013). Notably, EDNOS was the most common eating disorder, with upwards of 70% of individuals receiving this diagnosis (Fairburn & Bohn, 2005). The lifetime prevalence of EDNOS has been estimated to be 3.84% (Le Grange et al., 2012).

In this chapter, we first discuss the relationship between eating disorders and suicidal ideation, nonfatal attempts, and death by suicide, noting limitations in the extant literature along the way. We conclude with a discussion of the relationship between eating disorders and suicidal behavior in the context of the interpersonal–psychological theory of suicide (IPTS; Joiner, 2005; Van Orden et al., 2010).

Suicidal ideation

Suicidal ideation is an important precursor to nonfatal and fatal suicide attempts and is far more common than either of these behaviors, yet the literature examining its relationship with eating disorders is limited. Studies of adults with current eating disorder diagnoses found that 22–32% of those with AN, 22–34% of those with BN, 21–28% of those with BED, and 21–23% of those with EDNOS endorse current suicidal ideation (Favaro & Santonastaso, 1997; Milos et al., 2004; Swanson et al., 2011; Carano et al., 2012). These studies demonstrate that a notable proportion of people with eating disorders experience suicidal ideation and that all eating disorders have similar rates of suicidal ideation. However, because they lack a comparison group, these studies do not allow for conclusions regarding the relative risk for suicidal ideation conferred by eating disorders compared to people with similar demographic characteristics. One recent study did include a comparison group (Swanson et al., 2011), finding that 31% of those with a lifetime diagnosis of AN, 53% of those with a lifetime diagnosis of BN, and 34.4% of those with a lifetime diagnosis of BED reported lifetime suicidal ideation, compared to 11% of those with no eating disorder diagnosis. A key limitation of this study is that it did not examine *current* suicidal ideation. Additionally, due to crossover issues (Eddy et al., 2008), we are

A Concise Guide to Understanding Suicide, ed. Stephen H. Koslow, Pedro Ruiz, and Charles B. Nemeroff. Published by Cambridge University Press.

unable to determine if suicidal ideation occurred during an episode of AN or BN, before the onset of either disorder, or after remission. Moreover, the relative risk for suicidal ideation conferred by eating disorders compared to other mental disorders is unclear.

None of the aforementioned studies investigated the influence of comorbid conditions. Research examining this issue with continuous measures of eating disorder symptoms is mixed, with some studies (e.g., Miotto et al., 2003) finding that the relationship between suicidal ideation and eating disorder symptoms persists after controlling for depressive symptoms, and some finding that it is fully accounted for by depressive and aggressive symptoms (e.g., Miotto & Preti, 2007). Another limitation of this literature is that all of the aforementioned studies used brief measures of suicidal ideation, which can underestimate suicidal ideation's prevalence, compared to more detailed assessment instruments (Glenn & Klonsky, 2012).

In sum, more research is needed to determine the precise nature of the apparent eating disorder–suicidal ideation relationship. Suicidal ideation, non-fatal suicide attempts, and fatal suicide attempts have different demographic and clinical risk factors, and some theoretical models of suicide (e.g., the IPTS) propose different underlying causal processes for each.

Non-fatal suicide attempts

Franko and Keel (2006) conducted a comprehensive, systematic review of non-fatal suicide attempts. The authors concluded that individuals with AN and BN are equally likely to have a history of non-fatal suicide attempt (i.e., 3–20% for AN; 25–35% for BN). Franko and Keel (2006) also cited individual studies demonstrating that individuals with AN and BN have similar likelihood of past attempt compared to individuals with major depressive disorder (Bulik et al., 1999). Prospective studies demonstrate that eating disorders in general predict non-fatal suicide attempt (Johnson et al., 2002), and that current AN is a stronger predictor of non-fatal suicide attempt at follow-up than current BN (Franko et al., 2004).

Among those with eating disorders who attempt suicide, individuals with AN make more serious suicide attempts than individuals with other eating disorders. Bulik et al. (1999) found that individuals with AN reported greater suicide intent during past attempts than individuals with BN, although the groups did not differ in terms of medical lethality of attempt. A more recent study (Guillaume et al., 2011) found that those with a lifetime diagnosis of AN had substantially greater intent and lethality compared to individuals with BN and individuals without an eating disorder diagnosis.

Few studies have examined suicide attempts in individuals with BED and EDNOS. Two studies found rates between 13 and 15% for non-fatal suicide attempts in individuals with BED (Swanson et al., 2011; Carano et al., 2012). Grucza et al. (2007) reported that individuals with BED were 3.7 times more likely to have made a past suicide attempt than obese individuals without BED. Further, one study found that alexythmia (i.e., difficulty identifying and processing emotional states) is associated with suicidal ideation and attempt among those with BED (Carano et al., 2012).

Fatal suicide attempts

Cohort studies

Cohort designs prospectively examine suicide risk in a sample of individuals with a particular diagnosis, comparing their suicide risk to that of individuals with similar demographic characteristics. AN confers a high-risk of premature mortality due to all causes of death, as confirmed by a recent meta-analysis (Arcelus et al., 2011). Among those who died prematurely, one in five had died by suicide. This finding converges with an earlier meta-analysis that established suicide as one of the leading causes of death in people with AN (Sullivan, 1995). A recent meta-analysis of 40 cohort studies (Preti et al., 2011)[1] found that individuals with AN were 31 times more likely to make a fatal suicide attempt than females age 15–34 in the general population.

Preti et al.'s (2011) meta-analysis found that people with BN are seven times more likely to die by suicide than females aged 15–34 in the general population. This conclusion should be viewed with caution, however, given the small number of suicide decedents with BN included in the meta-analysis (i.e., 4 out of 1768).

There were only three studies of individuals with BED included in the Preti et al. (2011) meta-analysis, resulting in a sample of 246 individuals, who were followed on average for 5.3 years. There were no suicides reported in any of these individuals. Currently

[1] The studies included in this meta-analysis overlapped with but were not entirely redundant with Arcelus et al.'s (2011) meta-analysis.

there are too few data available to draw conclusions regarding the rate of completed suicide in individuals with BED.

In the first large-scale examination of mortality in individuals with EDNOS, Crow and colleagues (2009) found suicide rates in EDNOS that were comparable to AN and BN, though the standardized mortality ratio (SMR) for AN was lower (4.7) than in other published studies (e.g., 31; Preti et al., 2011). The authors suggested that the lower rate of completed suicide in the AN sample may have been due to the inclusion of individuals with a current (rather than lifetime) diagnosis, which resulted in a smaller number of AN patients (N = 177) as compared to BN (N = 906) and EDNOS (N = 802) patients.

A limitation of the Preti et al. (2011) meta-analysis is that the majority of the individuals included were in treatment. In a review of 14 studies examining treatment-seeking behavior in an eating disorder population, less than a quarter of individuals with diagnosable eating disorders reported seeking appropriate mental health treatment (Hart et al., 2011). Thus, studies examining suicidal behavior in treatment-seeking populations may not be representative. This is important, given the evidence that patient status is an important moderator of the link between death by suicide and mental disorder diagnosis, with those in treatment – and particularly inpatient treatment – tending to have higher rates of suicide (e.g., Bostwick & Pankratz, 2000). Thus, the suicide rates derived from cohort studies may overestimate the risk for suicide conferred by eating disorders. However, it is also possible that these results underestimate suicide risk, if treatment serves to prevent suicide. Alternatively, delayed ED case-finding may miss suicide cases, leading to prevalence underestimates.

Postmortem studies

Postmortem designs compare diagnostic prevalence among suicide decedents to the prevalence in a group of matched community members, living or deceased. A mental disorder diagnosis is considered to be a risk factor for suicide if it is over-represented among those who have died by suicide. There are few postmortem studies of the relationship between eating disorders and suicide. One study (Coren & Hewitt, 1998) examined the death records of over five million women in the USA. The researchers identified 571 individuals whose death certificate mentioned AN, either as a cause of death or as a diagnosis present at the time of death. Only 1% of these deaths were suicides; in contrast, 4% of the matched control group had died by suicide. This finding is inconsistent with findings from cohort studies, which suggest a strong link between suicide and AN. The explanation offered by Coren and Hewitt (1998) is that suicide decedents in their study would only be included in the AN group if they had a diagnosis of AN at the time of death. In contrast, cohort studies typically include anyone with a lifetime diagnosis at AN. Coren and Hewitt (1998) proposed that the relationship between AN and suicide may be spurious and accounted for by the high comorbidity between AN and mood disorders, given that AN did not appear to be a proximal risk factor for suicide in their study. Another possibility is that AN is a distal risk factor for suicide, and therefore may not need to be present at the time of death to increase risk for suicide.

The psychological autopsy is a type of postmortem study that involves intensive record review of suicide decedents, along with interviews with one or more informants who are knowledgeable about a decedent's state of mind near the time of death. A meta-analysis of 27 psychological autopsy studies (Arsenault-Lapierre et al., 2004), which included 3275 suicide decedents, did not mention eating disorders at all. This may be because eating disorders are rare in the general population, and thus, it is statistically improbable for individuals in psychological autopsy studies. Another explanation is that researchers do not provide sufficiently detailed information on eating disorder prevalence in published psychological autopsy studies, thereby hindering the inclusion of eating disorders in meta-analyses. An additional explanation, proposed by Hjelmeland and colleagues (2012), is that informants may be influenced by the knowledge that a decedent has died by suicide when recalling his/her mental disorder symptoms. Thus, informants may be particularly prone to assigning certain mental disorder symptoms to suicide decedents (e.g., depressive symptoms) rather than others (e.g., eating disorder symptoms).

Interpersonal theory of suicide

We chose to examine suicidality among individuals with eating disorders through the lens of the IPTS (Joiner, 2005; Van Orden et al., 2010), which is a theory of suicidal ideation and behavior with robust empirical support (e.g., Joiner et al., 2009; Van Orden et al., 2008). The IPTS identifies three essential variables (thwarted belongingness, perceived burdensomeness, the acquired capability for suicide) that must be in place before one can enact a lethal suicide attempt. Thwarted belongingness refers to a sense of not belonging, and is hypothesized to be comprised of both loneliness and the absence of reciprocal care. Both liability (i.e., the mental miscalculation that one's death is worth more to others than one's life) and self-hate contribute to perceived burdensomeness. The theory posits that either of these psychological states can lead to passive suicidal ideation; further, when both are experienced simultaneously they produce active suicidal ideation. However, a third factor, an acquired sense of fearlessness about death and high pain tolerance (i.e., acquired capability for suicide), is necessary for individuals to act on suicidal thoughts.

Perceived burdensomeness and eating disorders

To our knowledge no studies have directly measured perceived burdensomeness in eating disorder samples. However, it is likely that at least some individuals with eating disorders experience perceived burdensomeness. Factors that may contribute to perceived burdensomeness include: the cost of eating disorder treatment (adequate care treatment is estimated to be $119 200 per patient; Crow & Nyman, 2003), often needing family members to be responsible for treatment (Eisler, 2005), the course of treatment (i.e., treatment is often lengthy and relapse is common), and the sequelae of having an eating disorder (i.e., medical problems in need of ongoing care). In support of this hypothesis, multiple studies have found that caregivers of individuals with eating disorders report a high level of burden (see Zabala et al., 2009 for review). For instance, AN was found to have more associated caregiver burden than schizophrenia (Treasure et al., 2001), and there is some evidence that caregiver burden is higher among relatives of individuals with AN as compared to BN (Santonastaso et al., 1997). Of course, the aforementioned studies focus on burdensomeness as perceived by caregivers, which is not the same thing as perceptions of burdensomeness among individuals with eating disorders. It is possible to acknowledge that an individual's eating disorder symptoms and treatment are associated with real struggles among their family members while still vehemently opposing the notion that family members would be better off without him or her.

Burdensomeness can also be inferred from studies that measure quality of life, level of impairment, and related variables. In their review of studies assessing for quality of life issues in eating disorder patients, Hay and Mond (2005) found that eating disorders were associated with poorer quality of life and greater levels of impairment as compared to healthy controls and other patient populations. Further, Mond et al. (2004) found that almost half of people with eating disorders in the community reported that their eating disorder symptoms caused severe impairment. With respect to the amount of impairment caused by specific eating disorder behaviors, one study reported that binge eating was associated with more impairment than other weight control behaviors (Hay, 2003), and another study found that, in addition to objective overeating, self-induced vomiting was highly associated with impairment and psychological distress among community cases of eating disorders (Mond et al., 2004).

Van Orden and colleagues (2010) have proposed that the self-hate component of perceived burdensomeness is comprised of both shame and low self-esteem. Notably, there is strong research support for positive relationships between levels of disordered eating and shame (for a review see Goss and Allan, 2009) and low self-esteem (e.g., Fairburn et al., 2003). For example, research has found that women with BED experience more shame than women with sexual dysfunction (Masheb et al., 1999), that shame predicted the number of vomiting episodes in a group of individuals with BN, and that external versus internal shame was uniquely associated with anorexia and bulimia, respectively.

Low belongingness and eating disorders

There is robust evidence that people with eating disorders experience factors related to low belongingness pre-morbidly, during their illness, and sometimes even after recovery. For instance, attachment research has found that both people with AN and BN are more likely than controls to report both separation anxiety as children and insecure attachment styles as adults (Troisi et al., 2005). Further, impairments in interpersonal functioning, such as body image-related teasing and social difficulties, have been noted prior to the onset of BED and AN, respectively (Råstam and Gillberg, 1992; Fairburn et al., 1998). Of note, in the Råstam study (1992), half of the AN participants reported having no friends (compared to 17% of the control group).

With respect to the social interactions of currently ill AN individuals, overall the research suggests that individuals with AN feel as if they have fewer social supports, more negative interactions, and less social competence (see Zucker et al., 2007 for a review). Additionally, observers perceive women with current BN as less socially effective than healthy controls (e.g., Grisset & Norvell, 1992). Further, some individuals report that their identity begins to be subsumed by their eating disorder, thereby leaving few resources left to devote to interpersonal relationships (Lamoureux and Bottorff, 2005).

It appears that these interpersonal deficits may persist after recovery. For example, Holliday and colleagues (2006) found that individuals with AN not only had marked social isolation while ill, but that they continued to exhibit more social isolation after recovery than control participants. The effects stemming from these interpersonal deficits, like social isolation and social withdrawal, are likely even more pronounced in people with eating disorders given their high desire for social acceptance (Shafran et al., 2002). Sadly, social impairment has been found to negatively impact eating disorder treatment (Goodwin & Fitzgibbon, 2002), and thus may serve to maintain the disorder (Keel et al., 2005).

Acquired capability for suicide and eating disorders

The IPTS posits that the acquired capability for suicide (ACS), which is comprised of pain tolerance and fearlessness about death, is built up over the course of one's life through experience with events that are either painful (e.g., accidents, self-injury) or provocative (e.g., getting a tattoo, shooting a gun). In general, the weight control methods used by individuals with eating disorders could be considered to be both provocative and painful. Thus, the recurrent engagement in these behaviors may serve to elevate ACS. This construct may help resolve conflicting findings regarding the relationship between AN and suicide. Specifically, engagement in painful eating disorder behaviors and the attendant increase in acquired capability may serve as a distal risk factor for suicide. Thus, an individual would not need to be currently ill to have increased risk for death by suicide.

Three studies have tested the association between painful eating disorder behaviors and suicidality. Crow and colleagues (2009) examined whether unhealthy weight control behaviors (e.g., skipping meals, smoking more cigarettes), extreme weight control behaviors (e.g., self-induced vomiting, using laxatives), body dissatisfaction, and BMI predicted suicidal ideation and/or suicide attempts 5 years later. In accordance with the IPTS only extreme weight control behaviors predicted suicidal ideation and attempts in women; this relationship held even when controlling for depression and other demographic variables. Selby and colleagues (2010) found that pain-inducing behaviors (e.g., self-induced vomiting), linked BPAN to suicidal behavior and that dietary restraint linked RAN to suicidal behavior. Finally, in a sample of women with BN, Smith et al. (2012) found that over-exercise emerged as a stronger predictor of suicide attempts and gestures than self-induced vomiting, laxative abuse, or dietary restraint.

So far only one study has directly tested the association between painful eating disorder behaviors and ACS (Smith et al., 2012). In a collegiate sample, the authors also found that over-exercise was the only disordered eating behavior that was associated with ACS; further, they found that ACS mediated the relationship between over-exercise and suicidal behavior.

Future directions

From the research reviewed in this chapter, it appears that individuals with AN have greater suicide intent and lethality than individuals with BN (Bulik et al., 1999; Guillaume et al., 2011). Further, it appears that people with eating disorders, and particularly those with AN, may experience one or more of three of the IPTS constructs. It will be important for future research to investigate whether this increased risk among AN individuals is explained by elevations on IPTS constructs. We also believe it would be useful to examine the relationship between eating disorder symptoms and associated features (e.g., shame, body dissatisfaction, dietary restriction) and the components of the IPTS. Because the IPTS proposes separate causal processes underlying suicidal intent (i.e., fearlessness about death) and lethality (i.e., pain tolerance) it would also be worthwhile to examine whether some eating disorder behaviors are differentially associated with the different facets of acquired capability.

In conclusion, further investigation is needed on the prevalence of suicidal behavior among people with eating disorders and on the utility of IPTS constructs in predicting suicidal ideation and attempts in these individuals. Such information would prove informative for suicide risk assessments and treatment development.

References

American Psychiatric Association. (2000). *Diagnostic and Statistical Manual of Mental Disorder*, 4th ed., Text Revision. Washington, DC: American Psychiatric Association.

American Psychiatric Association. (2013). *Diagnostic and Statistical Manual of Mental Disorder*, 5th ed. Washington, DC: American Psychiatric Association.

Arcelus, J., Mitchell, A. J., Wales, J., et al. (2011). Mortality rates in patients with anorexia nervosa and other eating disorders. *Archives of General Psychiatry*, **68**, 724–731.

Arsenault-Lapierre, G., Kim, C., & Turecki, G. (2004). Psychiatric diagnoses in 3275 suicides: A meta-analysis. *BMC Psychiatry*, **4**, 37. doi:10.1186/1471-244X-4-37.

Bostwick, J. M., & Pankratz, V. S. (2000). Affective disorders and suicide risk: A reexamination. *American Journal of Psychiatry*, **157**, 1925–1932.

Bulik, C. M., Sullivan, P. F., & Joyce, P. R. (1999). Temperament, character and suicide attempts in anorexia nervosa, bulimia nervosa and major depression. *Acta Psychiatrica Scandinavica*, **100**, 27–32.

Carano, A., De Berardis, D., Campanella, D., et al. (2012). Alexithymia and suicide ideation in a sample of patients with binge eating disorder. *Journal of Psychiatric Practice*, **18**, 5–11.

Coren, S., & Hewitt, P. L. (1998). Is anorexia nervosa associated with elevated rates of suicide? *American Journal of Public Health*, **8**, 1206–1207.

Crow, S., & Nyman, J. A. (2003). The cost-effectiveness of anorexia nervosa treatment. *International Journal of Eating Disorders*, **35**, 155–160.

Crow, S., Peterson, C., Swanson, S., et al. (2009). Increased mortality in bulimia nervosa and other eating disorders. *American Journal of Psychiatry*, **166**, 1342–1346.

Eddy, K. T., Dorer, D. J., Franko, D. L., et al. (2008). Diagnostic crossover in anorexia nervosa and bulimia nervosa: Implications for DSM-V. *American Journal of Psychiatry*, **165**, 245–250.

Eisler, I. (2005). The empirical and theoretical base of family therapy and multiple family day therapy for adolescent anorexia nervosa. *Journal of Family Therapy*, **27**, 104–131.

Fairburn, C. G., & Bohn, K. (2005). Eating disorder NOS (EDNOS): An example of the troublesome "not otherwise specified" (NOS) category in DSM-IV. *Behaviour Research and Therapy*, **43**, 691–701.

Fairburn, C. G., Doll, H. A., Welch, S. L., et al. (1998). Risk factors for binge eating disorder. *Archives of General Psychiatry*, **55**, 425–432.

Fairburn, C. G., Cooper, Z., & Shafran, R. (2003). Cognitive behavior therapy for eating disorders: a "transdiagnostic" theory and treatment. *Behavior Research and Therapy*, **41**, 509–528.

Favaro, A., & Santonastaso, P. (1997). Suicidality in eating disorders: Clinical and psychological correlates. *Acta Psychiatrica Scandinavica*, **95**, 508–514.

Franko, D. L., & Keel, P. K. (2006). Suicidality in eating disorders: Occurrence, correlates, and clinical implications. *Clinical Psychology Review*, **26**, 769–782.

Franko, D. L., Keel, P. K., Dorer, D. J., et al. (2004). What predicts suicide attempts in women with eating disorders? *Psychological Medicine*, **34**, 843–853.

Glenn, C. R., & Klonsky, D. E. (2012). Factors to consider in the assessment of suicidal thoughts and behaviors in adolescents. In C. L. Bagge & C. R. Glenn (Co-chairs) *Measurement Matters: Roadblocks and Innovations in the Assessment of Suicide*. Symposium conducted at the meeting of the Association for Behavioral and Cognitive Therapy, November, 2012, National Harbor, Maryland.

Goodwin, R. D., & Fitzgibbon, M. L. (2002). Social anxiety as a barrier to treatment for eating disorders. *International Journal of Eating Disorders*, **32**, 103–106.

Goss, K., & Allan, S. (2009). Shame, pride and eating disorders. *Clinical Psychology & Psychotherapy*, **16**, 303–316.

Grisset, N. I., & Norvell, N. K. (1992). Perceived social support, social skills, and quality of relationships in bulimic women. *Journal of Consulting and Clinical Psychology*, **60**, 293–299.

Grucza, R. A., Przybeck, T. R., & Cloninger, C. R. (2007). Prevalence and correlates of binge eating disorder in a community sample. *Comprehensive Psychiatry*, **48**, 124–131.

Guillaume, S., Jaussent, I., Olie, E., et al. (2011). Characteristics of suicide attempts in anorexia and bulimia nervosa: A case-control study. *PLoS ONE*, **6**, e23578.

Hart, L. M., Granillo, M. T., Jorm, A. F., et al. (2011). Unmet need for treatment in the eating disorders: A systematic review of eating disorder specific treatment seeking among community cases. *Clinical Psychology Review*, **31**, 727–735.

Hay, P. (2003). Quality of life and bulimic eating disorder behaviors: Findings from a community based sample. *International Journal of Eating Disorders*, **33**, 434–442.

Hay, P. J., & Mond, J. (2005). How to 'count the cost' and measure burden? A review of health-related quality of life in people with eating disorders. *Journal of Mental Health*, **14**, 539–552.

Hay, P. J., Mond, J., Buttner, P., et al. (2008). Eating disorder behaviors are increasing: Findings from two sequential community surveys in South Australia. *PLoS ONE*, **3**, e1541.

Hjelmeland, H., Dieserud, G., Dyregrov, K., et al. (2012). Psychological autopsy studies as diagnostic tools: Are they methodologically flawed? *Death Studies*, **36**, 605–626.

Holliday, J., Uher, R., Landau, S., et al. (2006). Personality pathology among individuals with a lifetime history of anorexia nervosa. *Journal of Personality Disorders*, **20**, 417–430.

Hudson, J. I., Hiripi, E., Pope, H. G., et al. (2007). The prevalence and correlates of eating disorders in the National Comorbidity Survey Replication. *Biological Psychiatry*, **61**, 348.

Johnson, J. G., Cohen, P., Kasen, S., et al. (2002). Eating disorders during adolescence and the risk for physical and mental disorders during early adulthood. *Archives of General Psychiatry*, **29**, 545–552.

Joiner, T. E. (2005). *Why People Die by Suicide*. Cambridge, MA: Harvard University Press.

Joiner, T. E., Van Orden, K. A., Witte, T. K., et al. (2009). Main predictions of the interpersonal-psychological theory of suicidal behavior: Empirical tests in two samples of young adults. *Journal of Abnormal Psychology*, **118**, 634–646.

Keel, P. K., Dorer, D. J., Franko, D. L., et al. (2005). Postremission predictors of relapse in women with eating disorders. *American Journal of Psychiatry*, **162**, 2263–2268.

Lamoureux, M. M., & Bottorff, J. L. (2005). "Becoming the real me": Recovering from anorexia nervosa. *Health Care for Women International*, **26**, 170–188.

Le Grange, D., Swanson, S. A., Crow, S. J., & Merikangas, K. R. (2012). Eating disorder not otherwise specified presentation in the US population. *International Journal of Eating Disorders*, **45**(5), 711–718.

Masheb, R. M., Grilo, C. M., & Brondolo, E. (1999). Shame and its psychopathologic correlates in two women's health problems: binge eating disorders and vulvudynia. *Eating and Weight Disorders*, **4**, 187–193.

Milos, G., Spindler, A., Hepp, U., et al. (2004). Suicide attempts and suicidal ideation: Links with psychiatric comorbidity in eating disorder subjects. *General Hospital Psychiatry*, **26**, 129–135.

Miotto, P., & Preti, A. (2007). Eating disorders and suicide ideation: the mediating role of depression and aggressiveness. *Comprehensive Psychiatry*, **48**, 218–224.

Miotto, P., De Coppi, M., Frezza, M., et al. (2003). Eating disorders and suicide risk factors in adolescents: An Italian community-based study. *The Journal of Nervous and Mental Disease*, **191**, 437–443.

Mond, J., Rodgers, B., Hay, P., et al. (2004). Disability associated with community cases of commonly occurring eating disorders. *Australian and New Zealand Journal of Public Health*, **28**, 246–251.

Preti, A., Rochi, M. B. L., Siti, D., et al. (2011). A comprehensive meta-analysis of the risk of suicide in eating disorders. *Acta Psychiatrica Scandinavica*, **124**, 6–17.

Råstam, M., & Gillberg, C. (1992). Background factors in anorexia nervosa: A controlled study of 51 teenage cases including a population sample. *European Child and Adolescent Psychiatry*, **1**, 54–65.

Santonastaso, P., Saccon, D., & Favaro, A. (1997). Burden and psychiatric symptoms in key relatives of patients with eating disorders: a preliminary study. *Eating and Weight Disorders*, **2**, 44–48.

Selby, E., Smith, A. R., Bulik, C. M., et al. (2010). Habitual starvation and provocative behaviors: Two potential routes to extreme suicidal behavior in anorexia nervosa. *Behavior Research and Therapy*, **48**, 634–645.

Shafran, R., Cooper, Z., & Fairburn, C. G. (2002). Clinical perfectionism: A cognitive-behavioural analysis. *Behaviour Research and Therapy*, **40**, 773–791.

Smith, A. R., Fink, E. L., Anestis, M. D., et al. (2012). Exercise caution: Over-exercise is associated with suicidality in bulimia nervosa. *Psychiatry Research*. http://dx.doi.org/10.1016/j.psychres.2012.11.004

Sullivan, P. F. (1995). Mortality in anorexia nervosa. *American Journal of Psychiatry*, **152**, 1073–1074.

Swanson, S. A., Crow, S. J., Le Grange, D., et al. (2011). Prevalence and correlates of eating disorders in adolescents: Results from the National Comorbidity Survey Replication Adolescent Supplement. *Archives of General Psychiatry*, **68**, 714–723.

Treasure, J., Murphy, T., Szmukler, T., et al. (2001). The experience of caregiving for severe mental illness: a comparison between anorexia nervosa and psychosis. *Social Psychiatry and Psychiatric Epidemiology*, **36**, 343–347.

Troisi, A., Massaroni, P., & Cuzzolaro, M. (2005). Early separation anxiety and adult attachment style in women with eating disorders. *British Journal of Clinical Psychology*, **44**, 89–97.

Van Orden, K. A., Witte, T. K., Gordon, K. H., et al. (2008). Suicidal desire and the capability for suicide: Tests of the interpersonal-psychological theory of suicidal behavior among adults. *Journal of Consulting and Clinical Psychology*, **76**, 72–83.

Van Orden, K. A., Witte, T. K., Cukrowicz, K. C., et al. (2010). The interpersonal theory of suicide. *Psychological Review*, **117**, 575–600.

Zabala, M. J., Macdonald, P., & Treasure, J. (2009). Appraisal of caregiving burden, expressed emotion and psychological distress in families of people with eating disorders: A systematic review. *European Eating Disorders Review*, **17**, 338–349.

Zucker, N. L., Losh, M., Bulik, C. M., et al. (2007). Anorexia nervosa and autism spectrum disorders: Guided investigation of social cognitive endophenotypes. *Psychological Bulletin*, **133**, 976–1006.

Chapter 16

Suicidality and epilepsy: a complex relationship

Andres M. Kanner

Introduction

Suicidality, which encompasses passive and active suicidal ideation, suicide attempt and completed suicide, is a relatively frequent psychiatric comorbidity in patients with epilepsy (PWE) (Barraclough, 1987; Nilsson et al., 1997; Rafnsson et al., 2001; Christensen et al., 2007). Yet, PWE with current and/or past suicidal ideation and/or history of suicide attempts remains under-recognized and untreated. An alert from the FDA in the USA in 2008, suggesting that exposure to antiepileptic drugs (AEDs) is associated to an increased suicidal risk, began to kindle some interest in this problem. The relationship between epilepsy and suicidality is complex and multi-factorial. The aim of this article is to review the psychiatric, neuropsychobiological, pharmacologic, and epilepsy-related variables associated with increased suicidality risk in PWE and provide practical strategies that can be used in Neurology clinics to identify these patients.

Epidemiologic data

Completed suicide: Population-based studies have demonstrated a higher incidence of completed suicide in PWE than the general population. A review of 21 published studies that investigated the cause of death in PWE found suicide to account for a mean of 11.5% of all reported deaths (Jones et al., 2003). In fact, the overall standardized mortality ratio (SMR) resulting from completed suicide following a diagnosis of epilepsy has been found to range from 3.5 to 5.0 (Nilsson et al., 1997; Rafnsson et al., 2001). In a Danish population-based study, the SMR of completed suicide in PWE was 2.0 (95% CI = 1.7–2.3) after excluding people with psychiatric comorbidity and adjusting for various factors (Christensen et al., 2007). This risk increased by 32-fold in the presence of comorbid mood disorders and by 12-fold in the presence of anxiety disorders and schizophrenia. An SMR of 20.0 was found when including all known psychiatric diagnoses (95% CI = 12.7–31.2).

Suicide attempts are also significantly more frequent in PWE. In a cross-sectional study, Jones et al. (2003) found a 20.8% lifetime prevalence of suicide attempts among 139 outpatients followed in five tertiary epilepsy centers in the USA. In a more recent study of 208 patients with treatment-resistant focal epilepsy, suicide attempt within the last 4 weeks was endorsed by 4.6% patients, while a lifetime suicide attempt was identified in 21.1% of patients (Hesdorffer et al., 2013).

Suicidal ideation is a relatively frequent occurrence in PWE. In a Canadian population-based study, a lifetime history of suicidal ideation was found in 25% of PWE, compared to 12.2% of controls (Tellez-Zenteno et al., 2007). In the study of patients with treatment-resistant focal epilepsy, suicidal ideation in the previous month was endorsed by 18.5%, while a lifetime history of suicidal ideation was reported by 46.1%.

While a timely identification of PWE with suicidal ideation is of the essence, it is more imperative that clinicians recognize those with history of suicide *attempt* as it is the strongest predictor of a future completed suicide. For example, Harris and Barraclough (1989) found that PWE who attempted suicide had a 38.4% increased risk for later completed suicide compared with the general population. Likewise, in a Swedish population-based study, a previous suicide attempt was identified in 46.2% of people with epilepsy who eventually committed suicide (Rafnsson et al., 2001). The increased risk for completed suicide after epilepsy onset may represent recurrence of premorbid suicidality, but this has never been studied.

A Concise Guide to Understanding Suicide, ed. Stephen H. Koslow, Pedro Ruiz, and Charles B. Nemeroff. Published by Cambridge University Press.

Suicidality and epilepsy: a complex relation

As stated above, suicidality in PWE is complex and multi-factorial. The potential pathogenic mechanisms include: (i) epilepsy-related variables; (ii) personal and familial psychiatric history (particularly of mood disorders and/or suicidality); (iii) iatrogenic mechanisms; and (iv) common neurobiologic pathogenic mechanisms that are operant in suicide (and/or the psychiatric disorders leading to suicide) and epilepsy. The existence of such common pathogenic mechanisms may explain the existence of a bidirectional relation between suicidality and epilepsy, identified in recent population-based studies, whereby not only are PWE at higher risk of developing suicidality, but patients with a history of suicidal attempts have been found to be at greater risk of developing epilepsy (Hesdorffer et al., 2006, 2012).

Bidirectional relation between epilepsy and suicidality

Two population-based studies have demonstrated this bidirectional relation. The first study conducted in Iceland identified a five-fold higher risk for developing epilepsy among individuals who exhibited suicidality prior to the onset of the seizure disorder (Hesdorffer et al., 2006). This risk was independent of a history of major depressive disorder and alcohol abuse. The second study consisted of a matched, longitudinal cohort study conducted in the United Kingdom using the General Practice Research Database (Hesdorffer et al., 2012). It compared the incidence rate ratio (IRR) and prevalence ratio (PR) of suicidality for the 3 years preceding and following the onset of epilepsy between 3773 subjects with epilepsy (between the ages of 10 and 60 years) and 14 025 controls matched by year of birth, sex, general practice, and years of medical records before the index date of the onset of eczema and acute surgery. The IRR of suicidality before epilepsy diagnosis was higher during the 3 years before (IRR, 3.1–4.5) and 1 year after diagnosis of epilepsy (IRR, 5.3) than that of the control group. The PR was increased for suicide attempt before and after onset of epilepsy (PR, 2.6–5.2 and 2.4–5.6, respectively). Of note, the IRR of psychosis, depression, and anxiety were also significantly increased for all 3 years before (IRR, 1.5–15.7) and after the diagnosis of epilepsy (IRR, 2.2–10.9) compared to that of the control group. Similarly, three other population-based studies found that people with a history of depression have a two- to seven-fold higher risk of developing epilepsy (Hesdorffer et al., 2000, 2006; Adelow et al., 2012). Furthermore, the co-occurrence of migraine with aura (but not migraine without aura), major depression, and suicidality increase the risk of unprovoked seizures by more than six-fold (Hesdorffer et al., 2007).

Common pathogenic mechanisms

The bidirectional relation between epilepsy and suicidality (and/or associated psychiatric comorbidities) does not imply causality. Instead it may be explained by the existence of common neurobiologic pathogenic mechanisms operant in these conditions (for a detailed review see Kanner, 2006, 2012; Hecimovic et al., 2011). They include disturbances of several neurotransmitters, in particular serotonin (5HT), norepinephrine (NE), glutamate (GTE), and gamma-amino-butyric acid (GABA) as well as disturbances of the hypothalamic–pituitary–adrenal axis (HPAA) which, in turn, can result in abnormal secretion of some of these neurotransmitters.

The pathogenic roles of these neurotransmitters in mood disorders and suicidality have been well recognized and are reviewed in Chapter 11 of this book. Indeed, the monoamines 5HT and NE are known to play a fundamental pathogenic role in mood and anxiety disorders and in suicidality. In epilepsy, 5HT, NE, and GABA have been found to play an inhibitory effect of cortical hyperexcitability and to block the development of seizures in various animal models of epilepsy performed in rats, mice, rabbits, cats, and rhesus monkeys (for reviews see Kanner, 2006, 2012; Jobe et al., 2006). In humans, decreased serotonergic activity in patients with temporal lobe epilepsy (TLE) and juvenile myoclonic epilepsy has also been identified with functional neuroimaging studies using positron emission tomography targeting the binding of the $5HT_{1A}$ receptor. For example, in patients with TLE, a decreased binding was identified in hippocampi, amygdala, cingulate gyrus, and raphe nuclei (Toczek et al., 2003; Theodore et al., 2006). Of note, decreased $5HT_{1A}$ binding has been found in the same structures of patients with major depressive disorder (Sargent et al., 2000; Hasler et al., 2007).

Glutamate and GABA are the excitatory and inhibitory neurotransmitters "par excellence," respectively, which plays a pivotal role in epileptogenesis. Likewise, excessive glutamatergic and decreased GABAergic activity have been recognized in mood disorders and suicide. For example, Sequeira et al. performed gene expression analysis on 17 cortical and subcortical brain regions from 26 male subjects that committed suicide and 13 controls with and without major depression and controls (Sequeira et al., 2009). Independent brain samples from 34 subjects and animal studies were used to control for the potential confounding effects of comorbidity with alcohol. These investigators found abnormalities in glutamatergic- and GABAergic-related genes with the highest number of suicide-specific alterations identified in prefrontal cortex and hippocampus.

A pathogenic role of hyperactive HPAA resulting in high serum cortisol concentrations has been demonstrated for a long time in major depressive disorders and suicidality as well as in animal models of epilepsy and in humans with TLE (see Kanner, 2012 for a detailed review). For example, Kumar et al. demonstrated that the administration of corticosterone accelerated the electrical amygdala kindling in female non-epileptic Wistar rats 10–13 weeks of age. It has been shown that compared to a control group infused with water, rats treated with steroids required a significantly lower number of stimulations to reach a full kindled state (45.2 vs. 86.5, $p<0.01$). Likewise, a pathogenic role of hyperactive HPAA in suicide has been suggested in studies dating back to the 1960s, which reported high serum cortisol levels in patients who went on to commit suicide (Bunney and Fawcett, 1965). Likewise, in a study of 36 patients hospitalized with a mood disorder, non-suppression to dexamethasone was identified twice as frequently (36% vs.11%) in patients with suicide attempts (Jokinen and Nordström, 2009). Also, in a prospective study that followed 76 inpatient depressed patients over 5 years, non-suppressors to the dexamethasone suppression test were more likely to commit suicide (Coryell, 1990). These findings have been reported by other investigators (Norman et al., 1990).

Epilepsy-related risk factors

Postictal suicidal ideation has been investigated in one study of patients with treatment-resistant focal epilepsy (Kanner et al., 2004). Among 100 consecutive patients, 13% experienced suicidal ideation after more than 50% of their seizures, with a median duration of 24 hours. These patients were significantly more likely to have had a past history of bipolar or major depressive disorders as well as of psychiatric hospitalization. Suicidal behavior also has been reported in the context of postictal psychotic episodes. For instance, in a study of patients with TLE, Kanemoto et al. reported that suicide attempts were more frequent during postictal psychotic episodes (7%) than during either acute interictal psychosis (2%) or postictal confusion (0%) (Kanemoto et al., 1999).

Type of epilepsy syndrome

TLE has been associated with a 6- to 25-fold increased suicide risk (Currie et al., 1971; Robertson, 1997; Fukuchi et al., 2002); however, not all studies supported this finding (Nilsson et al., 1997, 2002).

Psychiatric risk factors

After controlling for comorbid socioeconomic status and psychiatric comorbidities, the Danish population-based study previously mentioned found that the PWE had twice the risk of committing suicide (RR = 1.99; 95% CI: 1.71–2.32) than controls (Christensen et al., 2007). However, the risk increased almost 14-fold when comorbid psychiatric disorders were present, in particular, mood (32-fold) and anxiety (12-fold) disorders. Of note, the study found that the risk of suicide was greatest during the first 6 months after the diagnosis of epilepsy (RR 5.4; 95% CI: 4.4–8.3) and was even higher in the presence of comorbid psychiatric disorders (RR = 29.2; 95% CI: 16.4–51.9) during this early period. Similarly, a Swedish study demonstrated that comorbid psychiatric disorders were associated with a nine-fold increase in the risk of suicide and a 10-fold increase for patients also using antipsychotic drugs (Nilsson et al., 2002). In the previously discussed study by Jones et al. (2003), the highest risks for a suicide attempt were correlated with a lifetime history of major depressive episode (OR, 5.9; 95% CI: 2.4–14.3) and lifetime manic episode (OR, 12.6; 95% CI: 1.3–125.9). Likewise, a lifetime history of a mood or anxiety disorder was identified as significantly associated with a risk of suicidal ideation.

Iatrogenic processes

There is a complex relation between seizure control and the occurrence (remission and de novo development) of psychiatric disorders. While PWE with poorly controlled seizures are at increased risk of psychiatric comorbidities, the sudden remission of epileptic seizures in patients with previously poorly controlled epilepsy has been associated with an increased risk of de novo or recurrence of mood, anxiety, and psychotic disorders. This phenomenon is known as alternative psychopathology or "forced normalization" (Wolf, 1991). This phenomenon has been associated with the use of several AEDs and surgical treatment of intractable epilepsy.

Do antiepileptic drugs increase the risk of suicide?

Psychiatric adverse events, including symptoms of depression and anxiety, have been reported with the use of several AEDs, particularly barbiturates (phenobarbital and primidone), topiramate, tiagabine, zonisamide, vigabatrin, and levetiracetam (Brent et al., 1987; Trimble et al., 2000; Mula et al., 2003; Mula and Sander, 2007). The incidence of suicidal phenomena linked to specific AEDs has not been systematically or well studied. In fact, only one study could be found; it showed that 0.7% of patients exposed to levetiracetam reported suicidal ideation (Mula and Sander, 2007). In another observational study of 224 consecutive patients treated with levetiracetam, the drug was discontinued in four (1.8%) individuals because of episodes of major depression, with suicidal ideation. All four patients had a prior history of a depressive disorder (AM Kanner, MD, unpublished data, December, 2006).

In all of these studies, psychiatric adverse events were identified in a subset of PWE who have a predisposition for the development of psychiatric comorbidities. These include patients with a past and/or a family history of psychiatric disorders. Thus, the development of psychiatric adverse events may reflect either the natural course of an underlying recurrent psychiatric illness with no real effect from AEDs, or it could suggest that AEDs lower the threshold for manifesting psychiatric symptoms in individuals who are vulnerable because of a genetic or historical predisposition to psychiatric disorders. Furthermore, if psychiatric symptoms follow the remission of seizures associated with the addition of an AED, the psychiatric symptoms are not the expression of AED toxicity.

In January of 2008, the FDA issued an alert regarding the association between suicidality and AEDs, which was based on results of a meta-analysis that included data from 199 randomized clinical trials of 11 AEDs: carbamazepine, felbamate, gabapentin, lamotrigine, levetiracetam, oxcarbazepine, pregabalin, tiagabine, topiramate, valproate, and zonisamide (US Department of Health and Human Services, Food and Drug Administration, Center for Drug Evaluation and Research, Office of Translational Sciences, Office of Biostatistics, 2008). The meta-analysis encompassed a total of 43 892 patients treated for epilepsy, psychiatric disorders, and other disorders, predominantly pain. The FDA concluded that there was a statistically significant 1.80-fold increased risk of suicidality with exposure to AEDs. Suicidality occurred in 4.3 per 1000 patients treated with AEDs in the active arm, compared with 2.2 per 1000 patients in the comparison arm. Of all the suicidality reported, suicidal ideation accounted for 67.6%, preparatory acts for 2.8%, attempts for 26.8%, and completed suicide for 2.8%. AEDs were associated with a greater risk for suicidality with epilepsy (OR, 3.53; 95% CI: 1.28–12.10) than with psychiatric disorders (OR, 1.51; 95% CI: 0.95–2.45) or other disorders (OR, 1.87; 95% CI: 0.81–4.76). Yet, the validity of the results of this meta-analysis has recently been questioned because of methodological problems (Hesdorffer & Kanner, 2009). These include:

(1) The assessment of suicidality was based on "spontaneous" reports of patients and not gathered in a systematic prospective manner.

(2) The FDA associated the increased risk of suicide with *all* AEDs, despite the fact that statistical significance was found in only 2 (i.e., topiramate and lamotrigine) of the 11 AEDs studied. Furthermore, inclusion of three additional studies of lamotrigine resulted in the loss of statistical significance for this AED. Two other AEDs, valproic acid and carbamazepine, actually yielded a "small protective effect." The FDA's decision to present the risk as involving all AEDs stemmed from a concern that singling out specific AEDs might only change prescribing practices, rather than emphasize the suicide risk. Clearly, their reasoning is not scientifically based.

(3) Most epilepsy trials (92%) include patients on adjunctive therapy (compared with 14% of psychiatric trials and 15% of other medical trials). It is unclear whether the higher suicidality rates in the epilepsy trials were due to drug interactions, given the high proportion of epilepsy trials designed with polytherapy, or whether they potentially were due to the low suicidality risk associated with carbamazepine and valproate – both drugs are protective for suicidality and are the most common comparison drugs in these trials.

(4) Suicidal behavior was greater in certain geographic regions. For example, the odds ratio of suicidality

was 1.38 (95% CI: 0.9–2.13) in North American studies and 4.53 (95% CI: 1.86–13.18) in studies done elsewhere. Such differences strongly suggest serious methodological errors in data gathering.

Furthermore, since the publication of the FDA alert, eight retrospective cohort and case–control studies, using observational study methodology, investigated the potential association between exposure to AEDs and suicidality in PWE or patients in whom AEDs were prescribed for the treatment of primary psychiatric disorders (Gibbons et al., 2009; Andersohn et al., 2010; Arana et al., 2010; Gibbons et al., 2010; Olesen et al., 2010; Patorno et al., 2010; Redden et al., 2011, VanCott et al., 2010). Reviews of these studies demonstrated contradictory results, which were attributed to serious methodologic problems. These included, in particular, failure to adjust for past suicidal behaviors (Andersohn et al., 2010; Olesen et al., 2010), or recognizing past suicidality but over an unspecified period of time (VanCott et al., 2010) or exclusion of subjects with a past history, or family history of suicidality before the study entry (Arana et al., 2010; Patorno et al., 2010). Since suicide attempts tend to be recurrent (between 14% and 17% after 1 year and more than 30% over 10 years) (Owens et al., 2002), they are likely to influence the clinicians' choice of AED in patients with such a history, whereby AEDs with positive psychotropic properties are likely to be prescribed and those with negative properties may be avoided in such patients. Clearly, such failure to adjust for prior suicidal behavior is likely to bias the findings of such studies.

In conclusion, the results of the FDA meta-analysis must be considered with great caution. In fact, to determine whether a specific AED increases or decreases the suicidal risk, it is necessary to conduct studies in which suicidality data are collected in a systematic and prospective manner. In the opinion of this author, some AEDs (barbiturates, levetiracetam, topiramate, zonisamide, and vigabatrin) can increase the suicidal risk in a subset of PWE who have a predisposition to develop psychiatric disorders.

Epilepsy surgery

Epilepsy surgery has become a recommended treatment for patients with focal epilepsy whose seizures fail to remit after two to three AEDs, given at optimal doses. Temporal lobectomy is the most frequent type of surgical procedure, consisting of 75% of all types of surgeries in adults and yielding a 50% seizure remission. While remission of presurgical comorbid mood and anxiety disorders can be found in one-third to one-half of patients, particularly when they become seizure-free, suicide has been a complication of severe post-surgical depressive episodes, accounting for 24% of all deaths, whether or not seizure-freedom was achieved (Pompili et al., 2006). Future studies with larger numbers of subjects are necessary to clarify these data, however.

How to identify patients at risk?

Neurologists are not expected to manage the psychiatric disorders associated with increased suicidal risk. Yet, they should identify PWE with an increased suicidal risk by screening for the three most frequent risks associated with suicidality: (i) current or past history of mood and anxiety disorders; (ii) family psychiatric history of mood disorders, particularly of suicidal behavior; and (iii) past suicidal attempts.

The use of self-report screening instruments aimed at identifying major depressive episodes and generalized anxiety disorders are available. These instruments include a six-item, self-rating instrument called the Neurological Disorders Depression Inventory for Epilepsy (NDDI-E), which was developed to identify major depressive episodes, specifically for people with epilepsy (Gilliam et al., 2006). The NDDI-E takes less than 3 minutes to complete; a score of >15 is *suggestive* of a major depressive episode with a specificity of 90% and a sensitivity of 80% and serves as a red-flag referral to a psychiatrist for further evaluation.

No self-rating instrument to identify symptoms of generalized anxiety disorder has been validated for people with epilepsy. Yet, The Patient's Health Questionnaire, Generalized Anxiety Disorder-7 (GAD-7), can be extremely helpful (Kroenke et al., 2007). It is a seven-item, self-rating instrument that takes 3 minutes to administer; a score of greater than 10 is suggestive of a generalized anxiety disorder.

Screening for suicidality in the outpatient Neurology clinic can be done with two instruments. The first one is the Suicidality Module of the Mini International Neuropsychiatric Interview (MINI) (Sheehan et al., 1998). It has six questions, which are answered with a YES or NO and provide information on any suicide attempt, active and passive suicidal ideation, and suicidal plans. The second instrument is the Columbia-Suicide-Severity Rating Scale (C-SSRS), which is the prospective counterpart to the FDA-commissioned Columbia Classification Algorithm for Suicide Assessment (C-CASA) adverse event system. C-CASA classification is requested in all psychiatry and obesity trials (Posner et al., 2011).

Concluding remarks

Suicidality is a relatively frequent comorbidity in PWE, and has a complex relation with epilepsy. Its pathogenic mechanisms are multiple, with prior or current psychiatric history and family psychiatric history being the most important risk factors. The degree to which AEDs cause an increased suicidal risk is not yet determined, and that assessment will require future studies that are methodologically sound. Nonetheless, caution must be used when prescribing certain AEDs in PWE with current or past and/or family psychiatric history.

References

Adelow, C., Anderson, T., Ahlbom, A., & Tomson, T. (2012). Hospitalization for psychiatric disorders before and after onset of unprovoked seizures/epilepsy. *Neurology*, **78**, 396–401.

Andersohn, F., Schade, R., Willich, S. N., & Garbe, E. (2010). Use of antiepileptic drugs in epilepsy and the risk of self-harm or suicidal behavior. *Neurology*, **75**, 335–340.

Arana, A., Wentworth, C. E., Ayuso-Mateos, J. L., & Arellano, F. M. (2010). Suicide-related events in patients treated with antiepileptic drugs. *New England Journal of Medicine*, **363**, 542–551.

Barraclough, B. M. (1987). The suicide rate of epilepsy. *Acta Psychiatrica Scandinavica*, **76**, 339–345.

Brent, D. A., Crumrine, P. K., Varma, R. R., Allan, M., & Allman, C. (1987). Phenobarbital treatment and major depressive disorder in children with epilepsy. *Pediatrics*, **80**, 909–917.

Bunney, W. E., & Fawcett, J. A. (1965). Possibility of a biochemical test for suicidal potential: An analysis of endocrine studies prior to three studies. *Archives of General Psychiatry*, **13**, 232–239.

Christensen, J., Vestergaard, M., Mortensen, P., Sidenius, P., & Agerbo, E. (2007). Epilepsy and risk of suicide: a population-based case–control study. *Lancet Neurology*, **6**, 693–698.

Coryell, W. (1990). DST abnormality as a predictor of course in major depression. *Journal of Affective Disorders*, **19**, 163–169.

Currie, S., Heathfield, K. W., Henson, R. A., & Scott, D. F. (1971). Clinical course and prognosis of temporal lobe epilepsy: a survey of 666 patients. *Brain*, **94**, 173–190.

Forsgren, L., & Nystrom, L. (1990). An incident case-referent study of epileptic seizures in adults. *Epilepsy Research*, **6**, 66–81.

Fukuchi, T., Kanemoto, K., Kato, M., et al. (2002). Death in epilepsy with special attention to suicide cases. *Epilepsy Research*, **51**, 233–236.

Gibbons, R., Hur, K., Brown, C. H., & Mann, J. J. (2009). Relationship between antiepileptic drugs and suicide attempts in patients with bipolar disorder. *Archives of General Psychiatry*, **66**, 1354–1360.

Gibbons, R. D., Hur, K., Brown, C. H., & Mann, J. J. (2010). Gabapentin and suicide attempts. *Pharmacoepidemiology and Drug Safety*, **19**, 1241–1247.

Gilliam, F. G., Barry, J. J., Hermann, B. P., et al. (2006). Rapid detection of major depression in epilepsy: a multicentre study. *Lancet Neurology*, **5**, 399–405.

Harris, E. C., & Barraclough, B. (1989). Suicide as an outcome for mental disorders: A meta-analysis. *Archives of Neurology*, **46**(10), 1065–1068.

Hasler, G., Bonwetsch, R., Giovacchini, G., et al. (2007). 5-HT(1A) receptor binding in temporal lobe epilepsy patients with and without major depression. *Biological Psychiatry*, **62**(11), 1258–1264.

Hecimovic, H., Salpekar, J., Kanner, A. M., & Barry, J. J. (2011) Suicidality and epilepsy: A neuropsychobiological perspective. *Epilepsy and Behavior*, **22**(1), 77–84.

Hesdorffer, D. C., & Kanner, A. M. (2009). The FDA alert on suicidality and antiepileptic drugs: Fire or false alarm? *Epilepsia*, **50**, 978–986.

Hesdorffer, D. C., Hauser, W. A., Annegers, J. F., & Cascino, G. (2000). Major depression is a risk factor for seizures in older adults. *Annals of Neurology*, **47**, 246–249.

Hesdorffer, D. C., Hauser, W. A., Ludvigsson, P., Olafsson, E., & Kjartansson, O. (2006). Depression and suicide attempt as risk factors for incident unprovoked seizures. *Annals of Neurology*, **59**, 35–41.

Hesdorffer, D. C., Lúdvígsson, P., Hauser, W. A., Olafsson, E., & Kjartansson, O. (2007). Co-occurrence of major depression or suicide attempt with migraine with aura and risk for unprovoked seizure. *Epilepsy Research*, **75**(2–3), 220–223.

Hesdorffer, D. C., Ishihara, L., Mynepalli, L., et al. (2012). Epilepsy, suicidality, and psychiatric disorders: a bidirectional association. *Annals of Neurology*, **72**(2), 184–191.

Hesdorffer, D. C., French, J. A., Posner, K., et al. (2013). Suicidal ideation and behavior screening in intractable focal epilepsy eligible for drug trials. *Epilepsia*, **54**(5), 879–887.

Jobe, P. C. (2006). Affective disorder and epilepsy comorbidity in the genetically epilepsy prone-rat (GEPR). In: F. Gilliam, A. M. Kanner, & Y. I. Sheline (Eds.) *Depression and Brain Dysfunction* (pp. 121–157). London: Taylor & Francis.

Jokinen, J., & Nordström, P. (2009). HPA axis hyperactivity and attempted suicide in young adult mood disorder inpatients. *Journal of Affective Disorders*, **116**(1–2), 117–120.

Jones, J. E., Hermann, B. P., Barry, J. J., et al. (2003). Rates and risk factors for suicide, suicidal ideation, and suicide attempts in chronic epilepsy. *Epilepsy and Behavior*, **4**, S31–S38.

Kanemoto, K., Kawasaki, J., & Mori, E. (1999). Violence and epilepsy: a close relation between violence and postictal psychosis. *Epilepsia*, **40**(1), 107–109.

Kanner, A. M. (2006). Epilepsy, suicidal behavior, and depression: do they share common pathogenic mechanisms? *Lancet Neurology*, **5**(2), 107–108.

Kanner, A. M. (2012). Can neurobiologic pathogenic mechanisms of depression facilitate the development of seizure disorders? *Lancet Neurology*, **11**, 1093–1102.

Kanner, A. M., Soto, A., & Gross-Kanner, H. (2004). Prevalence and clinical characteristics of postictal psychiatric symptoms in partial epilepsy. *Neurology*, **62**, 708–713.

Kroenke, K., Spitzer, R. L., Williams, J. B., Monahan, P. O., & Löwe, B. (2007). Anxiety disorders in primary care: prevalence, impairment, comorbidity, and detection. *Annals of Internal Medicine*, **146**, 317–325.

Mula, M., & Sander, J. W. (2007). Suicidal ideation in epilepsy and levetiracetam therapy. *Epilepsy and Behavior*, **11**, 130–132.

Mula, M., Trimble, M. R., Yuen, A., Liu, R. S., & Sander, J. W. (2003). Psychiatric adverse events during levetiracetam therapy. *Neurology*, **61**, 704–706.

Nilsson, L., Tomson, T., Farahmand, B. Y., et al. (1997). Cause-specific mortality in epilepsy: a cohort study of more than 9,000 patients once hospitalized for epilepsy. *Epilepsia*, **38**, 1062–1068.

Nilsson, L., Ahlbom, A., Farahmand, B. Y., Asberg, M., & Tomson, T. (2002). Risk factors for suicide in epilepsy: a case control study. *Epilepsia*, **43**, 644–651.

Norman, W. H., Brown, W. A., Miller, I. W., Keitner, G. I., & Overholser, J. C. (1990). The dexamethasone suppression test and completed suicide. *Acta Psychiatrica Scandinavica*, **81**, 120–125.

Olesen, J. B., Hansen, P. R., Erdal, J., et al. (2010). Antiepileptic drugs and risk of suicide: a nationwide study. *Pharmacoepidemiology and Drug Safety*, **19**, 518–524.

Owens, D., Horrocks, J., & House, A. (2002). Fatal and non-fatal repetition of self-harm: Systematic review. *British Journal of Psychiatry*, **181**, 193–199.

Patorno, E., Bohn, R. L., Wahl, P. M., et al. (2010). Anticonvulsant medications and the risk of suicide, attempted suicide, or violent death. *JAMA*, **303**, 1401–1409.

Pompili, M., Girardi, P., Tatarelli, G., Angeletti, G., & Tatarelli, R. (2006). Suicide after surgical treatment in patients with epilepsy: a meta-analytic investigation. *Psychological Reports*, **98**(2), 323–338.

Posner. K., Brown, G. K., Stanley, B., et al. (2011). The Columbia-Suicide Severity Rating Scale: initial validity and internal consistency findings from three multisite studies with adolescents and adults. *American Journal of Psychiatry*, **168**, 1266–1277.

Rafnsson, V., Ólafsson, E., & Hauser, W. A. (2001). Cause-specific mortality in adults with unprovoked seizures: A population-based incidence cohort study. *Neuroepidemiology*, **20**, 232–236.

Robertson, M. M. (1997). Suicide, parasuicide, and epilepsy. In: J. Engel, & T. A. Pedley (Eds.) *Epilepsy: A Comprehensive Textbook* (pp. 2141–2151). Philadelphia: Lippincott–Raven.

Sargent, P. A., Kjaer, K. H., Bench, C. J., et al. (2000). Brain serotonin 1A receptor binding measured by positron emission tomography with [11C]WAY-100635: effects of depression and antidepressant treatment. *Archives of General Psychiatry*, **57**, 174–180.

Sequeira, A., Mamdani, F., Ernst, C., et al. (2009). Global brain gene expression analysis links glutamatergic and GABAergic alterations to suicide and major depression. *PLoS One*, **11** Aug;4(8):e6585.

Sheehan, B. V., Lecrubier, Y., Sheehan, K. H., et al. (1998). The Mini International Neuropsychiatric Interview (MINI): The development and validation of structured diagnostic psychiatric interview for DSM-IV and ICD-10. *Journal of Clinical Psychiatry*, **59**(Suppl 20), 22–33.

Tellez-Zenteno, J. F., Patten, S. B., Jetté, N., Williams, J., & Wiebe, S. (2007). Psychiatric comorbidity in epilepsy: a population-based analysis. *Epilepsia*, **48**, 2336–2344.

Theodore, W. H., Giovacchini, G., Bonwetsch, R., et al. (2006). The effect of antiepileptic drugs on 5-HT-receptor binding measured by positron emission tomography. *Epilepsia*, **47**(3), 499–503.

Toczek, M. T., Carson, R. E., Lang, L., et al. (2003). PET imaging of 5-HT1A receptor binding in patients with temporal lobe epilepsy. *Neurology*, **60**, 749–756.

Trimble, R. M., Rüsch, N., Betts, T., & Crawford, P. M. (2000). Psychiatric symptoms after therapy with new antiepileptic drugs: Psychopathological and seizure related variables. *Seizure*, **9**, 249–254.

US Department of Health and Human Services, Food and Drug Administration, Center for Drug Evaluation and Research, Office of Translational Sciences, Office of Biostatistics (2008). Statistical review and evaluation: Antiepileptic drugs and suicidality. May 21, 2008.

VanCott, A. C., Cramer, J. A., Copeland, L. A., et al. (2010). Suicide-related behaviors in older patients with new anti-epileptic drug use: data from the VA hospital system. *BMC Medicine*, **8**, 4

Wolf, P. (1991). Acute behavioral symptomatology at disappearance of epileptiform EEG abnormality. Paradoxical or 'forced' normalization. *Advances in Neurology*, **55**, 127–142.

Chapter 17 Suicidal ideation and behavior during pregnancy and the postpartum period

Jessica Coker and Zachary N. Stowe

Introduction

Maternal mortality has steadily declined over the past 50 years largely secondary to advances in medical care. In contrast, the rates of violent maternal deaths including suicide and homicide during the perinatal period have remained essentially unchanged (Shadigian & Bauer, 2005). Currently, maternal mortality secondary to suicide and homicide outnumber all other indirect and direct causes of maternal death including hemorrhage, preeclampsia/eclampsia, and amniotic fluid embolism (Palladino et al., 2011). Maternal suicide is an important public health issue that receives limited educational attention among the public and health care providers. Suicidal ideation and/or suicide attempts during pregnancy pose potential adverse effects to the health and well-being of the fetus (Gandhi et al., 2006). The loss of a mother in the early postpartum period can also have long-term adverse impacts on the infant and family (Comtois et al., 2008). In the most devastating circumstances, filicide is highly correlated with postpartum suicide increasingly demonstrating the impact suicidal behaviors can impose on public health (Friedman & Resnick, 2007). The risk factors for maternal suicidal ideation, suicidal attempt, and completed suicide during the perinatal period are most certainly multifactorial. A major contributor to the risk for suicidal thoughts and behavior in multiple patient populations is the presence and/or history of mental illness. Despite the 'lay' perception that the perinatal period is uniformly a time of emotional well-being and happiness, there is sparse data supporting this misperception. Briefly, as many as 70% of women will endorse depressive symptoms during pregnancy and up to 16% fulfill diagnostic criteria for major depression (O'Hara et al., 1984; Affonso et al., 1990; Beck, 1995; Weissman & Olfson, 1995; Evans et al., 2001). Two large studies, collectively comprising 122 400 women, found a 14–20% incidence of prenatal MDD (Marcus et al., 2003; Oberlander et al., 2006).

Postpartum (PP) mental illness has been documented since Hippocrates and confirmed in numerous studies across multiple cultural/ethnic groups. The most common illness is postpartum depression, which affects 10–22% of adult women, and up to 26% of adolescent mothers (Troutman & Cutrona, 1990; Stowe & Nemeroff, 1995). Notably, 11% of women presenting for evaluation of postpartum depression (PPD) report symptom onset before delivery (Stowe et al., 2005).

There has been considerable discussion and debate in the literature regarding treatment issues during pregnancy and lactation, particularly in the context of pharmacology. While the majority of articles have focused on the potential impact of treatment and/or illness there is remarkably limited discussion of the risk for maternal death during this vulnerable period.

In this chapter we examine the extant literature on suicide, suicide attempts, and suicidal ideation during the perinatal period. Expanding the health care provider's familiarity with risk factors and potential protective factors is a requisite step in identifying women at increased risk of self-harm and implementing prevention strategies for such a devastating event.

Epidemiology

The prevalence of maternal mental illness during the perinatal period underscores the need to further scrutinize the rate of suicidal ideation, attempts, and completed suicides. There are limited investigations documenting the rate of thoughts of death and dying as well as thoughts of self-harm during pregnancy. The prevalence of suicidal ideation across the perinatal

A Concise Guide to Understanding Suicide, ed. Stephen H. Koslow, Pedro Ruiz, and Charles B. Nemeroff. Published by Cambridge University Press.

period (pregnancy and the first year postpartum) found the rate of suicidal ideation to be 2.7–3.2% when controlling for confounding factors during a 12-month time period (Wisner et al., 2013). This is comparable to the 2.8–3.3% in the general population (Gavin et al., 2011). In clinical populations with a history of mental illness, up to 35% of pregnant women endorsed thoughts of self-harm (Newport et al., 2007) which is remarkably consistent with the rate of suicidal ideation (35%) in pregnant women with post-traumatic stress disorder and comorbid substance abuse (Eggleston et al., 2009). In another review article, Lindahl and colleagues noted that 10.2–14.6% of women endorse thoughts of self-harm over the course of pregnancy(Lindahl et al., 2005). The variation noted in the incidence of suicidal ideation appears to be largely dependent on the population being surveyed.

Although women may experience suicidal ideation during the perinatal period at relatively high rates, that are at the minimum consistent with the general population, the research evaluating suicide attempts among pregnant and postpartum women indicates a lower rate of attempt. Two recent studies in the USA found that women are not as likely to attempt suicide during the perinatal period. Briefly, a study in Maryland found that pregnant women had half the rate of all hospitalizations due to suicide attempts than non-pregnant women of reproductive age (Greenblatt et al., 1997). A similar study in Pennsylvania showed that pregnant women were 62% less likely to be hospitalized for self-inflicted injury (Weiss, 1999). In Washington State from 1987 to 2001, postpartum women were hospitalized for a suicide attempt approximately one-third the rate of the general female population (Schiff & Grossman, 2006). This is consistent with previous investigations in a small sample from the United Kingdom looking at data from a catchment area "Casualty Department", which demonstrated postpartum women are approximately 43% less likely to attempt suicide (Appleby and Turnbull, 1995). All of these studies, with the exception of the Appleby investigation, evaluated all hospitalizations after a suicide attempt thereby excluding many women that: (1) were not evaluated by medical professionals; (2) were misclassified on the basis of an event being viewed as not being a suicide attempt; and/or (3) were not hospitalized following a suicide attempt. This raises important questions in how health care professionals approach pregnant women at high risk for suicidal behavior. There is limited discussion of how 'involuntary commitment laws' may apply differentially to pregnant women if one views the care and well-being of the fetus as representing "potential harm to others." Is there a reluctance to hospitalize pregnant women in psychiatric facilities and does pregnancy mobilize social support that further reduces the chance of hospitalization? The rate of mental illness, prevalence of suicidal ideation, and the suicide attempt data above underscore the potential that clinicians will encounter treatment issues for pregnant and postpartum women at risk for suicidal behavior.

Fortunately, completed suicide during pregnancy and postpartum is far less common than both suicidal ideation and suicide attempts. The perinatal period is unique when considering the potential protective factors against suicide. The higher rate of contact with medical professionals, potentially enhanced engagement of social support, and the psychological and biological constructs of maternal instinct may all play a role. In the United Kingdom, pregnant women are found to have 1/20th the risk of suicide compared to non-pregnant counterparts while postpartum have approximately 1/5th the risk (Appleby, 1991). The initial studies in the USA revealed pregnancy-associated suicide is estimated to be one-third the general female population (Marzuk et al., 1997). These studies have limitations regarding methods of collecting data and reliance on death certificates that were matched to birth records. This likely underestimates the number of suicides during this period as it has been estimated that up to 65% of death certificates do not have correct information when it comes to perinatal status (Dannenberg et al., 1995; Shadigian & Bauer, 2005).

To improve the surveillance of suicides in the USA, the National Violent Death Reporting System (NVDRS) was created in 2003. This database provides more in-depth information regarding violent deaths across 17 states. Data collected comes from four major sources: (1) death certificates; (2) coroner/medical examiner reports; (3) police reports; and (4) crime laboratories (Centers for Disease Control and Prevention – National Violent Death Reporting System, 2013). The NVDRS data found that only 5% of all suicides in reproductive aged women occurred during the perinatal period. Two percent of these were during pregnancy while the remaining 3% were in the postpartum period (Gold et al., 2012). The NVDRS data is remarkably consistent with the previous studies noted above. The rate of completed antenatal and postnatal suicide is 2.0–2.77 per 100 000 live births compared to the rate of 6.57 per 100 000 live births in reproductive aged women (Palladino et al., 2011).

The disparity between the rates of suicidal ideation and suicide attempt/completion is at some level reassuring when considering treatment. However, the methods employed during suicide attempts/completion during the perinatal period warrant discussion. Those women who succumb to suicidal thoughts and intention tend to have a propensity to use methods with a high degree of lethality including firearms and asphyxiation. Specifically, pregnant women are more likely to use firearms while postpartum women are more likely to use asphyxia and all other women of reproductive age are likely to choose poisoning or blunt trauma (Appleby, 1991; Gold et al., 2012). Ironically, these methods of suicide are more commonly associated with suicidal behavior in males. In contrast, pregnancy-associated suicide attempts remain consistent with non-pregnant women and involve overdose (Schiff & Grossman, 2006). Regardless of the method chosen, suicidal behavior has potentially severe adverse consequences to the fetus including preterm labor, cesarean delivery, low birth weights, and respiratory distress (Gandhi et al., 2006).

Studies of suicidal behavior – ideation, attempt, and completion – are summarized in Table 17.1.

Table 17.1. Studies of suicidal behavioral during pregnancy and the postpartum period

Reference	Sample size/type	Study design	Results	Risk factors	Comments
Suicidal ideation (SI)					
Newport et al., 2007	N = 383 Pregnant	Prospective, clinician (HRSD) and self-rated measures (BDI)	+SI in 16.7% on Ham-D +SI in 27.8% on BDI	Unmarried, never attended college, unplanned pregnancy, lifetime history of mood disorder, anxiety disorder, substance use disorder, current major depressive episode	All participants were referred to tertiary clinic for neuropsychiatric evaluation
Eggleston et al., 2009	N = 105 Pregnant	Prospective multiple rating scales	+SI in 35% in comorbid SUD and PTSD +SI in 9% of women with SUD and other Axis I disorder +SI in 3% of women with SUD only	Comorbid substance abuse and PTSD	All participants had diagnosis of SUD
Benute et al., 2011	N = 268 Pregnant	Prospective PRIME-MD structured interview	+SI in 5% of sample	Lack of religious belief	Interviewed at university hospital
Gavin et al., 2011	N = 2159 Pregnant	Prospective PHQ short form	+SI in 2.7%	Comorbid major depression, comorbid panic disorder, 12 or less years of education, living without a spouse or partner, high level of psychosocial stress, current smoker, positive domestic violence, non-white	Represents 12-month prevalence

Table 17.1. (cont.)

Reference	Sample size/type	Study design	Results	Risk factors	Comments
Suicidal ideation (SI)					
Wisner et al., 2013	N = 10 000 Postpartum	Prospective EPDS rating scale and follow-up SCID	+SI in 3.2%	Higher EPDS scores >10, comorbid psychiatric disorder	Majority of women had primary mood disorders
Suicide attempts (SA)					
Appleby and Turnbull, 1995	N = 131 Postpartum	Retrospective	43% odds ratio of hospitalization due to SA among postpartum	NA	Included only women seen at casualty department following parasuicide
Greenblatt et al., 1997	N = 80 311 Pregnancy	Retrospective discharge summaries in Maryland hospital from 1979 to 1990	~50% rate of hospitalizations among pregnant women compared to non-pregnant	NA	
Weiss, 1999	N = 16 722 Pregnancy	Retrospective records review	62% less hospitalizations for SA during pregnancy vs. non-pregnant	Non-white women, younger age	All hospitalizations
Schiff and Grossman, 2006	N = 520 Postpartum	Case–control	43.9 per 100 000 hospitalized SA among postpartum	<20 years old, single, non-white, <12 years of education, Medicaid, infant death	1/3 the rate of hospitalization among all women when adjusted for age
Comtois et al., 2008	N = 1775 Postpartum	Case–control	2% (N = 355) hospitalized for SA during postpartum	Younger, non-white, unmarried, greater gravidity and parity, public insurance	All hospitalizations
Completed suicides					
Appleby, 1991.	N = 14 Pregnancy & Postpartum	Retrospective records review	Pregnant = 0.05 mortality ratio Postpartum = 0.17 mortality ratio	Unmarried, past or current psychiatric disorder, stillbirth	Limited sample
Dannenberg et al., 1995	N = 115 Pregnancy & Postpartum	Retrospective records review of women who died in New York from 1987 to 1991	13% of injury-related deaths in perinatal period were due to suicide	NA	Office of Vital Statistics.
Gissler et al., 1996	N = 9192 Postpartum	Retrospective Linkage of birth and death certificates in Finland	5.4% completed suicide postpartum	2 months postpartum, single, mental disorders	
Marzuk et al., 1997	N = 315 Pregnancy	Retrospective records review	0.33 mortality ratio for pregnancy-associated suicide	NA	~1/3 rate of suicide in general female population
Oates, 2003	N = 378 Postpartum	Retrospective cohort, records review	10% (N = 28) suicide-associated postpartum deaths	NA	Small sample size from CEMD data

Table 17.1. (cont.)

Reference	Sample size/type	Study design	Results	Risk factors	Comments
Suicidal ideation (SI)					
Palladino et al., 2011	N = 223 Pregnancy & Postpartum	Retrospective cohort, records review	2.0 per 100 000 pregnancy-associated suicide rate	White or American Indian decent, intimate partner problems	45.7% occurred during pregnancy and the remaining during postpartum. Evaluated data from NVDRS
Samandari et al., 2011	N = 348 Pregnancy & Postpartum	Retrospective cohort, records review	2.77 per 100 000 pregnancy-associated suicide rate	Younger (14–29), never married	Data from North Carolina VDRS
Gold et al., 2012	N = 2083 Pregnancy & Postpartum	Retrospective cohort, records review	5% were pregnant/ postpartum at time of suicide	Current depressed mood, substance abuse, intimate partner problems	Postpartum women had higher risk of suicide via asphyxiation

N = sample size. NA: not available.
BDI: Beck Depression Inventory; CEMD: Confidential Enquiries into Maternal Deaths; EPDS: Edinburgh Postnatal Depression Scale; Ham-D: Hamilton Rating Scale for Depression; NVDRS: National Violent Death Reporting System; PHQ: Patient Health Questionnaire; PRIME-MD: Primary Care Evaluation of Mental Disorders; PTSD: post-traumatic stress disorder; SCID: Structured Clinical Interview for DSM-IV for Axis I primary and secondary diagnoses; SUD: substance use disorder; VDRS: Violent Death Reporting System.

Risk factors for suicidal behavior in pregnancy and the postpartum period

In several of the studies reviewed above, investigators have sought to delineate the risk factors for suicidal ideation, suicidal behavior, and completed suicide. Expanding the knowledge base of the identified risk factors provides the foundation to develop and enhance preventive strategies.

A significant, if not the most consistently reported, risk factor for suicide across multiple populations is past psychiatric history. Reports from the UK indicate that more than 60% of perinatal suicides occur in women with a past or current psychiatric disorder, with half of these women having a psychiatric admission following a previous childbirth (Appleby, 1991; Oates, 2003). In the USA, the relationship between past psychiatric history with pregnancy-associated suicides has not been fully examined. As discussed previously, women with psychiatric illness are shown to have a ten-fold increased risk of suicidal ideation. Research indicates that women with suicidal ideation and suicide attempts during pregnancy and the postpartum period also have higher rates of comorbid psychiatric illness including substance dependence, anxiety disorders, and eating disorders (Newport et al., 2007; Gavin et al., 2011; Wisner et al., 2013). An impediment to delineating the role(s) of individual psychiatric history is the difficulty in obtaining records regarding past psychiatric history at the time of reviewing birth/death certificates. For example, the reports from the UK were based on neuroleptic medications identified at autopsy as a proxy for psychiatric illness. Approximately 50% of reproductive aged women are not correctly diagnosed and/or treated with psychiatric medications; as such the presence of psychiatric illness is almost certainly underestimated in studies relying on available medical records (Farr et al., 2010). Despite this potentially confounding factor, controlling for psychiatric illness within the current data suggests that the prevalence of psychiatric illness remains similar among women who commit suicide regardless of their perinatal status. Best estimates reveal that 56% of all women committing suicide have a known mental health problem with mood disorder being most common followed by anxiety disorder and psychotic disorders; 32% of these women have a history of previous suicide attempt. Postpartum women are shown to have higher rates of reporting "depressed mood" within the 2 weeks prior to suicide compared to pregnant women (Gold et al., 2012). Notably, 32% of these women had a history of previous suicide attempt. Postpartum women were statistically more likely to be in a current depressed mood compared to pregnant women when the suicide was committed (Gold et al., 2012; Wisner et al., 2013).

Women under the age of 30 years constitute the majority of cases of suicidal ideation, attempts, and suicide completions during pregnancy and the postpartum period (Schiff & Grossman, 2006; Gold et al., 2012; Wisner et al., 2013). Conversely, in the non-perinatal group, women over 30 years of age have a higher rate of completed suicide. It has been argued that the group over 30 years of age would have fewer total pregnancies accounting for this increased rate of completed suicide (Gissler et al., 1996; Palladino et al., 2011; Samandari et al., 2011).

Single women have higher rates of suicide, with up to half of all suicides in the perinatal period occurring in single women (Palladino et al., 2011; Samandari et al., 2011; Gold et al., 2012). This is consistent with the suicide attempt and suicidal ideation studies that have also demonstrated higher rates among single women (Schiff & Grossman, 2006; Newport et al., 2007). A risk factor potentially related to being single is the influence of unplanned pregnancies. In contrast to this, a small study in Brazil showed no association between unplanned pregnancy and completed suicide; however, the investigators did report increased suicidal ideation associated with unintended pregnancies (Benute et al., 2011). This replicated an earlier report in a clinical population with psychiatric illness showing a postive association between unplanned pregnancy and suicidal ideation (Newport et al., 2007).

Similar to studies in non-perinatal populations, the role of social support and the presence of significant interpersonal relationships appear to influence suicidal behavior among both pregnant and postpartum women. Friction or conflict with a current or former intimate partner appears to be a contributing factor in perinatal suicide (Gold et al., 2012). For example, approximately half of women completing suicide had a history of conflict with a current or former intimate partner that was determined to play an influential role in the suicide (Palladino et al., 2011). Due to the inability to determine significance of the interpersonal conflict in postmortem studies, these figures may underestimate the role intimate partner conflict plays in the risk for perinatal suicide. The potentially adverse impact of losing social support secondary to intimate partner conflict may intensify suicidal behavior. Women with suicide attempts during the postpartum period report a history of domestic violence within 1 year preceding their attempt, supporting the importance of this factor (Gavin et al., 2011). Domestic violence occurs in 4–8% of pregnancies (Gazmararian et al., 1996), and while a definitive study is lacking, we have noted a high rate in pregnant and postpartum women admitted to our hospital (Stowe, personal observation).

Additional factors that may increase the risk for suicidal behavior during pregnancy and the postpartum period include African American or American Indian races, women with less than 12 years of education, public sponsored insurance, history of fetal/infant death within the past year, smoking, substance abuse, and high levels of psychosocial stress (Marzuk et al., 1997; Schiff & Grossman, 2006; Comtois et al., 2008; Samandari et al., 2011; Palladino et al., 2011; Gold et al., 2012; Wisner et al., 2013).

In addition, women infected with *Toxoplasma gondii* during the perinatal period have higher rates of self-directed violence. *Toxoplasma gondii* is a neurotropic protozoan parasite typically transmitted via raw/undercooked meat, the soil, and felines including most commonly contact with contaminated sandboxes/litter boxes. The parasite can also be congenitally acquired leading to a potentially adverse outcome for the infant (Jones et al., 2001). The parasite spreads to the neuronal cells of the brain, mainly in the prefrontal cortex and amygdala, and has been shown to increase self-directed violence behaviors in patients with psychiatric illness, including mood disorders and schizophrenia. In a Danish study, women who were seropositive for *T. gondii* IgG at delivery had a 1.53 increased relative rate of self-directed violence compared with seronegative counterparts over a 4-year study (Pedersen et al., 2012).

In contrast, several factors that have been examined and show no significant correlation with perinatal suicidal behaviors include a history of spontaneous/therapeutic abortions, maternal complications during labor or delivery, maternal parity, and "precipitating circumstances." These precipitating circumstances included "crisis within the last 2 weeks; the death or suicide of a friend or family member within the past 5 years; problems with finances, physical health, school or job; recent criminal/legal problems; and having a relationship problem other than an intimate partner" (Schiff & Grossman, 2006; Gavin et al., 2011; Gold et al., 2012).

The role of breastfeeding as either a protective or vulnerability factor for suicidal behavior has not been adequately investigated. There has been limited evidence that women who breastfeed tend to have better moods with decreased inflammation and lower rates of depression (Kendall-Tackett, 2007). The role of oxytocin and pitocin in this process has not been fully established but has the potential of offering suicide protection similar to possible increased serotonin levels in late pregnancy. Additional research in this area could be beneficial for both increased risk new mothers and possibly psychiatric patients in general.

In summary, the vulnerability factors for suicidal ideation and behavior during pregnancy and the postpartum period include: (1) current and/or past psychiatric history; (2) unplanned pregnancy; (3) less than 30 years of age; (4) single; and (5) intimate partner conflict. It is important to consider how these risk factors can be utilized in furthering our development of prevention strategies and in furthering understanding of the etiopathogenesis of suicidal behaviors in the perinatal period.

Prevention

Identifying a single risk factor with adequate sensitivity and specificity for suicidal ideation and behavior during pregnancy and the postpartum period is difficult. Typically women in the perinatal period have the highest rate of contact with health care providers providing significant opportunities for screening, identification of at risk groups, and the development of preventive strategies.

It is recommended by the American College of Obstetricians and Gynecologists (ACOG) to screen every patient for "barriers to care, unstable housing, unintended pregnancy, communication barriers, nutrition, tobacco use, substances use, depression, safety, intimate partner violence and stress" (American College of Obstetricians and Gynecologists Committee on Care for Underserved Women, 2006). The initial step in prevention is the screening process for identifying those at risk with multiple structured methods of screening for depression and suicidal ideation available. Arguably, sensitivity being more important than specificity, it is crucial to provide the most sensitive results to lower false negative results. As Newport et al. suggested, "the consequences of undetected suicidality can be devastating for both maternal and fetal well-being. Even an unsuccessful suicide attempt (e.g., drug overdose, carbon monoxide poisoning, etc.) can harm a fetus and have long-term adverse consequences for child development" (Newport et al., 2007). There is remarkably limited data comparing screening methods/instruments in perinatal women. Comparison of self-rated instruments (The Beck Depression Inventory [BDI] and Edinburgh Postnatal Depression Scale [EPDS]) to a clinician-rated scale (Hamilton Rating Scale for Depression [HRSD]) yielded a broad range of suicidal ideation in a clinical population of pregnant women (Newport et al., 2007). The self-rated scales consistently demonstrated a higher proportion of women with thoughts of passive and active suicidal ideation compared to the clinician-rated scale, 29.2% and 16.9%, respectively. A variety of factors may account for these findings including: (1) the "wording" of the question; and (2) greater patient comfort of endorsement on self-rated scales. In busy clinical settings, the self-rated measures may be more applicable and have the benefit of higher sensitivity. This is consistent with studies in non-perinatal populations that show clinician-rated scales underestimate suicidal ideation in approximately 20% of cases compared to self-rated reports (Yigletu et al., 2004). This was also suggested by previous authors who reported that select patients are more comfortable answering these types of personal questions in a self-reported measure such as computer interviews (Greist et al., 1973; Erdman et al., 1987).

It may not be practical in the busy clinical setting to consistently screen for mental illness and suicidal behavior at every visit. While the data is limited, there is evidence that the first 2 months postpartum pose the highest risk for completed suicide (Appleby, 1991; Gissler et al., 1996). In addition, suicide attempts occur more frequently at 1 and 12 months postpartum (Schiff & Grossman, 2006). Screening proximate to these windows of heightened vulnerability should be a requisite component of clinical assessment.

Similarly, screening for intimate partner conflict/violence is an additional modifiable risk factor for suicidal behaviors during the perinatal period. The three-question Abuse Assessment Screen completed by health care providers has shown both sensitive and specific results and is recommended in identifying women at increased risk of domestic violence (McFarlane et al., 1992). Once identified, referral to needed services such as mental health, violence, and legal services can be recommended (Martin et al., 2007). This area remains a relatively understudied topic and additional research is needed to determine the most effective intervention methods. Interventions may influence not only the risk for suicide, but also lower the rate of maternal homicide. This would have dramatic effects on maternal mortality as homicide is currently the leading cause of maternal death (Palladino et al., 2011).

Following the screening and identification of high-risk groups, it is difficult to determine best steps of intervention. All interventions should be driven by "safety first"; however the treatment of pregnant and postpartum women presents some challenges. The typical inpatient psychiatry milieu may not be the best or even safest environment for many pregnant and postpartum women, and hospitalization may have limited direct access to obstetrical care (e.g., free standing psychiatric facilities) and will invariably influence the ability to breastfeed for postpartum women.

Regardless, intervention measures may necessarily include "involuntary commitment" of the mother and pregnant women. Due to their perinatal status, these women are often evaluated differently when discussing this sensitive issue. A complete suicide risk assessment is crucial in developing further prevention and treatment plans. Authors have suggested that it is important to avoid the tempting debate of determining the primary patient, mother or fetus, and instead base decisions on level of emergency of the situation and competency of the mother (Nau et al., 2011).

The reproductive safety concerns for psychotropic medications have led some to suggest that alternative treatments are better options (Domar et al., 2013). However, to be effective, a treatment option must be available and affordable for the individual. The risk/benefits of psychotropic medications during pregnancy and lactation continue to stimulate vigorous debate. Women who are more likely to commit suicide have discontinued medication for their psychiatric illness due to concern over these potentially adverse side effects. The majority of women will discontinue the medications independently once pregnancy is known and others are stopped by primary physicians secondary to safety concerns (Austin et al., 2007). In women with mood disorders, discontinuation of pharmacotherapy is associated with a high risk for symptom recurrence (Viguera et al., 2000; Cohen et al., 2006). The association of discontinuing treatment during pregnancy with suicide is unclear; however, non-perinatal patients with bipolar disorder have shown a 20-fold increased rate of suicide within 1 year of discontinuing lithium, raising considerable concern (Baldessarini et al., 1999). For women with a history of suicidal behavior and/or multiple risk factors for suicidal behavior, additional care must be taken as stopping pharmacological treatment may make these women more vulnerable. Guidelines are available by the ACOG on management of psychiatric medications during pregnancy and postpartum (Obstetricians ACOG Committee on Practice Bulletins, 2008). Individual evaluations by a professional for women currently taking psychotropic medication must occur to weigh the risk of teratogenicity against the risk of not treating a psychiatric disorder (Dell, 2003). The risks, including relapse, teratogenicity, perinatal syndromes, and postnatal behavioral sequelae, must be weighed against the potential benefits, including prevention of relapse, suicide, substance use, and poor nutrition, before decision to stop or continue medication can be made (Altshuler et al., 1996). The same holds true for postpartum women during breastfeeding. Women should be encouraged not to stop any medications before first consulting with a physician. Preferably, counseling regarding psychiatric medications should be performed antenatally in order to prepare for pregnancy with least amount of risk (Austin et al., 2007).

Future directions

Although research into suicidal behaviors (ideation, attempts, completion) during the pregnant and postpartum period continues to grow, many questions remain unanswered. Arguably, it provides a unique opportunity to access vulnerability and resilience factors in a population that undergoes similar biological challenges, acute psychosocial changes, and potential activation of instinctive maternal drives. Studies continue to support the observation that pregnant women have slightly greater protection against suicide compared to postpartum women. Protection of the fetus and resulting responsibilities of becoming a mother may alleviate any suicidal thoughts that occur during this time. The pregnant woman may not be concerned about her own life but instinctively protects the life of her child (Samandari et al., 2011). Once the child is delivered, these fears of harming the fetus likely abate and suicide may again become an option as seen with increased risk among postpartum women. The question is then raised, what happens when these instincts fail or what precipitating factors cause suicide during pregnancy and the postpartum period? In our clinical experience, women that have attempted suicide during pregnancy and the postpartum period do not uniformly view the act as "harming the child" but in some instances "protecting the child."

The lay community and many academics continue to support a role(s) for gonadal steroids in the development of mental illness during the perinatal period, though study of these steroids in perinatal suicidal behavior is lacking. Whether or not the progressive and/or acute alterations in steroid levels seen in the perinatal period contribute to the risk is unclear. The clinical literature has not consistently demonstrated an increased vulnerability to suicide for women at other times such as menopause (albeit natural, surgical, or chemical/pharmacological). The rapidly growing use of exogenous progesterone in women at risk for preterm delivery may provide a natural comparative investigation with respect to how hormones may influence vulnerability. Previous studies have supported a potential role(s) for sex steroids in risk for mood disorders (Rapkin, 1999; Bloch et al., 2000; Society for Maternal-Fetal Medicine Publications Committee, with the assistance of Vincenzo Berghella, 2012), which by extension influence the risk for suicidal behaviors. The existing knowledge on the interaction of sex steroids with neurotransmitters, neuroendocrine systems, and genetic modulation is complex and bidirectional precluding a meaningful synopsis within the scope of this chapter.

Changes in hormones affect the HPA axis and may mimic alterations seen in major depression (Newport et al., 2007; Brummelte and Galea, 2010). Additionally, inflammation markers rise during the later stages of pregnancy as protection against infection. This rise in inflammation correlates with greater risks of depression during the last trimester of pregnancy and in the postpartum period (Stowe et al., 2005; Kendall-Tackett, 2007; Brummelte & Galea, 2010). Notably, many of the natural maternal changes seen during pregnancy mirror some of the biological findings reported in non-gravid samples with major depression, including: (1) hypercortisolemia; (2) non-suppression on the dexamethasone challenge; (3) elevated corticotropin-releasing hormone; (4) shortened REM latency on sleep polysonography; and (5) blunted TRH stimulation test. The interaction, if any, of such widespread neuroendocrine and immune changes with maternal instinct in the context of suicidal behaviors warrants further attention.

The role(s) of serotonin neurotransmission/metabolism in suicidal behaviors has undergone scrutiny. Overall there is evidence that pregnant women may have increased serotonin levels. Pregnant women have higher levels of urine serotonin and its metabolite in late gestation compared to non-pregnant women (Gujrati et al., 1985). As a natural defense mechanism, increased serotonergic state theoretically may inhibit women from acting on suicidal thoughts. Interestingly, the developing fetus has been targeted as a source of increased serotonin, which raises interesting questions about "self-preservation" (Marzuk et al., 1997).

The majority of researchers agree that suicidal behavior in the community is multi-factorial. Closer examination of the perinatal period may provide insights into the biopsychosocial interactions associated with both vulnerability and resilience for suicidal behavior.

Conclusions

Clinical research on suicidal behaviors during the perinatal period has produced remarkably consistent results with respect to the incidence and role of mental illness, although, like research in non-perinatal populations, it is often hampered by methodological considerations. The majority of evidence indicates a lower rate of completed suicide during pregnancy relative to non-gravid populations; however, there is evidence supporting considerable risk for suicidal ideation in women with mental illness during the perinatal period. A variety of risk factors such as mental illness, intimate partner violence, and unplanned pregnancy lend themselves to screening procedures to identify high-risk groups. The unique biological and psychosocial environment of the typical perinatal period provides an opportunity to scrutinize other variables, as of yet unexplored, that increase vulnerability to suicidal behavior. Similarly, closer examination of obstetrical variables such as fetal abnormalities, fetal/neonatal loss, breastfeeding, and extended bed rest will enhance our ability to detect vulnerable groups in those with and those without a history of mental illness.

The potentially devastating effects of maternal suicide during pregnancy and the postpartum period underscore the need to effectively screen this population and implement intervention strategies that include both active treatment and prevention.

References

Affonso, D. D., Lovett, S., Paul, S. M., et al. (1990). A standardized interview that differentiates pregnancy and postpartum symptoms from perinatal clinical depression. *Birth*, **17**, 121–130.

Altshuler, L. L., Cohen, L., Szuba, M. P., et al. (1996). Pharmacologic management of psychiatric illness during pregnancy: dilemmas and guidelines. *The American Journal of Psychiatry*, **153**(5), 592–606.

American College of Obstetricians and Gynecologists Committee on Care for Underserved Women. (2006). ACOG Committee Opinion No. 343: psychosocial risk factors: perinatal screening and intervention. *Obstetrics and Gynecology*, **108**(2), 469–477.

Appleby, L. (1991). Suicide during pregnancy and in the first postnatal year. *BMJ*, **302**, 137–40.

Appleby, L., & Turnbull, G. (1995). Parasuicide in the first postnatal year. *Psychological Medicine*, **25**, 1087–1090.

Austin, M., Kildea, S., & Sullivan, E. (2007). Maternal mortality and psychiatric morbidity in the perinatal period: challenges and opportunities for prevention in Australian setting. *Medical Journal of Australia*, **186**(7), 364-367.

Baldessarini, R., Tondo, L., & Hennen, J. (1999). Effects of lithium treatment and its discontinuation on suicidal behavior in bipolar manic-depressive disorders. *The Journal of Clinical Psychiatry*, **60**(suppl 2), 77–84.

Beck, C. T. (1995). Screening methods for postpartum depression. *Journal of Obstetric, Gynecologic and Neonatal Nursing*, **24**, 308–312.

Benute, G. R., Nomura, R. M., Jorge, V. M., et al. (2011). Risk of suicide in high-risk pregnancy: an exploratory study. *Revista da Associação Médica Brasileira*, **57**(5), 570–574.

Bloch, M., Schmidt, P., Danaceau, M., et al. (2000). Effects of global steroids in women with a history of postpartum depression. *American Journal of Psychiatry*, **157**, 924–930.

Brummelte, S., & Galea, L. (2010). Depression during pregnancy and postpartum: Contribution of stress and ovarian hormones. *Progress in Neuro-Psychopharmacology & Biological Psychiatry*, **34**, 766–776.

Centers for Disease Control and Prevention – National Violent Death Reporting System. (2013, February 14). Retrieved March 12, 2013, from http://www.cdc.gov/violenceprevention/nvdrs/

Cohen, L., Altshuler, L., Harlow, B., et al., (2006). Relapse of major depression during pregnancy in women who maintain or discontinue antidepressant treatment. *JAMA*, **295**, 499–507.

Comtois, K. A., Schiff, M. A., & Grossman, D. C. (2008). Psychiatric risk factors associate with postpartum suicide attempt in Washington State, 1992-2001. *American Journal of Obstetrics and Gynecology*, **120**, e1–120.e5.

Dannenberg, A. L., Carter, D. M., Lawson, H. W., et al. (1995). Homicide and other injuries as causes of maternal death in New York City, 1987-1991. *American Journal of Obstetrics and Gynecology*, **172**, 1557–1564.

Dell, D. O. (2003). Suicide in pregnancy. *The American College of Obstetricians, and Gynecologists*, **102**(6), 1306–1309.

Domar, A., Moragianni, V. A., Ryley, D. A., & Urato, A. C. (2013). The risks of selective serotonin reuptake inhibitor use in infertile women: a review of the impact on fertility, pregnancy, neonatal health and beyond. *Human Reproduction*, **28**(1), 160–171.

Eggleston, A. M., Calhoun, P. S., Svikis, D. S., et al. (2009). Suicidality, aggression, and other treatment considerations among pregnant, substance-dependent women with post-traumatic stress disorder. *Comprehensive Psychiatry*, **50**, 415–423.

Erdman, H., Greist, J. H., Gustafson, D. H., Taves, J. E., & Klein, M. H. (1987). Suicide risk prediction by computer interview: A prospective study. *Journal of Clinical Psychiatry*, **48**, 464–467.

Evans, J., Heron, J., Francomb, H., et al. (2001). Cohort study of depressed mood during pregnancy and after childbirth. *British Medical Journal*, **323**, 257–260.

Farr, S. L., Bitsko, R. H., Hayes, D. K., & Dietz, P. M. (2010). Mental health and access to services among US women of reproductive age. *American Journal of Obstetrics and Gynecology*, **203**, 542.e1-9.

Friedman, S., & Resnick, P. (2007). Child murder by mothers: patterns and prevention. *World Psychiatry*, **6**(3), 137–141.

Gandhi, S., Gilbert, W. M., & McElvy, S. S., et al. (2006). Maternal and neonatal outcomes after attempted suicide. *Obstetrics and Gynecology*, **107**(5), 984–990.

Gavin, A., Tabb, K. M., Melville, J. L., Guo, Y., & Katon, W. (2011). Prevalence and correlates of suicidal ideation during pregnancy. *Archives of Women's Mental Health*, **14**, 239–246.

Gazmararian, J. A., Lazorick, S., Spitz, A. M., et al. (1996). Prevalence of violence against pregnant women: a review of the literature. *JAMA*, **275**, 1915–1920.

Gissler, M., Hemminki, E., & Lönnqvist, J. (1996). Suicides after pregnancy in Finland, 1987–94: register linkage study. *BMJ*, **313**, 1431–1434.

Gold, K., Singh, V., Marcus, S. M., & Palladino, C. L. (2012). Mental Health, substance use and intimate partner problems among pregnant and postpartum suicide victims in the National Violent Death Reporting System. *General Hospital Psychiatry*, **34**, 139–145.

Greenblatt, J., Dannenberg, A. L., & Johnson, C. J. (1997). Incidence of hospitalized injuries among pregnant women in Maryland, 1979–1990. *American Journal of Preventative Medicine*, **13**(5), 374–379.

Greist, J., Gustafson, D. H., Stauss, F. F., et al. (1973). Computer interview for suicide-risk prediction. *American Journal of Psychiatry*, **130**, 1327–1332.

Gujrati, V., Shanker, K., Parmar, S. S., Vrat, S., Chandrawati, & Bhargava, K. P. (1985). Serotonin in toxaemia of pregnancy. *Clinical & Experimental Pharmacology and Physiology*, **12**, 9–18.

Jones, J., Kruszon-Moran, D., Wilson, M., et al. (2001). *Toxoplasma gondii* infection in the United States: seroprevalence and risk factors. *American Journal of Epidemiology*, **154**(4), 357–365.

Kendall-Tackett, K. (2007). A new paradigm for depression in new mothers: the central role of inflammation and how breastfeeding and anti-inflammatory treatments protect maternal mental health. *International Breastfeeding Journal*, **2**, 6.

Lindahl, V., Pearson, J. L., & Colpe, L. (2005). Prevalence of suicidality during pregnancy and the postpartum. *Archives of Women's Mental Health*, **8**, 77–87.

Marcus, S. M., Flynn, H. A., Blow, F. C., et al. (2003). Depressive symptoms among pregnant women screened in obstetrics settings. *Journal of Women's Health (Larchmt)*, **12**, 373–380.

Martin, S. L., Macy, R. J., Sullivan, K., & Magee, M. L. (2007). Pregnancy-associated violent deaths: the role of intimate partner violence. *Trauma, Violence & Abuse*, **8**(2), 135–148.

Marzuk, P. M., Tardiff, K., Leon, A. C., et al. (1997). Lower risk of suicide during pregnancy. *American Journal of Psychiatry*, **154**(1), 122–123.

McFarlane, J., Parker, B., Soeken, K., & Bullock, L., (1992). Assessing for abuse during pregnancy: severity and frequency of injuries and associate entry into prenatal care. *JAMA*, **267**(23), 3176–3178.

Nau, M., Bender, E., & Street, J. (2011). Psychotic denial of pregnancy: legal and treatment considerations for clinicians. *Journal of the American Academy of Psychiatry and the Law*, **39**, 31–39.

Newport, D., Levey, L. C., Pennell, P. B., Ragan, K., & Stowe, Z. N. (2007). Suicidal ideation in pregnancy: assessment and clinical implications. *Archives of Women's Mental Health*, **10**, 181–187.

Oates, M. (2003). Suicide: the leading cause of maternal death. *The British Journal of Psychiatry*, **183**, 279–281.

Oberlander, T. F., Warburton, W., Misri, S., et al. (2006). Neonatal outcomes after prenatal exposure to selective serotonin reuptake inhibitor antidepressants and maternal depression using population based linked health data. *Archives of General Psychiatry*, **63**, 898–906.

Obstetricians ACOG Committee on Practice Bulletins. (2008). ACOG Practice Bulletin: Clinical management of guidelines for obstetricians-gynecologists number 92, April 2008. Use of psychiatric medications during pregnancy and lactation. *Obstetrics and Gynecology*, **111** (4), 1001–1020.

O'Hara, M., Neunaber, D., & Zekoski, E. (1984). Prospective study of postpartum depression: Prevalence, course and predictive factors. *Journal of Abnormal Psychology*, **93**(2), 158–171.

Palladino, C. L., Singh, V., Campbell, J., Flynn, H., & Gold, K. J. (2011). Homicide and suicide during the perinatal period: findings from the National Violent Death Reporting System. *Obstetrics and Gynecology*, **118**(5), 1056–1063.

Pedersen, M. G., Mortensen, P. B., Norgaard-Pedersen, B., & Postolache, T. T. (2012). *Toxoplasma gondii* infection and self-directed violence in mothers. *Archives of General Psychiatry*, **69**(11), 1123–1130.

Rapkin, A. J. (1999). Progesterone, GABA and mood disorders in women. *Archives of Womens Mental Health*, **2**, 97–105.

Samandari, G., Martin, S. L., Kupper, L. L., et al. (2011). Are pregnant and postpartum women at increased risk for violent death? Suicide and homicide findings from North Carolina. *Maternal and Child Health Journal*, **15**, 660–669.

Schiff, M., & Grossman, D. (2006). Adverse perinatal outcomes and risk for postpartum suicide attempt in Washington State, 1987–2001. *Pediatrics*, **118**, e669–675.

Shadigian, E., & Bauer, S. (2005). Pregnancy-associated death: a qualitative systematic review of homicide and suicide. *Obstetrical and Gynecological Survey*, **50**(3), 183–190.

Society for Maternal-Fetal Medicine Publications Committee, with assistance of Vincenzo Berghella. (2012). Progesterone and preterm birth prevention: translating clinical trials data into clinical practice. *American Journal of Obstetrics & Gynecology*, **206**(5), 376–386.

Stowe, Z., & Nemeroff, C. (1995). Women at risk for postpartum-onset major depression. *American Journal of Obstetrics and Gynecology*, **173**(2), 639–645.

Stowe, Z. N., Hostetter, A. L., & Newport, D. J. (2005). The onset of postpartum depression: Implications for clinical screening in obstetrical and primary care. *American Journal of Obstetrics and Gynecology*, **192**, 522–526.

Troutman, B., & Cutrona, C. (1990). Nonpsychotic postpartum depression among adolescent mothers. *Journal of Abnormal Psychology*, **99**(1), 69–78.

Viguera, A., Nonacs, R., Cohen, L., et al. (2000). Risk of recurrence of bipolar disorder in pregnant and nonpregnant women after discontinuing lithium maintenance. *American Journal of Psychiatry*, **157**, 179–184.

Weiss, H. (1999). Pregnancy-related injury hospitalizations in Pennsylvania. *Annals of Emergency Medicine*, **34**(5), 626–636.

Weissman, M. M., & Olfson, M. (1995). Depression in women: implications for health care research. *Science*, **269**, 799–801.

Wisner, K. L., Sit, D. K., McShea, M. C., et al. (2013). Onset timing, thoughts of self-harm, and diagnoses in postpartum women with screen-positive depression findings. *JAMA Psychiatry*, **70**(5), 490–498.

Yigletu, H., Tucker, S., Harris, M., & Hatlevig, J. (2004). Assessing suicidal ideation: comparing self-report versus clinician report. *American Psychiatric Nurses Association*, **10**(1), 9–15.

Chapter 18

Childhood and adolescence

Tina R. Goldstein, Jeffrey A. Bridge, and David A. Brent

In this chapter, we provide an overview on the epidemiology, risk factors, and treatment approaches for suicidal behavior in youth. Where appropriate, we cite review articles in which the reader can find comprehensive discussions of the epidemiology of youth suicide, risk factors, and clinical guidance for the assessment and treatment of youth suicidal behavior (Bridge et al., 2006).

Epidemiology

This section provides a brief review of the epidemiology of youth suicide and suicidal behavior with a specific focus on demographic subgroups at highest risk for suicidal behavior and suicide.

Descriptive epidemiology of youth suicide and suicidal behavior

Youth suicide is a global public health problem. In the USA, suicide is the third leading cause of death in young people aged 10–19 years, behind only unintentional injuries and homicide (Centers for Disease Control and Prevention, 2013). In 2010, the latest year for which data are available, suicide was the second leading cause of death for 1926 youths aged 10–19 years, more than deaths in this age group from cancer (1078), cardiovascular disease (459), stroke (129), influenza and pneumonia (82), septicemia (79), diabetes (68), and HIV (24) combined (Centers for Disease Control and Prevention, 2013). Non-fatal suicidal behaviors are more prevalent. In 2011, 15.8% of high school students in the USA seriously considered attempting suicide, 12.8% planned a suicide attempt, 7.8% attempted suicide, and 2.4% made a suicide attempt requiring medical attention (Eaton et al., 2012).

Age and sex

Suicide is extremely rare before the age of 10 years (Figure 18.1). During the past 25 years, the number of suicide deaths in US children younger than 10 years has not exceeded 10 deaths in any single year (Centers for Disease Control and Prevention, 2013). Suicide rates increase with each year of age during adolescence, with the increase being more marked for males than females (Centers for Disease Control and Prevention, 2013). Consequently, rates of suicide are approximately four times higher for young males than those for females. This is in contrast to non-fatal suicidal behaviors, in which females have much higher rates of suicidal ideation, planning, and suicide attempts compared to males. The gender difference in suicide and suicidal behaviors is most likely due to the greater likelihood of males having multiple risk factors such as comorbid mood and alcohol abuse disorders, greater levels of impulsive aggression (i.e., the tendency to react to provocation with hostility or aggression), and choice of more lethal suicide attempt methods, which make them more likely than females to make a lethal suicide attempt (Shaffer et al., 1996; Brent et al., 1999; Bridge et al., 2006).

Race and ethnicity

In the USA, suicide rates are highest among American Indian/Alaskan Native youths (Centers for Disease Control and Prevention, 2013). White youths historically have had higher suicide rates than non-white youths, although the gap narrowed during the 1990s because of an increasing suicide rate among young black males (Bridge et al., 2006). Hispanic youths in the USA have higher rates of non-fatal suicidal behaviors compared to non-Hispanic youths but are not disproportionately represented among young suicide completers (Eaton et al., 2012; Centers for Disease Control and Prevention, 2013).

Methods of suicide

During the past 20 years, significant changes have occurred in the methods used for suicide by

A Concise Guide to Understanding Suicide, ed. Stephen H. Koslow, Pedro Ruiz, and Charles B. Nemeroff. Published by Cambridge University Press.

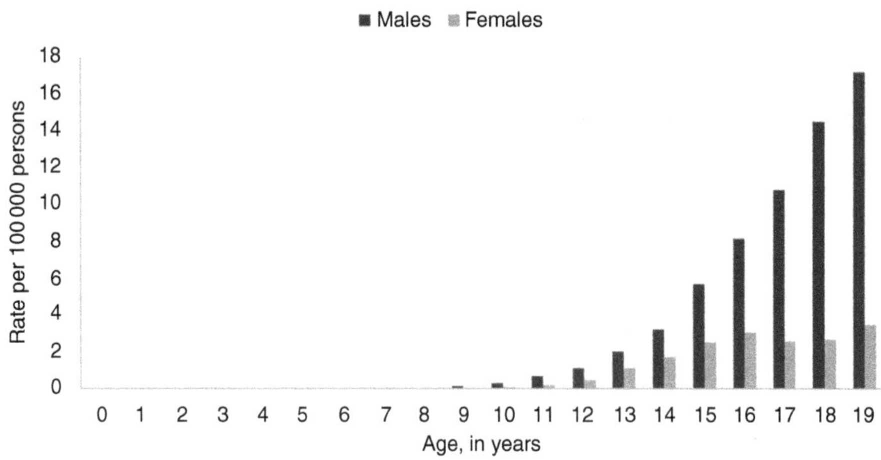

Figure 18.1. Suicide rates among males and females younger than age 20 in the USA, 2006–2010, by age.

youths, with an increase over time in suicide by hanging/suffocation and a concomitant decrease in suicide by poisoning and firearms, the predominant method of suicide in the USA (Centers for Disease Control and Prevention, 2013). Among US youths aged 10–19 years, the leading methods of suicide in 2010 were hanging/suffocation (48% of all suicide deaths), firearms (39%), and poisoning (6%) (Centers for Disease Control and Prevention, 2013). Although reasons for the change in suicide methods among US youths are unclear, the decline in suicides by firearms may be related to efforts to limit access to lethal means (e.g., enactment of youth-focused gun laws and national safe gun storage public awareness campaigns) (Bridge et al., 2010).

Recent trends in youth suicide rates

The suicide rate among US youth and young adults generally declined from the mid-1990s through the mid-2000s, except for a sharp increase from 2003 to 2004 (Bridge et al., 2010). From 2006 to 2010, the overall suicide rate for US youths aged 10–19 years increased by an average of 3.2% annually (Table 18.1). Among demographic subgroups, suicide rates increased from 2006 to 2010 for both males and females, white non-Hispanic youths, and Hispanic youths. Rates of suicide by hanging/suffocation increased during this period, whereas suicide rates by firearms and other methods did not change significantly during this period.

Risk factors

Numerous factors are associated with an increased risk of suicide and suicidal behavior in youths. In this section, we briefly review key risk factors by major domain including suicidality, psychiatric disorder, psychological factors, and psychosocial factors.

Suicidality

Those youth who exhibit suicidal ideation characterized by high severity (i.e., high intent, planning, frequency, and duration) are at greater risk of suicide attempt and completion (Brent et al., 1988). To illustrate, over half of youth with a suicide plan will attempt suicide within 1 year of ideation onset (Nock et al., 2013). Not surprisingly, the single most potent predictor of attempted and completed suicide is a history of attempted suicide (Brent et al., 1999). Up to 15% of youth who attempt suicide will reattempt within 1 year. The 3-month period following the initial attempt, as well as the period immediately following discharge from a psychiatric hospital, are particularly vulnerable periods for reattempt. Furthermore, those youth with a history of suicide attempts of high lethality are at greatest risk for subsequent completion (Bridge et al., 2006).

Adolescents who have been exposed to suicide and suicidal behavior are at greater risk themselves, although the effect is much stronger for suicidal behavior than for suicide, and stronger for more distant than for close friends (Ho et al., 2000). Studies show increased rates of suicide and suicidal behavior among adolescents following media attention to the topic. Furthermore, data support the phenomena of contagion

Table 18.1. Trends in suicide rates for youths aged 10–19 years in the USA, 2006 to 2010, overall and by demographic subgroups*

	2006	2007	2008	2009	2010	Average annual % change in suicide rate‡	*P*
Age group							
All	4.1	3.9	4.2	4.5	4.5	3.2	0.002
10–14	1.0	0.9	1.0	1.3	1.3	8.3	0.001
15–19	7.1	6.7	7.2	7.5	7.5	2.2	0.01
Gender							
Boys	6.4	6.1	6.5	6.8	6.9	2.4	0.004
Girls	1.7	1.5	1.9	2.1	2.0	6.6	0.003
Race/ethnicity							
White†	4.8	4.5	5.0	5.3	5.3	3.5	0.003
Black†	2.6	2.6	3.2	2.9	2.8	2.5	0.281
Other race†	5.4	4.6	5.0	5.0	5.3	0.1	0.831
Hispanic	2.8	2.8	2.6	3.3	3.3	5.1	0.01
Suicide method							
Hanging/suffocation	1.9	1.7	2.0	2.1	2.2	5.0	<0.001
Firearms	1.8	1.6	1.7	1.9	1.8	1.2	0.419
Other methods€	0.4	0.6	0.5	0.5	0.5	3.3	0.111

* Crude rates per 100 000 persons.
† Non-Hispanic.
‡ Trends in suicide rates were estimated by using negative binomial rate regression analyses.
€ Includes poisoning, fall, drowning, transportation-related, cut/pierce, fire/burn, other specified-classifiable, and unspecified methods.

and imitation of suicidal behavior such that adolescent suicidal behavior occurs in time/space clusters. Yet, prospective studies of adolescents exposed to a peer's suicide are mixed; some support increased risk for suicide attempt whereas others do not (Bridge et al., 2006).

Access to lethal means is a potent risk factor for youth suicide. A loaded firearm in the home of an adolescent has been associated with a 30-fold increased risk for suicide. Furthermore, among adolescent suicide completers, if a gun is available in the home, it is highly likely to be used as the method of suicide, whereas if there is no gun in the home then it is rarely the method employed. By limiting gun availability in the home through methods including storing guns unloaded and locked, and storing and locking ammunition separately decreases suicide risk in youth (Bridge et al., 2006).

Psychiatric disorder

Over 80% of adolescents who attempt suicide and 90% of adolescents who complete suicide have a diagnosable psychiatric disorder. The more severe and unremitting the psychiatric disorder, the greater the suicide risk posed. Psychiatric comorbidity is common among attempters and completers with nearly 70% of suicidal youth meeting criteria for multiple psychiatric diagnoses. Risk for completed suicide increases with each additional comorbid disorder in this population and while depression increases the risk for suicidal ideation, comorbidity with conduct disorder, PTSD, substance abuse, or panic disorder seems to facilitate the transition from ideation to actual behavior (Brent et al., 1999; Nock et al., 2013).

In terms of specific diagnostic categories that confer suicide risk in youth, mood disorders (including depression and bipolar disorder) are most strongly associated with suicidality. Over 80% of attempters and 60% of completers meet DSM criteria for a mood disorder. Mixed bipolar mood states confer particularly elevated risk for attempted and completed suicide in youth (Brent et al., 1988). Youth with disruptive behavior disorders are at 3–6 times greater risk for suicide. When comorbid with substance use disorders, especially among males, disruptive behavior disorders are more likely to result in completed suicide. Findings are mixed with respect to the unique risk for suicide associated with anxiety disorders in youth. Yet, panic disorder appears to render specific risk for suicide attempt in youth above and beyond its common comorbid presentation with mood and other psychiatric disorders. Girls who attempt suicide have greater rates of eating disorders than non-attempters, and some studies show greater rates of eating disorders among adolescents who die by suicide. Personality disorders in general are present at elevated rates among adolescent suicide completers, and even after controlling for comorbid Axis I conditions, Cluster B disorders elevate risk 8-fold (Brent et al., 1994). In the case of youth suicide completers who do not have a diagnosable psychiatric disorder, access to a loaded gun appears to be a potent risk factor (Brent & Bridge, 2003).

Psychological factors

Studies converge on several psychological factors associated with suicidal behavior in children and adolescents. Primarily, adolescents who attempt suicide demonstrate high rates of impulsive aggression (Melhem et al., 2007). Relatedly, impulsivity more generally also conveys risk for suicide attempt in youth. The unique contribution of hopelessness to suicide risk in youth may be partially accounted for by its role as a symptom of depression, although some studies have identified independent risk for reattempt and completed suicide associated with hopelessness. The tendency to experience prolonged and severe negative affect in response to stress, termed neuroticism, conveys increased risk for suicide attempts in youth. There are mixed findings regarding the association between perfectionism and suicidal behavior in youth, with some studies showing greater rates of suicide and attempt among youth displaying perfectionism, and others finding this association is better accounted for by psychopathology (Bridge et al., 2006).

Psychosocial factors

Family risk factors have been shown to be potent predictors of youth suicidal behavior. Studies provide strong support for the familiality of youth suicidal behavior via both genetic and environmental pathways. Rates of suicidal behavior in the first degree relatives of adolescent suicide completers and attempters are 2–6 times greater than in the general population. Although youth with a parent who exhibits mood disorder, substance use, and antisocial behaviors are at elevated risk for attempted and completed suicide, the heritability of suicidal behavior has been demonstrated to be independent of psychiatric disorder. To illustrate, offspring of mood-disordered parents with a history of suicide attempt are at 4–6 times greater risk for suicide attempt as compared with offspring of mood-disordered parents without a history of attempt (Melhem et al., 2007). Furthermore, suicidal behavior emerges at a younger age among those offspring with greater familial loading for suicidal behavior (Bridge et al., 2006).

Youth who come from a non-intact family of origin, and those who experience loss of a parent (due to death or physical/geographical separation) are at increased risk for attempted and completed suicide. Studies also demonstrate that the quality of the family environment contributes to suicide risk: family conflict, violence, poor communication (particularly with father), the perception that one's parents are not supportive, and overall low connection to family (as well as other support systems including friends, school, activities) have all been associated with elevated risk for attempted and completed suicide in youth (Bridge et al., 2006).

Rates of attempted and completed suicide are substantially elevated among youth with early traumatic experiences, including physical and sexual abuse. Early sexual abuse appears to convey particularly elevated risk for youth suicidality, and suicide risk is compounded with greater severity of sexual abuse (Bridge et al., 2006).

Population-based studies indicate sexual minority youth and same-sex attraction are associated with greater risk for suicidal behavior. However, the association may be mediated by higher rates of mood disorder, substance use, trauma, and family disconnection among youth who identify as non-heterosexual (Bridge et al., 2006).

Physical conditions, including diabetes and epilepsy, have been associated with youth suicidality above and beyond their association with psychiatric conditions. Similarly, illness or injury associated with functional impairment prospectively predicts suicide attempt in youth (Lewinsohn et al., 1996).

Interpersonal conflict or loss, primarily involving a parent or romantic partner, are among the most common psychosocial stressors associated with youth suicidal behavior. Stressors associated with school have been linked to youth suicidal behavior. Youth who report being bullied and/or bullying others at school are at elevated risk for suicidal behavior. Academic failure, risk for school dropout, and extended school absences are associated with increased suicide risk. Legal difficulties and other disciplinary actions have also been shown to precipitate suicidal behavior, particularly among those youth with behavioral and substance use disorders (Gould et al., 1996).

Adolescents who attempt suicide also display elevated rates of other health risk behaviors, including carrying a weapon, engaging in risky sex, and failing to use seat belts. This association may be understood by shared underlying risk factors (Bridge et al., 2006).

Treatment

We review intervention studies that focused on adolescent suicidal behavior. Some of these interventions also included participants who engaged in non-suicidal self-injury (NSSI). We organize these on the basis of those focused primarily on individual risk factors, those that targeted depression, and those that mainly focused on family or social processes.

Individually focused interventions

One of the best-studied interventions for adolescent "deliberate self-harm," a term that encompasses both suicide attempts and NSSI is developmental group therapy (DGT), an 8-session group intervention that focused on problem solving, emotion regulation, and social skills relevant to depression and self-harm in social settings of family, school, and with peers.

Two multi-site studies of DGT did not find an effect of DGT on deliberate self-harm. A 3-site study in Australia randomized 72 adolescents to either DGT + TAU vs. TAU alone (Hazell et al., 2009). Around half had engaged in suicidal behavior. The DGT group received 9 sessions of the experimental treatment and both groups received 10 sessions of TAU. At 6 months, DGT was associated with a higher rate of recurrent self-harm (88% vs. 68%), but this was in part accounted for by an imbalance between groups, insofar as the DGT group had a much higher rate of previous suicide attempts (71% vs. 43%), and after adjustment for this difference, there were no longer significant differences between groups. At 12 months, the rate of repeated attempts was 37% in DGT + TAU vs. 45% in TAU, which was non-significantly different, although there was a significantly greater improvement in global functioning in the DGT group.

An 8-site study of DGT in the UK examined 366 adolescents who had engaged in deliberate self-harm, of whom two-thirds had attempted suicide. Those in the experimental group received 10 sessions of DGT and nine sessions of TAU vs. 10 sessions of TAU in the comparison condition (Green et al., 2011). DGT when added to TAU was no more efficacious than TAU alone in reducing the rate of repetition of deliberate self-harm at 6 and 12 months (ORs 0.99 and 0.88, respectively), and this was true regardless of sample stratification (e.g., just attempts, just highly lethal attempts, etc.). Possible explanations for the disappointing performance of DGT in both of these replications offered by the investigators were improvement in the quality of TAU, greater dose of TAU which overwhelmed the effects of DGT, and lack of individualization of the DGT to needs of individual patients.

Treatments that focus on depression

Three large clinical trials in the past decade examined the roles of antidepressants and CBT, either alone or in combination, for the treatment of adolescent depression, and a meta-analysis of all studies found that combined treatment relative to monotherapy did not protect against suicidal events (Dubicka et al., 2010). A slow rate of decline in symptoms of depression and suicidal ideation, family conflict, alcohol and drug use, and a history of NSSI were predictive of future suicidal events and suicide attempts (Brent et al., 2009; Wilkinson et al., 2011).

Treatments that focus on family and social processes

Harrington et al. conducted an RCT with 162 adolescents who had made an overdose, comparing a 5-session home-based family intervention (focused on problem solving and communication) + TAU to TAU alone. There was no treatment effect of the reduction of either suicidal ideation or recurrence of suicide attempts or on family climate, although in the non-depressed subgroup, there was a greater decline in suicidal ideation in the group that received family therapy (Harrington et al., 1998).

King et al. (2006) developed an intervention, the Youth-nominated Support Team (YST), for adolescent inpatients hospitalized for either suicidal ideation or behavior to elicit and sustain support in the social network of these patients. YST helped the adolescent to identify supportive adults and coach those adults on how to respond to these youths' requests for support. In the first study, YST-1, 289 hospitalized adolescents were randomized to YST + TAU vs. TAU alone. The actual intervention was 1–2 hours in duration, and teens had an average of 39 contacts with members during the 6-month period of the trial. There were no main effects on suicide attempts or ideation, but girls who were assigned YST showed a greater reduction in suicidal ideation than those assigned to TAU alone. Only 35% of those adolescents eligible for the study agreed to participate, however.

King and colleagues (2009) then conducted a larger clinical trial, YST-2, with 448 hospitalized suicidal or suicide-attempting adolescents, and in this study, 43% of those eligible participated. YST-2 was a briefer intervention, 3 months in duration, and generated fewer contacts with social network members (around 10 per adolescent). Again, there were no main effects on suicide ideation or attempts, but in those adolescents with a history of multiple suicide attempts, YST-2 was associated with a more rapid decline in suicidal ideation over the first 6 months of follow-up, but not beyond that. The effects of YST-2 might have been overwhelmed by the amount of TAU that participants received, namely 34 psychotherapy or medication sessions in YST-2 + TAU vs. 31 sessions of TAU in the comparison group.

Huey et al. (2004) tested the efficacy of multisystemic therapy (MST) in reducing suicide attempts in patients presenting with a psychiatric emergency including suicidal ideation or attempts, but also homicidal ideation or behavior, and psychosis. 156 participants were randomized to either MST or hospitalization, although 44% of those in the MST cell were also hospitalized during the study. Of those randomized to MST, 31% had made an attempt prior to entry into the study vs. 19% in the TAU group. At the end of the study, 4% in both groups had reattempted, which was reported in the study as a significant effect in favor of MST, but may have been accounted for by regression to the mean.

Attachment-based family therapy (ABFT) is an intervention designed to heal discord between parent and child and generally improve the quality of parent–child attachment. Diamond et al. (Diamond et al., 2010) compared ABFT to brief clinical management (BCM) in 66 mostly African American low income adolescents with high levels of suicidal ideation. Participants in ABFT and BCM received on average 10 and 3 sessions, respectively. Participants who received ABFT were 4–6 times more likely to have their ideation reduced to below a clinically significant threshold as were those assigned to BCM. While it is encouraging that this treatment reduced the severity of suicidal ideation, it has not yet been demonstrated to prevent recurrent suicide attempts.

Esposito-Smythers et al. (2011) conducted a pilot study using "integrated CBT (iCBT)" for suicidal, alcohol or substance abusing adolescents. iCBT had many of the common elements of CBT, but additionally used motivational interviewing to target alcohol and substance abuse, and had a prominent family intervention component that focused on problem solving, contingency-management, parental monitoring, and parent–child communication. In this small (N = 36) RCT, participants were randomized to iCBT or TAU, which consisted of nearly 35 sessions and 20 sessions of treatment, respectively. The iCBT treatment had a much stronger family component. Despite the small sample, the study found a significant difference at the 18 month follow-up point with respect to repeat suicide attempts (5.3% vs. 35.3%), hospitalizations (15.8% vs. 52.9%), arrests, episodes of heavy drinking, and marijuana use.

Conclusions

Suicide in adolescents continues to be a leading cause of death and has increased in recent years. Psychiatric disorder, particularly mood disorders comorbid with substance abuse and/or conduct disorder, figure prominently in those who commit suicide. Impulsive aggression and emotional lability, whether attributable to a bipolar mixed state or a personality disorder are important risk factors and treatment targets for adolescent suicide prevention. Family discord, abuse, and peer victimization are among the most important social and environmental factors contributing to adolescent suicidal risk.

Elements of treatment that appeared efficacious include those that focused on improving family climate and social support and achieving sobriety. It is difficult to comment on the individually focused treatments in part because the dose of treatment may have been low relative to TAU and because the treatment could not be individualized to the needs of participants. Given that a large number of suicidal events occur early in treatment, front-loading of treatment may be beneficial. Although efficacious treatments for depression can result in reductions in suicidal ideation, which in turn may prevent recurrent suicidal events, treatments that enhance family cohesion and target sobriety are likely to be beneficial above and beyond the management of depression to prevent suicidal behavior.

References

Brent, D. A., & Bridge, J. (2003). Firearms availability and suicide: Evidence, interventions, and future directions. *American Behavioral Scientist*, **46**, 1192–1210.

Brent, D. A., Perper, J. A., Goldstein, C. E., et al. (1988). Risk factors for adolescent suicide: A comparison of adolescent suicide victims with suicidal inpatients. *Archives of General Psychiatry*, **45**, 581–588.

Brent, D. A., Johnson, B. A., Perper, J., et al. (1994). Personality disorder, personality traits, impulsive violence, and completed suicide in adolescents. *Journal of the American Academy of Child and Adolescent Psychiatry*, **33**, 1080–1086.

Brent, D. A., Baugher, M., Bridge, J., Chen, T., & Chiappetta, L. (1999). Age- and sex-related risk factors for adolescent suicide. *Journal of the American Academy of Child and Adolescent Psychiatry*, **38**(12), 1497–1505.

Brent, D. A., Emslie, G., Clarke, G., et al. (2009). Predictors of spontaneous and systematically assessed suicidal adverse events in the Treatment of SSRI-Resistant Depression in Adolescents (TORDIA) Study. *American Journal of Psychiatry*, **166**, 418–426.

Bridge, J. A., Goldstein, T. R., & Brent, D. A. (2006). Adolescent suicide and suicidal behavior. *Journal of Child Psychology and Psychiatry*, **47**, 372–394.

Bridge, J., Greenhouse, J. B., Sheftall, A., et al. (2010). Changes in suicide rates by hanging and/or suffocation and firearms among young persons aged 10–24 years in the United States: 1992–2006. *The Journal of Adolescent Health*, **46**(5), 503–505.

Centers for Disease Control and Prevention. (2013). National Center for Injury Prevention and Control. Web-based Injury Statistics Query and Reporting System (WISQARS) [online]. Last accessed, 2/06/2013. Source of data from WISQARS is the National Vital Statistics System from the National Center for Health Statistics. Available from: www.cdc.gov/ncipc/wisqars

Diamond, G. M., Wintersteen, M., Brown, G., Diamond, G. M., & Gallop, R. (2010). Attachment-based family therapy for adolescents with suicidal ideation: A randomized controlled trial. *Journal of the American Academy of Child and Adolescent Psychiatry*, **49**(2), 122–131.

Dubicka, B., Elvins, R., Roberts, C., et al. (2010). Combined treatment with cognitive-behavioral therapy in adolescent depression: a meta-analysis. *British Journal of Psychiatry*, **197**(6), 433–440.

Eaton, D. K., Kann, L., Kinchen, S., et al. (2012). Youth risk behavior surveillance – United States, 2011. *MMWR Surveillance Summary*, **61**(4), 1–162.

Esposito-Smythers, C., Spirito, A., Kahler, C. W., Hunt, J., & Monti, P. (2011). Treatment of co-occurring substance abuse and suicidality among adolescents: a randomized trial. *Journal of Consulting and Clinical Psychology*, **79**(6), 728–739.

Gould, M. S., Fisher, P., Parides, M., Flory, M., & Shaffer, D. (1996). Psychosocial risk factors of child and adolescent completed suicide. *Archives of General Psychiatry*, **53**, 1155–1162.

Green, J., Wood, A., Kerfoot, M., et al. (2011). Group therapy for adolescents with repeated self-harm: radnomized controlled trial with economic evaluation. *British Medical Journal*, **342**(7802), 859.

Harrington, R., Kerfoot, M., Dyer, E., et al. (1998). Randomized trial of a home-based family intervention for children who have deliberately poisoned themselves. *Journal of the American Academy of Child and Adolescent Psychiatry*, **37**(5), 512–518.

Hazell, P., Martin, G., Kay, T., et al. (2009). Group therapy for repeated deliberate self-harm in adolescents: failure of replication of a randomized trial. *Journal of the American Academy of Child and Adolescent Psychiatry*, **48**(6), 662–670.

Ho, T. P., Leung, P., Hung, S., & Tang, C. (2000). The mental health of the peers of suicide completers and attempters. *Journal of Child Psychology and Psychiatry*, **41**(3), 301–308.

Huey, S. J., Henggeler, S. W., Rowland, M. D., et al. (2004). Multisystemic therapy effects on attempted suicide by youths presenting psychiatric emergencies. *Journal of the American Academy of Child and Adolescent Psychiatry*, **43**(2), 183–190.

King, C. A., Kramer, A., Preuss, L., et al. (2006). Youth-nominated support team for suicidal adolescents: A randomized controlled trial. *Journal of Consulting and Clinical Psychology*, **74**(1), 199–206.

King, C., Klaus, N., Kramer, A., et al. (2009). The Youth-Nominated Support Team-Version II for suicidal adolescents: A randomized controlled intervention trial. *Journal of Consulting and Clinical Psychology*, **77**(5), 880–893.

Lewinsohn, P. M., Seeley, J. R., Hibbard, J., Rohde, P., & Sack, W. H. (1996). Cross-sectional and prospective relationships between physical morbidity and depression in older adolescents. *Journal of the American Academy of Child and Adolescent Psychiatry*, **35**, 9, 1120–1129.

Melhem, N. M., Brent, D. A., Ziegler, M., et al. (2007). Familial pathways to early-onset suicidal behavior: Familial and individual antecedents of suicidal behavior. *American Journal of Psychiatry*, **164**, 1364–1370.

Nock, M., Green, J., Hwang, I., et al. (2013). Prevalence, correlates, and treatment of lifetime suicidal behavior among adolescents: Results from the National Comorbidity Survey Replication Adolescent Supplement. *JAMA Psychiatry*, 1–11.

Shaffer, D., Gould, M. S., Fisher, P., et al. (1996). Psychiatric diagnosis in child and adolescent suicide. *Archives of General Psychiatry*, **53**, 339–348.

Wilkinson, P., Kelvin, R., Roberts, C., Dubicka, B., & Goodyer, I. (2011). Clinical and psychosocial predictors o suicide attempts and nonsuicidal self-injury in the Adolescent Depression Antidepressants and Psychotherapy Trial (ADAPT). *American Journal of Psychiatry*, **168**, 495–501.

Chapter 19

Indigenous/native populations

Deborah Goebert

This chapter looks at indigenous populations – those who have been colonized and have become a minority population in their homeland. Indigenous populations include, but are not limited to, American Indian, Alaska Natives, Australian Aboriginals, First Nations of Canada, Native Hawaiians, and New Zealand Maori. While an attempt is made at identifying approaches to suicide prevention, the tremendous diversity among indigenous communities and the unique strengths of each culture are acknowledged. Further, the power of each community to prevent suicide and to instill hope is recognized.

Epidemiology of indigenous suicide

Rates of death by suicide and suicide attempts vary vastly among communities, with the most indigenous groups experiencing the highest rates. Around the world, death by suicide and attempt rates for indigenous people are significantly higher than those of other ethnic groups.

Coupe (2005) cited increased suicide death rates among indigenous peoples compared to other ethnic groups in the same country. Suicide death rates were 1.7 times higher for American Indians and Native Alaskans, two to three times higher for Canadian Inuit and Metis, three to four times higher for Australian Aborigines, and 1.5 times higher for New Zealand Maori. Suicide rates have been steadily on the rise in Micronesia and Guam, with suicide being the leading cause of death; and the rate of suicide for Native Hawaiians is currently 12.9% as compared to 9.6% for non-Native Hawaiian residents (Else et al., 2007). While these rates are all consistently and significantly higher than other groups, not all indigenous communities experience high rates. Within indigenous groups, there is tremendous diversity in suicidal behaviors by place, tribe, history, age, gender, and spiritual practice. For example, suicide death rates among Alaska Natives range from 2.04 per 10 000 in the Southeastern Tribal Region to 9.23 per 10 000 in the Northwest Arctic Tribal Region (Streur et al., 2012).

For every suicide death, there are significantly more attempts. For example, the percentage of adults aged 18 or older having serious thoughts of suicide in the past year was 5% among American Indians and Alaska Natives, significantly higher than the overall US rate of 3.7% (SAMHSA, 2010a). Higher rates were found among First Nations adults with 15.8% reporting that they had made a suicide attempt in their lifetime and 1% reporting having made an attempt in the past year (First Nations Information Governance Committee, 2005). In Western Australia, suicide attempt rates among indigenous adults are two or three times higher than those of non-indigenous adults depending on sex and age (Silburn et al., 2012).

Indigenous youth suicide

In the last few decades, suicide has emerged as a youth phenomenon clustered among those between the ages of 13 and 24. While youth suicide remains a rare and tragic event, it is most prominent among indigenous peoples (Harder et al., 2012). The suicide death rate among American Indian and Alaska Native youth is 2.5 times higher than the national average. Suicide death rates for indigenous youth are 5 to 7 times that of non-indigenous youth in Canada, with the highest suicide death rates for Inuit youth at 11 times the national average. Throughout the Pacific Island region, suicide death and attempt rates are highest among youth. Since Hawaiʻi began collecting suicide statistics in 1908, suicide death rates for Native Hawaiians, especially Native Hawaiian youth, have been increasing (Else et al., 2007). In recent years, Native Hawaiian youth have been recorded to have the highest suicide death rates in the USA by ethnicity with rates 1.7 times higher than other ethnic groups.

A Concise Guide to Understanding Suicide, ed. Stephen H. Koslow, Pedro Ruiz, and Charles B. Nemeroff. Published by Cambridge University Press.

Suicide death rates among Micronesian youth began rising nearly 40 years ago and have been linked to a complex web of social and cultural factors.

Among indigenous peoples, adolescents are at higher risk of suicidality than adults. In Western Australia, suicide attempt rates among indigenous youth are around double those of their non-indigenous counterparts. Data from the CDC (2010) indicated that American Indian/Alaska Native high school students have significantly higher rates of suicidality compared to all students. For example 10% of American Indian/Alaska Native students reported having made a suicide attempt compared to 6.3% among all students; 17% reported having made a suicide plan compared to 10.9% among all students; and 19% reported having seriously considered attempting suicide compared to 13.8% among all students. Similarly, Native Hawaiian and other Pacific Islander high school students have significantly higher rates for suicide phenomena: 11.9% reported having made a suicide attempt; 13.2% reported having made a suicide plan; and 14.9% reported having seriously considered attempting suicide.

Risk and protective factors

Conventional researchers have framed the issue in terms of discrete risk factors that are similar across ethnocultural groups, such as neighborhood poverty, rural location, an unstable family situation, or teen alcohol use. They have also included loss of culture and acculturative stress among the contributory factors driving indigenous suicide (Collings & Beautrais, 2005). In their critical review of the suicide literature for indigenous populations, Harder and colleagues (2012) identified consistency in risk factors predisposing suicidal ideation, attempts, and deaths. Depression and having a friend or family member attempt or die by suicide were the strongest risk factors followed by other psychiatric disorders, and suffering from previous childhood abuse. Additionally, indigenous populations can suffer acculturation and oppression as a result of colonization including poverty, discrimination, and racism. Acculturative stress, psychocultural stress due to cultural differences between two or more cultures, refers to the psychological, somatic, and social difficulties that may occur during the acculturation processes. The term "walking in two worlds" is frequently used by indigenous groups to describe the dichotomous manner of simultaneously operating within the dominant group and the Native world, and reflects feelings of marginality and alienation. Several studies have concluded that disruption caused by dramatic cultural changes may account for the increased suicide rates among indigenous groups. For example, Yuen and colleagues hypothesized that key transitions in adolescence may be more difficult for them to negotiate (Yuen et al., 2000). They found that youth with high levels of indigenous cultural affiliation and low levels of assimilation were more likely to attempt suicide. Given these high rates of suicidality, their higher rates of mental illness, incarceration, interpersonal violence, substance use, teenage pregnancy, and high school dropouts among indigenous people are not surprising (Andrade et al., 2006; Mackin et al., 2012).

Unique to indigenous peoples, historical trauma can be an additional risk factor. Historical trauma is the cumulative emotional and psychological loss over the lifespan and across generations, emanating from considerable group trauma (Brave Heart, 2000). In a ground-breaking series of work, Brave Heart ties the plight of American Indians and other indigenous peoples to the Holocaust experience – genocide, ethnic cleansing, and policies of forced acculturation. Historical trauma theory posits that while contemporary Native life has adapted, a significant proportion of indigenous people have poor well-being, in large part due to massive traumas (physical, emotional, social, and spiritual genocide) occurring in the past. Historical trauma can result in patterns of symptoms in initial survivors and their families as well as subsequent generations. Evidence supporting this syndrome comes primarily from psychoanalytic clinical case studies of offspring and a few empirical studies. Whitbeck et al. (2004) developed scales to measure historical trauma and its effects. They found that American Indian adults frequently think about historical losses. Furthermore, these losses were associated with negative feelings of anxiety, depression, anger, and avoidance. The historical content of victimization is not limited to individuals since all indigenous families have a collective history of trauma and abuse (US Department of Health and Human Services, 2010b). Thus, there is a connection between historically traumatic events and contemporary stressors, impacting physical and emotional well-being.

Despite exposure to historical trauma, multiple risks, and adversity, most indigenous people do not exhibit suicidality or other behavioral problems and demonstrate resilience (Mmari et al., 2010; Mackin et al., 2012). Resiliency indicators connote the capacity for individuals, as well as communities, to withstand adversity and maintain health and well-being. Resilience research attempts to identify factors that predict positive outcomes for those who experience increased risk, emphasizing beneficial, rather than pathologic, processes and outcomes. A number of protective factors have been identified for preventing suicidality including talking with parents, higher levels of family cohesion, family organization, parental bonding, and community support (Else et al., 2007; Mmari et al., 2010; Mackin et al., 2012). In their review, Harder and colleagues (2012) found similar patterns among protective factors of suicide ideation and attempts with the strongest buffering effect from high levels of social or familiar support. Furthermore, the importance of culture was more profound for suicidal behavior than for ideation. A pioneering study of 11 666 indigenous adolescents identified three risk and three protective factors (Borowsky et al., 1999). The study showed that only 1% of youth with three protective factors and no risk factors had attempted suicide, compared to suicide attempts in 81% of girls and 75% of boys with three risk and no protective factors. Reducing risk factors was associated with reduced suicidality. However, more importantly, increasing protective factors were far more effective in reducing suicide attempts. More recent studies have demonstrated that communities that preserve their cultural heritage are dramatically more successful in preventing suicide (US Department of Health and Human Services, 2010b).

Indigenous researchers have advocated a more holistic approach where the primary intervention to reduce indigenous suicide is not to focus individual-level risk factors, but the restoration of culture at the group level. Interventions must encompass mental, physical, cultural, and spiritual health as well as the harmonized interrelations which comprise cultural well-being. From a Native perspective, strengths-based approaches enhance existing assets and relationships in these families and communities. They entail culturally proscribed norms in purposeful ways, facilitating a positive sense of belonging to a valued community (Maton et al., 2003; Kana'iaupuni, 2005). A number of studies have presented evidence that cultural affinity or engagement acts as a protective factor against the problems of trauma associated with historical loss and discrimination, as well as suicidal behaviors or ideation (Colquhoun & Dockery, 2012). This has been posited to function through the processes of enculturation (learning about one's traditional culture, cultural identity, resilience, and sense of community). Indigenous communities can unite around a common goal of suicide prevention, linking cultural meanings that support and strengthen their group, social morals, and ethics.

Strengths-based approaches

Mental health interventions and social services have been historically modeled on deficits – in upbringing, personality, socioeconomic status, neurobiology, and environment – that lead to stress, psychopathology, and problem behaviors. These interventions often under-value or conflict with indigenous cultures and lifestyles; and not surprisingly have had limited success (Kral et al., 2009). During the last decade, researchers and practitioners in mental health, social work, education, and child welfare have begun to apply a holistic, strengths-based model of development (Guerra & Bradshaw, 2008). Strength-based approaches identify positive resources and abilities in youth, their families and communities, then systematically create healing strategies (Lerner & Benson, 2003; Guerra & Bradshaw, 2008). Many suicide prevention programs employ gatekeeper training strategies educating natural helpers and trusted adults to recognize the warning signs for suicide and respond appropriately. There is relatively little empirical research, however, on the effects of these programs on youth, family, and community development. This lack of research is due to the wide variation of programs using a "strength-based" framework and the lack of empirical work in indigenous communities. To date, the only strengths-based program that has been evaluated is *Sources of Strength* (SoS), a universal, school-based suicide prevention approach (Wyman et al., 2010). SoS training builds on protective influences of peers, improving adaptive norms regarding suicide, their connectedness to adults, and school engagement among peer leaders. However, there are a number of promising cultural strategies that are based on community strengths but have not undergone scientific evaluation (US Department of Health and Human Services, 2010b). These programs are aligned with tradition, convention, belief, or anecdotal evidence.

Indigenous approaches

Several national efforts state goals to achieve health equity, eliminate disparities, and improve the health of all groups by preventing suicides and attempted suicides among indigenous people (Krysinska et al., 2009; SAMHSA, 2010b; US Department of Health and Human Services, 2010a; US Department of Health and Human Services, 2012). These efforts recommend engaging indigenous communities in identifying the cultural, historical, and spiritual factors which may influence suicide and suicidal behavior; promoting approaches to enhance self-esteem and capacity to enable individuals and communities to connect with a value system based on identity, place, people, and land; and developing partnership approaches with communities to strengthen local responses to complex issues.

Comprehension of local, traditional indigenous perspectives of suicide and well-being enhances the knowledge of existing evidence that suicide determinants are valid for indigenous peoples (Else et al., 2007; Wilson & Rosenberg, 2002). Earlier studies among indigenous peoples have shown a relationship between attenuated suicide rates and community ties to traditional values; and fewer suicides related to community involvement in health, education, and cultural services (Berlin, 1987; Chandler & Lalonde, 1998). Our qualitative work indicates that cultural adaptation influences among community members engaged in youth suicide prevention showed that youth programs that integrate cultural processes enhance youth participation, lead to improved self-concept, connectedness, and improved mental health and wellness (Goebert et al., 2012). Surface structures of cultural adaptation (e.g., local pictures and video) are helpful but not essential. Instead, programs need to include elements of deep structures of cultural adaptation that deal with feelings and attitudes that are learned by being a member of a particular group. It involves the thoughts, beliefs, values, and relationships as expressed in actions, words, and the intricacies of the way we live. These findings indicate that effective suicide prevention programs require sufficient time to form meaningful relationships to access, exchange and transform deep structures of cultural adaptation among program participants.

A review of prevention programs for Native American and Alaska Native communities concluded that programs work best if they are culturally relevant and developed with community input (Middlebrook et al., 2001). Community involvement in developing policies and programs makes a significant difference in well-being because it reinforces the contemporary discourse in many Native communities that *our culture is our treatment* (Kral et al., 2009). Placing indigenous epistemology and pedagogy at the center of suicide prevention programs encourages production and teaching of knowledge from the ground level (Trinidad, 2009). It engenders indigenization; and thereby empowers communities to tell their own story of past and present; and communities, cultures and social practices once seen as marginalized become sources of hope (Grande, 2004; Trinidad, 2009). Indigenization represents a paradigm shift in developing Native programs; it links intervention to a sense of community. Using this paradigm of indigenization, involved communities can evoke their history and traditions; then develop – with technical consultation from academic researchers and community advisers – culturally relevant, locally directed healing interventions which integrate scientific principles that determine effectiveness and efficacy.

Community engaged approaches

A key feature of community engaged approaches is "the process of working collaboratively with and through groups of people affiliated by geographic proximity, special interest, or similar situations to address issues affecting the well-being of those people" (CDC, 2011, p 7). As depicted in Figure 19.1 (Goebert et al., 2012), a common purpose of improving well-being through a suicide safe community is at its core. The process requires a supportive environment committed to knowledge sharing and collective self-determinism. Effective suicide prevention for indigenous peoples requires a broad-based community commitment and ownership. Innovative strategies rooted in community problem solving are needed. The need to look at resiliency and risk factors from a holistic point of view, along with communities whose rates of suicide are low to see what these communities are doing right, was thought to be a priority for prevention efforts. Community engagement can only be sustained by identifying and mobilizing community assets and strengths and by developing the community's capacity through partnerships, training, technical assistance, and resources to make decisions and take action.

The roles of researchers and community members also is being reframed, with researchers taking on the role of a facilitator of knowledge rather than an expert, working with community members on an equal basis. Community engaged research is defined as scientific inquiry conducted with communities and in partnership with researchers and community members. Community engaged research is a broad term to

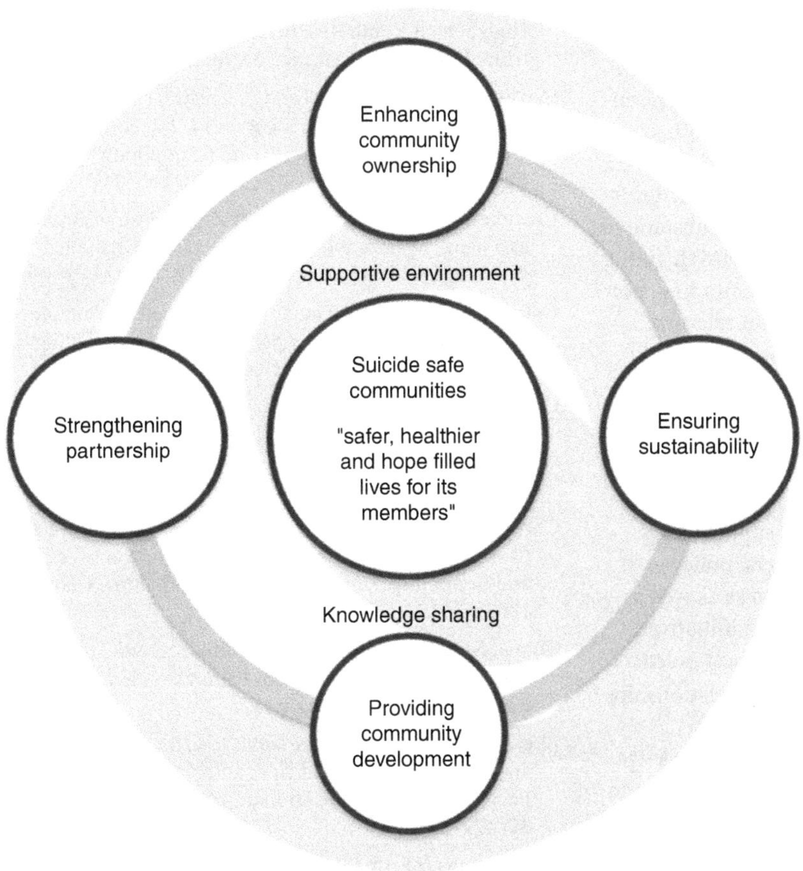

Figure 19.1. Community engaged process for suicide prevention.

refer to such approaches as community-based participatory research and participatory action research and is a relational method of sharing power throughout the research process that addresses an important problem in the community, oriented to social justice, and action oriented, rather than being a particular research method. This process will ensure opportunities for community members and key stakeholders in the community's health to be full participants in each phase of the research, from conception to dissemination and translation of results. Community engaged intervention research is based on strengths-based approaches (Wallerstein & Duran, 2006). Community engaged research also recognizes that health is determined by sociopolitical forces, often with disproportionate impact upon disenfranchised groups such as indigenous populations (Corbie-Smith et al., 2004). Ideally, community engaged research blends empirical support with key stakeholder feedback, resulting in culturally relevant interventions responding to the local community needs while generating meaningful and sustainable results. Recruiting participants from indigenous communities is challenging because they may be skeptical of research, particularly if direct benefits to the community are unclear. Research on recruitment indicates that recruiting subjects into intervention trials is difficult because placebos and randomization are viewed negatively (Yancey et al., 2006). Research that reduces respondent burden, expands community involvement, offers delayed or alternative interventions to control group participants, and assures that care will be delivered improves recruitment and retention in such communities. Community engaged research provides such assurances to the community by incorporating the knowledge, ideas, and concerns of community partners throughout all phases of the study.

Future directions

In 2014, the National Alliance for Suicide Prevention released its research agenda, emphasizing a need to understand community resilience and values. Specific priorities for native populations are in development (National Action Alliance for Suicide Prevention: American Indian/Alaska Native 2.0 Task Force, 2014). In 2006, an international conference brought representatives from research, service organizations, youth, community programs, and governments (countries, tribes, and villages) together to share the most current information on indigenous suicide, and to bring substantive research and prevention efforts forward (NIMH, 2006). They identified key directions in research, funding, policy, and prevention initiatives that remain relevant:

- Research: Suicide prevention research needs to examine suicide from a strengths-based, community engaged, indigenous perspective in order to develop practice-based evidence using mixed methods techniques.
- Funding: Financial resources must support long-term collaboration among researchers, policy makers, and community representatives as well as the development of community-based initiatives, professional recruitment, and cultural best practices.
- Health policy: Formal capacity building relationships need to be redefined to support networks, collaboration, and the lateral transfer of knowledge among indigenous communities; creating change in current policies that limit the roles and financial reimbursement for traditional healers and cultural experts in the areas of research and program support.
- Community Initiatives: Community engaged processes (planning, research, and prevention) need to be supported to strengthen cultural knowledge, promote cultural healing, and establish best practices regarding suicide prevention.

References

Andrade, N. N., Hishinuma, E. S., McDermott, J. F., Jr., et al. (2006). Prevalence of mental disorders in Native Hawaiian adolescents using the NIMH Diagnostic Interview Schedule for Children (DISC). *Journal of the American Academy of Child and Adolescent Psychiatry*, **45**, 26–36.

Berlin, I. N. (1987). Suicide among American Indian adolescents: An overview. *Suicide and Life-Threatening Behavior*, **17**, 218–232.

Borowsky, I., Resnick, M., Ireland, M., & Blum, R. (1999). Suicide attempts among American Indian and Alaska Native youth risk and protective factors. *Archives of Pediatrics and Adolescent Medicine*, **153**, 573–580.

Brave Heart, M. Y. H. (2000). Wakiksuyapi: Carrying the historical trauma of the Lakota. *Tulane Studies in Social Welfare*, **21–22**, 245–266.

Centers for Disease Control and Prevention (CDC). (2010). High School Youth Risk Behavior Survey Data. Retrieved from: http://apps.nccd.cdc.gov/youthonline.

Centers for Disease Control and Prevention (CDC). (2011). *Principles of Community Engagement*, 2nd edn. Atlanta, GA: CDC/ATSDR Committee on Community Engagement.

Chandler, M. J., & Lalonde, C. E. (1998). Cultural continuity as a hedge against suicide in Canada's first nations. *Transcultural Psychiatry*, **35**, 220–221.

Collings, S. C., & Beautrais, A. L. (2005). *Suicide Prevention in New Zealand: A Contemporary Perspective*. Wellington, New Zealand: Ministry of Health.

Colquhoun, S., & Dockery, A. (2012). *The Link between Indigenous Culture and Wellbeing: Qualitative Evidence for Australian Aboriginal Peoples*. Perth: Curtin University, Centre for Labour Market Research.

Corbie-Smith, G., Moody-Ayers, S., & Thrasher, A. (2004). Closing the circle between minority inclusion in research and health disparities. *Archives of Internal Medicine*, **164**, 1362–1364.

Coupe, N. (2005). *Whakamomori: Maori Youth Suicide Prevention*. PhD dissertation. Palmerston North, New Zealand: Massey University.

Else, I. R., Andrade, N. N., & Nahulu, L. B. (2007). Suicide and suicidal-related behaviors among indigenous Pacific Islanders in the United States. *Death Studies*, **31**, 479–501.

First Nations Information Governance Committee (2005). *First Nations Regional Longitudinal Health Survey (RHS) 2002/03: Results for Adults, Youth and Children Living in First Nations Communities*. Ottawa: First Nations Centre.

Goebert, D., Chung-Do, J., Sugimoto-Matsuda, J., et al. (2012). *Hawaii's Caring Communities Initiative: Community-Academic Partnerships for Youth Suicide Prevention*. Poster presented at the 2012 Science of Eliminating Health Disparities Summit in National Harbor, MD, December 17, 2012.

Grande, S. M. A. (2004). *Red Pedagogy: Native American Social and Political Thought*. Lanham, MD: Rowman & Littlefield Publishers, Inc.

Guerra, N. G., & Bradshaw, C. P. (2008). Linking the prevention of problem behaviors and positive youth development: Core competencies for positive youth development and risk prevention. In N. G. Guerra & C. P. Bradshaw (Eds.) *Core Competencies to Prevent Problem Behaviors and Promote Positive Youth Development. New Directions for Child and Adolescent Development*, **122**, 1–17.

Harder, H. G., Rash, J., Holyk, T., Jovel, E., & Harder, K. (2012). Indigenous youth suicide: a systematic review of the literature. *Pimatisiwin*, **10**, 125.

Kana'iaupuni, S. M. (2005). Ka'akālai Kū Kanaka: A call for strengths-based approaches from a Native Hawaiian perspective. *Educational Researcher*, **34**, 32–38.

Kral, M. J., Wiebe, P. K., Nisbet, K., et al. (2009). Canadian Inuit community engagement in youth suicide prevention. *International Journal of Circumpolar Health*, **68**, 292–308

Krysinska, K., Martin, G. & Sheehan, N. (2009). *Identity, Voice, Place: Suicide Prevention for Indigenous Australians – A Social and Emotional Wellbeing Approach.* Queensland, Australia: The University of Queensland.

Lerner, R. M., & Benson, P. I. (2003). *Developmental Assets and Asset-building Communities: Implications for Research, Policy, and Practice.* New York: Kluwer Academic/Plenum.

Mackin, J., Perkins, T., & Furrer, C. (2012). The power of protection: a population-based comparison of native and non-native youth suicide attempters. *American Indian and Alaska Native Mental Health Research (Online)*, **19**, 20–54.

Maton, K. I., Schellenbach, C. J., Leadbeater, B., & Solarz, A. (2003). *Investing in Children, Youth, Families and Communities: Strengths Based Research and Policy.* Washington, DC: American Psychological Association.

Middlebrook, D. L., LeMaster, P. L., Beals, J., Novins, D. K., & Manson, S. (2001). Suicide prevention in American Indian and Alaska Native communities: A critical review of programs. *Suicide and Life-Threatening Behavior*, **31**(Suppl), S132–S149.

Mmari, K. N., Blum, R. W., & Teufel-Shone, N. (2010). What increases risk and protection for delinquent behaviors among American Indian youth? Findings from three tribal communities. *Youth & Society*, **41**, 382–413.

National Action Alliance for Suicide Prevention: American Indian/Alaska Native 2.0 Task Force. (2014). American Indian/Alaska Native 2.0 Task Force. Available at: http://actionallianceforsuicideprevention.org/task-force/aian2.

National Action Alliance for Suicide Prevention: Research Prioritization Task Force. (2014). A prioritized research agenda for suicide prevention: An action plan to save lives. Rockville, MD: Natinal Institute of Mental Health and the Research Prioritization Task Force.

National Institute on Mental Health (NIMH). (2006). *Indigenous Suicide Prevention Research & Programs in Canada and the United States: Setting a Collaborative Agenda- Report and Recommendations.* Albuquerque, NM: National Institute on Mental Health.

Silburn, S., Glaskin, B., Henry, D., & Drew, N. (2012). *Preventing Suicide among Indigenous Australians.* Downloaded Dec 2012 from http://aboriginal.childhealthresearch.org.au/media/54877/chapter7.pdf.

Streur, W. J., McLaughlin, J., & Castrodale, L. (2012). Characteristics of suicide among Alaska Native and Alaska non-Native people, 2003–2008. *State of Alaska Epidemiology Bulletin: Recommendations and Reports*, **15**, 1–22.

Substance Abuse and Mental Health Services Administration (SAMHSA). (2010a). *Results from the 2009 National Survey on Drug Use and Health: Mental Health Findings.* Rockville, MD: SAMHSA.

Substance Abuse and Mental Health Service Administration (SAMHSA) (2010b). SAMHSA's 10 Strategic Initiatives. Washington, DC: SAMHSA. Available at: www.samhsa.gov/about/siDocs/prevention.pdf

Trinidad, A. M. O. (2009). Toward kuleana (responsibility): A case study of a contextually grounded intervention for Native Hawaiian youth and young adults. *Aggression and Violent Behavior*, **14**, 488–498.

US Department of Health and Human Services. (2010a). *Healthy People 2020.* Washington, DC: US Department of Health and Human Services.

US Department of Health and Human Services. (2010b). *To Live to See the Great Day That Dawns: Preventing Suicide by American Indian and Alaska Native Youth and Young Adults.* DHHS Publication SMA (10)-4480, CMHS-NSPL-0196, Printed 2010. Rockville, MD: Center for Mental Health Services, Substance Abuse and Mental Health Services Administration.

US Department of Health and Human Services, Public Health Service. (2012). *2012 National Strategy for Suicide Prevention: Goals and Objectives for Action.* Rockville, MD: US Department of Health and Human Services, Public Health Service.

Wallerstein, N. B., & Duran, B. (2006). Using community-based participatory research to address health disparities. *Health Promotion Practice*, **7**, 312–323

Whitbeck, L. B., Adams, G. W., Hoyt, D. R., & Chen, X. (2004). Conceptualizing and measuring historical trauma among American Indian people. *American Journal of Community Psychology*, **33**, 119–130.

Wilson, K., & Rosenberg, M. W. (2002). Exploring determinants of health for First Nations peoples in Canada: Can existing frameworks accommodate traditional activities? *Social Science and Medicine*, **55**, 2017–2031.

Wyman, P. A., Brown, C. H., LoMurray, M., et al. (2010). An outcome evaluation of the Sources of Strength suicide prevention program delivered by adolescent peer leaders in high schools. *American Journal of Public Health*, **100**, 1653–1661.

Yancey, A. K., Ortega, A. N., & Kumanyika, S. K. (2006). Effective recruitment and retention of minority research participants. *Annual Review of Public Health*, **27**, 1–28.

Yuen, N. Y. C., Nahulu, L. B., Hishinuma, E. S., & Miyamoto, R. H. (2000). Cultural identification and attempted suicide in Native Hawaiian adolescents. *Journal of the American Academy of Child and Adolescent Psychiatry*, **39**, 360–367.

Chapter 20

Bullying and suicidality in youth

Anat Brunstein Klomek and Madelyn S. Gould

Introduction

For years bullying was considered a routine part of growing up but nowadays it is a topic of concern for youths, parents, school staff, and mental health professionals. The CDC is currently trying to reach a consensus about the definition of bullying to address the problem of divergent definitions employed in different research studies. The most widely employed definition is: A person is bullied when he or she is exposed, repeatedly and over time, to negative actions on the part of one or more persons which are more powerful (Olweus, 1991). Bullying behavior involves four major roles – bully/perpetrator, victim, bully–victim (bullies in some situations and victims in others), and bystander (Rivers & Noret, 2010). Most of the existing research examining the association between bullying and suicide has focused on the first three groups.

Only in the last few decades have studies indicated that bullying among children is a pervasive problem and it is now recognized as an important public health issue. Population-based studies indicate that 20% to 30% of school children are frequently involved in bullying as bullies and/or victims (Nansel et al., 2001). Bullying behavior falls into four general categories: direct/physical (e.g., assaults or theft), direct/verbal (e.g., threats, insults, or nicknames), indirect/relational (e.g., social exclusion, spreading nasty rumors), and the newest form, cyberbullying (see section below on cyberbullying).

When examining the association between bullying and suicide it is important to differentiate the types of suicidality included in studies. Suicidal ideations are thoughts of suicide which can be passive ("I wish I was dead") and/or active ("I'm thinking of suicide"). These thoughts may or may not include intent to act on them and/or a plan. Suicidal attempts include behaviors that are self-directed and deliberately result in injury/potential for injury and for which there is evidence of some suicidal intent. At the end of the continuum, there is death by suicide. In a typical 12-month period, nearly 14% of American high school students seriously consider suicide, 11% make plans about how they will end their lives, 6.3% actually attempt suicide, and approximately 1 in 10 000 young individuals will die by suicide (CDC, 2010).

There are many risk factors for suicide among adolescents. Peer relationships are important ones and are now frequently studied around the world (e.g., Horesh et al. 2012).

Before we continue with the examination of the association of bullying with suicide it should be highlighted that most children involved in bullying do not harm or kill themselves. One aim of the research in the field is to identify which children/adolescents involved in bullying behaviors are at greatest risk for suicidal behavior. Much of the research attention has been given to understanding the impact of bullying on the *victims'* depression, suicidal ideation, and suicidal behavior. Until the past decade, the research on those who *bully others* has largely focused on its association with antisocial and violent behavior. It has now become clear that it is important to include an examination of depression, suicide ideation, suicide attempts, and death by suicide for bullies as well as victims.

Over the past few years, the media has focused public attention on instances of suicide among adolescents who have been bullied, and there are increasingly more anti-bullying policies and laws around the world. The significant increment in news reports concerning deaths associated with bullying may be the result of a rise in public awareness. However, one should be aware that the media message that bullying leads to suicide may not be accurate. There seems to be a very

A Concise Guide to Understanding Suicide, ed. Stephen H. Koslow, Pedro Ruiz, and Charles B. Nemeroff. Published by Cambridge University Press.

complex relationship between bullying and suicide and there could be mediating factors that are important to take into consideration. In this chapter we will try to explain this complex association between bullying and suicide among adolescents. We will include correlational studies, longitudinal studies, and a separate section about the newest form of bullying – cyberbullying.

Correlational studies

Most of the data to date about the association between bullying, depression, and suicide is based on cross-sectional studies. Kim and Leventhal (2008) and our group (Klomek et al., 2010) have published review papers summarizing many of these studies. Bullying and victimization have been found to be associated with depression (e.g., Kaltiala-Heino et al., 1999; Hawker & Boulton, 2000; Klomek et al., 2007). In studies examining the association between bullying and depression, victims are found to manifest more depressive symptoms and psychological distress compared to non-victims (e.g., Kumpulainen et al., 1998; Hawker and Boulton, 2000). Findings pertaining to bullies are less consistent. Some studies did not find an association between being a bully and depression (e.g., Fekkes et al., 2004); whereas other studies have found that bullies, and not merely victims, report high levels of depression (Kaltiala-Heino et al., 1999; Klomek et al., 2007). The inconsistent results may be explained by different studies, varying gender distributions, and definitions of bullying. Females and males appear to have a different threshold by which bullying is associated with depression (Klomek et al., 2007). For males, only frequent bullying is associated with depression; whereas, for females, even infrequent bullying is associated with depression. One possible explanation for depression in those who bully others, for both genders, may be that bullies engage in aggressive behaviors to compensate for negative feelings or low self-esteem (O'Moore & Kirkham, 2001). Those who are *both* victims and bullies are usually found to be at the highest risk for depression (e.g., Kaltiala-Heino et al., 1999; Fekkes et al., 2004; Klomek et al., 2007).

There also appears to be an association between bullying and suicidal ideation (e.g., Kaltiala-Heino et al., 1999; Kim et al., 2005; Klomek et al., 2007; 2008a) and suicide attempts (Kaltiala-Heino et al., 1999; Kim et al., 2005; Klomek et al., 2007, 2008a). Some studies have found that suicidal thoughts and behaviors are more strongly associated among victims than bullies (e.g., Hinduja & Patchin, 2010; Skapinakis et al., 2011), while others have emphasized that bullies are also at very high risk (Luukkonen et al., 2009; Hepburn et al., 2012; Klomek et al., 2013). These studies are different in the definition of suicidality and the bullying behaviors that are included.

Cui et al (2011) recently studied a large representative sample of Chinese adolescents (N = 8778) and found that being victimized was associated with suicide ideation and suicide attempts. Interestingly, feelings of loneliness acted as a moderator affecting the association between peer relationships and suicide ideation and attempts. Feeling lonely exacerbated the ill effect of peer problems on suicidal behavior, while the lack of feelings of loneliness acted as a buffer. Similarly, Skapinakis et al. (2011) examined 5614 students 16–18 years old who were attending 25 senior high schools in Greece. Victims of bullying behavior were more likely than students who were not victims of bullying to express that "life was not worth living" (passive suicidal ideation). This association was particularly strong for those who were bullied on a weekly basis. This association was independent of the presence of psychiatric morbidity, assessed by means of a very detailed structured interview, and a wide range of other socio-economic or family-related variables. In contrast, being a bully was not associated with passive suicide ideation after adjusting for these other factors. These findings were similar in both boys and girls; although the population impact of victimization on the prevalence of suicidal ideation was higher for boys.

In examining studies focusing on adolescents, Kaminski and Fang (2009) studied the association between victimization by peers and suicidal ideation and behavior in the USA. This study was a secondary analysis of data from three cohorts of adolescents: (1) a nationally representative survey of adolescents in grade 7 through 12, Wave I of the National Longitudinal Study of Adolescent Health, conducted by the Carolina Population Center in 1994–1995; (2) a nationally representative survey, the Youth Risk Behavior Surveillance System, conducted by the Centers for Disease Control and Prevention in 2005; and (3) a survey in a high-risk community conducted by the Centers for Disease Control and Prevention in 2004. They found that when controlling for differences in age, sex, race/ethnicity, and depressive symptomatology, adolescents reporting more frequent victimization by peers were still more likely to report suicidal ideation and suicidal behavior.

A population-based cohort study of 1526 Dutch children around age 12 (Herba et al., 2008) indicated that victims of bullying have an increased risk for suicide ideation if their parents have internalizing disorders or if they feel rejected by their parents at home.

As described above, some studies have found a higher risk of both suicide ideation and suicide attempts among bullies and not only victims. Hepburn et al. (2012) for example analyzed whether involvement in bullying as a bully, victim, or both bully and victim (bully–victim) was associated with a higher risk of suicidal ideation or suicide attempts among a multiethnic urban high school sample of 1838 youth in 9–12 grades in the USA. They found that students who reported having been involved in bullying as a bully, victim, or bully–victim were more likely than those who had not been involved in bullying to report having seriously considered or attempted suicide within the past year. When age, race/ethnicity, and gender were controlled, students who were bully–victims were at highest risk for both suicidal ideation and suicide attempt. Similarly, Luukkonen et al. (2009), investigated the association of bullying behavior with suicide attempts and self-mutilation among adolescents. The sample included 508 Finnish adolescents (age 12–17 years) admitted to psychiatric inpatient care. They found that after adjusting for age, school factors, family factors, and psychiatric disorders there was a higher risk of suicide attempts in girls who were victims or who bullied others compared with those not involved in bullying behavior. Corresponding associations were not found for boys; nor was any association of bullying behavior with self-mutilation found among either gender.

Bystanders hold a very important role since they are usually the majority of the children involved in the bullying and may have a lot of influence in social situations. Rivers and Noret (2010) have studied the role of bystanders in the association between bullying and suicidality. Their study included a cross-sectional survey of a representative sample of 2002 school students in England aged 12 to 16 years and found that those with multiple roles (victim, bully, and bystander) were significantly more likely to report having had thoughts of ending their life.

Long-term consequences of bullying

Longitudinal studies are crucial to the understanding of the temporal association between bullying behaviors and suicidality. Bullying and being bullied are found to be rather stable during child development. In a Finnish cohort, for example, almost all boys who were bullied at the age of 16 had been bullied already at age 8. Half of the boys who bullied at 16 had already been bullying when they were 8. Children and adolescents who are involved in bullying have a range of later psychological difficulties (e.g., Sourander et al., 2007). Bullying's long-term negative consequences can persist until adulthood (Sourander et al., 2007; Roeger et al., 2010). The number of longitudinal studies examining the association between bullying and suicidality is increasing, but results are still inconsistent. This may be due to the variability in the studies' protocols, including the age of the samples, definitions of suicidality and/or bullying behaviors, length of follow-up, and the extent to which mediating factors were controlled for (see section on critical view of the field below).

With regard to the age of the samples, some studies include children while others focus on pre-adolescents and/or adolescents. We will start with studies including younger children and adolescents and will proceed to those examining older participants. Fisher et al. (2012), for example, have recently assessed 2232 children at ages 5, 7, 10, and 12 and examined whether frequent victimization in childhood increases the likelihood of self-harm 6 months before their twelfth birthday. Results indicated that exposure to frequent bullying predicted higher rates of self-harm even after children's premorbid emotional and behavioral problems, low IQ, and family environmental risks were taken into account. In addition, compared with bullied children who did not self-harm, bullied children who self-harmed were distinguished by a family history of attempted/completed suicide, concurrent mental health problems, and a history of physical maltreatment by an adult.

Our study among 8-year-old Finnish boy students (Klomek et al., 2008b) examined the frequency of bullying behavior and its association with suicidal ideation at age 18. We found that bullying others *infrequently* among boys at age 8 was not associated with an elevated risk of depression (mild or severe) nor with suicidal ideation at age 18. This contrasted with the strong relationship between *frequent* bullying and later depression and suicide ideation. We hypothesized that infrequent bullying may be relatively normative behavior among boys, consistent with reports that the level of aggression is higher among males compared to females. Our results which found that frequent childhood bullying among boys predicted internalizing problems in adolescence questions previous reports that bullying is especially associated with externalizing problems while victimization is associated with internalizing problems (Sourander et al., 2007). Our findings add to those of a 10-month prospective study conducted by Kim et al. (2009). In her Korean study, Kim and her colleagues followed seventh- and eighth-grade students for 10 months and showed that problem behavior was a consequence rather than a cause of bullying experience (Kim et al., 2009). In another study from Finland we examined the association of bullying at age 8 and suicide attempts and completed suicides among both boys and girls (Klomek et al., 2009). We found that this association varied by gender. Among boys, frequent bullying and victimization at age 8 was not associated with later suicide attempts and completed suicides, after controlling for both childhood conduct and depression symptoms. Frequent victimization among girls at age 8, however, was associated with later suicide attempts and completed suicides, even after controlling for childhood conduct and depression symptoms.

In a recent study among 6043 children and preadolescents, Winsper et al. (2012) examined the prospective link between involvement in bullying at ages 4–10 and suicide ideation and suicide/self-injurious behavior at age 11.7. They found that chronic victims and bully–victims were at highest risk for suicide ideation and suicide/self-injurious behavior at age 11 after controlling for confounders (child abuse, maladaptive parenting, domestic violence, externalizing and internalizing symptoms). Both overt and relational victimization were associated with suicidal ideation and suicide/self-injurious behavior. In addition, "pure bullies" (according to child self-report at age 8 and teacher report) were likely to engage in suicidal/self-injurious behavior.

A recent study by our group examined high school students in New York who were involved in bullying behavior and followed 4 years later, when some of them were out of high school (Klomek et al., 2011). We compared three groups of high school students: students who were involved in frequent bullying behavior with no concurrent depression or suicidal ideation or behavior; students who were involved in frequent bullying behavior and also had depression, or suicidal ideation or behavior; students who experienced depression, suicide ideation/behavior, but who did not have bullying experiences. Our findings indicated that students who only reported bullying experience (as bullies, victims, or both) did not develop later depression or suicide ideation/behavior and had fewer psychiatric problems than students identified as at risk for suicide. However, students who reported bullying experience and depression and/or suicide ideation/behavior were more impaired 4 years later than those who only reported depression or suicide ideation/behavior.

In a retrospective study of 2907 adults in South Australia, who reported on their memories of bullying experiences, respondents with a history of being bullied were approximately three times more likely to report suicidal ideation compared with those who did not. This association remained after controlling for both depression and sociodemographic variables.

Cyberbullying

Cyberbullying is a growing and concerning phenomenon (Hinduja & Patchin, 2010; Sourander et al., 2010). Similar to traditional bullying, the definition of cyberbullying still varies between studies. A common definition of cyberbullying by Smith et al. (2008) is that it is an aggressive, intentional act carried out by a group or individual, using electronic forms of contact, repeatedly and over time against a victim who cannot easily defend him- or herself. The phenomenon only appeared a few years ago, as the use of electronic devices such as computers and mobile phones by young people increased. School surveys from the USA show that the rate of being a cyberbully or a victim of cyberbullying is 4% and 11%, respectively (Kowalski & Limber, 2007). Many cyberbullies and cybervictims are also traditional bullies and victims (Jose et al., 2012). Sourander et al. (2010) have found that both cyberbullying and cybervictimization are associated with psychiatric and psychosomatic problems.

Media has been reporting on adolescents' suicides resulting from peer cyber victimization. However, studies examining the association between suicidal ideation/behavior and experiences with cyber victimization or cyber-offending have only recently started, are still few in numbers, and are cross-sectional. Although the media tends to convey a clear message about a causal relationship between cyberbullying and suicide we still do not have evidence to support this conclusion. Hinduja and Patchin (2010) have examined the extent to which cyberbullying is associated with suicidal ideation among adolescents. Among a sample of 1963 US children in middle school, youth who experienced traditional bullying or cyberbullying, as either a bully or a victim, had more suicidal thoughts and were more likely to attempt suicide than those who had not experienced such forms of peer aggression. Similarly, in a cross-sectional study we conducted among high school students we found that being frequently victimized by email or Internet during high school was related to a high-risk of depression, ideation, and attempts compared to students not victimized. Infrequent victimization was also related to increased risk among females. Our results also indicated that the more types of victimization the higher the risk for depression and suicidality among both girls and boys (Klomek et al., 2008a).

Critical overview of the methodological variation in the research

The current literature on bullying and victimization and their association with depression, suicidal ideation, and suicide includes studies that vary markedly in methodology. How bullying and suicidality are conceptualized and assessed is the first source of variability. Studies use different scales for the assessment of bullying behavior. Some rely on self-reports (e.g. Klomek et al., 2007), peer nominations (Bouman et al., 2012), parent reports, teacher reports, or multiple informants (e.g., child and mother: Fisher et al., 2012; child, mother, and teacher: Winsper et al., 2012). Moreover, most studies use questionnaires (Kim et al., 2009); whereas some use interviews (Fisher et al., 2012).

Other sources of variation include the frequency and the duration of the bullying behavior. Some studies include any involvement in bullying behavior while others focus on frequent involvement (Klomek et al., 2011; Fisher et al., 2012). Few studies have examined the duration of the bullying. In a recent study Winsper et al. (2012) studied the duration and found differences between those who were involved chronically and those who were not. Moreover, only some studies examined specific types of bullying (e.g. Klomek et al., 2008a).

Another variation in studies is the outcomes that are investigated. While some studies examine passive suicidal ideation (Skapinakis et al., 2011) others have examined any active suicidal ideation (Winsper et al., 2012) or severe active suicidal ideation (Klomek et al., 2007). In the study by Skapinakis et al. (2011) suicidal ideation was assessed with a question on "tiredness of life." They did not include questions about more severe forms of suicidal ideation (death wishes or actual ideas of harming oneself) and therefore their results cannot be generalized to more severe forms of suicidal ideation. These ideation outcomes may be different clinically since infrequent passive suicidal ideation may be normative during adolescence while more severe active suicidal ideation may be very concerning. Moreover, studies also vary in the definition of suicidal behavior. Most previous studies did not focus on suicide attempts requiring hospitalization and did not include completed suicides. A recent study (Fisher et al., 2012) has even included different self-harm behaviors including biting arms, banging head, hair pulling, etc.

Another factor which is crucial to take into consideration is the age of the children involved in bullying. While some studies focus on elementary school children (Klomek et al., 2010), others focus on pre-adolescents (Winsper et al., 2012) or adolescents (Klomek et al., 2011). In addition, many studies have not controlled for suicide-related risk factors which may be important mediating factors (depression, externalizing disorders, family and school factors, etc.) (Kim & Leventhal, 2008).

Lastly, only some of the studies have examined gender differences (e.g., Klomek et al., 2007, 2009; Winsper et al., 2012), which is an important moderating factor for both bullying and the risk for suicide.

These methodological differences between the studies may explain some of the inconsistent results in the field. Variation in the assessments and definitions of bullying behaviors (including the variation in the frequency of involvement), outcomes, and moderating and confounding factors examined may explain why some studies find an association between bullying behavior with suicidality while others do not.

Recommended future research

Both bullying behavior and suicide are complex phenomena moderated by many factors, including personal individual characteristics, parent characteristics, family dynamics, school factors, and cultural aspects. Future studies examining the association between bullying and suicide should aim to take more of these aspects into account, and examine how these moderate or mediate the link between bullying and suicide risk. These factors may also be resilience, as well as risk factors for both bullying and suicidality. An important question to study is how to promote resilience factors among children and adolescents, which may help to prevent subsequent sequelae, including suicidal behavior.

Lastly, more evidence-based interventions aimed at decreasing both bullying and suicidal risk should be developed. These should include skills to develop healthy relationships, adaptive communications, improving emotion regulation, etc. One option may be Interpersonal Psychotherapy (IPT-A) which has been found to be effective among depressed adolescents (Mufson et al., 2004) and is currently being adapted to work with victimized teens.

Conclusion

Despite methodological and other limitations described above, it is clear that there is a relationship between bullying and suicide risk. Studies support the conjecture that bullying and peer victimization puts adolescents at increased risk of suicidal ideation and behavior, especially when other psychopathology is present. The idea that psychiatric conditions are expected to have a strong moderating effect that needs to be taken into account when examining the influence of bullying behavior among children and adolescents is not surprising since suicidal ideation and behavior cannot be attributed to just one event or factor. Studies have shown that bullies, victims, and bully–victims are different groups and all should be targeted for interventions, especially those who are frequently involved in these behaviors. It is also clear that each gender has a markedly different risk profile that should be taken into consideration when building prevention and intervention programs. Community-based suicide prevention programs and clinical interventions should be particularly attentive to youth exhibiting symptoms of psychopathology who are also involved in frequent bullying.

References

Bouman, T., van der Meulen, M., Goossens, F. A., et al. (2012). Peer and self-reports of victimization and bullying: Their differential association with internalizing problems and social adjustment. *Journal of School Psychology*, **50**(6), 759–774.

Centers for Disease Control and Prevention (CDC). (2010). Youth risk behavior surveillance – United States, 2009. Surveillance summaries. *Morbidity and Mortality Weekly Report*, **59**, SS-5.

Cui, S., Cheng, Y., Xu, Z., Chen, D., & Wang, Y. (2011). Peer relationships and suicide ideation and attempts among Chinese adolescents. *Child Care Health Development*, **37**(5), 692–702.

Fekkes, M., Pijpers, F. I., & Verloove-Vanhorick, S. P. (2004). Bullying behavior and associations with psychosomatic complaints and depression in victims. *The Journal of Pediatrics*, **144**, 17–22.

Fisher, H. L., Moffitt, T. E., Houts, R. M., et al. (2012). Bullying victimization and risk of self harm in early adolescence: longitudinal cohort study. *British Medical Journal*, **344**, e2683.

Hawker, D. S. J., & Boulton, M. J. (2000). Twenty years' research on peer victimization and psychosocial maladjustment: A meta-analytic review of cross-sectional studies. *Journal of Child Psychology and Psychiatry*, **41**, 441–455.

Hepburn, L., Azrael, D., Molnar, B., & Miller, M. (2012). Bullying and suicidal behaviors among urban high school youth. *Journal of Adolescent Health*, **51**(1), 93–95.

Herba, C. M., Ferdinand, R. F., Stijnen, T., et al. (2008). Victimization and suicide ideation in the TRAILS study: specific vulnerabilities of victims. *Journal of Child Psychology and Psychiatry*, **49**(8), 867–876.

Hinduja, S., & Patchin, J. W. (2010). Bullying, cyberbullying, and suicide. *Archives of Suicide Research*, **14**(3), 206–221.

Horesh, N., Levi, Y., & Apter, A. (2012). Medically serious versus non-serious suicide attempts: relationships of lethality and intent to clinical and interpersonal characteristics. *Affective Disorders*, **136**(3), 286–293.

Jose, P. E., Kljakovic, M., Scheib, E., & Notter, O. (2012). The joint development of traditional bullying and victimization with cyber bullying and victimization in adolescence. *Journal of Research on Adolescence*, **22**(2), 301–309.

Kaltiala-Heino, R., Rimpela, M., Marttunen, M., Rimpela, A., & Rantanen, P. (1999). Bullying, depression, and suicidal ideation in Finnish adolescents: school survey. *British Medical Journal*, **319**, 348–351.

Kaminski, J. W., & Fang, X. (2009). Victimization by peers and adolescent suicide in three US samples. *The Journal of Pediatrics*, **155**(5), 683–688.

Kim, Y. S., & Leventhal, B. (2008). Bullying and suicide. A review. *International Journal of Adolescent Medicine and Health*, **20**(2), 133–154.

Kim, Y. S., Koh, Y. J., & Leventhal, B. (2005). School bullying and suicidal risk in Korean middle school students. *Pediatrics*, **115**, 357–363.

Kim, Y. S., Leventhal, B. L., Koh, Y. J., & Boyce, W. (2009). Bullying increased suicide risk: prospective study of Korean adolescents. *Archives of Suicide Research*, **13**, 15–30.

Klomek, B. A., Marrocco, F., Kleinman, M., Schonfeld, I., & Gould, M. S. (2007). Bullying, depression and suicidality in adolescents. *Journal of the American Academy of Child and Adolescent Psychiatry*, **46**(1), 40–49.

Klomek, A. B., Marrocco, F., Kleinman, M., Schonfeld, I., & Gould, M. S. (2008a). Victimization, depression and suicidality in adolescents. *Suicide and Life-Threatening Behavior*, **38**(2), 166–180.

Klomek, A. B., Sourander, A., Kumpulainen, K., et al. (2008b). Childhood bullying as a risk for later depression and suicidal ideation among Finnish males. *Journal of Affective Disorders*, **109**, 47–55.

Klomek, A. B., Sourander, A., Niemelä, S., et al. (2009). Childhood bullying behaviors as a risk for suicide attempts and completed suicides: a population-based birth cohort study. *Journal of American Academy of Child Adolescent Psychiatry*, **48**, 254-261.

Klomek, A. B., Sourander, A., & Gould, M. (2010). The Association of Suicide and Bullying in Childhood to Young Adulthood: a review of cross-sectional and longitudinal research findings. *Canadian Journal of Psychiatry*, **55**(5), 282–288.

Klomek, A. B., Kleinman, M., Altschuler, E., et al. (2011). High school bullying as a risk for later depression and suicidality. *Suicide and Life-Threatening Behavior*, **41**(5), 501–516.

Klomek, B. A., Kleinman, M., Altschuler, A., et al. (2013). Suicidal adolescents' experiences with bullying perpetration and victimization during high school as risk factors for later depression and suicidality. *International Journal of Adolescent Health*, **53**, 37–42.

Kowalski, M. R., & Limber, P. S. (2007). Electronic bullying among middle school students. *Journal of Adolescent Health*, **41**, S22–S30.

Kumpulainen, K., Rasanen, E., Henttonen, I., et al. (1998). Bullying and psychiatric symptoms among elementary school-age children. *Child Abuse and Neglect*, **22**, 705–717.

Luukkonen, A. H., Räsänen, P., & Hakko, H., et al. (2009). Bullying behavior is related to suicide attempts but not to self-mutilation among psychiatric inpatient adolescents. *Psychopathology*, **42**, 131–138.

Mufson, L., Dorta, K. P., Wickramaratne, P., et al. (2004). A randomized effectiveness trial of interpersonal psychotherapy for depressed adolescents. *Archives of General Psychiatry*, **61**(6), 577–584.

Nansel, T. R., Overpeck, M., Pilla, R. S., et al. (2001). Bullying behaviors among U.S. youth: Prevalence and association with psychosocial adjustment. *Journal of the American Medical Association*, **285**(16), 2094–2100.

Olweus, D. (1991). Bully/victim problems among school children: Basic facts and effects of a school based intervention program. In D. Pepler & K. Rubin (Eds.) *The Development and Treatment of Childhood Aggression* (pp. 411–448). Hillsdale, NJ: Erlbaum.

O'Moore, M., & Kirkham, C. (2001). Self-esteem and its relationship to bullying behavior. *Aggressive Behavior*, **27**(4), 269–283.

Rivers, I., & Noret, N. (2010). Participant roles in bullying behavior and their association with thoughts of ending one's life. *Crisis*, **31**(3), 143–148.

Roeger, L., Allison, S., Korossy-Horwood, R., Eckert, K. A., & Goldney, R. D. (2010). Is a history of school bullying victimization associated with adult suicidal ideation? A South Australian population-based observational study. *Journal of Nervous and Mental Disease*, **198**(10), 728–733.

Skapinakis, P., Bellos, S., Gkatsa, T., et al. (2011). The association between bullying and early stages of suicidal ideation in late adolescents in Greece. *BMC Psychiatry*, **11**: 22.

Smith, P. K., Mahdavi, J., Carvalho, M., et al. (2008). Cyberbullying: its nature and impact in secondary school pupils. *Journal of Child Psychology and Psychiatry*, **49**, 376–385.

Sourander, A., Jensen, P., Rönning, J. A., et al. (2007). What is the early adulthood outcome of boys who bully or are bullied in childhood? The Finnish "From a Boy to a Man" study. *Pediatrics*, **120**, 397–404.

Sourander, A., Brunstein Klomek, A., Ikonen, M., et al. (2010). Psychosocial risk factors associated with cyberbullying among adolescents: a population-based study. *Archives of General Psychiatry*, **67**(7), 720–728.

Winsper, C., Lereya, T., Zanarini, M., & Wolke, D. (2012). Involvement in bullying and suicide-related behavior at 11 years: A prospective birth cohort study. *Journal of the American Academy of Child and Adolescent Psychiatry*, **51**, 271–282.

Chapter 21

College students

Amanda L. McMillan and Steven J. Garlow

Epidemiology

Suicide is the third leading cause of death among adolescents and young adults in the USA. Only accidents and homicides claim more young lives in any given year (Centers for Disease Control and Prevention, 2013). There are no systematic mortality data collected specifically on young adults enrolled in colleges and universities across the country, however many argue that suicide may actually be the second leading cause of death on college campuses due to much lower risk of homicide for college students than young adults in the general population (Suicide Prevention Resource Center (SPRC), 2004).

A landmark study of suicide rates among college students conducted by the Big Ten Suicide Prevention Research Group reported on suicides at 12 midwestern universities from 1980 to 1990. The overall student suicide rate across all campuses during the study period was 7.5/100 000 (Silverman et al., 1997). This rate was 50% of the US national rate (15/100 000) matched for age, gender, and race. But the Big 10 Student Suicide Study also revealed that risk for suicide increased dramatically with age of the students. For those under age 25 the rate was 5.8/100 000, which was significantly lower than the national rate for age-matched controls, while the rate for those over age 25 was 10.7/100 000, which did not differ significantly from the national rate. Suicide rates appear to increase for students enrolled in graduate school as well. Undergraduate women had a suicide rate of 3.4/100 000 compared to their male counterparts at 9.1/100 000. However, among graduate students, the rate for women (9.1/100 000) approached that of men (11.6/100 000) and the two groups were not significantly different.

The most recent data from the American College Health Association-National College Health Assessments (ACHA-NCHA) reports statistics on 90 000 students at 141 schools. This survey indicates that among those polled, 7.1% of respondents have "seriously considered suicide" in the past 12 months and 1.2% have made a suicide attempt in the past year (ACHA, 2012). Interestingly, only 34.2% of students reported having been provided with information on suicide prevention from their college or university.

Another source of current data on college student suicide-related behaviors is the annual National Survey of College Counseling (NSCC), which assess a variety of topics related to mental health need and services provided at a diverse range of colleges and universities in the USA. The survey results include responses from directors of 293 college counseling centers responsible for 2.7 million students eligible for counseling services at these institutions (Gallagher, 2012). Of these students, 278 000 or 10.4% participated in counseling center services during the survey year. Of the counseling center directors surveyed, 88% report a recent increase in students with severe psychiatric or psychological problems on campus including students taking psychotropic medications, and students with alcohol and drug abuse and addiction issues, self-injurious behaviors, and eating disorders. Respondents consequently noted a dramatic rise in student psychiatric hospitalizations, which have more than tripled since 1994. Perhaps the most striking and disturbing statistic relates directly to the 106 reported student suicides, of which only 21% were current or former clients of their respective counseling centers. Additionally, in 68% of suicides, the student gave no warning of suicidal intent.

Mental illness in college students and access to care

Mental illness, particularly depression and substance use disorders, are risk factors for suicide-related

A Concise Guide to Understanding Suicide, ed. Stephen H. Koslow, Pedro Ruiz, and Charles B. Nemeroff. Published by Cambridge University Press.

behaviors among college students. Identification of those students with mental illnesses and providing them with appropriate psychiatric and psychological treatment is one potential method to reduce suicide risk. However, as demonstrated in the NSCC, psychiatric disorders appear to often be undiagnosed and untreated among college students. This mismatch between student need and service utilization is particularly striking as many college campuses provide students with universal access to free short-term psychotherapy and health care services. A 2007 survey of mental health care access and help-seeking behaviors among university students found that of those with positive screens for depression and anxiety, 37% to 84% did not receive any services, depending on the underlying psychiatric disorder (Eisenberg et al., 2007).

A survey of college students living with mental illnesses conducted by the National Alliance on Mental Illness (NAMI) provides more data illuminating the limitations of access to treatment on college campuses and some insights into reasons for students not utilizing services. Responses from 765 students indicate that only 50% disclosed their mental illness to the college (Gruttadaro & Crudo, 2012). Students who chose to disclose often did so to secure academic accommodations. Of those who did not disclose, many cited fear of stigma, particularly those in mental health degree programs. Just over half of respondents had sought mental health treatment on campus, and of those who did not, a subset reported not knowing if their college provided such services. A large number of students reported having experienced a mental health crisis while in college (73%), but 35% of these reported that their college was never aware of the crisis.

An American Foundation for Suicide Prevention (AFSP) sponsored screening effort conducted at one university campus sought to identify students with depression and suicide ideation and encourage them to enter into mental health treatment. Secondarily, the rates of depression and suicidal ideation among the students who responded to the web-based questionnaire were recorded. Of the 729 students who participated, 11.1% endorsed current suicidal ideation and 16.5% endorsed a lifetime history of suicide attempt or self-injurious behavior (Garlow et al., 2008). Not surprisingly, more severe current depression was associated with greater risk for suicidal ideation in this population. Consistent with previous screening efforts, 85% of students with moderately severe to severe depression and 84% with current suicidal ideation were not receiving any mental health treatment at the time of assessment.

A similar project of suicide risk screening was undertaken at 15 university campuses across the USA and data was collected on a total of 8487 students. Among these students, 6.7% reported having had suicidal ideation, 1.6% having a suicide plan, and 0.5% having made a suicide attempt in the previous year (Downs & Eisenberg, 2012). Of the students with suicidal ideation, plan, or attempt history, 51.5% reported utilizing some type of psychiatric treatment during the previous year, but only 31.6% were engaged in current treatment. The investigators sought to further assess help-seeking behaviors among this group and identified several barriers to treatment engagement including minimization of perceived need, normalizing student stress, stigma, time, financial reasons, and beliefs about the effectiveness of treatment.

Risk and protective factors

The number of students on college campuses dealing with psychological or psychiatric issues continues to rise and with it, concern about the problem of college student suicide. Much energy has been put into research to identify both factors that heighten risk for suicide as well as those that may serve to protect against such actions. Increased knowledge about risk factors for student suicide may lead to earlier and more accurate identification of students who would benefit from crisis intervention and mental health services. Services could be structured to better meet the needs of the at risk students and to minimize barriers to care. Similarly, better understanding of protective factors will allow for the fostering and reinforcement of such coping strategies and behaviors to enhance resilience and lower risk.

Risk factors

The move from high school to college and with it the end of childhood and the beginning of adulthood marks a significant life transition. Often, this transition is accompanied by the first time of true physical and social independence from parents and other primary supports in an individual's life. Though often met with excitement and anticipation, it can also bring feelings of isolation and lack of support. Importantly, this transitional period to young adulthood coincides with a heightened age-defined risk window for onset of many major mental illnesses including major depressive disorder, bipolar disorder, and schizophrenia. All of these major mental illnesses are associated with an increased risk for suicide when compared to the general population.

Depression has consistently been recognized as a major risk factor for suicide and suicide-related ideas and behaviors in teens and young adults in the general population. The relationship between depression and suicide also manifests in college and university students. Of 106 reported student suicide deaths reported in the National Survey of College Counseling, 80% of the victims were depressed (Gallagher, 2012). In the AFSP sponsored screening project, there was a direct relationship between depression severity and suicide ideations, with students who had significantly higher mean depression scores having the greatest rate of endorsement of suicidal ideation (Garlow et al., 2008). Further, suicide ideations were more common in those students with other strong, negative emotional states including anxiety, irritability, rage, desperation, and being out of control.

Intoxicating substance use and abuse are another significant risk factor associated with suicide in adolescents and young adults. A review on this topic reports that both general substance use and substance use disorders were often significantly higher among adolescents and young adults with suicidal ideation, history of suicide attempts, and, assessed retrospectively through psychological autopsy, suicide victims (Esposito-Smythers & Spirito, 2004). Specifically, adolescents who died by suicide were 6 to 8.5 times more likely to be diagnosed with any substance use disorder. Similarly, substance use disorders were associated with a 3 to 4 times increase in suicide attempts. Lifetime depressive episodes and lifetime cocaine use were associated with suicidal behaviors in African American males and females in a prospective study that followed participants from childhood through adolescence and into young adulthood (Juon & Ensminger, 1997). Finally, both general alcohol and illicit drug use appear to be associated with increasing severity of suicide-related behaviors; rates of drug and alcohol use are higher among those who die by suicide than those who attempt and higher among those who attempt compared to those with suicide ideation.

In a study examining the prevalence of cocaine and alcohol use immediately preceding suicide, it appears that among adolescents, white suicide victims are far more likely to have used alcohol and/or cocaine immediately prior to suicide than their African American counterparts (Garlow et al., 2007). Strikingly, this relationship reverses among adult suicide victims. Although these results are representative of adolescents and young adults in general, they can certainly be generalized to college students. The relationship between maladaptive alcohol use and suicide is particularly concerning for college students, considering that college students often engage in binge drinking, an activity that increases impulsivity, a characteristic of many adolescent and young adult suicides. The NSCC reported that over the past 5 years college counseling center directors have noted an increase in substance use disorders among students. Specifically, 48% of directors reported an increase in illicit drug use and 36% noted an increase in alcohol abuse among students on campus (Gallagher, 2012). Relevant also, of the 106 student suicides reported, 74% were white students and only 2% were African Americans.

New and concerning patterns of drug use are emerging in college students, parallel to the general adolescent and young adult population. In particular the diversion of prescription pharmaceutical agents such as stimulants, opiates, and sedative hypnotics for recreational use is rampant and accelerating in this age group. A study of college students scrutinized the relationship of depressive symptoms and suicidal ideation to the growing phenomenon of non-medical use of prescription drugs (Zullig & Divin, 2012). The data utilized was collected from the ACHA-NCHA and showed that 13% of students surveyed admitted to using opiates, stimulants, sedatives, or antidepressants that were not prescribed to them. Further analyses revealed that those students who reported feeling hopeless, sad, depressed, or had considered suicide were 1.2 to 1.4 times more likely to be using prescription drugs for non-medical purposes.

Certain groups within the college student population appear to face higher risk for suicide and have fewer resources available for addressing this risk. Subsets of the larger student population with different characteristics and needs such as commuter students, older students including graduate and professional school students, international students, and gay, lesbian, bisexual and transgender students have different vulnerabilities and often less adequate means for addressing those risks (SPRC, 2004). The mental health and suicide prevention resources on campus may not be tailored to the specific needs and characteristics of these subgroups of students.

Commuter students are more often enrolled in 2-year or community colleges, which are often underfunded and have limited resources for student health and mental health services. A nurse or other midlevel provider is often the only provider available in student health services at these institutions. Health programs on these campuses are often entirely supported by student fees, as local college districts allocate less money to these institutions than to their 4-year counterparts (Brindis & Reyes, 1997). Commuter students in general differ from their campus-based counterparts in that they rarely identify with their school and often spend a limited amount of time on campus. These students are more difficult to reach with traditional student health outreach and campus-based programs (SPRC, 2004). Often commuter students have other risk factors such as being older and having to attend school part-time while working to support themselves and their family members, which leads to financial stress and strain.

Older students are becoming more prevalent on college campuses and in graduate and professional school programs across the country. As noted earlier in the Big Ten study, students 25 and older had a significantly higher suicide risk than those younger than 25 (Silverman et al., 1997). Additionally, female graduate students appear to be at the highest risk, with 39% of all female suicides occurring among graduate students. This is notable because female graduate students constitute only 19% of the female university student population. Suicide rates among females on college campuses skyrocket to above national rates during the graduate school years. The results of a survey, The Nature of Suicidal Crises in College Students, in 2006 further elucidated the risk among older students, specifically graduate students (Brownson et al., 2011). Results indicate that more undergraduates than graduate students think about suicide but older students are likelier than younger students to actually die by suicide. These data further indicate that female graduate students were over twice as likely as graduate men to report a recent suicide attempt.

Medical students represent another group of older students with apparently elevated risk for suicide. Medical students have demonstrated higher risk of both suicidal ideation and suicide (Schwenk et al., 2010). Reportedly, 3% to 15% of medical students have suicidal ideation at any time during training, medical students have significantly lower quality of life than age-matched populations, and burnout affects up to 50% of medical students (Dyrbye et al., 2008). Further, medical students are less likely than their peers to receive appropriate treatment despite being situated in an environment that would suggest better access to care (Schwenk et al., 2010). This is often largely due to stigma, which is frequently perceived as worse among those who are suffering with depression, and generally leads to a limited view of available options for treatment (Moutier et al., 2012).

Similar to commuter students, older students often live off campus, have marked financial strain, and competing responsibilities such as part-time work and children and families to support. There is frequently a significant amount of both financial and personal investment in the decision to return to school, which may help to make this population a higher risk for suicide (Silverman et al., 1997). Older female students, frequently pursuing graduate and professional level training, may suffer from additional stresses when moving into these traditionally male domains in addition to the strain inherent to these roles. Moreover, they may be faced with greater pressure to balance work and home commitments (Stephenson et al., 2005; Brownson et al., 2011).

International students experience significant and unique academic and social challenges. Often English is not their native language, and this complicates academic performance. Additionally, they have diminished options for financial aid and are frequently restricted from working in the USA, making finances tight and limiting their access to health care and mental health services (Mori, 2000). International students are farther from home and more socially and culturally isolated than their fellow domestic student colleagues. Additionally, in many cultures outside of the USA, there is a significant stigma associated with mental illness and this may limit their ability to access services if and when they are needed (Yi et al., 2003).

Gay, lesbian, bisexual, and transgender (GLBT) students are often exposed to specific types of prejudice and harassment that other students do not experience, solely based on their sexual orientation. It has been hypothesized that this would lead to an increased risk for suicide among this group of students, as it has certainly been shown to increase suicide risk among other populations of GLBT individuals. One study looked at a group of 70 GLBT students from five midwestern colleges and compared them to a matched heterosexual control group of 141 students (Westefeld et al., 2001). The results indicate that among GLBT students, there is a positive correlation between feelings of depression and loneliness, and that both of these measures negatively correlate with scores on the College Student Reasons for Living Inventory (CSRLI). Both of these conditions have been previously found to independently increase risk for suicide. The study also found that GLBT students were significantly more depressed, lonely, and had fewer reasons for living than the control group students.

One final risk factor, impulsivity, appears to be more heavily related to youth than adult suicide. Often this can be exacerbated by previously discussed factors such as alcohol and illicit drug use or other mental illnesses, or strong negative emotional states. The National Violent Injury Statistics System (NVISS), developed by the Harvard Injury Control Research Center (HICRC) and other collaborating partners, is a pilot study designed to advocate for a federally supported, ongoing data collection system for homicide and suicide (HICRC, 2001). The database reports that 47% of youth aged 18–24 years old experienced a precipitating event or life crisis on the same day or within 2 weeks of suicide. This is compared to 36% in the total sample and far exceeds all older adult age ranges. One in five young adults committed suicide on the same day as a life crisis and one in four within 2 weeks. The life crises experienced by these 18- to 24-year-olds who died by suicide included intimate partner relationship problems (49%), legal issues (20%), financial problems (12%), and conflict with family or friend (13%) (HICRC, 2001). Consistent with these statistics on young adults in general, of the 106 student suicides reported by directors of college counseling centers in the NSCC: 47% had relationship problems, 22% had academic problems, and 18% had financial problems precipitating their suicide (Gallagher, 2012).

Protective factors

Far less research has focused on protective factors, or factors mitigating college student suicide risk. Instead, most have chosen to invest in identifying factors that increase the likelihood of students completing suicide. This may be a limiting factor, as protective factors research helps to identify those adaptive characteristics that may limit suicidal potential and inhibit suicidal behaviors. This may provide fertile ground for targeted prevention interventions, especially if these skills or characteristics can be taught, encouraged, or supplemented.

An overview of extant protective factors research among college students has identified a few salient characteristics of students who are better able to cope with stressful situations and may contribute to an individual's ability to persevere in spite of thinking about suicide (Westefeld et al., 2006). One consistently identified protective factor for college students is social support. This social support may come from having an emotional connection to family, friends, and to the college or university which they attend. Another strong indicator of having social support is through involvement in extracurricular activities, which is an important protective factor for college students.

Another important factor is having a reason for living. Specifically identified reasons for living include: feelings of responsibility toward family, fear of social disapproval, moral objections to suicide, survival and coping skills, college and future related concerns, and a fear of suicide (Westefeld et al., 2006). It appears that having a reason to live is more important than having a reason not to die among college students considering suicide.

Prevention

The problem of college student suicide is not a new one. However, the efforts to address this problem in the form of awareness, education, and prevention are all relatively new. There are few college suicide prevention programs that have been systematically tracked and tested for effectiveness. While the suicide rate among college students is thankfully low when compared to the non-college-attending peers, the problem still presents an enormous public health crisis. And, college campuses represent an environment that is particularly well suited to prevent it. The application of community mental health and public health principles and practices can be effectively deployed in the relatively closed and homogeneous environment of a college campus. Another important concept in college suicide prevention is in developing a coalition of stakeholders from all areas and domains of the college community, students, faculty, athletic staff, support staff, and others to be included in and empowered to contribute to this goal.

Colleges are relatively small, planned communities with a strong social network. These communities are often quite liberal in their understanding and discourse surrounding such issues as stigma of mental illness and utilization of treatment resources such as psychotherapy. College campuses also have the unique arrangement of students living, working, and playing in one place; universal access to students' residential, social, and academic lives. This feature of college campuses especially as it impacts undergraduates affords a tremendous opportunity to apply community and public mental health strategies toward comprehensive suicide prevention. Suicide prevention efforts can be seamlessly integrated into various aspects of the student experience. One additional benefit of this approach is that awareness and coping strategies and behaviors can be introduced to the student early and repeatedly, potentially modifying suicide risk in future years after they leave college. Finally, college campuses have final jurisdiction over students conduct and attendance at the institution and can set up requirements in behavior, treatment compliance, and many other restrictions in the hopes of ensuring safety.

However, few colleges are taking a systematic approach toward suicide prevention. One possible reason is the relative difficulty in assessing the efficacy of an intervention due to low suicide rates both before and after implementation of such programs (Westefeld et al., 2006). This makes program evaluation efforts difficult, and without such documentation, it is hard to know if interventions are indeed making a difference at all. Another possible impediment to universal, coordinated college campus suicide prevention efforts may be linked to a fairly new occurrence. Over the course of the last decade, there have been a handful of legal cases concerning institutional liability in the case of student suicide on campus. The perception of enhanced liability may make college administrators reluctant to delve too deeply into suicide prevention efforts for fear of adverse legal action if the system fails to prevent a suicide death.

These cases, *Jain v. State of Iowa*, *Schieszler v. Ferrum College*, and *Shin v. Massachusetts Institute of Technology*, as well as the more recent case of George Washington University student Jordan Nott, all provide examples of the anxiety surrounding campus response to student suicide (Appelbaum, 2006; Westefeld et al., 2006). These cases visit the question of whether a special relationship exists between a college/university and a student who attempts/completes suicide. The difficulty for college administrators arises in that the precedents are unclear at best and different jurisdictions often arrive at opposite findings in cases with quite similar circumstances (Westefeld et al., 2006).

Problems arise when college campuses begin responding to these concerns of liability with new policies which range anywhere along the spectrum from prohibiting the collection of identifiable information on students who manifest suicide-related behaviors, due to concerns that this may create a duty to protect, all the way to requiring mandatory leave of absence or the signing of a gag order by students who voice suicidal ideation (Appelbaum, 2006). This climate of fear of litigation and liability often creates an atmosphere that is counter to logic and certainly counter to the much hoped for suicide prevention efforts. While it could be argued that college campuses have an invested interest in ensuring that suicidal students receive appropriate treatment, these responses seem far more likely to dissuade students from seeking treatment. The fear of perceived adverse consequences, such as expulsion or informing parents may keep students quiet, often until it is too late. Too often, the inaccurate assumption that students would be better off seeking treatment at home leads to worse outcomes when students are separated from their social network and only source of self-esteem.

Despite the paucity of suicide prevention programs being pioneered on college campuses, work is being done to further this goal. One example of such a program exists at the University of Illinois, with empirical evidence to support its effectiveness in reducing suicide rates (Joffe, 2008). This program instituted an administrative policy that mandated assessments for all students who met a set of criteria, which triggered the completion of a Suicide Incident Report Form. Identified students were obligated to attend and participate in four assessment sessions with a mental health professional or suffer the consequence of possible withdrawal from the university.

Subjective reports of increased openness on the campus relative to suicidal students as well as a feeling of having resources and recourse when engaging students who expressed suicide ideations were initial consequences. Objective results indicate that the program increased student contact with mental health resources and decreased suicide rates on campus. In the 8 years prior (1976–1983) to program implementation, the suicide rate at the university was 6.91/100 000. The rate calculated during the 21 years of program implementation (1984–2005) was 3.78/100 000 students, a 45.3% reduction in deaths by suicide. Importantly, none of the students identified by suicide incident reports died by suicide. Also, this program was deployed during a period of time in which national suicide rates remained stable, and strikingly, during a period of time in which suicide rates at similar institutions were increasing (Joffe, 2008).

The SPRC and Jed Foundation outline a comprehensive coordinated approach to suicide prevention which emphasizes key elements that must be addressed to ensure effective program application and suicide prevention including: leadership to promote mental health and suicide prevention, screening, crisis management, educational programs, mental health services, life skills development, means restriction, social marketing, and social network promotion (SPRC, 2004). This approach would engage all relevant members of the college community, not just the counselors and mental health centers, which allows for universal application and availability to more students. Importantly, this approach emphasizes that implementation should cross multiple social spheres accessing students' whole lives including residence, academics, employment, and extracurricular activities.

Many of the key elements outlined in this comprehensive approach have been addressed by various prevention projects and research investigations individually or in combination. For example, the importance of screening in suicide prevention is clear; if at risk students are not identified, then they cannot be helped. The AFSP piloted a Web-based screening program to assess for and identify students at high-risk for suicide (Haas et al., 2008). Students were then engaged in online dialogues with counselors and were invited to attend in-person evaluation sessions. Of the students invited (undergraduates at two universities) who chose to complete the initial screening, 84.4% were deemed high or moderate risk. Of those identified, 19.4% attended in-person evaluation sessions and 13.5% entered treatment. Students who engaged in online dialogues with a counselor were three times more likely to come for in-person evaluation and enter treatment. This prevention program in addition to addressing screening and identification of at risk students also addresses such important factors as barrier reduction, increasing student awareness to available resources and encouraging students to access such care.

A similar program, employing the screening and assessment program developed by AFSP, was deployed at the medical school of University of California, San Diego (UCSD) (Moutier et al., 2012). This program was developed to address a specific high-risk population, physicians and physicians-in-training, through a two pronged approach of screening, assessment, and referral as well as a broad sweeping education effort across multiple specialties Grand Rounds. The program aimed to increase awareness of depression and suicide and to de-stigmatize treatment seeking among a population that traditionally promotes "toughing it out" and routinely believes that professional consequences will result from seeking help.

Yet another important component of comprehensive prevention programming involves campus education and training to facilitate awareness, identification, and appropriate intervention, often in a crisis situation. A study of the Question, Persuade and Refer (QPR) training program observed a group of residence advisers (RAs) and assessed their level of suicide prevention knowledge and attitudes prior to and following training (Tompkins & Witt, 2009). The trained RAs were compared to a control group who did not undergo training, and demonstrated significant gains in these domains, which were retained upon re-evaluation in the following semester.

Yet another important component of suicide prevention involves means restriction. This can be accomplished through university policy limiting or restricting access to firearms on campus. Similarly, risk management officers should concern themselves with controlling student access to lethal chemicals found in science laboratories, as well as restricting access to locations on campus where students could jump or fall including windows, bridges, or roofs (SPRC, 2004).

With the knowledge that few colleges and universities were addressing suicide prevention programing in any systematic way, the Garrett Lee Smith (GLS) Memorial Act was passed and signed into law in 2004 with the goal of providing federal funding for youth and young adult suicide prevention programing (Goldston et al., 2010). To date, 74 college campus grants have been funded to implement suicide prevention programs in the context of educational seminars, crisis hot lines, preparation of informational materials, preparation of educational materials for families of students to increase awareness of potential mental health issues, gatekeeper training programs for students and staff, and creation of networks for accessing mental health resources on college campuses. The goal of the GLS grants on college campuses is to develop sustainable programs of suicide prevention that will endure well after the 3-year funding period expires. One requirement of all GLS campus grantees is to engage in rigorous local and cross-site evaluation of the suicide prevention programing. The hope is that this will address the paucity of data on suicide prevention program successes and will provide information on necessary modifications so that programs may better reach their goals.

College and university campuses are a unique setting in which to implement suicide prevention strategies. The relatively closed and homogeneous community is ideal for application of public health and community mental health approaches across all domains of the community. A comprehensive approach that develops a coalition of various stakeholders invested in suicide prevention will ultimately lead to a culture of reduced stigma for mental illness and lower barriers to treatment engagement. Another beneficial consequence is that inculcation of some of these behaviors, attitudes, and coping strategies during the formative college years may continue to protect against suicide-related behaviors in future years.

References

American College Health Association (ACHA). (2012). *American College Health Association-National College Health Assessment II: Reference Group Data Report Spring 2012*. Hanover, MD: American College Health Association.

Appelbaum, P. S. (2006). "Depressed? Get out!": dealing with suicidal students on college campuses. *Psychiatric Services*, **57**(7), 914–916.

Brindis, C., & Reyes, P. (1997). At the crossroads: options for financing college health services in the 21st century. *Journal of American College Health*, **45**(6), 279–288.

Brownson, C., Drum, J. D., Smith, S. E., & Denmark, A. B. (2011). Differences in suicidal experiences of male and female undergraduate and graduate students. *Journal of College Student Psychotherapy*, **25**, 277–294.

Centers for Disease Control and Prevention. (2013). *WISQARS Leading Causes of Death Reports, 1999–2007.* Available at: http://webappa.cdc.gov/sasweb/ncipc/leadcaus10.html (accessed January 4, 2013).

Downs, M. F., & Eisenberg, D. (2012). Help seeking and treatment use among suicidal college students. *Journal of American College Health*, **60**(2), 104–114.

Dyrbye, L. N., Thomas, M. R., Massie, F. S., et al. (2008). Burnout and suicidal ideation among U.S. medical students. *Annals of Internal Medicine*, **129**, 334–341.

Eisenberg, D., Golberstein, E., & Gollust, S. E. (2007). Help-seeking and access to mental health care in a university student population. *Medical Care*, **45**(7), 594–601.

Esposito-Smythers, C., & Spirito, A. (2004). Adolescent substance use and suicidal behavior: a review with implications for treatment research. *Alcoholism: Clinical and Experimental Research*, **28**(5), 77S–88S.

Gallagher, R. P. (2012). National Survey of College Counseling. *Monograph Series Number 9T.* Alexandria, VA: International Association of Counseling Services.

Garlow, S., Purselle, D., & Heninger, M. (2007). Cocaine and alcohol use preceding suicide in African American and white adolescents. *Journal of Psychiatric Research*, **41**, 530–536.

Garlow, S. J., Rosenberg, J., Moore, J. D., et al. (2008). Depression, desperation, and suicidal ideation in college students: results from the American Foundation for Suicide Prevention college screening project at Emory University. *Depression and Anxiety*, **25**, 482–488.

Goldston, D. B., Walrath, C. M., McKeon, R., et al. (2010). The Garrett Lee Smith memorial suicide prevention program. *Suicide and Life-Threatening Behavior*, **40**(3), 245–256.

Gruttadaro, D., & Crudo, D. (2012). *College Students Speak: A Survey Report on Mental Health.* Arlington, VA: National Alliance on Mental Illness.

Haas, A., Koestner, B., Rosenberg, J., et al. (2008). An interactive web-based method of outreach to college students at risk for suicide. *Journal of American College Health.* **57**(1), 15–22.

Harvard Injury Control Research Center (HICRC). (2001). *National Violent Injury Statistics System Pilot.* Cambridge, MA: Harvard University.

Joffe, P. (2008). An empirically supported program to prevent suicide in a college student population. *Suicide and Life-Threatening Behavior*, **38**(1), 87–103.

Juon, H., & Ensminger, M. (1997). Childhood, adolescent, and young adult predictors of suicidal behaviors: a prospective study of African Americans. *Journal of Child Psychology and Psychiatry*, **38**(5), 553–563.

Mori, S. (2000). Addressing the mental health concerns of international students. *Journal of Counseling and Development*, **78**, 137–143.

Moutier, C., Norcross, W., Jong, P., et al. (2012). The suicide prevention and depression awareness program at the University of California, San Diego School of Medicine. *Academic Medicine*, **87**, 320–326.

Schwenk, T. L., Davis, L., & Wimsatt, L. A. (2010). Depression, stigma, and suicidal ideation in medical students. *Journal of the American Medical Association*, **304**(11), 1181–1190.

Silverman, M. M., Meyer, P. M., Sloane, F., Raffel, M., & Pratt, D. M. (1997). The big ten student suicide study: a 10-year study of suicides on midwestern university campuses. *Suicide and Life-Threatening Behavior*, **27**(3), 285–303.

Stephenson, J. H., Belesis, M. P., & Balliet, W. E. (2005). Variability in college student suicide: age, gender, and race. *Journal of College Student Psychotherapy*, **19**(4), 5–33.

Suicide Prevention Resource Center (SPRC). (2004). *Promoting Mental Health and Preventing Suicide in College and University Settings*. Newton, MA: Education Development Center.

Tompkins, T. L., & Witt, J. (2009). The short-term effectiveness of a suicide prevention gatekeeper training program in a college setting with residence life advisors. *Journal of Primary Prevention*, **30**, 131–149.

Westefeld, J., Maples, M., Brian, B., & Taylor, S. (2001). Gay, lesbian, and bisexual college students: the relationship between sexual orientation and depression, loneliness, and suicide. *Journal of College Student Psychotherapy*, **15**(3), 71–82.

Westefeld, J. S., Button, C., Haley, J. T., et al. (2006). College student suicide: a call to action. *Death Studies*, **30**, 931–956.

Yi, J., Lin, J., & Kishimoto, Y. (2003). Utilization of counseling services by international students. *Journal of Instructional Psychology*, **30**(4), 333-342.

Zullig, K., & Divin, A. (2012). The association between non-medical prescription drug use, depressive symptoms and suicidality among college students. *Addictive Behaviors*, **37**, 890–899.

Chapter 22

Suicide in older adults

Yeates Conwell and Kimberly Van Orden

Suicide among older adults is a far more common occurrence than among youth in the USA (Centers for Disease Control and Prevention, 2013), and worldwide older people are the group with highest rates of completed suicide (World Health Organization, 2002). Given that older adults are the fastest growing segment of our population (Kinsella et al., 2009), the total number of older adults who take their own lives is expected to rise dramatically in coming decades. Suicide deaths are, therefore, a major public health challenge.

In this chapter we first review the scope of the problem of older adult suicide. Then we discuss characteristics and correlates of suicide in older adulthood and the implications each has for the reduction of late life suicide-related morbidity and mortality.

Scope of the problem

Data from the Centers for Disease Control indicate that in 2010 almost 6000 people over the age of 65 took their own lives in the USA (Centers for Disease Control and Prevention, 2013). Figure 22.1 illustrates the great variation in rates of completed suicide as a function of age, race, and gender. In general, suicide rates are higher for men than for women of all races. Among women overall, midlife is a period of relatively greater risk. For ethnic minority men rates are highest at younger and middle age, while for white men there is an early peak in midlife followed by a dramatic rise in the old old age group to rates that are 4 to 5 times higher than that of the US population. In many other countries of the world, the inexorable rise of suicide with age for men seen in the USA holds true for women as well (World Health Organization, 2002).

In addition to age effects, suicide rates vary by birth cohort over time. The large post-World War II "Baby Boom" cohort, the leading edge of which reached age 65 in 2011, have experienced relatively higher suicide rates at all ages than preceding or later birth cohorts (Phillips et al., 2010). Given that the Baby Boomers will swell the ranks of the oldest-old age group in the USA by an additional 13.2 million between 2010 and 2050 (i.e., from 5.8 million in 2010, projected to 19 million in 2050) (Vincent & Velkoff, 2010), the total number of older adults who die by suicide is expected to rise dramatically in that time frame. The public health mandate to find effective prevention strategies is clear.

The nature of suicidal ideation and behavior in older adults

In contrast to completed suicide, population-based studies of suicidal ideation indicate that prevalence rates are lower among older adults than middle-aged and younger people (e.g., Gallo et al., 1994). It is unclear whether this difference reflects cohort or aging related differences in willingness to express suicidal thoughts, for example, or whether it can be accounted for by difficulties in measurement of death and suicidal ideation at different points in the life course. As a consequence, however, to the extent that suicidal thoughts expressed to others are a signal of the need to intervene, older people may be disadvantaged.

Similarly, studies have repeatedly found that lifetime prevalence rates of attempted suicide are lower in older than middle-aged and younger adults (Centers for Disease Control and Prevention, 2013). The estimated ratio of attempted to completed suicides in the general population is approximately 10–20:1 and as high as 200:1 in young women, while the estimated ratio among older adults is 1 to 4 suicide attempts for each completed suicide (Hawton & Harriss, 2008). This pronounced difference reflects several characteristics of older adults who become suicidal. They are frailer due to increased physical illness burden,

A Concise Guide to Understanding Suicide, ed. Stephen H. Koslow, Pedro Ruiz, and Charles B. Nemeroff. Published by Cambridge University Press.

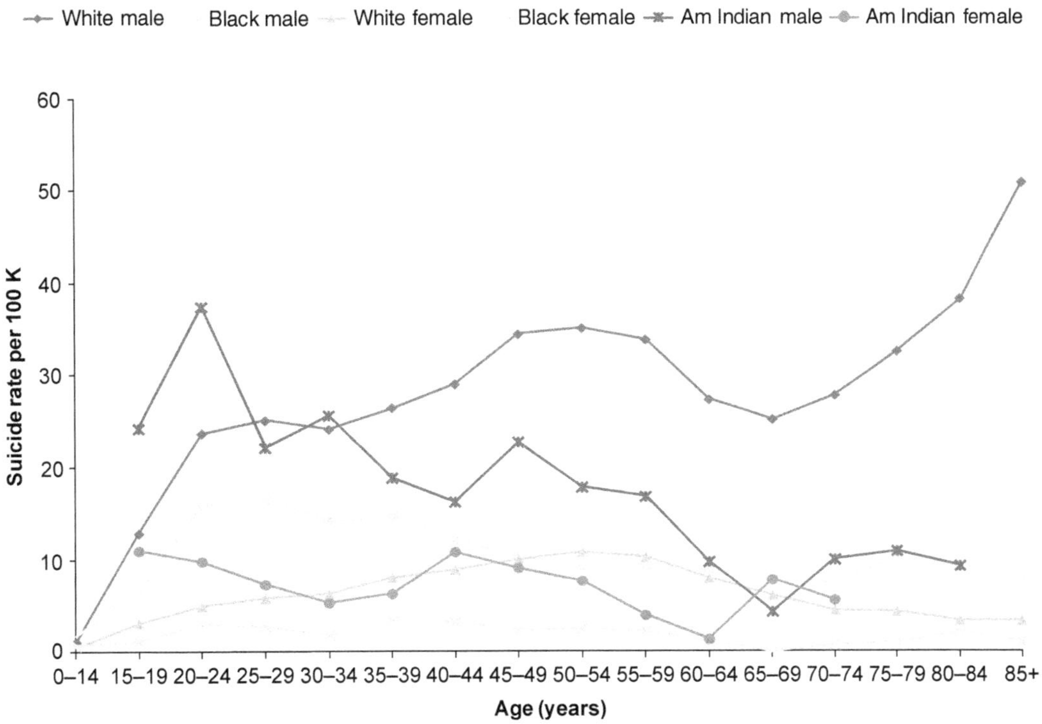

Figure 22.1. Suicide rates in the USA, 2010, by age, race, and sex. See plate section for color version. Source: Centers for Disease Control and Prevention, Web-based Injury Statistics Query and Reporting System (WISQARS).

making them less likely to survive a self-destructive act. Second, older adults tend to be more isolated, making discovery and rescue less likely (Conwell et al., 1998). And perhaps most important, the older adult attempting suicide is far more likely to use a gun. In 2010 in the USA 46.7% of suicides among those under age 65 were by firearm whereas among older adults, 71.4% died of self-inflicted gun-shot wounds (Centers for Disease Control and Prevention, 2013). While older adults are more likely to die on their first attempt, a history of a non-lethal attempt remains a potent risk factor in this age group. Among older adults who presented to a general hospital with self-harm, the risk of dying by suicide after a future attempt was 67 times greater compared to older adults in the general population (Murphy et al., 2012).

Implications for prevention: Because suicidal states are more difficult to detect among older adults, and because self-destructive acts once initiated are far more often lethal in this age group, preventive intervention strategies that target high-risk individuals ("indicated interventions"), while necessary, are unlikely to have a significant impact on the overall suicide rate in later life. Certainly when an older person is recognized to be suicidal, aggressive intervention is indicated. From a public health and prevention perspective, however, interventions that reduce the likelihood of an older person becoming suicidal ("selective" and "universal preventive interventions") will have the greatest impact.

Settings in which to prevent late life suicide

A smaller proportion of older adults with diagnosable psychiatric illness seek care from mental health specialty providers than is the case for younger and middle-aged adults. Instead, they are more likely to see their primary care providers. The same is true of individuals who took their own lives. One-third to a half of older people who died by suicide had seen their primary care provider in the last week of life and up to three-quarters within the last month (Luoma et al., 2002; Chiu et al., 2004). Although one-third had seen a mental health provider at some point, very few were in active treatment at the time of death. Primary care offices, therefore, as well as specialty medical practices, are the most important settings on which to focus efforts to detect and intervene in reducing suicide in older adults (Bartels et al., 2002; Bruce et al., 2004; Unutzer et al., 2006).

Other service settings in which older adults at risk for suicide are frequently encountered should be considered as well. Bruce and colleagues have demonstrated high rates of depressive symptoms and suicidal ideation in elderly patients receiving visiting nurse services (Raue et al., 2007). Clients of aging services network agencies, which are mandated to provide non-medical services and supports to maintain independent functioning of older adults, have a high prevalence of mood disorders and suicidal ideation as well. Richardson et al., for example, found that 27% of aging services care management clients had symptoms consistent with current major depression; almost half had one or more lifetime episodes (Richardson et al., 2011a, b), and 14% had current death or suicidal ideation (O'Riley et al., 2013).

Implications for prevention: Consistent with the earlier observation that indicated prevention has a small role to play in late life suicide, mental health specialty settings will likely play less of a role than primary and specialty medical care and other relevant community-based long-term care services and supports. Effective prevention strategies will require integration of mental health expertise with providers of other disciplines, and implementation in alternative settings better suited to detection and management of risk in older adults.

Risk factors and implications for preventive interventions

Mental illness

Carefully controlled psychological autopsy studies examining the role that psychiatric illness plays in late life suicide have consistently reported that 80–100% of older adults who died by suicide had a diagnosable Axis I disorder at death (Harwood et al., 2001; Beautrais, 2002; Waern et al., 2002; Chiu et al., 2004; Conwell et al., 2010). More specifically, they showed significant associations between suicide and substance use disorders, anxiety disorders, and non-affective psychoses in older adults, albeit with odds ratios that vary widely between studies. Far stronger and more consistent are the observed associations between mood disorders and suicide, with the odds of diagnosable major depression in older adult suicide decedents approximately 50 to 60 times greater than in controls. Mood disorders, in particular single episode major depression, also were present in a higher proportion of older adults who died by suicide than decedents at younger ages (Conwell et al., 1996), suggesting the hypothesis that age-related changes in the brain may help explain increased risk for suicide in this age group.

Alexopoulos and colleagues have described the "depression-executive dysfunction syndrome" of late life in which fronto-striatal dysfunction associated with microvascular lesions leads to late onset mood disorder characterized by cognitive deficits, poor treatment response, relapse, and recurrence (Alexopoulos et al., 2002). Both structural neuroimaging (Ahearn et al., 2001) and neuropsychological studies reinforce this possibility of age-related brain changes underlying suicide in later life (for example, Dombrovski et al., 2010). Age at onset of affective illness is difficult to establish among older adults who died by suicide because data must be obtained by proxy and because relatively few suicides had prior contact with mental health providers where documentation of symptoms and their course is more consistently available. It is well established that both single episode and recurrent major depression are associated with increased risk for suicide in this age group (Waern et al., 2002b; Conwell et al., 2010). However, single episode, late onset depression may have an especially close link. Conwell and colleagues reported a significant age by gender interaction among suicides in which the frequency of single episode major depression at death rose significantly with age for men, but not for women (Conwell et al., 1996), consistent with the observed gender difference in risk for suicide in later life.

Both vascular disease and depression are risk factors for dementia (Gracia-Garcia et al., 2013), which in turn has a devastating impact on cognitive coping and problem solving, affect regulation, functional capacity, and social networks. One would expect therefore that dementia would be associated with suicide in later life. However, findings from the few published studies are mixed. One study using postmortem tissue found significantly greater Alzheimer's-type pathology in the hippocampus of older adult suicides than controls (Rubio et al., 2001), but another found no such differences (Peisah et al., 2007). Due most likely to difficulty making proxy-based diagnoses of mild cognitive impairment or early dementia (the time of dementing illness in which affective symptomatology tends to be most pronounced), no psychological autopsy study has yet found elevated risk associated with dementia

(Harwood et al., 2001; Waern et al., 2002a; Chiu et al., 2004; Conwell et al., 2010). Record linkage studies, however, do indicate increased risk for suicide among individuals diagnosed with dementia, particularly in the first several years after diagnosis (Erlangsen et al., 2008).

The observation that risk of suicide increases in many countries with diverse cultures raises the possibility that age-related changes in the brain may contribute. However, virtually no research has examined genetic determinants of late life suicide, and few studies have addressed other neurobiological factors. Barriers to such investigations include the low base rate of suicide attempts and suicidal ideation in later life as well as methodological challenges posed by comorbid medical illness and its treatments for the interpretation of findings. Additional research in these areas is sorely needed.

Implications for prevention: The presence of clinically significant affective symptomatology and cognitive impairment indicate the need for clinicians to inquire further about suicidal ideation and intent in their older patients. Early diagnosis and aggressive treatment of late life mood disorders is likely to be an important component of comprehensive late life suicide prevention. Table 22.1 lists studies the primary outcomes of which were suicidal ideation, attempts, or completed suicide in older adults. Mood disorders were the clinical target in the majority of interventions tested.

Numerous ecological analyses have shown a significant inverse correlation between antidepressant prescription rates and suicide rates at the population level, suggesting that aggressive treatment of depression will reduce suicide deaths. Concern over inducing suicidal states with antidepressant exposure seem not to apply to the elderly. Stone and colleagues analyzed proprietary data submitted to the US FDA from 372 double-blind, randomized placebo-controlled trials of antidepressants in adults (see Table 22.1). They found that while the relative risk for suicidal ideation or behavior emerging during antidepressant treatment was elevated for participants under age 25, it was no different than placebo for those aged 25 to 64 years, and significantly reduced for those over age 65 who received antidepressant treatment (Stone et al., 2009). In an analysis of individual-level Danish registry data, Erlangsen and Conwell found that among individuals over 50 years of age who were treated with an antidepressant, risk for suicide decreased significantly with greater age in both men and women (Erlangsen & Conwell, 2014). These findings suggest that antidepressants may be more effective in preventing suicide in later life than at younger ages. At the same time, however, a greater proportion of individuals who died by suicide in older adulthood than at younger ages had an affective illness (Conwell et al., 1996), and a smaller proportion of old old adults dying by suicide had received antidepressant treatment (Erlangsen & Conwell, 2014). It appears, therefore, that more aggressive efforts to identify and treat depression in later life are needed to reduce suicide deaths.

Given the frequency with which older adults see their primary care providers, primary care-based collaborative depression care management is the preferred clinical approach to identification and treatment of older adults at risk for suicide. Although insufficiently powered to determine their impact on suicide attempts or suicide in older adults, both the IMPACT (Unutzer et al., 2002) and PROSPECT (Bruce et al., 2004; Alexopoulos et al., 2009) studies are notable. They were rigorously conducted randomized controlled trials testing whether primary care-based collaborative depression care management was more effective than enhanced care as usual in reducing depressive symptoms and suicidal ideation. Both studies found significantly greater improvements in those who received the care management intervention than enhanced care as usual, with significant differences observed among subjects with major depression through 24 months of follow-up.

Physical illness and disability

Physical illness and functional impairment have such a high base rate in older adults that their predictive value in identifying individuals at risk is low. Nonetheless, significant associations have been found between suicide in later life and a variety of disorders. These include malignancies; central nervous system disorders including spinal cord trauma, epilepsy, and Huntington's disease; chronic pain; congestive heart failure; and chronic obstructive pulmonary disease (Harris & Barraclough, 1994; Quan et al., 2002; Juurlink et al., 2004). Furthermore, comorbidity appears to increase relative risk. Juurlink and colleagues showed, for example, that relative risk of suicide increased linearly with the number of illnesses from approximately 1.7 for one condition to over 8 in individuals with seven or more physical illnesses (Juurlink et al., 2004).

Table 22.1. Studies reporting on interventions associated with suicide risk reduction in later life

Study (site)	Study design; Prevention approach	Participants (controls)	Age	Intervention	Outcome	Results
Suicidal ideation						
Unützer et al., 2006 (USA)	RCT; Indicated	906 (895) with major depression/ dysthymia	≥ 60	IMPACT: Primary care-based depression care management; tx algorithms; patient, family, provider education; duration 12 months	SI	Significantly lower rates of SI in intervention subjects than controls (care as usual [CAU]) at 6 and 12 months; improvements retained at 18 and 24 month follow-up
Alexopoulos et al., 2009; Bruce et al., 2004 (USA)	RCT; Indicated	320 (279) with mood disorders	≥ 60	PROSPECT: Primary care-based depression care management; tx algorithms; patient, family, provider education	SI	Significantly greater depression treatment outcomes in intervention subjects than controls (enhanced CAU). More rapid reduction in SI, and 2.2 times greater reduction in SI over 24 months
Stone et al., 2009 (USA)	Meta-analysis; Indicated	372 randomized, placebo-controlled trials. 99 231 randomized subjects with affective disorders (50%) or other psychiatric conditions (50%)	≥ 18	Antidepressant medications	SI (or behavior [14%])	Odds ratios (CI 95%) for emergence of suicidality while on medication decreased with increasing age: <25 yrs = 1.62 (0.97–2.71) 5–64 yrs = 0.79 (0.64–0.98) ≥65 yrs = 0.37 (0.18–0.76)
Completed or attempted suicide						
Erlangsen & Conwell, 2014 (Denmark)	Population-based cohort study; Indicated	All residents of Denmark, 1996–2006 ♂: 1 215 524 ♀: 1 343 568	≥ 50	Antidepressant prescriptions redeemed at pharmacies nationwide; individual-level data from linked registries	Suicide	Men and women receiving antidepressants had a 2% and 3% decline in suicide rate respectively with each additional year of age over 50 An opposite trend was found for persons not in treatment. Fewer persons aged 80 dying by suicide had received antidepressant prescriptions during the last months of life than younger persons
Oyama et al., 2008 (Japan)	Meta-analysis; Multi-level	5 quasi-experimental studies comparing regions with and without intervention. ♂: 20 598 person-years ♀: 28 437 person-years	≥ 65	Depression screening, psychoeducation workshops, referral, follow-up, treatment by psychiatry or primary care (PC)	Suicide	With screening + psychiatric follow-up, combined incidence rate ratios (IRR; CI 95%) for suicide were lower for both men (0.3 [0.1–0.7]) and women (0.3 [0.2–0.6]). For screening + PC follow-up, IRRs were significantly lower for women (0.4 [0.2–0.6]) but not for men,

Table 22.1. (cont.)

Study (site)	Study design; Prevention approach	Participants (controls)	Age	Intervention	Outcome	Results
						suggesting gender difference in effectiveness
De Leo et al., 2002 (Italy)	Observational study; Selective	♂: 2983 ♀: 15 658	≥ 65	24 hr access to supports as needed; weekly phone contact	Suicide	Significantly reduced standardized mortality ratio in women receiving the intervention (16.7% [2.0%–59.9%]); no change for men
Chan et al., 2011 (Hong Kong)	Cohort study; Indicated	351 suicide attempters received intervention (66 pre-intervention), all diagnoses	≥ 65	Primary care-based gatekeeper training, referral to geropsychiatry, care management, active aftercare for suicide attempters	Suicide and suicide attempt	7.6% of subjects completed suicide in 2 years prior to initiation of the intervention. In the 2 years following initiation, 2.0% of subjects died by suicide ($P = 0.028$). There was no difference in reattempt rates between the two periods

The relationship between physical illness and suicide is likely to be multi-factorial. For example, an illness may have direct impact on both an individual's cognitive function and affective state leading to impaired problem solving abilities and clinically significant depression. It may also disrupt social networks, alter self-image and coping capacity, and impose financial burden.

Finally, physical illness that is associated with functional disability appears to have an important influence as well. Waern et al. (2002a) observed a significant association between suicide and need for help with activities of daily living in old suicides relative to controls, and others report similar findings (Conwell et al., 2010).

Implications: Physical illness alone is of little practical use in identifying individuals at risk. However, more complex and comorbid conditions, particularly those associated with pain and disability, indicate the need for vigilance for the emergence of hopelessness, depression, suicidal ideation, and suicidal intent in later life. As well, they indicate the potential importance of interventions designed to optimize functioning and minimize pain in older adults with physical illness as a selective preventive approach for suicide in later life. For example, while no studies have yet examined the association between palliative care interventions and suicide-related outcomes in older adults, one would expect them to be potent selective preventive interventions. Similarly, rehabilitation services, community-based programs to mitigate the impact of disability on independent functioning in the community, and policy interventions designed to assure early and adequate access to routine health care and preventive services represent selective and universal approaches that should be expected to reduce suicide in later life.

Social connectedness

Another domain in which variables have been shown in many studies to be linked to suicidal behavior in later life is social connectedness (for a review, see Fassberg et al., 2012). The construct can be conceptualized and measured in a number of ways, including functional (e.g., instrumental and perceived social support), structural (marital status, whether one is alone or with others, or more complex mapping of social network density and size), and psychological connectedness (e.g., loneliness or feeling like a burden on others). It is clear that being socially disconnected has a marked adverse impact on health, including all-cause mortality (Holt-Lunstad et al., 2010).

Numerous controlled psychological autopsy studies have found close associations between suicide case status and living alone, family discord, and reduced social support (Van Orden & Conwell, 2011). Individuals who report strong family connections are less likely to have suicidal ideation, while in other studies older adults who took their own lives were significantly less likely to have had a confidante than controls, and less likely to participate in community activities or have a hobby (Conwell et al., 2011; Van Orden & Conwell, 2011).

Implications for prevention: Interventions designed to increase social connections, decrease social isolation, and improve social supports of older adults may serve many beneficial purposes. For individuals in or near suicidal crises, they may reduce the likelihood of action; mobilizing family and environmental supports is a fundamental aspect of crisis management for a suicidal patient. Equally important, however, is the role that such interventions might play in preventing the onset of depression and/or suicidal states. De Leo and colleagues reported results of the Telehelp/Telecheck intervention in Padua, Italy in which older adults at risk for adverse physical and mental health outcomes were equipped with voice activated telephone links to supportive services (De Leo et al., 2002) (Table 22.1). Staff members responded to clients' calls as needed, but also initiated contacts with them in order to anticipate their needs and reduce their isolation. Over 11 years of intervention delivery, there were significantly fewer suicides among Telehelp/Telecheck clients than would have been expected in a comparable population (standardized mortality ratio of 0.167).

Although not specific to older adults, other studies indicate that even minimal supportive contacts may save lives. Motto and Bostrom (2001), for example, sent letters four times a year to high-risk patients following discharge. The letters expressed concern and best wishes, and invited the subjects to respond if they wished. Survival analysis revealed a significantly lower rate of completed suicide in the contact group compared to those randomly assigned to receive no follow-up letters. Carter and colleagues (Carter et al., 2007) mailed a series of eight postcards over 1 year to individuals over 16 years of age who had been evaluated in the emergency department following an overdose. Compared to those who received usual care only, the postcard recipients had almost 50% fewer repeat suicide attempts on average.

Despite the low cost of such interventions, a greater likelihood of social isolation in later life, and the empirical association of social disconnectedness and suicide in elders, we are aware of no studies in which a "caring letter" approach has specifically targeted older adults. Potential recipients of caring letters might include those who were recently bereaved, known to be depressed, or disconnected socially due to physical illness and associated functional impairment (e.g., post stroke or with progressive sensory impairments).

Multi-level preventive intervention

There is no single "cause" of suicide in later life. Rather, it results from a complex combination of factors that come together at a particular point in time for an individual older adult and lead to the assessment that life is no longer worth living. At a population level, therefore, the greatest impact to reduce the rate and total number of older adult suicides will likely be achieved by coordinated programs that integrate clinical and community-based preventive interventions across the range of available indicated, selective, and universal approaches.

Two studies provide preliminary evidence of the effectiveness of such a multi-level approach (Table 22.1). Chan et al. tested the effectiveness of a multi-component program for late life suicide prevention in Hong Kong that includes gatekeeper training in primary care and community sites, care management, psychiatric referral, and depression treatment (Chan et al., 2011). Comparing outcomes for older adults with histories of suicide attempts, they found that rates of completed suicide were significantly lower over 2 years after initiation of the program than during the 2-year period preceding its implementation. In a series of quasi-experimental studies in rural Japanese villages with high rates of older adult suicide, Oyama and colleagues found that community education, depression screening and referral, and engagement of older adults in group activities resulted in significantly lower late life suicide rates than in demographically similar regions elsewhere in Japan. Merging five such studies using the meta-analytic methods (Oyama et al., 2008), they showed that when follow-up was conducted by a psychiatrist, the suicide incidence rate ratios were significantly reduced for both men and women; when follow-up for depression was provided by general practitioners, however, the significant effect was found only for older female participants. Given that rates of suicide in later life are substantially higher among men than women, additional research is needed on how best to understand the factors that place older men at risk, the selective and universal interventions best suited to their needs, and how best to engage and retain them in care.

Conclusions

The covert and highly lethal nature of suicidal ideation and behavior in older adults make the goal of reducing death by suicide in older people especially challenging. The rapid increase in the size of the older adult population with the emergence into later life of the Baby Boom cohort makes meeting this challenge an especially pressing one. At the same time, the fact that late life suicide is multi-determined suggests that there are numerous potential targets for prevention efforts. No single factor is sufficient to explain an individual's decision to end his or her life. Risk factors influence that calculus in combination, and changes in the relative impact of any one factor may in turn change the individual's outlook on life, allowing time to make even more substantive and permanent changes to lower overall risk. Effective diagnosis and treatment of depression, management of pain, engagement of older patients and their families as partners in care, optimizing function and minimizing disability, and assuring that the older person maintains social connections and meaning in life are all important avenues to pursue.

References

Ahearn, E. P., Jamison, K. R., Steffens, D. C., et al., (2001). MRI correlates of suicide attempt history in unipolar depression. *Biological Psychiatry*, **50**, 266–270.

Alexopoulos, G. S., Kiosses, D. N., Klimstra, S., Kalayam, B., & Bruce, M. L. (2002). Clinical presentation of the "depression-executive dysfunction syndrome" of late life. *American Journal of Geriatric Psychiatry*, **10**(1), 98–106.

Alexopoulos, G. S., Reynolds, C. F., 3rd, Bruce, M. L., et al. (2009). Reducing suicidal ideation and depression in older primary care patients: 24-month outcomes of the PROSPECT study. *American Journal of Psychiatry*, **166**(8), 882–890.

Bartels, S. J., Coakley, E., Oxman, T. E., et al., (2002). Suicidal and death ideation in older primary care patients with depression, anxiety, and at risk alcohol use. *American Journal of Geriatric Psychiatry*, **10**(4), 417–427.

Beautrais, A. L. (2002). A case control study of suicide and attempted suicide in older adults. *Suicide & Life-Threatening Behavior*, **32**(1), 1–9.

Bruce, M. L., Ten Have, T., Reynolds, C. F., III, et al., (2004). Reducing suicidal ideation and depressive symptoms in depressed older primary care patients: a randomized controlled trial. *JAMA: Journal of American Medical Association*, **291**(9), 1081–1091.

Carter, G. L., Clover, K., Whyte, I. M., Dawson, A. H., & D'Este, C. (2007). Postcards from the EDge: 24-month outcomes of a randomised controlled trial for hospital-treated self-poisoning. *British Journal of Psychiatry*, **191**, 548–553.

Centers for Disease Control and Prevention. (2013). *Web-based Injury Statistics Query and Reporting System (WISQARS). Leading Causes of Death Reports*. Atlanta, GA: National Center for Injury Prevention and Control. http://www.cdc.gov/injury/wisqars/index.html

Chan, S. S., Leung, V. P., Tsoh, J., et al., (2011). Outcomes of a two-tiered multifaceted elderly suicide prevention program in a Hong Kong Chinese community. *American Journal of Geriatric Psychiatry*, **19**(2), 185–196.

Chiu, H. F., Yip, P. S., Chi, I., et al., (2004). Elderly suicide in Hong Kong – a case-controlled psychological autopsy study. *Acta Psychiatrica Scandinavica*, **109**(4), 299–305.

Conwell, Y., Duberstein, P. R., Cox, C., et al., (1996). Relationships of age and axis I diagnoses in victims of completed suicide: A psychological autopsy study. *American Journal of Psychiatry*, **153**(8), 1001–1008.

Conwell, Y., Duberstein, P. R., Cox, C., et al. (1998). Age differences in behaviors leading to completed suicide. *American Journal of Geriatric Psychiatry*, **6**(2), 122–126.

Conwell, Y., Duberstein, P. R., Hirsch, J. K., et al. (2010). Health status and suicide in the second half of life. *International Journal of Geriatric Psychiatry*, **25**(4), 371–379.

Conwell, Y., Van Orden, K., & Caine, E. D. (2011). Suicide in older adults. *The Psychiatric Clinics of North America*, **34**(2), 451–468.

De Leo, D., Dello Buono, M., & Dwyer, J. (2002). Suicide among the elderly: the long-term. *Journal of Psychiatry*, **181**, 226–229.

Dombrovski, A. Y., Clark, L., Siegle, G. J., et al. (2010). Reward/Punishment reversal learning in older suicide attempters. *American Journal of Psychiatry*, **167**(6), 699–707.

Erlangsen, A., & Conwell, Y. (2014). Age-related response to redeemed antidepressants measured by completed suicide in older adults: a nationwide cohort study. *American Journal of Geriatric Psychiatry*, **22**(1), 25–33. http://dx.doi.org/10.1016/j.jagp.2012.08.008

Erlangsen, A., Zarit, S. H., & Conwell, Y. (2008). Hospital-diagnosed dementia and suicide: a longitudinal study using prospective, nationwide register data. *American Journal of Geriatric Psychiatry*, **16**(3), 220–228.

Fassberg, M. M., van Orden, K. A., Duberstein, P., et al. (2012). A systematic review of social factors and suicidal behavior in older adulthood. *International Journal of Environmental Research and Public Health*, **9**(3), 722–745.

Gallo, J. J., Anthony, J. C., & Muthen, B. O. (1994). Age differences in the symptoms of depression: A latent trait analysis. *Journals of Gerontology*, **49**(6), P251–P264.

Gracia-Garcia, P., de-la-Camara, C., Santabarbara, J., et al. (2013). Depression and incident Alzheimer disease: the impact of disease severity. *American Journal of Geriatric Psychiatry*, http://dx.doi.org/10.1016/j.jagp.2013.02.011

Harris, E. C., & Barraclough, B. M. (1994). Suicide as an outcome for medical disorders. *Medicine*, **73**(6), 281–296.

Harwood, D., Hawton, K., Hope, T., & Jacoby, R. (2001). Psychiatric disorder and personality factors associated with suicide in older people: a descriptive and case-control study. *International Journal of Geriatric Psychiatry*, **16**(2), 155–165.

Hawton, K., & Harriss, L. (2008). How often does deliberate self-harm occur relative to each suicide? A study of variations by gender and age. *Suicide & Life-Threatening Behavior*, **38**(6), 650–660.

Holt-Lunstad, J., Smith, T. B., & Layton, J. B. (2010). Social relationships and mortality risk: a meta-analytic review. *PLoS Medicine*, **7**(7), e1000316.

Juurlink, D. N., Herrmann, N., Szalai, J. P., Kopp, A., & Redelmeier, D. A. (2004). Medical illness and the risk of suicide in the elderly. *Archives of Internal Medicine*, **164**(11), 1179–1184.

Kinsella, K., Wan, H., & U.S. Census Bureau. (2009). An Aging World: 2008. *International Population Reports, P95/09-1.* Washington, DC: US Census Bureau.

Luoma, J. B., Martin, C. E., & Pearson, J. L. (2002). Contact with mental health and primary care providers before suicide: A review of the evidence. *American Journal of Psychiatry*, **159**(6), 909–916.

Motto, J. A., & Bostrom, A. G. (2001). A randomized controlled trial of postcrisis suicide prevention. *Psychiatric Services*, **52**(6), 828–833.

Murphy, E., Kapur, N., Webb, R., et al., (2012). Risk factors for repetition and suicide following self-harm in older adults: multicentre cohort study. *British Journal of Psychiatry*, **200**, 399–404.

O'Riley, A. A., Van Orden, K. A., He, H., et al. (2013). Suicide and death ideation in older adults obtaining aging services. *American Journal of Geriatric Psychiatry.* doi: S1064-7481(12)00100-5 [pii] 10.1016/j.jagp.2012.12.004

Oyama, H., Sakashita, T., Ono, Y., et al. (2008). Effect of community-based intervention using depression screening on elderly suicide risk: a meta-analysis of the evidence from Japan. *Community Mental Health Journal*, **44**(5), 311–320.

Peisah, C., Snowdon, J., Gorrie, C., Kril, J., & Rodriguez, M. (2007). Investigation of Alzheimer's disease-related pathology in community dwelling older subjects who committed suicide. *Journal of Affective Disorders*, **99**(1–3), 127–132.

Phillips, J. A., Robin, A. V., Nugent, C. N., & Idler, E. L. (2010). Understanding recent changes in suicide rates among the middle-aged: period or cohort effects? *Public Health Reports*, **125**(5), 680–688.

Quan, H., Arboleda-Florez, J., Fick, G. H., Stuart, H. L., & Love, E. J. (2002). Association between physical illness and suicide among the elderly. *Social Psychiatry & Psychiatric Epidemiology*, **37**(4), 190–197.

Raue, P. J., Meyers, B. S., Rowe, J. L., Heo, M., & Bruce, M. L. (2007). Suicidal ideation among elderly homecare patients. *International Journal of Geriatric Psychiatry*, **22**(1), 32–37.

Richardson, T. M., Friedman, B., Podgorski, C., et al. (2011a). Depression and its correlates among older adults accessing aging services. *American Journal of Geriatric Psychiatry*, **20**(4), 346–354.

Richardson, T. M., Simning, A., He, H., & Conwell, Y. (2011b). Anxiety and its correlates among older adults accessing aging services. *International Journal of Geriatric Psychiatry*, **26**, 31–38.

Rubio, A., Vestner, A. L., Stewart, J. M., et al. (2001). Suicide and Alzheimer's pathology in the elderly: a case-control study. *Biological Psychiatry*, **49**(2), 137–145.

Stone, M., Laughren, T., Jones, M. L., et al. (2009). Risk of suicidality in clinical trials of antidepressants in adults: analysis of proprietary data submitted to US Food and Drug Administration. *British Medical Journal*, **339**, b2880. doi: 10.1136/bmj.b2880

Unutzer, J., Katon, W., Callahan, C. M., et al. (2002). Collaborative care management of late-life depression in the primary care setting: a randomized controlled trial. *JAMA*, **288**(22), 2836–2845.

Unutzer, J., Tang, L., Oishi, S., et al. (2006). Reducing suicidal ideation in depressed older primary care patients. *Journal of the American Geriatrics Society*, **54**(10), 1550–1556.

Van Orden, K., & Conwell, Y. (2011). Suicides in late life. *Current Psychiatry Reports*, **13**(3), 234–241.

Vincent, G. K., & Velkoff, V. A. (2010). The Next Four Decades: The Older Population in the United States: 2010 to 2050. *Current Population Reports, P25-113.* Washington, DC: US Census Bureau.

Waern, M., Rubenowitz, E., Runeson, B., et al. (2002a). Burden of illness and suicide in elderly people: case-control study. *British Medical Journal*, **324**(7350), 1355.

Waern, M., Runeson, B. S., Allebeck, P., et al. (2002b). Mental disorder in elderly suicides: a case-control study. *American Journal of Psychiatry*, **159**(3), 450–455.

World Health Organization. (2002). Distribution of suicides rates (per 100,000), by gender and age, 2000. Retrieved April 19, 2010 from: http://www.who.int/mental_health/prevention/suicide/suicide_rates_chart/en/index.html

Chapter 23

Armed forces

James A. Naifeh, Matthew K. Nock, and Robert J. Ursano

Suicide is currently a major public health concern for the US armed forces, and its emotional, operational, and financial costs are substantial (Tanielian & Jaycox, 2008). The purpose of this chapter is to provide an overview of suicidal events within the armed forces, including epidemiology, screening and surveillance efforts, risk and protective factors, prevention, and treatment considerations. We will focus primarily on the US military, which has received increased scrutiny over the past decade due to rising suicide rates amid ongoing combat operations.

Epidemiology of suicidal events in the armed forces

Since the 2001 launch of Operation Enduring Freedom (OEF) in Afghanistan, followed by Operation Iraqi Freedom (OIF) in 2003, the US military has been continuously engaged in what is now the longest war in the Nation's history. Suicides historically have occurred at a lower rate among Service members than the US general population, adjusting for demographic differences (Eaton et al., 2006). This likely has been due to the military's efforts to screen out individuals with a significant psychiatric or criminal history, as well as Service members' universal access to health care, steady employment, and strong military social support network. Shortly after the commencement of OIF, however, the suicide rate of the US military began to rise (Figure 23.1). This upward trend was most pronounced in the Army and Marines (Ramchand et al., 2011). In 2008, Army and Marine suicide rates surpassed the US general population rate for the first time in decades (Department of the Army, 2012). Rates in the US Navy and Air Force also rose during this time, eventually reaching rates comparable to that of the general population. In 2012 suicide resulted in more deaths than combat (Hoge & Castro, 2012).

Medical records reveal a similar upward trend in non-fatal suicidal events. Following the introduction of "suicide ideation" as a diagnostic code in the International Classification of Diseases (ICD-9-CM) in October 2005, there has been a sharp and steady annual increase in the number of military hospitalizations with primary diagnoses of suicidal ideation, from 5 in 2006 to 355 in 2010. Hospitalizations with non-primary diagnoses of suicidal ideation substantially increased during this period, as well, reaching approximately 3200 in 2010 (Armed Forces Health Surveillance Center, 2011d; Department of the Army, 2012).

Unlike suicide deaths, which are investigated and closely tracked by the Office of the Armed Forces Medical Examiner, there is no "gold standard" system for documenting non-fatal suicidal events. As a result, estimates for suicidal ideation and suicide attempts are less reliable. A major challenge in interpreting available data involves separating true increases in non-fatal suicidal events from increases based on greater awareness, identification, and reporting among unit commanders and medical staff. Supplementing medical records with self-report data from Service members may prove useful in this regard. For example, a representative, anonymous survey of active U.S. military personnel (N = 28 546), found that 4.6% of Service members reported "seriously considering suicide" in the past year (Army: 4.9%; Navy: 5.1%; Marine Corps: 5.5%; Air Force: 3.1%), similar to the 2005 version of the same survey (Bray et al., 2009). However, the overall rate of reported suicide attempt in the past year more than doubled, from 0.8% in 2005 to 2.2% in 2008, with all military branches reporting significantly higher rates in 2008 (Army: 1.1% vs. 2.0%; Navy: 0.9% vs. 2.8%; Marine Corps: 0.9% vs. 2.3%; Air Force: 0.3% vs. 1.6%).

A Concise Guide to Understanding Suicide, ed. Stephen H. Koslow, Pedro Ruiz, and Charles B. Nemeroff. Published by Cambridge University Press.

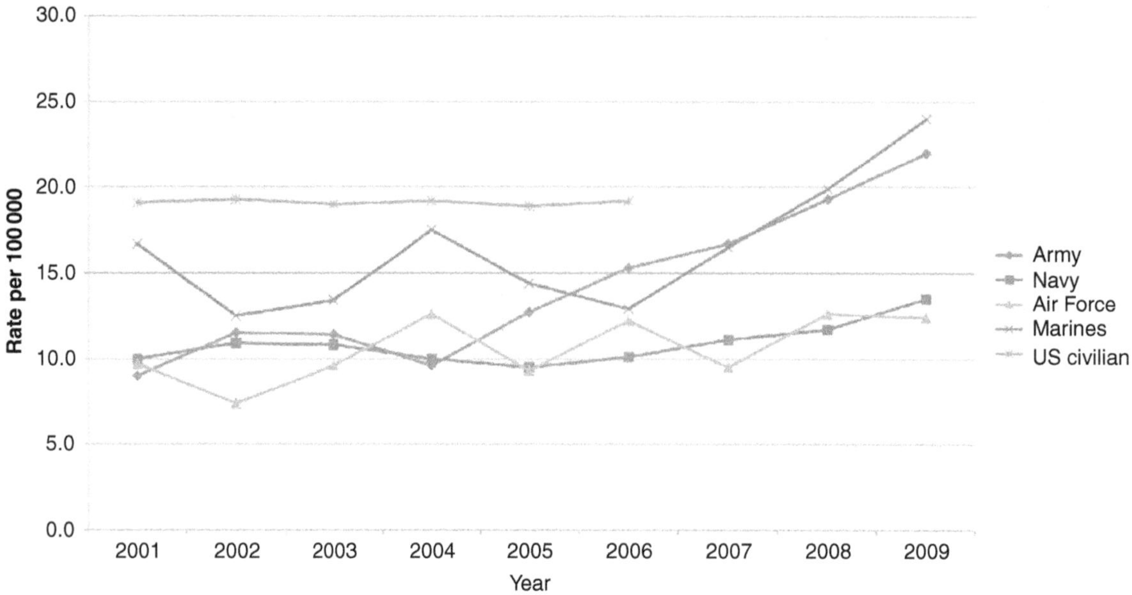

Figure 23.1. Suicide Rates by US Military Service, 2001 to 2009; 2001–2008 suicide rates from Ramchand et al. (2011); 2009 suicide rates from Luxton et al. (2010). *US civilian rate adjusted based on Department of Defense-wide demographic characteristics (Ramchand et al., 2011). See plate section for color version.

Method of injury and lethality

From 2008 to 2010, firearms were the most common method of US armed forces suicides, including both non-military issue firearms (44% of deaths) and military issue firearms (17% of deaths). Hanging was the second most common method of suicide (23%), followed by drugs (4%). By comparison, drugs were the most common method of injury used in suicide attempts (58%), followed by use of a sharp or blunt object (14%), and hanging (9%) (Bush et al., 2013). Compared to the civilian population, the ratio of suicide attempts to suicide deaths is smaller in the military, suggesting a higher degree of lethality among Service members (Anestis & Bryan, 2013). It appears this cannot be attributed solely to firearms, to which Service members have considerable access and are well trained to use. Although a greater proportion of military suicides and suicide attempts involve firearms compared to the general population, the smaller attempt to death ratio remains even after use of firearms is excluded.

Pre-enlistment suicidal history

An important research and policy question is the extent to which military service is associated with first-onset suicidal thoughts and behaviors. There is limited evidence from which to draw conclusions, but available data underscore the importance of the issue. A representative US Department of Defense (DoD) survey found that 3.8% of Service members reported that they "seriously considered suicide" before joining the military (Army: 4.4%; Navy: 3.8%; Marine Corps: 4.0%; Air Force: 2.8%), whereas 2.5% reported a pre-military suicide attempt (Army: 3.3%; Navy: 2.2%; Marine Corps: 3.0%; Air Force: 1.3%) (Bray et al., 2009).

Additionally, a recent simulation study estimated a variety of mental health outcomes using survey data from the US general population that was matched to the profile of US Army personnel on key sociodemographic variables (Gadermann et al., 2012). Even after excluding individuals who reported making a serious suicide attempt prior to their expected age of enlistment (based on the assumption that these individuals would have been ineligible for military service), it was estimated that the majority of individuals endorsing lifetime suicidal thoughts (82.4%), suicide plan (68.4%), or suicide attempt (72.8%) would have had their first onset prior to enlistment. Similarly, among those endorsing suicidal thoughts, plans, or attempts in the past 12 months, 59.5%, 73.1%, and 55.8%, respectively, were estimated to have a pre-enlistment onset (Gadermann et al., 2012). Together, these findings suggest that a substantial number of Service members have likely experienced suicidal thoughts and behaviors prior to military service, and that their risk of suicidal outcomes may persist after enlistment.

Surveillance and screening

In response to the recent upward trends in suicidality, the US military has increased its mental health surveillance and screening efforts. In 2004, the Army implemented the Army Suicide Event Report (ASER), a form intended to be completed by medical providers in order to document suicide-related events that resulted in death, hospitalization, or evacuation, as well as the risk factors surrounding the event (Gahm, 2005). The form underwent several revisions in subsequent years, expanding in scope and evolving in its definition of non-fatal suicidal events. In 2008, a similar reporting system, the Department of Defense Suicide Event Report (DoDSER), was implemented across all US military branches. The DoDSER replaced all previous reporting systems and, for the first time, allowed aggregated analyses of suicide-related events across the DoD (Gahm et al., 2012). Despite the utility of the DoDSER as a surveillance tool, a major challenge with this type of reporting systems is that it relies on consistent and widespread compliance by busy providers. Although use of the ASER was inconsistent in its initial years, particularly for non-fatal events (Gahm, 2005; Gahm & Lucenko, 2006), compliance with the DoDSER reporting system appears to be improving.

In order to provide mental health surveillance in combat zones, the Office of the Surgeon General of the Army implemented the Mental Health Advisory Team (MHAT) survey in 2003. The MHAT is an anonymous self-report questionnaire administered to randomly selected OEF/OIF units to assess the behavioral health of land combat forces. In 2010 the program was expanded to include Joint representation of other US military branches. The DoD has also implemented widespread mental health screening programs for those returning from overseas operations. The Post-Deployment Health Assessment (PDHA) and Post-Deployment Health Reassessment (PDHRA) are designed to identify health and mental health problems in Service members who have returned from an operational deployment (McCarthy et al., 2012). The PDHA is completed within 30 days of redeployment and the PDHRA is completed within 90 to 180 days. These screening programs include both face-to-face evaluation by medical providers and self-administered surveys inquiring about a range of psychosocial and mental health difficulties.

A challenge for screening programs is that the detection of mental health concerns, including suicidality, depends largely on Service members' willingness to disclose such problems. This willingness may be affected by perceptions of social stigma or concerns over how it might negatively impact one's military career (Warner et al., 2011). Research suggests that anonymity increases self-reported mental health problems among Service members (e.g., Gadermann et al., 2012), including PDHA questions about suicidal ideation, depression, PTSD, and willingness to seek care (Warner et al., 2011). Unfortunately, anonymity in mental health screening may itself create a barrier to providing distressed Service members with appropriate referrals and follow-up care.

Risk factors

A very limited body of research has identified associations between various risk factors and military suicides, and the results are somewhat mixed across studies. Descriptive statistics based on DoDSER records (Bush et al., 2013) suggest that US military Service members who died by suicide or attempted suicide from 2008 to 2010 were most typically male, Caucasian, under 25 years old, junior enlisted rank (E1-E4), and had at least a high school education. Both deaths and attempts most commonly occurred in the USA and in the Service member's own residence. There was also DoDSER evidence of prior self-injury in 15% of suicides and 34% of suicide attempts (Bush et al., 2013). By comparison, an examination of US Army medical records found that 4.6% of suicides had a previous code for suicide attempt and 4.0% had a previous code for suicidal ideation (Black et al., 2011).

These descriptive findings are generally supported by univariate analyses of suicide risk, which have implicated male gender (Black et al., 2011; Bachynski et al., 2012), having ever deployed (Black et al., 2011; Hyman et al., 2012), junior enlisted rank (Bachynski et al., 2012), reduction in rank (Hyman et al., 2012), and divorce or separation (Hyman et al., 2012). History of inpatient and outpatient treatment for a mental disorder (Black et al., 2011; Bachynski et al., 2012; Hyman et al., 2012), and prescription for SSRIs and sleep medications (Hyman et al., 2012) also demonstrated significant univariate associations with suicide.

Such risk factors have rarely been examined in a multivariate model. One recent case–control study of medical and administrative records from all US military Services found that, after adjusting for covariates, suicide was associated with mental disorder diagnosis, history of OEF/OIF deployment, and SSRI prescription (Hyman et al., 2012). Another study examining risk factors for non-fatal suicidal events in a multivariate model found several significant risk factors that differed by gender (Snarr et al., 2010). This large, online survey of active duty members of the US Air Force found that risk of past year suicidal ideation was predicted by female gender, lower enlisted rank, and non-Christian religion. Being unmarried increased risk of suicide ideation among men, and risk of suicide attempt was increased for lower ranking men and Hispanic women (Snarr et al., 2010).

Mental disorders

As with civilian studies, mental health diagnoses are among the most consistent risk factors for military suicides (Black et al., 2011; Bachynski et al., 2012; Hyman et al., 2012), particularly mood, anxiety, and substance use disorders (Black et al., 2011; Bachynski et al., 2012). According to DoDSER records, 15% of suicides and 25% of suicide attempts involved a previous diagnosis of anxiety disorder, including PTSD (5% of suicides, 10% of attempts), whereas 21% of suicides and 40% of attempts involved a previous diagnosis of mood disorder, including major depression (8% of suicides, 20% of attempts).

Recent surveys have found that up to 25% of US military personnel report mental health problems upon returning from deployments to OIF/OEF (Hoge et al., 2004, 2006). The counts and rates of incident mental disorder diagnoses increased by approximately 65% from 2000 through 2011, with 936 283 active component members receiving at least one mental disorder diagnosis during this time (Armed Forces Health Surveillance Center, 2012). This upward trend was primarily attributable to increased diagnoses of adjustment disorders, depressive disorders, and PTSD and other anxiety disorders. PTSD is of particular relevance to armed forces populations, given its historical and empirical relationship to combat exposure, as well as its association with suicidal behaviors, particularly in the presence of comorbid depression (Panagioti et al., 2009).

In addition to increasing suicide risk, mental disorders among Service members are associated with greater organizational burden and other negative individual outcomes. In 2010, mental disorders among active component Service members were among the top reasons for medical encounters, accounting for 20.7% of all hospitalizations (Armed Forces Health Surveillance Center, 2011c) and 42.7% of all hospital bed days, more than any other major medical category (Armed Forces Health Surveillance Center, 2011a). Since 2001, there has been a greater than three-fold increase in the number of bed days attributable to substance abuse, mood, anxiety, and adjustment reaction (Armed Forces Health Surveillance Center, 2011a). Mental disorders were also among the most common reasons for ambulatory visits, accounting for 15.6% of all encounters, a 113.7% increase since 2006 (Armed Forces Health Surveillance Center, 2011b). Further, the presence of a mental disorder, whether identified through medical records or post-deployment health screening, is associated with increased likelihood of attrition from the military, including involuntary separation (Hoge et al., 2005, 2006). Within 6 months of first hospitalization, 45% of Army Soldiers with a primary mental disorder diagnosis and 27% with a secondary mental disorder diagnosis were separated from military service, versus only 11% of Soldiers diagnosed with other medical conditions (Hoge et al., 2005).

Another potential risk factor, traumatic brain injury (TBI), is one of the "signature wounds" of OEF/OIF, affecting many Service members with blast injuries (Hoge et al., 2008; Schneiderman et al., 2008). Despite evidence of a strong univariate association between TBI and military suicide (Hyman et al., 2012), a recent case–control study found no association between suicide and type or frequency of TBI in this population (Skopp et al., 2012). However, TBI is associated with other risk factors for suicidality, including mental disorders, such as PTSD and depression (Hoge et al., 2008; Schneiderman et al., 2008), as well as increased aggression, disinhibition, and impulsivity (Rao & Lyketsos, 2000; Kim, 2002).

Stressful events

While Service members must contend with many of the life stressors and potentially traumatic events experienced by the general population, including sexual and physical assault, accidents, serious illness and disasters, there are numerous stressors that are unique to military service. When Service members are exposed to stressors, those with underlying biological, cognitive, and emotional vulnerabilities may be at greatly increased risk for suicidal thoughts and behaviors (Nock et al., 2013).

Integration into military culture can be a very stressful experience, particularly during basic training, which is physically and mentally taxing and involves near complete separation from previous social support networks. Overseas deployment is both a phasic and multidimensional stressor. In anticipation of deployment, Service members must make numerous preparations, particularly those who will be leaving a spouse and children behind. While deployed, Service members may be exposed to extreme and chronic stress during combat or humanitarian crises. For those serving in front-line combat roles, there is the frequent threat of death or serious injury from enemy fire and improvised explosive devices, witnessing the death or injury of others, as well as the possibility of having to kill other human beings. In this high stress environment, Service members may experience significant hyperarousal, agitation, and sleep deprivation for extended periods of time, increasing their suicide risk (Bryan et al., 2010).

The difficulty of being separated from loved ones during deployment may be exacerbated by problems on the home front, including financial strain, child disciplinary issues, marital discord, infidelity, and romantic breakups. Combat deployments, such as those during OEF and OIF, often last a year or more. The possibility that one's deployment will be extended is a stressor for both the Service member and his or her family. For those Service members with a history of multiple deployments, a shorter length of time between deployments, or dwell time, may be a risk factor for mental health problems (MacGregor et al., 2012). Despite these factors, most suicides and suicide attempts in recent years did not occur during OEF/OIF deployment. In fact, there was no history at all of OEF/OIF deployment or combat exposure in over half of those cases according to DoDSER data (Bush et al., 2013).

Returning from combat deployment requires readjustment to the pace and responsibilities of life outside a war zone. During this time, many Service members have to adapt to life with severely disabling and/or disfiguring injuries, as advances in medical technology have increased the survival rate following injuries that would have historically been fatal (Tanielian & Jaycox, 2008). Finally, separation from the armed forces brings with it the challenges of reintegrating into civilian life as a veteran (Institute of Medicine, 2010).

The most commonly identified situational stressors in cases of US military suicides and suicide attempts are military work stress, relationship problems, and legal history, with stressors such as substance abuse, physical health problems, abuse history, and financial stress generally occurring at lower rates (Department of the Army, 2012). Financial problems may be particularly relevant to members of the National Guard and Reserve. The part-time nature of their service obligation, combined with repeated mobilizations, leaves them especially vulnerable to unemployment and economic downturns.

Protective factors

Very little research has been done on factors that protect against suicide in the armed forces. There is some evidence of lower risk among US Army Soldiers 25–34 years old (Bachynski et al., 2012) and those of African American race (Black et al., 2011; Bachynski et al., 2012), but many other potential protective factors have yet to be thoroughly examined. For example, social support is a likely protective factor that may be particularly relevant within the structure and culture of the military. Research suggests that perceptions of strong unit cohesion, including support from leadership and peers, may help protect Service members from mental health problems, including PTSD (Halverson, 1995; Brailey et al., 2007). Among Soldiers, unit cohesion has also been associated with greater perceptions of combat readiness and decreased likelihood of leaving the Army (Halverson, 1995; Griffith, 2002). Thus, the benefits of strong social support, particularly within one's own unit, may protect Service members from psychiatric problems that put them at greater risk for suicide, while also helping them carry out their mission more effectively. Interestingly, marital status, which is often a proxy for familial social support, has not been found to be associated with suicide (Black et al., 2011; Bachynski et al., 2012).

Suicide prevention programs

The US military has greatly increased its suicide prevention efforts, yet published findings on the effectiveness of existing programs is lacking and generally inconsistent (Bagley et al., 2010). Current programs are varied in their scope and methods, ranging from universal (primary), to selected (secondary), to indicated (Ramchand et al., 2011), and often incorporating elements from more than one approach. Many universal prevention programs, which aim to teach basic information and/or skills, are delivered online. These programs are typically accessible via the Suicide Outreach website maintained by the US DoD and Department of Veterans Affairs (VA) (http://www.suicideoutreach.org/), or on the suicide prevention websites of individual Services. For example, the Marine Corps' suicide prevention website includes the telephone number for the National Suicide Prevention Lifeline (http://www.mccsmcrd.com/MarineAndFamilyPrograms/BehavioralHealth/SuicidePrevention/index.html). Other universal prevention programs are delivered in person, such as the Marine Corps' Entry Level Training in Suicide Prevention, which is given to all Marines during boot camp, officer candidate school, and basic school.

Some prevention programs involve both selected and indicated approaches by targeting high-risk groups, then intervening when suicidality is detected. For example, the Army's Applied Suicide Intervention Skills Training (ASIST) aims to teach chaplains, behavioral health professionals, and other gatekeepers who often come into contact with Soldiers seeking help (selected prevention) to identify suicidal thoughts, assess risk, create a safety plan, and follow-up with Soldiers (indicated prevention) (Ramchand et al., 2011). Similarly, Assessing and Managing Suicide Risk (AMSR) is a 1-day Air Force training program for behavioral health providers. AMSR focuses on 24 competencies within seven categories: (a) Working with individuals at risk for suicide: Attitudes and approach, (b) Understanding suicide, (c) Collecting accurate assessment information, (d) Formulating risk, (e) Developing a treatment and services plan, (f) Managing care, (g) Documenting, and (h) Understanding legal and regulatory issues related to suicidality (http://www.sprc.org/traininginstitute/amsr/clincomp.asp).

Treatment considerations

From 2001 to 2010, 45% of US Service members who died by suicide and 73% of those with an intentionally self-inflicted injury or poisoning (based on inpatient or outpatient diagnosis) had an outpatient medical visit within the previous 30 days, most frequently to primary care (Trofimovich et al., 2012). These Service members generally used health care at similar rates to matched controls up until around 60 days prior to their suicidal or self-injurious event, at which point their rate of outpatient visits intensified. Based on DoDSER records, there was prior inpatient mental health care in 13% of suicides and 24% of suicide attempts, and prior outpatient behavior health care in 39% of suicides and 60% of suicide attempts. Furthermore, 23% of Service members who died by suicide and 43% of those who made an attempt were known to have been prescribed psychotropic medication at some point (Bush et al., 2013).

There are several challenges to the prevention and treatment of suicide-related outcomes within the US military mental health system. First, despite near universal access to military health care, many Service members may not utilize those resources. Most Service members are young and male, demographic characteristics associated with decreased help-seeking behavior in the general population (Wang et al., 2005). Additionally, stoicism and autonomy are individual characteristics that the military generally values and encourages. While these traits may help to protect against a host of mental health problems, they may also diminish the likelihood of help seeking. Indeed, the primary reason that suicidal individuals from around the world give for not seeking treatment is the belief that they can handle it on their own (Bruffaerts et al., 2011).

Many Service members at risk for suicide may be unwilling to seek treatment due to perceived stigma, particularly those who are experiencing mental health problems (Hoge & Castro, 2012). Studies have found that Service members who screen positive for PTSD, depression, and other psychiatric difficulties are more likely than those who screen negative to perceive barriers to care (e.g., "My unit leadership would have less confidence in me," "Members of my unit would view me differently," "I would be seen as weak," "It would harm my career") (Hoge et al., 2004; Warner et al., 2011). Perceived stigma takes on even greater importance in light of the structure of the military health care system. Whereas protected health information is subject to strict privacy regulations in the civilian world, US law contains an armed forces exemption permitting commanders to access, without consent, the medical and mental health records of subordinates under certain circumstances, such as to aid in making determinations about fitness for duty. Concerns over how this might impact one's military career and status among supervisors and peers may deter Service members from fully disclosing mental health problems, including suicidality, or from seeking help altogether

(Warner et al., 2011; Department of the Army, 2012). Perhaps unsurprisingly, available evidence suggests that the majority of Service members who make a suicide attempt or die by suicide do not communicate their intent to anyone beforehand (Bush et al., 2013).

Another challenge is maintaining continuity of care, a problem which has been highlighted by the Department of Defense Task Force on the Prevention of Suicide by Members of the Armed Forces (2010). Transition is a common aspect of military life, with Service members moving between different phases of training, military installations, units, and deployments, as well as from civilian to military life and vice versa. Of particular relevance to Service members at risk is recent discharge from inpatient treatment (Department of Defense Task Force on the Prevention of Suicide by Members of the Armed Forces, 2010). With each transition, Service members may encounter new providers and treatment facilities, with available resources differing markedly from one environment to the next. For example, a Service member who has attended regular appointments with a team of providers in a large military medical center will have far fewer mental health resources once he deploys to a combat zone (Bryan et al., 2010). In every instance, the patient's mental health history must be adequately communicated to new providers and supervisors, particularly for those with a history of suicidal thoughts and behaviors.

Lastly, weapons management is uniquely challenging for military treatment providers. In this population, possession of firearms is commonplace and may even be an operational requirement for some Service members. This is particularly true for Service members in a combat environment (Bryan et al., 2010). Indeed, in 2010, firearms were more commonly used in both suicides and suicide attempts among deployed Service members than among those not deployed (Kinn et al., 2011). In addition to their military issued firearms, non-deployed Service members may have access to others' weapons, and many keep personal firearms at home. This is a key safety consideration, as 72% of firearms suicides in the US armed forces involved a non-military issue weapon (Bush et al., 2013).

Ready access to weapons obviously poses a serious threat to the safety of suicidal patients. Effectively restricting access to lethal means in this population requires coordination between mental health providers, unit leadership, and the Service member's family. Command leadership must also be involved in such decisions due to their potential operational impact. Similar levels of coordination are also necessary when restrictions on weapons access are being lifted. For some Service members, firearms restriction may be especially stigmatizing. In these situations it may be necessary to consider alternatives, such as allowing the Service member to maintain possession of the weapon but removing the firing pin. However, in a combat zone, where firearms restriction may be virtually impossible, clinicians may need to consider medical evacuation as a necessary safety measure (Bryan et al., 2010).

There are ongoing efforts to improve mental health care for US Service members. A collaboration between the US DoD and VA has resulted in the development of clinical practice guidelines for a variety of physical and psychiatric conditions, including suicidality (available online at http://www.healthquality.va.gov). For clinicians seeking DoD-relevant guidance and resources, the *Air Force Guide for Managing Suicidal Behavior* may be accessed online (http://www.airforcecounseling.com/downloads/misc-guides/air-force-guide-for-managing-suicidal-behavior/). Additionally, in an effort to address some of the challenges described above, and in recognition of the important role that primary care plays in Service members' access to the military medical system, the US Army has implemented a program called Re-Engineering Systems of Primary Care Treatment in the Military (RESPECT-Mil; Engel et al., 2008). RESPECT-Mil is a systems-level collaborative care approach to improving the identification and clinical management of PTSD and depression in military primary care settings.

Conclusion

Armed forces personnel in the USA and around the world encounter many challenges and stressors in the course of their service, some of which are similar to those faced by other unique populations, such as first responders (e.g., police, firefighters, and emergency medical services personnel) and victims of disasters and terrorist attacks. The rising rate of suicides in the US military over the past decade of war has led to an unprecedented focus on research and prevention. One notable effort is the Army Study to Assess Risk and Resilience in Service-members (Army STARRS; www.ArmySTARRS.org), the largest study of suicide and mental health risk and resilience ever conducted in the US military. Army STARRS was initiated in 2008 by the Department of the Army and the National Institute of Mental Health to inform data-driven approaches to reducing suicidal behaviors among Soldiers and improving mental health and functioning. Its contributions, along with those of numerous other studies currently underway, are a major step toward reducing suicides among Service members.

References

Anestis, M. D., & Bryan, C. J. (2013). Means and capacity for suicidal behavior: A comparison of the ratio of suicide attempts and deaths by suicide in the US military and general population. *Journal of Affective Disorders*, **148**(1), 42–47.

Armed Forces Health Surveillance Center. (2011a). Absolute and relative morbidity burdens attributable to various illnesses and injuries, U.S. Armed Forces, 2010. *Medical Surveillance Monthly Report*, **18**(4), 2–7.

Armed Forces Health Surveillance Center. (2011b). Ambulatory visits among members of the active component, U.S. Armed Forces, 2010. *Medical Surveillance Monthly Report*, **18**(4), 16–21.

Armed Forces Health Surveillance Center. (2011c). Hospitalizations among members of the active component, U.S. Armed Forces, 2010. *Medical Surveillance Monthly Report*, **18**(4), 8–15.

Armed Forces Health Surveillance Center. (2011d). Surveillance snapshot: Hospitalizations for suicidal ideation. *Medical Surveillance Monthly Report*, **18**(4), 23.

Armed Forces Health Surveillance Center. (2012). Mental disorders and mental health problems, active component, U.S. Armed Forces, 2000–2011. *Medical Surveillance Monthly Report*, **19**(6), 11–17.

Bachynski, K. E., Canham-Chervak, M., Black, S. A., et al. (2012). Mental health risk factors for suicides in the US Army, 2007–8. *Injury Prevention*, **18**, 405–412.

Bagley, S. C., Munjas, B., & Shekelle, P. (2010). A systematic review of suicide prevention programs for military or veterans. *Suicide and Life-Threatening Behavior*, **40**, 257–265.

Black, S. A., Gallaway, M. S., Bell, M. R., & Ritchie, E. C. (2011). Prevalence and risk factors associated with suicides of army soldiers 2001–2009. *Military Psychology*, **23**, 433–451.

Brailey, K., Vasterling, J. J., Proctor, S. P., Constans, J. I., & Friedman, M. J. (2007). PTSD symptoms, life events, and unit cohesion in U.S. soldiers: Baseline findings from the Neurocognition Deployment Health Study. *Journal of Traumatic Stress*, **20**, 495–503.

Bray, R. M., Pemberton, M. R., Hourani, L. L., et al. (2009). *2008 Department of Defense Survey of Health Related Behaviors Among Active Duty Military Personnel: A Component of the Defense Lifestyle Assessment Program (DLAP)*. Research Triangle Park, North Carolina: RTI International.

Bruffaerts, R., Demyttenaere, K., Hwang, I., et al. (2011). Treatment of suicidal people around the world. *British Journal of Psychiatry*, **199**, 64–70.

Bryan, C. J., Kanzler, K. E., Durham, T. L., West, C. L., & Greene, E. (2010). Challenges and considerations for managing suicide risk in combat zones. *Military Medicine*, **175**, 713–718.

Bush, N. E., Reger, M. A., Luxton, D. D., et al. (2013). Suicides and suicide attempts in the U.S. military, 2008–2010. *Suicide and Life-Threatening Behavior*, **43**(3), 262–273.

Department of Defense Task Force on the Prevention of Suicide by Members of the Armed Forces. (2010). *The Challenge and the Promise: Strengthening the Force, Preventing Suicide and Saving Lives*. Washington, DC: Department of Defense.

Department of the Army. (2012). *Army 2020: Generating Health & Discipline in the Force Ahead of the Strategic Reset*. Washington, DC: Department of the Army.

Eaton, K. M., Messer, S. C., Wilson, A. L. G., & Hoge, C. W. (2006). Strengthening the validity of population-based suicide rate comparisons: An illustration using U.S. military and civilian data. *Suicide and Life-Threatening Behavior*, **36**, 182–191.

Engel, C. C., Oxman, T., Yamamoto, C., et al. (2008). RESPECT-Mil: Feasibility of a systems-level collaborative care approach to depression and post-traumatic stress disorder in military primary care. *Military Medicine*, **173**, 935–940.

Gadermann, A. M., Engel, C. C., Naifeh, J. A., et al. (2012a). Prevalence of DSM-IV major depression among U.S. military personnel: Meta-analysis and simulation. *Military Medicine*, **177**, 47–59.

Gadermann, A. M., Gilman, S. E., McLaughlin, K. A., et al. (2012b). Projected rates of psychological disorders and suicidality among soldiers based on simulations of matched general population data. *Military Medicine*, **177**, 1002–1010.

Gahm, G. A. (2005). *Army Suicide Event Report (ASER): Calendar Year 2004*. Tacoma, WA: Suicide Risk Management and Surveillence Office, Army Behavioral Health Technology Office, Madigan Army Medical Center.

Gahm, G. A., & Lucenko, B. A. (2006). *Army Suicide Event Report (ASER): Calendar Year 2005*. Tacoma, WA: Suicide Risk Management and Surveillance Office, Army Behavioral Health Technology Office, Madigan Army Medical Center.

Gahm, G. A., Reger, M. A., Kinn, J. T., et al. (2012). Addressing the surveillance goal in the National Strategy for Suicide Prevention: The Department of Defense Suicide Event Report. *American Journal of Public Health*, **102**(Suppl 1), S24–S28.

Griffith, J. (2002). Multilevel analysis of cohesion's relation to stress, well-being, identification, disintegration, and perceived combat readiness. *Military Psychology*, **14**(3), 217–239.

Halverson, R. R. (1995). *Psychological Well-Being and Physical Health Symptoms of Soldiers Deployed for Operation Uphold Democracy*. A Summary of Human Dimensions Research in Haiti: DTIC Document.

Hoge, C. W., & Castro, C. A. (2012). Preventing suicides in US service members and veterans: Concerns after a decade of war. *Journal of the American Medical Association*, **308**, 671–672.

Hoge, C. W., Castro, C. A., Messer, S. C., et al. (2004). Combat duty in Iraq and Afghanistan: Mental health problems and barriers to care. *New England Journal of Medicine*, **351**, 13–22.

Hoge, C. W., Toboni, H. E., Messer, S. C., et al. (2005). The occupational burden of mental disorders in the U.S. military: Psychiatric hospitalizations, involuntary separations, and disability. *American Journal of Psychiatry*, **162**, 585–591.

Hoge, C. W., Auchterlonie, J. L., & Milliken, C. S. (2006). Mental health problems, use of mental health services, and attrition from military service after returning from deployment to Iraq or Afganistan. *Journal of the American Medical Association*, **295**, 1023–1032.

Hoge, C. W., McGurk, D., Thomas, J. L., et al. (2008). Mild traumatic brain injury in U.S. soldiers returning from Iraq. *New England Journal of Medicine*, **358**, 453–463.

Hyman, J., Ireland, R., Frost, L., & Cottrell, L. (2012). Suicide incidence and risk factors in an active duty US military population. *American Journal of Public Health*, **102**(Suppl 1), S138–S146.

Institute of Medicine. (2010). *Returning Home from Iraq and Afghanistan: Preliminary Assessment of Readjustment Needs of Veterans, Service Members, and their Families*. Washington, DC: The National Academies Press.

Kim, E. (2002). Agitation, aggression, and disinhibition syndromes after traumatic brain injury. *NeuroRehabilitation*, **17**(4), 297–310.

Kinn, J. T., Luxton, D. D., Reger, M. A., et al. (2011). *DoDSER: Department of Defense Suicide Event Report: Calendar Year 2010 Annual Report*. Joint Base Lewis-McChord, WA: National Center for Telehealth & Technology, Defense Centers of Excellence for Psychological Health & Traumatic Brain Injury.

Luxton, D. D., Skopp, N. A., Kinn, J. T., et al. (2010). *Department of Defense Suicide Event Report (DoDSER): Calendar Year 2009 Annual Report*. Joint Base Lewis-McChord, WA: National Center for Telehealth & Technology, Defense Centers of Excellence for Psychological Health & Traumatic Brain Injury.

MacGregor, A. J., Han, P. P., Dougherty, A. L., & Galarneau, M. R. (2012). Effect of dwell time on the mental health of US military personnel with multiple combat tours. *American Journal of Public Health*, **102**(Suppl 1), S55–S59.

McCarthy, M. D., Thompson, S. J., & Knox, K. L. (2012). Use of the Air Force Post-Deployment Health Reassessment for the identification of depression and posttraumatic stress disorder: Public health implications for suicide prevention. *American Journal of Public Health*, **102**(Suppl 1), S60–S65.

Nock, M. K., Deming, C. A., Fullerton, C. S., et al. (2013). Suicide among soldiers: A review of psychosocial risk and protective factors. *Psychiatry: Interpersonal and Biological Processes*, **76**, 97–125.

Panagioti, M., Gooding, P., & Tarrier, N. (2009). Post-traumatic stress disorder and suicidal behavior: A narrative review. *Clinical Psychology Review*, **29**, 471–482.

Ramchand, R., Acosta, J., Burns, R. M., Jaycox, L. H., & Pernin, C. G. (2011). *The War Within: Preventing Suicide in the U.S. Military*. Santa Monica, CA: RAND Corporation.

Rao, V., & Lyketsos, C. (2000). Neuropsychiatric sequelae of traumatic brain injury. *Psychosomatics*, **41**, 95–103.

Schneiderman, A. I., Braver, E. R., & Kang, H. K. (2008). Understanding sequelae of injury mechanisms and mild traumatic brain injury incurred during the conflicts in Iraq and Afghanistan: Persistent postconcussive symptoms and posttraumatic stress disorder. *American Journal of Epidemiology*, **167**, 1446–1452.

Skopp, N. A., Trofimovich, L., Grimes, J., Oetjen-Gerdes, L., & Gahm, G. A. (2012). Relations between suicide and traumatic brain injury, psychiatric diagnoses, and relationship problems, active component, U.S. armed forces, 2001–2009. *Medical Surveillance Monthly Report*, **19**(2), 7–11.

Snarr, J. D., Heyman, R. E., & Smith, A. M. (2010). Recent suicidal ideation and suicide attempts in a large-scale survey of the U.S. Air Force: Prevalences and demographic risk factors. *Suicide and Life-Threatening Behavior*, **40**, 544–552.

Tanielian, T., & Jaycox, L. H. (2008). *Invisible Wounds of War: Psychological and Cognitive Injuries, Their Consequences, and Services to Assist Recovery*. Santa Monica, CA: RAND Corporation.

Trofimovich, L., Skopp, N. A., Luxton, D. D., & Reger, M. A. (2012). Health care experiences prior to suicide and self-inflicted injury, active component, U.S. Armed Forces, 2001–2010. *Medical Surveillance Monthly Report*, **19**(2), 2–6.

Wang, P. S., Berglund, P., Olfson, M., et al. (2005). Failure and delay in initial treatment contact after first onset of mental disorders in the National Comorbidity Survey Replication. *Archives of General Psychiatry*, **62**(6), 603–613.

Warner, C. H., Appenzeller, G. N., Grieger, T., et al. (2011). Importance of anonymity to encourage honest reporting in mental health screening after combat deployment. *Archives of General Psychiatry*, **68**, 1065–1071.

Chapter 24

Medical illness

Gary J. Kennedy and Anne Rohs

Introduction

Although suicide is most commonly associated with affective and psychotic disorders, there is a growing body of evidence that serious physical illnesses increase risk as well. And because suicidal deaths are comparatively rare, efforts to improve risk reduction have proven difficult. As a result studies indicating that specific physical illness may increase risk are of interest, even more so with the highest rates of completed suicide occurring among older adults who are more likely to exhibit a profile of multi-morbidity. Collaborative protocols to reduce suicidal ideation among primary care patients are effective. But what is the evidence to support a similar collaboration between mental health professionals and specialty care providers such as oncologists, cardiologists, or infectious disease specialists? Do commonalities emerge across the array of physical disorders which are associated with suicide and which might make this defined clinical population more accessible for interventions? Are the more commonly used depression screening instruments sufficient to detect suicidality? If not, how should screening procedures be altered to identify vulnerable physically ill individuals without burdening patients and providers when risk is negligible?

Physical illness is a genuine risk factor for suicidal behavior

Large cross-national studies show that there is an association between physical illness and physical conditions with suicide attempts and deaths. The world mental health survey examined data from 14 countries, controlling for demographic and socioeconomic status as well as psychiatric disorders. Most physical conditions were associated with suicidal ideation. Hypertension, stroke, myocardial infarction, arthritis, chronic pain, and respiratory problems were most strongly associated with attempts. Epilepsy was most strongly associated with suicidal outcomes. As the number of physical conditions increased so too did the risk of suicide. However each additional illness added but a small increment. Factoring in the presence of a mental disorder added little to risk prediction. Physical conditions were associated with elevated risk regardless of the economic status of the country (Scott et al., 2010).

Kishi et al. (2001) found patients with acute, life-threatening physical illness are also at increased risk of suicidal plan and attempts and that risk is mitigated by treatment of comorbid depressive disorders. They examined 496 patients admitted to Baltimore city hospital for stroke, traumatic brain injury, myocardial infarction, or spinal cord injury for the presence of a suicidal plan or history of an attempt. More than 7% of the cohort mentioned a plan or attempt with the highest frequency occurring among those with spinal cord injury. Those with a plan or an attempt were younger, less likely to be married, more likely to have psychiatric or substance abuse history with a higher frequency of generalized anxiety and major depressive disorders. A total of 21% were diagnosed with major depressive disorder and of those 25% had suicidal plans. If patients were depressed, there was a strong correlation between improvement in depressive symptoms and recanting of their suicidal plan at follow-up. Untreated depression correlated with continued suicidal plan. The reliability of findings from this study is limited due to sample size and difficulties with follow-up following hospitalization.

However, the relationship of depression to suicidality among acutely ill patients may not hold in studies of primary care samples where physician contact and presumably the opportunity for risk reduction is more common. In an 8-year-long nested case–control study

A Concise Guide to Understanding Suicide, ed. Stephen H. Koslow, Pedro Ruiz, and Charles B. Nemeroff. Published by Cambridge University Press.

of 593 family medicine practices in the UK, 873 cases of suicidal death were compared to 17 460 patients matched by age and gender. Patients without any one of 11 specific diagnoses served as the reference group for relative risk estimates of death made possible by linkage to the national mortality records. The authors sought to identify conditions associated with an increased risk of suicide, determine the extent to which depression might explain risk elevation, and examine differences in risk by gender and advanced age. Unnatural deaths due to undetermined causes (medical examiner's open verdicts), generally thought to be suicides, were included. Conditions thought to be associated with depression or suicide were chosen based on review of the literature. Conditions associated with greater burden of care for practitioners were also selected based on consensus conference. Illnesses chosen a priori for examination included cancer, coronary heart disease, hypertension, stroke, diabetes, asthma, chronic obstructive pulmonary disease (COPD), osteoarthritis, osteoporosis, back pain, and epilepsy. Any current or past episode of depressive disorder unless coded as "remitted" at the time of death was used to classify the patient as "depressed." Although younger patients would be expected to be healthier and less burdened by the illnesses in question, age matching precluded the potential confounding effect of youth. However, gender-specific interaction terms were formally tested after time-specific illness prevalence estimates had been obtained for cases and controls. Logistic regression models provided relative risk estimates.

Among men and women combined, elevated relative risk of suicide appeared with four conditions: coronary heart disease, stroke, COPD, and osteoporosis with mean ages of 74, 79, 66, and 77 respectively. The magnitude of risk ranged from an odds ratio of 1.53 (95% CI 1.14–2.04) for coronary heart disease to 2.33 (95% CI 1.46–3.72) for osteoporosis. However, when the investigators adjusted the analyses for the presence of depression, risks remained significantly elevated for these four conditions but fell considerably ranging from 1.09 (95% CI 0.81–1.46) for coronary heart disease to 1.62 (95% CI 0.99–2.63) for osteoporosis. Women who committed suicide (mean age 54) were significantly older than men who did so (mean age 48). Among women but not men the relative risk of suicide increased significantly and substantially with the level of multi-morbidity as measured by the number of 11 illnesses present at the time of death. Women with three or more of the specific illnesses experienced an odds ratio of 2.27 (95% CI 1.35–3.84) and were aged a mean of 77 years. Also among women but not men the relative risk of suicide was significantly and substantially elevated for cancer (OR 2.23 [195% CI 0.28–3.86]), coronary heart disease (OR3.10 [95% CI 1.81–5.29]), and COPD (OR 3.23 [95% CI 1.57–6.66]) with nearly two-fold elevation in risk remaining with cancer and heart disease after controlling for depression. The authors conclude that prior or current episodes of depression did not explain the association of suicide with cancer or coronary heart disease among older women. Moreover depression explained only a minority of risk seen among younger women and those with multiple physical illnesses. They challenge the notion that physical illness leads to suicide via depression. Lacking measures of household composition, social support, economic status, and disability they could not examine alternative hypotheses among men or women. And lacking data on the use of alcohol and tobacco, which are more prevalent among males and are also related to cancer, heart disease, osteoporosis, depression and suicide, the contribution of unhealthy behaviors to risk could not be estimated (Webb et al., 2012).

Specific illnesses associated with suicide

The 2012 Surgeon General's report, National strategy for Suicide Prevention lists a number of specific medical illnesses thought to be associated with heightened risk of suicide. Most are either life threatening or chronically disabling but those caused by traumatic injury or HIV infection are wholly preventable. Certain degenerative diseases of the central nervous system are associated with either increased frequency of suicidal ideation or suicide attempts. In a review of more than 120 publications on suicidality and dementia, Haw et al. (2009) found elevated rates only for Huntington's disease in which suicide occurred three times more often than the population at large. For most persons with other dementias the risk of suicide appeared to be the same or less than for the general population when matched for age. However, risk was increased during the period immediately after diagnosis and in the setting of hospitalization. Wishing for death is not uncommon but suicide attempts are rare. Putative risk factors include depression, hopelessness, preserved insight, younger age, and failure to respond to anti-dementia drugs. Among persons with Huntington's disease risk of suicide decreased immediately after patients were given an unequivocal diagnosis. Risk increased in early stages of illness, whereas it diminished later in the course of disease (Paulsen et al., 2005). These findings suggest that suicide risk can be stratified based on two critical periods of increased suicidality: immediately before diagnosis, and in early stages of the disease.

Although the dementias are not associated with elevated risk of suicide, multiple sclerosis is with rates elevated several-fold. Risk factors associated with increased risk include male gender, social isolation, major depressive disorder, severity of depressive symptoms, alcohol abuse, and younger age. Disease characteristics associated with suicide included early onset and progressive subtype. Risk of suicide appeared to decline after the first year following diagnosis (Pompili et al., 2012). Potentially preventable traumatic injuries to the spinal cord and to the brain are associated with elevated attempted and completed suicide. Patients with traumatic brain injury including minor head trauma such as concussion, are at increased risk of suicide. There are several hypothetical explanations. First injury and or the resulting disability may precipitate depression which may progress to hopelessness and suicidality. Second both suicide and traumatic brain injury share many premorbid risk factors such as male gender, substance abuse, and history of aggressiveness. Indeed the majority of patients with TBI had a premorbid psychiatric disorder. Third the injury may impact cognitive domains such as executive function (frontal lobe trauma) which can inhibit response to antidepressant medications as well as interfere with planning and problem solving and finding alternatives to self-destructive solutions. There does not appear to be a window of risk (Wasserman et al., 2008). However when injury is repetitive and induces a chronic traumatic encephalopathy, the risk of suicide may be strikingly elevated yet unappreciated (McKee et al., 2009). Suicide among military combatants and professional athletes, particularly football players, is the most salient example.

Epilepsy is also associated with suicide. Some have suggested that anxiety and depression and suicidality may be due to burden of epilepsy or side effects of anticonvulsants. Hesdorffer et al. (2012) examined the incidence of psychiatric disorders in patients with epilepsy before and after diagnosis within the General Practice Research Database in the UK. They compared 3773 cases of epilepsy with 14 000 controls matched for gender, year of birth, and practice location cataloging diagnoses of psychosis, depression and anxiety, and suicidality in the 3 years before and after the diagnosis of epilepsy. Control cases were chosen from patients with either a diagnosis of eczema or acute surgery to make the range of illness severity comparable. The incident rate ratio of anxiety, depression, and psychosis was significantly increased for all years before the diagnosis (IRR, 1.5–15.7) as well as after the diagnosis (IRR, 2.2–10.9). The incidence of suicidality was elevated before the diagnosis (IRR, 3.1–4.5) and 1 year after diagnosis (IRR, 5.3). The prevalence ratio for a suicide attempt was increased both before the onset of epilepsy (PR, 2.6–5.2) and afterwards (PR, 2.4–5.6). Epilepsy was associated with an increased onset of psychiatric disorders and suicide before and after epilepsy diagnosis. The findings demonstrated a bidirectional relationship of between psychiatric disorders and epilepsy in the 3 years preceding and for 2 years following the diagnosis. They did not support the hypothesis that increased risk of suicide could be explained by anticonvulsant use in epileptic patients. The authors conclude that shared underlying pathophysiological mechanisms both lower the seizure threshold and increase the risk for psychiatric disorders and suicidality.

HIV/AIDS

Lack of a cure, stigma, and discrimination make the burden of living with this disease potentially higher than other medical illnesses suggesting an elevated risk of suicide as well. In a national record linkage study of Denmark spanning the years 1986–2006 investigators identified 9900 men who died from suicide. Compared with age-matched controls, suicide cases were more often living as single, with lower income, and in the capital area. A history of psychiatric illness was present in 43.81% of suicide cases, compared to 5.60% of controls. Of the suicides 0.44% had a diagnosis of AIDS or HIV while the rate was 0.05% in controls. Among all 144 individuals with AIDS or HIV infection, persons who completed suicide were more likely to have received inpatient hospital treatment for AIDS/HIV. They were also more likely to have received the diagnosis in the previous 2 years suggesting that increased time from diagnosis decreases risk. HIV/AIDS constituted a significant risk for subsequent suicide with an IRR of 8.73 in crude analysis, 4.81 adjusted for psych history and specific psychiatric diagnosis, and 3.84 when further adjusted for marital status, annual gross income, place of residence, citizenship, and presence of other physical illnesses. Thus risk increased for patients who required hospitalization, those with a hospital admission in the previous year or with multiple hospitalizations, and those who had received a diagnosis in the last 2 years. Both AIDS/HIV and psychiatric illness increased the risk of suicide, but when combined the two illnesses had a substantially stronger effect than presence of either one alone. The increased suicide risk associated with AIDS/HIV infection was somewhat higher before the introduction in 1997 of highly active antiretroviral therapy (HAART) but remained highly significant after the advent of HAART (Jia et al., 2012)

Other illnesses associated with suicide

A number of additional medical illnesses are listed as potentially associated with heightened risk of suicide because of associated pain or the burdensome nature of treatment (Surgeon General, 2012). Arthritis is thought to be associated with suicide as a result of comorbid depression, disability, and pain. Chronic renal disease is also listed with the risk of suicidality compounded by affective and other psychiatric disorders occurring in excess compared to otherwise healthy adults. Patients who express symptoms of depressive disorder are more likely to request withdrawal from life-saving hemodialysis. This situation highlights the likelihood that an untold number of deaths among persons, particularly those of advanced years and multi-morbidities, may be the result of self-neglect or suicide by cessation of life-sustaining medications such as insulin or antiarrhythmics. And finally there may also be an increased risk of suicide associated with obesity. Obesity is probably the most prevalent chronic illness in the USA and is often comorbid with other medical and psychiatric illnesses. There has been controversy regarding the association of obesity and suicide, with some groups suggesting a paradoxical protective effect of increased BMI on fatal self-injury. Further clouding the picture is evidence suggesting an increased risk of suicide associated with patients who have undergone bariatric surgery. On balance patients who are overweight are at risk for suicide (Heneghan, 2012).

Cancer

Fang and associates (2012) conducted a historical cohort study of 6 073 250 Swedes examining proximate risk of suicide or cardiovascular death among persons recently diagnosed with cancer. Relative risk estimates were calculated in comparison to cancer-free patients from the week following diagnosis to 53 weeks thereafter or longer. Compared to cancer-free-patients, the relative risk of suicide was 12.6 (95% CI 8.6–17.8) during the first week and 3.1 (95% CI 2.7–3.5) during the first year following the cancer diagnosis. The relative risk of cardiovascular death was 5.6 (95% CI 5.2–5.9) during the first week and 3.3 (95% CI 3.1–3.4) during the fourth week following diagnosis.

Over the 1991–2006 period of observation there were 13 284 suicides among cancer-free patients, an incidence rate of 0.18 per 100 person-years. There were 786 suicidal deaths among persons diagnosed with cancer, an incidence rate of 0.36 per 1000 person-years. There were 29 persons with cancer who killed themselves within a week of diagnosis; 110 had done so by the 12th week of observation. The highest relative risks were observed for the worst cancers including esophagus, liver, pancreas followed by lung cancer. Risk fell after the first week but remained elevated beyond the first year for all cancers including prostate, breast, colorectal anatomy, lymphatic or hematopoietic, and CNS as well. The incidence rates of suicide were higher among patients with pre-existing psychiatric diagnoses whether or not they had received a recent diagnosis of cancer. But in comparison, relative risks of suicide following a cancer diagnosis were higher among persons without a pre-existing mental disorder. As expected the incidence rates and relative risks of suicide among men exceeded those among women both with and without the diagnosis. The relative risk of suicide among those with a diagnosis did not differ by age with the exception of the 65–74 year age group whose relative risk at 3.7 (95% CI 2.9–4.5) was noticeably larger.

This study is noteworthy for the sample size, range of cancers included, unequivocal outcomes, and comparison of two causes of death, cancer and suicide with similar behavioral risk factors, namely, smoking, excessive alcohol intake, and depression. Because risk of death was most elevated during the first week following diagnosis, the emotional impact of having cancer rather than the progression of the disease seems more likely to account for the phenomenon. Curiously, those with prior psychiatric diagnoses were not more vulnerable to the aftershock of diagnosis suggesting prior emotional stress may have inoculated them against being overwhelmed. However, the authors did not (have yet to) investigate outcomes of morbidity such as non-fatal hospitalization due to suicide attempts, cardiovascular diseases, or mental illness. As a result their findings likely underestimate the stressful effects of receiving a diagnosis of cancer. Among cancer patients recently discharged from hospital, admissions within the previous year are associated with elevated risk of subsequent suicide within 90 days post discharge. Half of the suicides occurred within the first month after discharge (Lin et al., 2009). However, among persons discharged from psychiatric units of whom as many as 3% will commit suicide, risk stratification has provided little value in efforts to decrease the number of patients who will kill themselves after discharge (Large et al. 2011).

Screening

Among adults aged 55 and older who take their lives 77% have seen their primary care provider within 1 year and 58% within a month of their deaths (Luoma et al., 2002). As a result screening for suicidal ideation among primary care patients seems appealing as a model to examine the potential benefits of screening patients in specialty care or with illnesses associated with risk of suicide. However, there is controversy over the extent to which passive thoughts of death predict risk of active suicidal ideation. Thoughts of death may represent a realistic appraisal in the context of life-threatening illness or extreme old age, so that care must be taken to distinguish death ideation from suicidal thought. Yet in a study of antidepressant treatment for recurrent depressive disorder, Szanto et al. (1996) found patients with passive suicidal thoughts were as pessimistic about the future as those with active thoughts but denied intent to harm themselves. As treatment continued, active suicidal thoughts became passive before disappearing entirely suggesting a continuum of risk and the utility of questions for passive thoughts of death.

Collaborative studies in primary care settings have used passive suicidal ideation as a target of intervention. PROSPECT, The Prevention of Suicide in Primary Care Elderly: Collaborative Trial (Bruce et al., 2004) and IMPACT, the Improving Mood: Promoting Access to Collaborative Treatment for Depression in Primary Care (Unützer et al., 2006) studies identified patients as having suicidal ideation if they endorsed a "weak desire to live today," the first item from the Scale for Suicidal Ideation (Beck et al., 1979). This threshold was chosen in light of Brown et al.'s (2000) finding that psychiatric patients aged 55 and older with "weak desire to live today" exhibited a 15.5-fold increased risk of suicide compared to those who did not. The intervention which integrated specially trained mental health personnel into the primary care setting, monitored adherence to antidepressant guidelines, and made psychotherapy and psychiatric consultation readily available significantly reduced but did not eliminate depression and suicidality.

Bauer et al. (2013) examined a primary care population of more than 11 000 disadvantaged "safety-net" primary care patients, persons with an elevated prevalence of substance abuse and other mental disorders. They found more than 45.5% exhibited suicidal ideation as defined by a positive response to the ninth item of the Patient Health Questionaire-9 (PHQ-9). The ninth item of the PHQ-9 asks about "thoughts that you would be better off dead, or of hurting yourself in some way" in the previous 2 weeks and does not mention suicide explicitly. More than 10% of the patients studied had admitted to suicidal ideation almost every day. Of those who experienced suicidal ideation "nearly every day," only 2% did not endorse clinically significant mood disturbance or anhedonia and only 3% scored less than the clinically significant symptom threshold score of 10. Of those with suicidal ideation at least "several days" during the previous 2 weeks, 12.3% scored below 10. However, they did not report the number of patients who were found to have active thoughts of suicide as assessed during follow-up clinical encounters.

Walker and associates (2011) performed follow-up telephone interviews of 330 cancer center patients who with the self-report version of the PHQ-9 acknowledged "thoughts you might be better off dead or harming yourself." When contacted by telephone one-third of the group denied those thoughts, one-third acknowledged them but denied thoughts of "suicide," and the remaining third reported explicit thoughts of suicide. Persons who indicated they had "thoughts you might be better off dead or harming yourself" more than half the days in the last 2 weeks were more likely to express explicit suicidal ideation. However, 23% of those (54/235) who confirmed the thoughts had occurred for "several days" and as a result scored only one on the item were also found to have suicidal thoughts. In short one-third of persons reporting passive thoughts of death will acknowledge active suicidal ideation when interviewed and the more frequent the passive thoughts of death the more likely they are to express thoughts of suicide.

To determine if death ideation was associated with other markers of elevated risk for suicide, Van Orden et al. (2013) used latent class analyses within a population-based cross-sectional study of community residents aged 85 and older in Gothenberg, Sweden. Both death ideation and thoughts of suicide were measured with the scale of Paykel et al. (1974) which reads:

> Have you ever felt that life was not worth living? 2) Have you ever wished you were dead? – for instance, that you could go to sleep and not wake up? 3) Have you ever thought of taking your life, even if you would not really do it? 4) Have you ever reached the point where you seriously considered taking your life or perhaps made plans how you would go about doing it? 5) Have you ever made an attempt to take your life?

Two distinct groups of older persons expressing thoughts of death emerged. First were those with high present levels of depressive symptoms and anxiety. The second group included persons with more distant histories of suicidal thought. As such both groups with death ideation exhibited risk factors associated with suicidal behavior.

In summary, most older persons with passive thoughts of death will not acknowledge thoughts of suicide but are at risk nonetheless. Thoughts of death may represent the patient's relative status on a continuum of risk. The PHQ-9, which is widely used in primary care, seems a reasonable screen for depression, thoughts of death, and suicidal ideation in specialty care settings as well.

Conclusion

Physically ill persons particularly those with cancer, HIV/AIDS, Huntington's disease, traumatic injury to the central nervous system, and epilepsy are at increased risk for suicidality. Nonetheless the overwhelming majority of persons with these conditions are never suicidal. And while mental disorders may be prevalent comorbid conditions, their relationship to suicidality in the context of physical illness is not straightforward. Neither a psychosocial nor biomedical theory of how physical illness elevates risk of suicide seems common to the illnesses described. However, TBI with its antecedent behavioral risk factors as well as disrupted neural circuitry is a useful example for both universal and selective preventive interventions. Use of tobacco and excess alcohol, accident prone behaviors, head trauma, and unprotected sex are legitimate targets of universal preventive interventions that would indirectly lower the risk of suicide associated with physical illnesses. Screening physically ill persons with a depressive symptom assessment such as the PHQ-9 which has a query approximating suicidality seems a reasonable selective intervention. Adding a history of hospitalization would further refine the selection process. Nonetheless as demonstrated by both the PROSPECT and IMPACT studies, sizeable efforts will be required to achieve detectable benefits.

References

Bauer, A. M., Chan, Y.-F., Huang, H., Vannoy, S., & Unützer, J. (2013). Characteristics, management, and depression outcomes of primary care patients who endorse thoughts of death or suicide on the PHQ-9. *Journal of General Internal Medicine*, **28**(3), 363–369. doi: 10.1007/s11606-012-2194-2

Beck, A. T., Kovacs, M., & Weissman, A. (1979). Assessment of suicidal intention: The scale for suicidal ideation. *Journal of Consulting and Clinical Psychology*, **47**, 343–352.

Brown, G. K., Beck, A. T., Steer, R. A., & Grisham, J. R. (2000). Risk factors for suicide in psychiatric outpatients: a 20-year prospective study. *Journal of Consulting Clinical Psychology*, **68**, 371–377.

Bruce, M. L., Ten Have, T. R., Reynolds, C. F., 3rd, et al. (2004). Reducing suicidal ideation and depressive symptoms in depressed older primary care patients: a randomized controlled trial. *JAMA*, **291**(9), 1081–1091.

Fang, F., Fall, K., Mittleman, M. A., et al. (2012). Suicide and cardiovascular death after a cancer diagnosis. *New England Journal of Medicine*, **366**(14), 1310–1318.

Haw, C., Harwood, D., & Hawton, K. (2009). Dementia and suicidal behavior: a review of the literature. *International Psychogeriatrics*, **21**(3), 440–453.

Heneghan, H. M., Heinberg, L., Windover, A., Rogula, T., & Schauer, P. R. (2012). Weighing the evidence for an association between obesity and suicide risk. *Surgery of Obesity and Related Disorders*, **8**(1), 98–107.

Hesdorffer, D. C., Ishihara, L., Mynepalli, L., et al. (2012). Epilepsy, suicidality, and psychiatric disorders: a bidirectional association. *Annals of Neurology*, **72**(2), 184–191.

Jia, C. X., Mehlum, L., & Qin, P. (2012). AIDS/HIV infection, comorbid psychiatric illness, and risk for subsequent suicide: a nationwide register linkage study. *Journal of Clinical Psychiatry*, **73**(10), 1315–1321.

Kishi, Y., Robinson, R. G., & Kosier, J. T. (2001). Suicidal ideation among patients with acute life-threatening physical illness: patients with stroke, traumatic brain injury, myocardial infarction, and spinal cord injury. *Psychosomatics*, **42**(5), 382–390.

Large, M., Sharma, S., Cannon, E., Ryan, C., & Nielssen, O. (2011). Risk factors for suicide within a year of discharge from psychiatric hospital: a systematic meta-analysis. *Australia and New Zealand Journal of Psychiatry*, **45**(8), 619–628.

Lin, H. C., Wu, C. H., & Lee, H. C. (2009). Risk factors for suicide following hospital discharge among cancer patients. *Psychooncology*, **18**(10), 1038–1044.

Luoma, J. B., Martin, C. E., & Pearson, J. L. (2002). Contact with mental health and primary care providers before suicide: a review of the evidence. *American Journal of Psychiatry*, **159**(6), 909–916.

McKee, A. C., Cantu, R. C., Nowinski, C. J., et al. (2009). Chronic traumatic encephalopathy in athletes: progressive tauopathy following repetitive head injury. *Journal of Neuropathology Experimental Neurology*, **68**(7), 709–735.

Paulsen, J. S., Nehl, C., Hoth, H. F., et al. (2005). Depression and stages of Huntington's disease. *Journal of Neuropsychiatry & Clinical Neurosciences*, **17**(4), 496–502.

Paykel, E. S., Myers, J. K., Lindenthal, J. J., et al. (1974). Suicidal feelings in the general population: a prevalence study. *British Journal of Psychiatry*, **124**, 460–469.

Pompili, M., Forte, A., Palermo, M., et al. (2012). Suicide risk among patients with MS: a systematic review of the current literature. *Journal of Psychosomatic Research*, **73**(6), 411–417.

Scott, K. M., Hwang, I., Chiu, W.-T., et al. (2010). Chronic physical conditions and their association with first onset of suicidal behavior in the world mental health surveys. *Psychosomatic Medicine*, **72**(7), 712–719.

Surgeon General. (2012). *National Strategy for Suicide Prevention: Goals and Objectives for Action: A Report of the US Surgeon General and of the National Action Alliance for Suicide Prevention.* Editors: Office of the Surgeon General (US); National Action Alliance for Suicide Prevention (US). Washington, DC: US Department of Health & Human Services (US), Publications and Reports of the Surgeon General.

Szanto, K., Reynolds, C. F., Frank, E., et al. (1996). Suicide in elderly depressed patients: Is active vs. passive suicidal ideation a clinically valid distinction? *American Journal of Geriatric Psychiatry*, **4**(3), 197–207.

Unützer, J., Tang, L., Oishi, S., et al. (2006). Reducing suicidal ideation in depressed older primary care patients. *Journal of the American Geriatric Society*, **54**, 1550–1556.

Van Orden, K. A., Simning, A., Conwell, Y., Skoog, I., & Waern, M. (2013). Characteristics and comorbid symptoms of older adults reporting death ideation. *American Journal of Geriatric Psychiatry*. **21**(8), 803–810.

Walker, J., Hansen, C. H., Butcher, I., et al. (2011). Thoughts of death and suicide reported by cancer patients who endorsed the "suicidal thoughts" item of the PHQ-9 during routine screening for depression. *Psychosomatics*, **52**(5), 424–427.

Wasserman, L., Shaw, T., Vu, M., et al. (2008). An overview of traumatic brain injury and suicide. *Brain Injury*, **22**(11), 811–819.

Webb, R. T., Kontopantelis, E., Doran, T., et al. (2012). Suicide risk in primary care patients with major physical diseases. a case-control study. *Archives of General Psychiatry*, **69**(3), 256–264.

Chapter 25

Suicide in the criminal justice system

Steve Leifman and Tim Coffey

Introduction

On August 24, 2011, the Civil Rights Division of the United States Department of Justice (DOJ) notified officials in Miami-Dade County, Florida of findings from a more than 3-year investigation into conditions in county correctional facilities (Department of Justice, 2011). The investigation was initiated pursuant to the Civil Rights of Institutionalized Persons Act (CRIPA) following a series of troubling reports calling into questions the health and safety of individuals in the custody of the Miami-Dade Corrections and Rehabilitation Department (MDCR). Concerns over dangerous conditions in the jail, including repeated instances of suicide and serious self-injury, had been profiled by numerous local, national, and international media outlets. In addition, in 2005 the Miami-Dade County Grand Jury issued a scathing report detailing the crisis of people with serious mental illnesses who become entangled in the criminal justice system (Miami-Dade County Grand Jury, 2005). As part of their investigation, the Grand Jury toured the psychiatric unit of the jail, including the area housing individuals deemed to be acutely suicidal. Conditions were described as follows:

> The setting and the cells were cold and stark. Plexiglas covered the doors to allow correctional officers full, direct and unobstructed views into the cells at all times. The persons detained in these cells were at risk for suicide and were under almost constant watch with bed checks every 15 minutes. The lights are on in the cells 24 hours a day and many of us found the area to be extremely cold. The beds are made of metal. To help prevent suicides, the cells are devoid of any items that could assist in that effort. Thus, no sheets, mattresses, toiletries or clothing is allowed. Neither are books, pens, papers or recreational activities. There is absolutely nothing for these inmates to do as they are confined to their cells. The inmates are offered [safety] garments, if they choose to wear them. Notwithstanding all of these precautions, the seriously disturbed inmates still find ways to harm themselves. These include diving off the bed onto the concrete floor and banging one's head against the wall.
>
> (p. 12)

The outcome of the DOJ investigation confirmed many of the findings of the Grand Jury and went on to conclude that conditions within MDCR violated inmates' constitutional rights to be protected from harm and serious risk of harm. Furthermore, it was found that because of these violations, inmates had suffered grievous bodily harm, including death. Among the primary findings of the DOJ was that, "MDCR is deliberately indifferent to the suicide risks and serious mental health needs of its prisoners. At least eight prisoners have committed suicide since 2007, and thousands of prisoners have suffered from inadequate mental health crisis services" (Department of Justice, 2011, p. 1).

The investigation identified numerous areas of deficiency including inadequate screening and assessment at the time of booking, poor communication among correctional officers and health care staff, failure to properly observe and assess individuals at risk of suicide, and failure to provide adequate suicide prevention training. In addition, the physical environments within areas of the jail designated to house inmates identified to be acutely suicidal were found not only to be counter-therapeutic, but in some cases conducive to self-harm. For example, cells designated to house females on suicide watch contained fixtures and protrusions from which ligatures could easily be attached, and blind spots prevented continuous observation of acutely suicidal individuals.

A Concise Guide to Understanding Suicide, ed. Stephen H. Koslow, Pedro Ruiz, and Charles B. Nemeroff. Published by Cambridge University Press.

In some respects the DOJ's findings in Miami-Dade County were not surprising in that they simply validated what had been widely reported by the media and what many, particularly those who work in the criminal justice system, already knew. Had this been an isolated occurrence, limited to the shortcomings of a single local jail system, it would have been no less alarming, but at least it could have been regarded simply as an outlier system in much need of remediation. Unfortunately, this investigation was just one of the more recent examples of correctional systems across the USA which fail to adequately recognize and anticipate the heightened risks of suicidal behavior and self-harm that are disproportionately characteristic of detention populations.

Since 1998, the DOJ's Civil Rights Division has conducted at least 34 investigations of adult and juvenile correctional facilities in which findings revealed inadequate suicide prevention and/or deliberate indifference to suicide risk (US Department of Justice, n.d.). Furthermore, these investigations appear to be occurring with increasing frequency. In most cases, investigations reveal patterns of systemic failures to adequately screen for suicide risk upon admission to facilities and over the course of detention, provide appropriate referral and treatment for individuals identified to be at risk of suicide, and to provide requisite training in suicide assessment and prevention for correctional officers and correctional health care staff.

According to the DOJ (Department of Justice, 2011), constitutional requirements and generally accepted professional standards for correctional mental health care mandate the development of suicide prevention standards in correctional settings. These standards require eight critical components of suicide prevention policies: (1) suicide prevention education and training for all correctional officers and correctional health care personnel; (2) appropriate screening measures to assess suicide risk; (3) appropriate housing placement for individuals identified to be at risk of suicide; (4) appropriate assessment, observation, and monitoring of individuals identified to be at risk; (5) referrals to mental health providers and facilities; (6) appropriate communication between correctional officers and correctional health care personnel; (7) appropriate intervention measures addressing procedures for how to respond to suicide attempts; and (8) appropriate notification, reporting, and review if a suicide does occur.

Prevalence and characteristics of suicide in correctional settings

The impact of suicide in a correctional setting goes far beyond the tragedy visited upon the victim. It is a traumatic event in an already stressful environment that can have lasting impacts on those who work in correctional settings and other detainees or inmates who may witness or be in proximity to the victim. Beyond the correctional setting, there can be long reaching effects including impacts on family members and friends of the victim, civil actions and lawsuits brought against institutions and governments, scrutiny by the media, civil rights organizations, and regulatory bodies, and even political scandal. For these reasons, there is considerable interest in ensuring correctional facilities implement appropriate screening and prevention measures to protect both detainees and the institutions in which they are housed.

Suicide is one of the most common causes of death in correctional settings (US Department of Health and Human Services (DHHS), 2012), and is more common among people with histories of involvement in the criminal justice system than among the general population (Pratt et al., 2006; Kariminia et al., 2007; Webb et al., 2011). In local jails, which are typically operated by counties or local municipalities and house individuals newly arrested, those awaiting arraignment, trial, or other court hearings, and those sentenced to relatively short periods of incarceration (generally one year or less), suicide is the leading cause of death. In prisons, which are operated by state and federal governments and house individuals convicted of felonies and sentenced to greater than 1 year of incarceration, suicide is the fifth leading cause of death.

Factors that may influence suicidal thoughts or behaviors in correctional settings can be thought of as including a broad array of individual and environmental influences (Hassan, 1996; WHO, 2007; US DHHS, 2012). These influences include personal risk factors that the individual brings into the correctional setting such as age, gender, psychiatric and substance use disorders, past suicide attempts, and social disenfranchisement. In addition, elements of the physical layout of correctional settings, as well as policies and procedures that may be in place to screen for and respond to individuals at risk of suicide, can influence the likelihood of individuals engaging in acts of self-harm. Environmental and institutional stressors may include undesirable housing placement or work assignment, disciplinary actions, conflicts with staff or other inmates, and legal problems or setbacks (Daniel, 2006).

There is considerable variability across correctional settings, both with respect to the physical environment and the custodial population housed, which may influence suicide risk (WHO, 2007). The size and location of the correctional facility (e.g., large state prison vs. small town jail, urban county lockup vs. rural work camp), legal status of detainees (e.g., pretrial defendants vs. sentenced prisoners), length of incarceration (e.g., short-term detainees in local jails vs. inmates serving long prison terms), criminal history of the population, physical environment (e.g., sanitation, crowding, isolation, availability of purposeful activities), access to health care and mental health services, staffing patterns, and psychosocial factors all have an influence on the likelihood individuals may attempt to harm themselves (US DHHS, 2012). In addition, by the very nature of the population served in correctional settings (i.e., predominantly younger males with high rates of substance abuse, mental illnesses, antisocial personality traits, poor family/social support, histories of violence and/or trauma, self-injurious behaviors, impulsive aggression, and risk-taking behaviors), custodial populations tend to experience many more risk factors for suicide than does the general population (Blaauw et al., 2005; Daniel, 2006).

The experience of being arrested and incarcerated is highly stressful and deprives individuals of important resources, which may intensify existing vulnerabilities (Felthous, 1994; Daniel, 2006). In addition to loss of freedom, incarceration may result in real or perceived loss of family and social support. Incarceration also often instills fear and uncertainty about the future, and the possibility of being victimized physically or sexually. Arrest and incarceration may also trigger an overwhelming sense of shame and embarrassment. Combined with environmental stressors such as single cell isolation or overcrowding in hostile surroundings, these stressors may exceed one's capacity to cope (WHO, 2007). Furthermore, prolonged periods of incarceration increase the likelihood of experiencing conflict with other inmates or the institution, victimization, and/or legal frustration, which may lead to physical or emotional breakdown.

Most suicides in correctional settings occur by hanging or asphyxiation during night and weekend shifts when staffing levels are often reduced (Daniel, 2006; WHO, 2007; Hayes, 2010). Materials that may be used as ligatures include bedding, shoelaces, belts, socks, elastic waistbands, and bandages. Blood flow to the brain can be disrupted with less than 5 pounds of pressure applied to the neck. As such, death by asphyxiation can be accomplished while kneeling, sitting, standing, or lying (Daniel, 2006). Permanent brain damage can occur in as little as 3 minutes, with death occurring in as little as 5 to 7 minutes.

Suicide risk is also strongly related to placement in single cell housing (Daniel, 2006; Hayes, 2010). One study of 48 suicides occurring in the New York City Department of Correction over an 8-year period found that 91% of deaths occurred in cells in which inmates were housed alone (Marcus & Alcabes, 1993). Placement in single cell housing appears to be particularly conducive to suicide risk if it involves isolation from others for long periods of time, such as administrative segregation where individuals are often confined alone in cells for 23 hours per day (Daniel, 2006).

Psychosocial factors associated with suicide risk include lack of family or social support, history of attempted suicide (particularly within the past 2 years), history of mental illness, history of substance abuse, history of trauma or victimization, recent inmate to inmate conflict, recent disciplinary action, and adverse information such as loss of gain time or disruption of family or social support outside of the correctional facility (Way et al., 2005; Daniel, 2006).

The first national study of suicides in county and local jails was completed by the National Center on Institutions and Alternatives (NCIA) using data collected in 1979 (Hayes & Rowan, 1988). Findings documented 419 suicides nationwide. Average age of victims was 28 years, 67% were white, 97% were male, and 54% were single. Seventy-four percent of victims were charged with non-violent offenses, and 30% were charged with alcohol- and/or drug-related offenses. Ninety-one percent of victims were held in pre-trial detention. At the time of death, 59% of victims were under the influence of drugs or alcohol and 68% were held in isolation. Fifty percent of victims died within the first 24 hours, with 27% occurring within the first 3 hours. Thirty percent had a known history of a mental illness and 17% had a known history of suicide attempt. Ninety-six percent of deaths were the result of hangings or asphyxiation.

Since the problem of suicide in correctional settings was first examined more than 30 years ago, considerable effort has been devoted to promoting awareness of suicide in jails and prisons, and developing more effective screening tools, prevention measures, and interventions. More recent investigations suggest these efforts have had an impact on some aspects of correctional suicide, while other aspects have remained more or less enduring.

Examining data from 2005 and 2006, the NCIA replicated their previous investigations and documented a total of 696 (366 in 2005 and 330 in 2006) suicides in county and local jails (Hayes, 2010). Similar to previous findings, 76% of victims were white, 93% were male, 91% were held in pre-trial detention, and 93% of deaths were the result of hanging or asphyxiation. Unlike previous findings, the average age of victims was somewhat older at 35 years. Previous research indicated more than half of victims were single, however more recent findings revealed only 42% of victims were single. Whereas previous findings indicated roughly three-quarters of victims were charged with non-violent offenses, updated findings revealed that 43% of victims, the largest segment of offense categories, were charged with violent offenses, whereas just over half were charged with non-violent offenses. Nineteen percent were charged with drug or alcohol-related offenses. At the time of death, 20% of victims were under the influence of drugs- or alcohol, as compared to roughly 60% in previous investigations. While two-thirds of suicides previously documented occurred while victims were housed in isolation, 38% of suicides occurred under such placement in the updated sample. Previous findings indicated that roughly half of suicides occurred within the first 24 hours. Current findings indicate that 23% of suicides occurred within the first 24 hours, with 27% occurring within the first 2–14 days and 20% occurring during the first 1–4 months. Victims were also more likely to have a known history of mental illnesses and prior suicide attempts at 38% and 34% respectively.

More recent investigation has also developed additional estimates of suicides in correctional settings to include both local jails and state and federal prisons (Mumola, 2005; Noonan, 2012). Findings indicate that while the populations housed in these correctional settings are at increased risk of self-harm compared to the general population, there are important differences in rates and patterns of suicidal behavior. According to the Bureau of Justice Statistics (BJS), roughly 300 suicides occur in local jails annually accounting for nearly one-third of all fatalities. By contrast, roughly 200 suicides occur annually in state prisons accounting for approximately 6% of all fatalities.

Whereas the rate of suicide among the general population is estimated to be 12 per 100 000 (Hoyert & Xu, 2012), the rates of suicide in jails and state prisons are 42 per 100 000 and 16 per 100 000 respectively (Noonan, 2012). As such, suicide among jail detainees is nearly three and a half times that of the general population and more than two and a half times that of state prison inmates. Suicide among state prison inmates is approximately one-third more common than among the general population; however some of the difference between these rates is likely accounted for by demographic differences among these populations including age and gender.

Suicide rates in the general population are higher among certain age groups. For example adults aged 25 to 44 are observed to commit suicide at a rate of just under 15 per 100 000, one-quarter more often than the general population (Hoyert & Xu, 2012). Among state and federal prison inmates, 60% of all inmates are between the ages of 25 and 44 years old (Carson & Sabol, 2012). Likewise, 60% of individuals who commit suicide in local jails and state prisons are also between the ages of 25 and 44 years old (Noonan, 2012).

Similarly, rates of suicide in the general population among males are four times higher than among females, accounting for 79% of all suicide deaths in the USA (Centers for Disease Control, 2012). Within correctional settings, males constitute the vast majority of inmates in local jails (87%; Minton, 2013) and state and federal prisons (93%; Carson & Sabol, 2012). Males also account for the vast majority of suicide deaths in local jails (88%) and state prisons (96%; Noonan, 2012).

Care should be taken when interpreting difference in rates of suicide between jail and prison inmates. The average daily population of detainees in local jails in the USA is approximately 736 000, whereas the average daily population of inmates in state and federal prisons is 1.5 million (Glaze & Parks, 2012). During the 12-month period ending June 30, 2012, local jails admitted roughly 11.6 million individuals (Minton, 2013). By contrast, during 2011, state and federal prisons admitted 668 800 individuals (Carson & Sabol, 2012). As such, annual admissions to local jails are equal to nearly 16 times the average daily population of these facilities, each of which could be at risk of suicide while in custody, whereas annual admissions to state and local prisons are equal to only about 44% of the average daily population.

Considering the significant growth in correctional populations over the past 30 years, it is notable that the number of annual suicides in correctional settings appears to have decreased. The average daily population of individuals detained in local jails for the 12 months ending June 30, 1985 was 265 000 (Bureau of Justice Statistics, 1985). During the 1985 calendar year, the NCIA identified a total of 453 suicides occurring in local jails (Hayes & Rowan, 1988). This is equivalent to a suicide rate of 171 per 100 000 detainees. For the 12 months ending June 30, 2011, the average daily population of individuals detained in local jails was 736 000 (Minton, 2013). Had the rate of suicide in jails remained proportionate to the average daily population, we would expect to see roughly 1250 suicides occur annually. Instead, the average number of suicides in local jails between 2000 and 2010 was observed to be 290, with a slight increase in recent years. This represents a 75% decrease in the jail suicide rate and suggests that significant advances have been made in the areas of suicide assessment and prevention in correctional settings.

Interventions and suicide precautions

While the causes of suicide are complex and not well understood, and the ability to accurately and reliably predict who will attempt suicide is not possible, it is clear these incidents occur in the context of highly stressful life events and that some people are more vulnerable to self-harm in these situations than others (WHO, 2007). Using data from the first national study of jail suicide, the NCIA developed the very first risk profile describing the population observed to be at greatest risk for suicide in jail settings:

> The victim was most likely to be a 22-year-old White, single male. He would have been arrested for public intoxication, the only offense leading to his arrest, and would thereby be under the influence of alcohol and/or drugs upon incarceration. Further, the victim would not have had a significant history of prior arrests. He would have been taken to an urban county jail and immediately placed in isolation for his own protection and/or surveillance. However, less than three hours after incarceration, he would be dead. He would have hanged himself with material from his bed (i.e., sheet or pillowcase). The incident would have taken place on a Saturday night in September, between the hours of midnight and 1:00 a.m. Jail staff would have found the victim, they say, within 15 minutes of the suicide. Later, jail records would indicate that the victim did not have a history of mental illness or previous suicide attempts.
>
> (Hayes & Rowan, 1988, p. 12)

To date, most efforts to develop suicide prevention and risk assessment strategies in correctional settings have focused on identifying common characteristics among people who attempt or complete suicide while in detention; as well as common elements of situations and circumstances in which suicide attempts occur. As such, research has focused less on attempting to identify underlying causes of suicidal behavior, and more on identifying individual and situational indicators that may be used to generate risk profiles.

The use of such profiles has been criticized by some as quick fixes and superficial interventions that can be misleading, causing correctional personnel to believe that risk factors can reliably predict behavior and overlooking individuals who do not mirror the profile. Furthermore, in some instances risk profiles may simply reflect broader characteristics of the local detention population making reliance on such indicators less useful (Hayes, 2010).

Those who defend the use of risk profiles argue that they are not intended to predict behavior, but to sensitize correctional personnel to characteristics most frequently associated with the population of individuals known to engage in suicidal behavior. As such, risk profiles are intended to be tools to aid the identification of potentially at risk individuals, but not as a basis for such decisions (WHO, 2007; Hayes, 2010). Regardless of philosophy, numerous studies have demonstrated many risk factors to be highly consistent over time and across communities (Blaauw et al., 2005).

While research has been effective in identifying common characteristics among correctional populations known to attempt or complete suicide, the utility of these findings to predict individual suicide risk has proven elusive. Part of the problem is that many characteristics of detainees and inmates who engage in suicidal behavior are shared by many more individuals in correctional settings who do not engage in self-harm (WHO, 2007; Hayes, 2010). As such, while characteristics indicative of increased risk of suicide have been identified, our inability to more accurately and reliably measure these traits in a way that distinguishes those who are highly likely to engage in suicidal behavior from those who are not, necessarily results in risk assessments that are often overly inclusive and, therefore, of limited useful utility.

Current requirements for correctional facilities to implement programs and policies to screen individuals for suicide risk upon admission and to provide appropriate levels of care have resulted not only from research which has increased awareness of correctional suicide, but also from litigation which has helped to define constitutional requirements and professional standards for health care services provided to custodial populations. In 1980, the Fifth Circuit Court of Appeals ruled in the case of *Ruiz v. Estelle* that correctional facilities were required to screen for suicide and provide treatment for those found to be at risk (Ruiz v. Estelle, 1980). As a result, the National Commission for Correctional Health Care (NCCHC), which is the main accrediting body for correctional health care providers, now requires all correctional facilities to incorporate suicide prevention policies and programs as a requirement of accreditation.

In general, elements of suicide prevention policies and programs in correctional settings must include adequate screening and assessment, observation and monitoring of individuals found to be at risk, mental health treatment including use of psychotherapeutic medications, effective communication between correctional officers and correctional health care personnel, modification of physical environment to reduce opportunities for behavior, education and training for all staff, and processes for reporting and review of suicides or serious suicide attempts that occur (Hayes, 2010).

Initial screening for suicide can be the single most important measure taken to identify individuals at risk of suicide, especially in jail settings (Felthous & Holzer, 2006). Screening should always be conducted in such a way to ensure as much privacy as possible, and should include questions about both current and past thoughts of suicide and suicide attempts, any specific plan to harm oneself, past treatment for psychiatric needs, recent losses of a significant nature (e.g., job, family member, close friend), and family history of suicide (Hayes, 2010). Screening should also include notations about physical appearance and any previous admissions to the facility that involved concerns about suicide risk or mental health needs (Felthous, 1994; Hayes, 2010). In addition, whenever possible input from the law enforcement officer transporting the individual should be collected to determine if there were any behaviors or statements made suggesting possible suicide risk.

In many correctional settings, initial screening for suicide risk is completed by correctional officers as part of the booking or reception process. Often, this entails the use of a brief screening instrument which is scored based on the number of suicide risk factors endorsed. Referral for more in-depth assessment is made if the total score exceeds a predetermined threshold. It is important that correctional officers completing such screening measures also receive instruction to refer for further assessment if individuals endorse specific risk factors such as having current thoughts of suicide, even if the threshold score for referral is not reached (Felthous & Holzer, 2006).

Initial screening for suicide risk among all individuals entering correctional settings is critically important. Unfortunately, if this information is not well communicated to others, it may end up playing a relatively small role in the prevention of actual suicide attempts (WHO, 2007). The reason for this is that the purposes of screening tools are simply to identify individuals who may be at increased risk of attempting suicide at some point during their incarceration. They are not intended to predict when or under what circumstance attempts may occur. In many settings, lack of comprehensive suicide precautions across the continuum of incarceration creates gaps in care and opportunities to identify inmates and detainees who may be at risk of suicide. For example, a jail may assess for suicide at the time of booking; however, if there is inadequate follow-up for individuals identified to be at risk – poor communication among staff, lack of policies and procedures ensuring individuals are reassessed over time, staffing shortages, or lack of adequate staff training in suicide prevention – then there are opportunities for individuals to fall through the cracks. Beyond initial screening, it is important that effective policies and practices be in place for ongoing assessment, monitoring, observation, and treatment. Suicide screening and assessment should be ongoing. Because of the many factors which may influence suicidal thoughts or behavior in correctional settings, it is important to reassess individuals over time, particularly if changes are observed which suggest an individual may be experiencing increased levels of distress (Hayes, 2010).

Monitoring of individuals identified to be at high-risk of suicidal behavior in correctional settings can be particularly challenging, particularly in situations or at times of day when there may be more limited staff available. Ideally, a person considered to be at high risk of suicide should receive constant one-on-one monitoring. Unfortunately, the demands of a correctional setting and limited staffing resources often make this impossible. As an alternative, many institutions rely on frequent, but not constant, observation; usually at staggered intervals of at most every 15 minutes. However, given that a suicide attempt by hanging can result in permanent brain damage in as little as 3 minutes and death can occur in 5 to 7 minutes, this frequent, but not constant, monitoring may still be inadequate to effectively prevent suicides (Daniel, 2006).

Hayes (2010) recommends two levels of observation for suicidal inmates. The first involves close observation of individuals who are not acutely suicidal, but may have expressed suicidal thoughts, exhibited recent suicidal behavior, or may be exhibiting non-verbal signs of suicide risk despite denial of suicidal ideations. These individuals should be placed in a cell, free of protrusions, with frequent, staggered monitoring, not to exceed every 10 minutes. The second level of observation involves constant, one-on-one observation of individuals who are either actively threatening self-harm or are engaging in suicidal behavior. Hayes also points out that other aids such as cameras, inmate companions, and cellmates can be used to supplement monitoring of suicidal individuals, but should never serve as a substitute for staff observation.

Screening, assessment, and monitoring alone will not be sufficient to protect individuals from harming or attempting to harm themselves if adequate measures are not taken to ensure effective communication in correctional settings. Because indications of suicide risk may be transient and not readily apparent to all individuals who come into contact with a person contemplating self-harm, it is important that policies and procedures be in place to alert others who may be in a position to prevent a suicide attempt. Hayes (2010) identifies three critical areas where effective communication is necessary: communication between the arresting or transporting officer and correctional staff at booking or reception; communication between staff working within correctional facilities, including correctional officers, health care staff, and mental health staff; and communication between staff working in correctional facilities and individuals who are experiencing suicidal thoughts. Each of these types of interaction provides the opportunity to communicate key information which may prevent thoughts of suicide from escalating to a suicide attempt.

The physical environment of correctional settings also plays a critical role in facilitating or inhibiting suicidal behavior. Careful attention should be paid to ensure that cells designed to house inmates who are at risk of suicide do not contain protruding fixtures from which ligatures can be attached, or blind spots that may block observation. Housing units should also contain emergency response kits including first aid supplies and a rescue tool that can be used to cut through materials used as ligatures (Hayes, 2010).

In general, it is recommended that individuals identified to be acutely suicidal should not be placed in isolation or segregation units unless absolutely necessary for the physical safety of the individual or other inmates. Such placement does not promote improved mental health (Hayes, 2010). Ideally, an individual who is experiencing thoughts of suicide should be housed in a setting that provides opportunities for social contact and close observation.

Because of the high-risk of self-harm, inmates placed alone in segregation must always have constant observation, which includes direct visualization of an individual's head and neck (Felthous & Holzer, 2006). Such observation not only helps to ensure that individuals do not have the ability to harm themselves when no one is looking, but it also provides social contact for the individual which may lessen feelings of isolation, alienation, and loss of social support (Felthous, 1994). It is important that staff interact with suicidal individuals in these situations, and not just observe (Hayes, 2010).

It is also important that decisions about what privileges and property individuals are allowed to have are based on clinical justifications and made on a case by case basis. While there may be times when concerns for an individual's safety mean that any and all properties, including clothing and bedding, must be removed, doing so without adequate clinical support can serve to exacerbate an already critical situation. Such measures should be taken only as a last resort when there is an imminent risk of self-harm (Hayes, 2010).

It is recommended that all staff working in correctional settings – including correctional officers, mental health, and health care staff – receive initial training in suicide prevention, followed by annual refresher training (WHO, 2007). All training should include mock drills to ensure efficiency and mastery of response. At minimum, initial suicide prevention training should include the following components: staff and administration attitudes toward suicide and impact this has on prevention; elements of correctional environments that are conducive to suicide; potential predisposing factors for suicide; high-risk suicide periods; warning signs and symptoms; identification of suicidal individuals who deny risk; recent suicides and/or serious suicide attempts; components of the facility's suicide prevention policy, and liability issues (Hayes, 2010). In addition, all staff who have regular contact with inmates or detainees should receive training in basic first aid and cardiopulmonary resuscitation, as well as the use of emergency equipment located on housing units. It is also important to ensure adequate staffing to allow for ongoing in-service training, as well as correctional and clinical coverage.

Finally, it is important for correctional facilities to conduct multidisciplinary morbidity/mortality reviews for all suicides and serious suicide attempts. These reviews should focus on reviewing the circumstances in which the event occurred, the response of staff members to the event, statements from witnesses and others who had recent contact with the victim, review of mental health and health care records, and any recommendations for changes in policies or procedures to reduce the likelihood of a similar event occurring in the future (DHHS, Hayes, 2010).

Conclusion

Even in the best-run correctional systems, it is nearly impossible to identify and prevent all suicide attempts, and it is possible for a determined individual to kill or seriously harm him- or herself even when the appropriate suicide precautions are in place. That said, the layout, operations, and internal culture of correctional facilities can have a significant impact on the likelihood that an individual in custody will attempt self-harm. The fact that rates of suicide in correctional settings have dropped so precipitously over the past 30 years indicates that significant advances in screening and intervention have been achieved, but there is still more to be accomplished.

As is apparent from the spate of recent DOJ investigations into civil rights violations and suicide risk among individuals in correctional settings, the fact that there are constitutional requirements to protect individuals in custody from harm and risk of harm, along with supporting litigation and legal precedent, does not automatically ensure correctional systems are adequately equipped to respond to the risk of suicide and suicide attempts among detainees and inmates. Review of these investigations suggest that many times the problem is not simply a matter of deliberate indifference, but rather systemic failures to adopt comprehensive policies and procedures, across the continuum of incarceration, to identify and respond to individuals at risk of suicide. As a result, while many systems may do a perfectly adequate job of screening and identifying individuals at admission, the failure to effectively communicate this information to other parts of the system means that individuals are unnecessarily exposed to risk of self-harm.

While there are certain recognized elements to suicide prevention policies and programs in correctional settings, there is considerable variability across systems and levels of incarceration. Some of this is necessary in that programs and policies must be flexible and tailored to local needs and circumstances. That said, standard precautions such as the use of validated suicide and mental health screening tools should be adopted by all correctional systems. Once an individual at risk of suicide is identified, it is critical that policies and procedures be in place to ensure appropriate follow-up assessment and treatment is initiated, and that necessary information is communicated among correctional staff who are responsible for ensuring the individual's protection from harm. Finally, it is critical that correctional settings be designed and operated in such a way as to minimize opportunities for self-harm, and that policies and procedures regarding housing and restriction of privileges do not inadvertently exacerbate suicide risk.

References

Blaauw, E., Kerkhof, A. J., & Hayes, L. M. (2005). Demographic, criminal, and psychiatric factors related to inmate suicide. *Suicide and Life-Threatening Behavior*, **35**(1), 63–75.

Bureau of Justice Statistics. (1985). *Jail Inmates: 1985*. Washington, DC: Bureau of Justice Statistics, US Department of Justice.

Carson, E. A., & Sabol, W. J. (2012). *Prisoners in 2011*. Washington, DC: Bureau of Justice Statistics, US Department of Justice.

Centers for Disease Control and Prevention, National Center for Injury Prevention and Control. (2012). Suicide: Facts at a Glance [Fact sheet]. Retrieved from: http://www.cdc.gov/ViolencePrevention/pdf/Suicide_DataSheet-a.pdf

Daniel, A. E. (2006). Preventing suicide in prison: a collaborative responsibility of administrative, custodial, and clinical staff. *Journal of the American Academy of Psychiatry and the Law Online*, **34**(2), 165–175.

Department of Justice (2011). Investigation of the Miami-Dade County Jail [Findings letter]. Retrieved from: http://www.justice.gov/crt/about/spl/documents/Miami-Dade_findlet_8-24-11.pdf.

Felthous, A. R. (1994). Preventing jailhouse suicides. *Journal of the American Academy of Psychiatry and the Law Online*, **22**(4), 477–488.

Felthous, A. R., & Holzer, C. E. (2006). Commentary: carceral suicides – some exceptions and paradoxes. *Journal of the American Academy of Psychiatry and the Law*, **34**(2), 176–178.

Glaze, L. E., & Parks, E. (2012). *Correctional Populations in the United States, 2011*. Washington, DC: Bureau of Justice Statistics, US Department of Justice.

Hassan, R. (1996). Social factors in suicide in Australia. *Trends and Issues in Crime and Criminal Justice*, No. 52. Canberra: Australian Institute of Criminology.

Hayes, L. M. (2010). *National Study of Jail Suicide: 20 Years Later*. Washington, DC: Bureau of Justice Statistics, US Department of Justice.

Hayes, L. M., & Rowan, J. R. (1988). *National Study of Jail Suicides: Seven Years Later*. Alexandria, VA: National Center on Institutions and Alternatives.

Hoyert, D. L., & Xu, J. (2012). Deaths: preliminary data for 2011. *National Vital Statistics Reports*, **61**(6), 1–65.

Kariminia, A., Law, M. G., Butler, T. G., et al. (2007). Suicide risk among recently released prisoners in New South Wales, Australia. *Medical Journal of Australia*, **187**(7), 387–390.

Marcus, P., & Alcabes, P. (1993). Characteristics of suicides by inmates in an urban jail. *Hospital & Community Psychiatry*, **44**(3), 256–261.

Miami-Dade County Grand Jury (2005). *Mental Illness and the Criminal Justice System: A Recipe for Disaster/A Prescription for Improvement*. Miami, FL: Author. Retrieved from: http://www.miamisao.com/publications/grand_jury/2000s/gj2004s.pdf

Minton, T. D. (2013). *Jail Inmates at Midyear 2012 – Statistical Tables (NCJ No. NCJ 241264)*. Washington, DC: Bureau of Justice Statistics, US Department of Justice.

Mumola, C. J. (2005). *Suicide and Homicide in State Prisons and Local Jails*. Washington, DC: Bureau of Justice Statistics, US Department of Justice.

Pratt, D., Piper, M., Appleby, L., Webb, R., & Shaw, J. (2006). Suicide in recently released prisoners: A population-based cohort study. *Lancet*, **368**, 119–123.

Ruiz v. Estelle. (1980). 503 F. Supp. 1265 (S.D. Texas).

US Department of Health and Human Services (DHHS) – Office of the Surgeon General and National Action Alliance for Suicide Prevention (2012). *2012 National Strategy for Suicide Prevention: Goals and Objectives for Action*. Washington, DC: Author.

US Department of Justice (n.d.). Civil Rights Division Special Litigation Section Cases and Matters. Retrieved from: http://www.justice.gov/crt/about/spl/findsettle.php

Way, B. B., Miraglia, R., Sawyer, D. A., Beer, R., & Eddy, J. (2005). Factors related to suicide in New York state prisons. *International Journal of Law and Psychiatry*, **28**(3), 207–221.

Webb, R. T., Qin, P., Stevens, H., et al. (2011). National study of suicide in all people with a criminal justice history. *Archives of General Psychiatry*, **68**(6), 591–599.

World Health Organization (WHO). (2007). *Preventing Suicides in Jails and Prisons*. Geneva: Author.

Chapter 26

Reduction of suicidal behavior in bipolar disorder patients during long-term treatment with lithium

Leonardo Tondo and Ross J. Baldessarini

Background

As many as 90% of suicides occur in persons with a diagnosable psychiatric disorder (Simon & Hales, 2012), often associated with precipitating events. Bipolar disorders as well as severe, recurrent major depression (especially involving psychiatric hospitalization) have the highest standardized mortality ratio (SMR) of any psychiatric disorders, averaging 20 times above the international general population rate of approximately 15/100 000/year (0.015%/year; Tondo et al., 2003; Simon & Hales, 2012). Depressive, and especially mixed (agitated-dysphoric), phases in bipolar disorder patients are far more likely to be associated with suicidal behaviors than depressive or manic periods; suicide is rare in hypomania and poorly evaluated in increasingly recognized, nonbipolar depression with agitation or mixed features (Swann et al., 2013; APA 2013). Moreover, rates of suicides and of suicide attempts (as well as "lethality" as reflected in their ratio [A/S]) are at least as high among type II bipolar disorder patients as in type I cases (Tondo & Baldessarini, 2007; Novick et al., 2010).

Despite the very limited assessment of effects of treatments for bipolar depression on suicidal risk, it remains plausible to expect that such risk can be reduced more effectively by preventing depressive morbidity in bipolar disorder patients rather than treating acute depressive episodes. In general, it is striking that depressive or dysphoric morbidity accounts for three-quarters of the 50% of follow-up weeks ill, even when bipolar disorder patients receive clinically appropriate treatments, and not only in the mid-course of the illness, but also from its onset (Table 26.1).

Effects of antidepressant treatment: the challenge of bipolar depression

Even though suicidal behavior occurs mainly in depressive or dysphoric states in bipolar disorders (Isometsä et al., 1994; Tondo et al. 1998), antidepressant treatments have not been studied for potential therapeutic or adverse effects on suicidal behavior in bipolar disorder patients. This state of knowledge is in keeping with the limited and inconsistent evidence of other clinical benefits of antidepressants in bipolar depression (Yatham et al., 2013; Vázquez et al., 2013; Pacchiarotti et al., 2013). Antidepressants exert a range of effects in depressed bipolar disorder patients that might be expected to worsen suicidal risk. Such an adverse outcome is especially likely in the presence of agitation, dysphoria, restlessness, irritability, anger, and insomnia, which can be induced or worsened by antidepressant treatment (Koukopoulos & Koukopoulos, 1999; Maj et al., 2006; Tondo et al., 2010). Such responses to serotonergic antidepressants may be associated with younger age (Baldessarini et al., 2005; Barbui et al., 2009).

Adverse effects on mood, including agitation, associated with antidepressant treatment may contribute to the high risk of suicidal behavior among type II bipolar disorder patients, many of whom are treated with antidepressants for the prominent depressive component of the disorder. Notably, based on a review by Novick et al. (2010), the meta-analytically pooled rates of suicide attempts among type I (31.9 [CI: 25.6–38.2]%) and type II bipolar disorder patients (30.7 [24.4–37.0]%) in 20 studies did not differ appreciably (random-effects meta-analytic RR = 1.08 [CI: 0.92–1.27], P = 0.33). A more detailed discussion on the

A Concise Guide to Understanding Suicide, ed. Stephen H. Koslow, Pedro Ruiz, and Charles B. Nemeroff. Published by Cambridge University Press.

Table 26.1 Long-term morbidity types in bipolar I disorder patients

Study	Subjects	Percent of time ill		
(year)	(n)	Manic	Depressed	Total
Judd et al., 2002	146	9.90	38.9	38.9
Post et al., 2003	258	11.0	34.1	44.2
Joffe et al., 2004	138	7.70	42.7	49.7
Paykel et al., 2006	204	10.2	43.7	50
Baldessarini et al., 2010	303	14.8	31.0	44.9
DeDios et al., 2010	296	8.60	26.4	34.8
Tondo et al., 2013	236	12.5	20.9	32.3
Vergunst et al., 2013	31	–	31.1	–
Total; weighted means [95% CI]	1612	10.8 [8.61–13.0]	32.5 [26.1–38.9]	43.3 [37.4–49.2]
Depression/total			75.1%	
Depression/mania ratio			3.01%	

Morbidity types: depressive-dysthymic, manic-hypomanic, and total (as percentage of time ill). Data are pooled from 8 studies involving a total of 1612 subjects being treated by accepted clinical community standards. One study involved patients followed prospectively from first-lifetime major episodes with hospitalization (Baldessarini et al., 2010); others represent morbidity in mid-course of bipolar I disorder illness. Note that, despite treatment, patients were unwell more than 43% of the time, and that depressive illness accounted for more than three-quarters of the total, with a ratio of mania-like/depressive illness of over 3:1. Findings include those reported and referenced previously (Baldessarini et al., 2010) plus more recent findings by DeDios et al. (2010), Vergunst et al. (2013), and new findings not reported previously (Tondo et al., 2013).

association between the use of antidepressants and suicidal behavior is presented in Chapter 28 by Ryan and Nemeroff.

Suggestive evidence concerning lithium treatment

Clinical observations in the early 1990s suggesting a role of antidepressants in triggering suicidal ideation in some depressed patients (Teicher et al., 1993) led to rapid, widespread discussion in both the scientific and lay press, despite reviews of evidence supporting and negating this hypothesis (Hammad et al., 2006; Baldessarini et al., 2007). Ironically, there has been much less evident interest in the far stronger evidence that lithium may be associated with reduction of suicidal behavior that has evolved since the 1970s. An early consideration of that hypothesis estimated that perhaps 21% of 64 suicides among patients diagnosed with a major affective disorder might have been prevented if lithium treatment had been used (Barraclough, 1972). In the following years, several reports contributed to the possibility that treatment with lithium may be associated with beneficial effects on suicidal behavior. A double-blind study (Prien et al., 1974) of 249 bipolar and 78 unipolar depressed patients found two suicides associated with placebo treatment (1.28%/year) and none with lithium or imipramine treatment during 24 months of follow-up. Kay and Petterson (1977) also found no suicides in 123 patients followed briefly in a specialized lithium clinic. Poole et al. (1978), in a *mirror* study of 5 years before versus during lithium treatment, found half as many suicide attempts during treatment of 100 patients with various mood disorders.

Another early study found a six-fold lower annual rate of suicide attempts among 95 patients with various recurrent major affective disorders, based on comparing rates before versus during an average of 5.1 years of lithium treatment. Lepkifker et al. (1985) compared the rate of suicide before versus during lithium maintenance treatment for an average of 8.3 years in 33 unipolar depressive disorder patients: 21.2% had made a suicide attempt before treatment (2.55%/year), compared to none during lithium treatment.

Coppen and his colleagues (Coppen et al., 1991) also found no suicides in 103 major affective disorder patients attending a lithium clinic for 11 years

(<0.088%/year). A later extension of this study identified one suicide in a total of 1519 patient-years (0.066%/year) with lithium maintenance treatment for major affective disorders (Coppen and Farmer, 1998). Moreover, a 13.8-fold higher rate (0.91%/year) was found in 27 untreated unipolar depressed patients, perhaps suggesting a protective action of lithium (Coppen and Farmer, 1998).

Müller-Oerlinghausen and collaborators (1992) designed an early case–control study of suicidal risk in 68 patients with various major affective disorder diagnoses and at least one suicide attempt, during an average of 8.0 years of lithium treatment and following its discontinuation, finding six suicides or attempts during treatment (1.10%/year) but 11 after lithium discontinuation (2.02%/year; $\chi^2 = 30.5$; $P < 0.0001$). Later, Nilsson (1999) found a 4.8 times (CI: 1.10–12.6; $P = 0.02$) higher rate of suicides in patients who discontinued lithium.

We studied the suicidal behaviors of 360 type I or II bipolar disorder patients before, during, and following discontinuation of long-term lithium monotherapy, and found rates of suicide and life-threatening attempts to be 6.4 times lower during lithium treatment than either before or long after treatment (Tondo et al., 1998). Notably, however, the risk of suicidal acts increased by 20-fold within several months after discontinuing lithium maintenance treatment, and later fell back to the same level encountered before lithium treatment had started. Moreover, this early suicidal risk following discontinuation of long-term treatment with lithium was twice as high following abrupt or rapid versus gradual discontinuation of lithium (≥14 versus <14 days). Also of interest, the ratio of attempts/suicides (A/S) was twice that during treatment with lithium, suggesting *reduced lethality* of suicidal behavior with this treatment, with fewer fatalities per attempt (Baldessarini et al., 2006).

Initial meta-analyses of studies of lithium treatment and suicidal risk

Up to 2001, we found 12 early studies providing data suitable for meta-analysis (Tondo et al., 2001). The observed, meta-analytically pooled rate of suicides and attempts without lithium was 1.02%/year, and nearly nine times lower during long-term lithium treatment, with a computed risk ratio (without versus with lithium treatment) of 8.85 (95% CI: 4.14–19.1; $P < 0.0001$). In line with earlier reports, in our later meta-analysis (Tondo et al., 2003) of 28 studies involving 823 suicides among 21 484 bipolar disorder patients at risk for an average of 9.93 years, the pooled, weighted mean annual incidence of suicide without lithium was 0.39%/year (390/100 000/year), or more than 20 times higher than the international suicide rate in the general population, of approximately 0.015%/year.

The very high risk of suicide among bipolar disorder patients also was supported by our subsequent review of the medical records of nearly 3000 outpatients diagnosed with DSM-IV major mood disorders (Tondo & Baldessarini, 2007). In that study, the risk of suicide among bipolar disorder patients was similar in types I and II bipolar disorder, and both rates were somewhat higher than among patients diagnosed with unipolar major depressive disorder, overall, but similar among patients of all three types whoever required psychiatric hospitalization. The annual risk of *suicide* among 843 bipolar I and II disorder patients in Sardinia was 150/100 000, or more than 15 times higher than in the Italian general population, and three times greater than among 1983 patients diagnosed with recurrent major depressive disorder, most of whom were outpatients. The annual rate of *suicide attempts* was 1.26% among bipolar disorder patients, versus 0.48% in unipolar depressive cases. The *index of lethality* (ratio of attempts/suicides, A/S) of suicidal behavior (Baldessarini et al., 2006) was 8.6 in bipolar disorder patients and 9.6 in unipolar patients, compared to an estimated A/S risk ratio of 20–30 in the general population (Kessler et al., 2005). These observations indicated relatively high lethality of suicide attempts among mood disorder patients generally, and particularly among bipolar disorder patients – presumably reflecting both intent and methods.

In addition, in a meta-analysis of eight studies on unipolar recurrent depression patients, we found that long-term lithium treatment was again associated with a substantial reduction of risk of suicides and attempts (by approximately 76%) among patients treated with lithium compared to other alternatives, mainly anticonvulsants (Guzzetta et al., 2007). There is also evidence from small numbers of long-term, randomized, placebo-controlled trials that lithium may limit deaths from all causes as well as suicides in recurrent unipolar depression (Cipriani et al., 2013).

Updated meta-analyses of available findings

To date, an association of reduced suicidal risk during long-term treatment with lithium in bipolar disorder patients is supported consistently by nearly three-dozen original studies, meta-analyses, and reviews (Tondo et al. 2001, 2003; Angst et al., 2005; Cipriani et al., 2005; Kessing et al., 2005; Müller-Oerlinghausen et al., 2006). Our most recent meta-analysis of 31 studies included eight trials randomized versus placebo or active-alternative treatments. In these trials, suicidal behavior was ascertained along with other adverse outcomes in an informal and incidental manner, as it has been in most randomized, controlled treatment trials, with the notable exception of the InterSePT trial of clozapine versus olanzapine in suicidal schizophrenia patients (Meltzer et al., 2003). The controlled trials involving lithium treatment provided data on suicidal behavior in mood disorder patients treated long-term with lithium, a comparator, or placebo, and involved more than 110 000 person-years of risk (Baldessarini et al., 2006). Averaged crude rates of suicidal acts were 0.56%/year (or per 100 person-years) with lithium and 2.64%/year without lithium, indicating a major overall, crude reduction of suicidal risk of about five-fold. Apparent reductions were similar for both suicides and attempts, and among purely bipolar disorder patients and samples of persons with various recurrent major mood disorders. Meta-analysis of all 31 available studies found an overall reduction of risk by approximately 80% (risk ratio = 4.91, CI: 3.82–6.31; P <0.0001). Results remained highly significant compared to placebo treatment when only the eight RCTs were considered (RR=1.76, CI: 1.65–1.88; P = 0.001; Table 26.2). When we further extended this analysis in 2008 to include 34 studies, we found similar reductions of risk and estimated a number-needed-to-treat (NNT) equal to 23 (CI: 21–25; Baldessarini & Tondo, 2008). A recent meta-analytical review included 48 randomized trials (6674 subjects) that compared long-term lithium treatment with placebo or active drugs in various types of mood disorder patients (Cipriani et al., 2013). Lithium was found to be more effective than placebo in reducing the number of suicides (OR=0.13, CI: 0.03–0.66) and in decreasing deaths from any cause (OR=0.38, CI: 0.15–0.95). Similar effects also were found in patients with recurrent unipolar major depression. In the few available comparisons to other treatments (including antidepressants, anticonvulsants, and antipsychotic drugs), lithium tended to provide superior reductions of suicidal or other mortal risks.

Since our 2008 meta-analysis (Baldessarini & Tondo, 2008), several additional studies have provided more data. One is a rare randomized, controlled trial (Lauterbach et al., 2008) which found a substantial but statistically non-significant difference in rates of

Table 26.2. Meta-analytic findings of studies of lithium vs. suicide risk

Conditions	Studies (n)	Risk ratio (RR) (95% CI)	*P*-value
All studies	35	3.77 (2.72–5.24)	<0.0001
Outcomes			
Suicides	15	4.03 (2.37–6.85)	<0.0001
Attempts	8	3.73 (1.50–9.33)	<0.005
Both	12	3.66 (2.28–5.87)	<0.0001
Diagnoses			
Bipolar	14	3.84 (2.34–6.30)	<0.0001
Major affective	21	3.72 (2.40–5.77)	<0.0001
Major depression	8	4.69 (1.66–13.3)	<0.0001
Trial types			
Open	29	3.95 (2.79–5.58)	<0.0001
Randomized, placebo-controlled	6	1.91 (0.89–4.08)	0.096
Comparator type			
vs. no lithium or placebo	27	4.22 (2.91–6.10)	<0.0001
vs. anticonvulsants	8	2.42 (1.15–5.10)	0.02

Analyses based on conservative, random-effects modeling, with stratification.
From Baldessarini et al. (2006), updated to include data from Guzzetta et al. (2007), Collins & McFarland (2008), Lauterbach et al. (2008), Smith et al. (2009), and Oquendo et al. (2011).

suicidal acts between patients treated for 12 months with lithium versus those randomized to placebo (adjusted hazard ratio [HR]: 0.52; CI: 0.18–1.43, favoring lithium). However, all completed suicides (n = 3) had occurred in the placebo-treated group. In another randomized comparison of lithium versus placebo added to citalopram treatment for 4 weeks (Khan et al., 2011), suicidal behavior and ideation were rated explicitly with the Montgomery-Åsberg Depression Rating Scale and the Sheehan Suicidality Tracking Scale, Beck Suicide Scale (BSS), and Beck Hopelessness Scale (BHS). No suicides or attempts occurred in either group in this brief trial, but all of the rating scale scores decreased significantly more with the combination of citalopram and lithium than with citalopram plus placebo. This effect may represent an added antidepressant effect of adding lithium to an antidepressant (Bauer et al., 2003) but the brief trial did not specifically indicate an antisuicidal action. In addition, a retrospective analysis of data from 161 bipolar disorder patients found that rates of non-lethal suicide-related events were lower during long-term lithium treatment than with other mood stabilizers given alone or with first- or second-generation antipsychotic drugs (Koek et al., 2012).

The evident beneficial effects of lithium in reducing mortality as well as morbidity associated with suicidal behaviors are even more remarkable given the potentially lethal toxicity of lithium in acute overdoses. However, recent analyses of outcomes of ingestions of potentially toxic substances reported by the US Centers for Disease Control and Prevention (CDCP) indicate that mortality from overdoses of lithium is similar to that associated with modern antidepressant or antipsychotic agents, or less than expected, possibly owing to protection from lethal effects by vomiting as well as timely treatment by hemodialysis (Watson et al., 2004; Baldessarini, 2013). Despite lithium's potential lethality, suicide attempts with lithium during long-term treatment have been reported to be uncommon (Waddington & McKensie, 1994), and we found none among more than 700 patients with major mood disorders treated with lithium for several years at the Lucio Bini Mood Disorders Center in Sardinia (unpublished observations, 2013). It is possible that suicide attempts using this agent are limited by its major antisuicidal effects.

Based on all these studies, a recent review by Lewitzka et al. (2013) and a report by the European Psychiatric Association (Wasserman et al., 2012) recommended the use of long-term lithium treatment to reduce risk of suicidal behavior in bipolar disorder patients.

Conditions other than mood disorders

There is very limited information about possible effects of lithium treatment in reducing suicidal risk in psychopathological conditions other than bipolar disorder or recurrent major depressive disorder. For prevention of suicidal behavior in schizophrenia, clozapine is a recommended and FDA-approved alternative (Meltzer et al., 2003; Hennen & Baldessarini, 2005). It is generally accepted that patients with borderline personality disorder are unresponsive to long-term lithium treatment, in addition to showing typically inconsistent adherence to any treatment (Kutcher et al., 1990). However, symptoms commonly found in personality disorder patients and often associated with suicidal behavior, such as emotional instability and aggressive or self-injurious behavior, may respond to lithium as well (Hori, 1998). Finally, a review found that treatment of borderline disorder patients with lithium, carbamazepine, valproate, low doses of antipsychotics, and serotonin reuptake or monoamine oxidase inhibitor antidepressants appeared to be useful in limiting affective instability and impulsive or aggressive behaviors, and possibly reducing self-injurious behaviors (Rothenhäusler & Kapfhammer, 1999).

Lithium in drinking water

A curious finding has been consistently lower rates of suicide and other violent behaviors in populations exposed to drinking water with relatively high concentrations of lithium salts, even though these concentrations yielded daily intakes far lower than those required for clinically effective treatment of mood disorder patients with lithium carbonate – measured in μEq/L compared to mEq/L plasma concentrations encountered clinically (Baldessarini, 2013). An early study on this topic found lower rates of hospital admissions and homicide in Texas counties with relatively high lithium levels in the drinking water (Dawson et al., 1972). A more recent Texas study also found significantly higher local incidences of suicide, homicide, rape, and other criminal behaviors among 27 counties with very low or undetectable lithium in drinking water than in counties with lithium concentrations of 10–25 μEq/L (Schrauzer & Shrestha, 1990). In addition, at least three international studies have reported lower rates of suicidal or other aggressive behaviors in association with relatively high concentrations of lithium ion in drinking water, typically ranging from about 0.1 to 32 μEq/L (Ohgami et al., 2009; Kapusta et al., 2011; Blüml et al., 2013).

The significance of these provocative findings is far from clear, especially since even the higher reported lithium exposures were far lower than exposures associated with the clinical use of lithium treatment. Estimated intakes are less than 0.10 mEq/day at a daily drinking water intake of 2–3 L, versus clinical doses of about 16 to 41 mEq/day of lithium ion (600–1500 mg/day of lithium carbonate [Li_2CO_3]) that yield daily minimum serum concentrations, typically of 0.6–0.6 mEq/L. Therefore, drinking water would be expected to generate serum concentrations not greater than 0.003 mEq/L, plus small additional amounts from locally grown foodstuffs (Baldessarini, 2013). Although such levels of daily ingestion of lithium are expected to yield very low serum concentrations of lithium ion by pharmacological standards for treatment of bipolar disorder, perhaps lifelong exposure to even low concentrations of lithium might have unrecognized biological effects.

Other mood-stabilizing treatments

There is little research that directly compares suicidal risks during treatment with mood-stabilizing agents other than lithium, and available findings have usually favored lithium (Baldessarini & Tondo, 2009; Cipriani et al., 2013). Two studies found nearly three-fold average lower suicidal risks with lithium than with either carbamazepine or valproate among bipolar or schizoaffective disorder patients (Thies-Flechtner et al., 1996; Goodwin et al., 2003). Although anticonvulsants may have some beneficial effects on suicidal behavior (Yerevanian et al., 2003), our meta-analysis of protective effects against suicidal behavior of lithium versus several proved or putative mood-stabilizing anticonvulsants (including carbamazepine, lamotrigine, and valproate) found lithium to be significantly superior (Baldessarini & Tondo, 2009). This meta-analysis was based on six studies with more than 30 000 patients treated for longer with lithium (31 months) than with an anticonvulsant (19 months). Half of the trials involved randomized assignment to treatments. The observed rate of suicidal acts averaged 0.3%/year during treatment with lithium versus 0.9%/year with anticonvulsants, to yield meta-analytically pooled risk ratio of 2.86 (CI: 2.29–3.57; $P < 0.0001$), or nearly three-fold superiority favoring lithium over the few anticonvulsants that have been tested in this way.

A Danish national pharmacoepidemiological cohort study of over 16 600 persons sampled for 6 years found significantly fewer suicides among patients receiving prescriptions for lithium or valproate in addition to an antipsychotic drug, compared to antipsychotic treatment alone (Smith et al., 2009). Another recent controlled and randomized, but underpowered trial found no difference in rates of suicidal behavior among 35 potentially suicidal bipolar disorder patients randomized to lithium or valproate (with or without other uncontrolled treatments) for up to 30 months (Oquendo et al., 2011). Finally, a study from the Veteran Administration System on more than 1000 patients found reduced incidence rates for attempted suicide ranking: lithium plus divalproex < divalproex alone < lithium alone (Ahearn et al., 2013). It remains unclear whether these studies support the hypothesis that both valproate and lithium exert similar antisuicidal effects, or are simply inconclusive.

Comments

The findings reviewed here were based on data from reports and meta-analyses of available studies reporting on associations of suicides and attempts with versus without long-term lithium treatment, including several randomized, placebo-controlled, trials. With few exceptions, usually involving inconclusive study designs, the findings indicate markedly lower rates of suicidal behavior with long-term lithium treatment in bipolar disorder patients, and suggestive or inconclusive evidence concerning comparisons of lithium versus anticonvulsant or antipsychotic drugs commonly used in the treatment of bipolar disorder (Table 26.2). These effects were particularly strong among bipolar disorder patients, but also among samples involving various recurrent major affective disorders, and possibly in unipolar, recurrent major depression. The available evidence suggests that this effect of lithium treatment may even be superior to that with anticonvulsants proposed as mood stabilizers or antipsychotic drugs, although these comparisons require further study in adequately designed comparisons, as does the validity of the impression that lithium treatment is effective in reducing suicidal risk. Whether antidepressant treatments affect suicidal risk in bipolar disorder patients remains unknown. Nevertheless, the clinical association of suicidal risk with dysphoria, agitation, anger, aggression, and impulsivity strongly suggests that treatment with lithium or other mood-stabilizing medicines, perhaps including antipsychotic drugs, is likely to be safer, if not more effective, than antidepressants in therapeutic efforts to reduce suicidal risk.

Methodological limitations of studies cited above include instances of reporting rates of suicidal acts that did not involve treated and untreated risk periods of similar length. Moreover, it is not clear how the timing of periods sampled might have influenced the results obtained. For example, some investigators (e.g., Jamison, 1986; Tondo et al., 1998) have proposed that suicidal acts are most likely to occur early in the course of bipolar illness among young patients. If this impression is valid, such temporal distribution might lead to an unrepresentatively low risk during treatment if lithium maintenance treatment is significantly delayed if treated subjects are sampled at older ages. Conversely, if suicidal behavior is an indication for treatment, there may be increased suicidal risk close to initiation of lithium or other candidate treatments. Another limitation of many of the studies reviewed above is marked variation in the availability of potentially relevant clinical details; they may include diagnostically heterogeneous cases, including some cases of schizoaffective disorder or recurrent unipolar depression, with varying suicidal risks. As a consequence it is not always clear that patients given different treatments are closely matched in potentially relevant clinical characteristics. Whereas mirror-image studies (with versus without a treatment) involve the same subjects, it is possible to confound such comparisons by mismatching on the clinical status of patients at different times, particularly in a complex and often-changing illness like bipolar disorder. It is even possible that patients who accept, tolerate, benefit from, and continue to take lithium may not be clinically identical to those who refuse or discontinue such treatment. Clearly, randomized and prospective trials involving explicit outcome measures relevant to suicidal risk are needed. On the other hand the clinical, ethical, and practical challenges of such trials are daunting (Meltzer et al., 2003), and commercial interest in lithium, in particular, has always been low.

Potential mechanisms by which lithium might reduce suicidal risk are not clear. Such effects may involve preventing recurrences of high-risk mood states (mixed states, dysphoria, depression) or represent a distinct action on suicidal and perhaps other aggressive or impulsive behaviors. Barraclough (1972) and Coppen and Farmer (1998) supported an association of antisuicidal effects with mood-stabilizing actions of lithium, and a recent study found superior antisuicidal effects among bipolar disorder patients who otherwise responded well to lithium treatment (Manchia et al., 2013). Others have found an imprecise correlation of mood-stabilizing and antisuicidal effects, or have emphasized clinical observations of increased suicidal behavior after stopping lithium, independent of the previous responsiveness of mood symptoms to lithium therapy, and suggested distinct antisuicidal or anti-aggressive actions of lithium (Müller-Oerlinghausen et al., 1992; Müller-Oerlinghausen & Lewitzka, 2010; Lenz et al., 1994; Ahrens & Müller-Oerlinghausen, 2001; Lewitzka et al., 2013).

Several findings suggest decreased physiological activity in serotonin-mediated neurotransmission in brain tissue of suicide victims, apart from effects of the means of suicide (such as poisoning and overdoses) that may confound the results. Increased abundance of serotonin 5-HT_2 receptor sites found in postmortem brain tissue of suicides may reflect their upregulation secondary to reduced presynaptic production or release of serotonin (Mann et al., 1986; Pandey et al., 2003; Savitz et al., 2009). Low concentrations of the main metabolite of serotonin, 5-hydroxyindoleacetic acid (5-HIAA), in cerebrospinal fluid of persons making violent suicide attempts also support a connection between deficient central serotonergic function and suicide (Moberg et al., 2011). In addition, Maes et al. (1995) found that seasonal variations in plasma concentrations of the serotonin precursor amino acid L-tryptophan correlated inversely with seasonal variations in the prevalence of violent suicide, complementing other findings of reduced tryptophan levels in depression. Finally, lithium treatment may tend to facilitate the production, release, and actions of serotonin in brain tissue (Müller-Oerlinghausen, 1985; Price et al., 1990; Baldessarini, 2013). Additional evidence supportive of that proposal may be arising from modern genomic research, including findings of associations between clinical responses to lithium treatment and genetic variants involved in regulating the production of the serotonin transporter protein (Tharoor et al., 2013). Taken together, these observations may support the hypothesis that a decrease of cerebral serotonergic function may contribute to suicidal risk and might be countered selectively by lithium treatment (Kovacsics et al., 2009; Saunders & Hawton, 2009; Müller-Oerlinghausen & Lewitzka, 2010). However, a beneficial effect of increased serotonergic function is at odds with the apparent lack of an antisuicidal effect of serotonergic antidepressants in bipolar disorder. An alternative possibility is decreased cerebral dopaminergic activity (Malhi et al., 2013).

Conclusions

The findings summarized above pertaining to research focusing on the hypothesis that lithium treatment may have a special role in reduction of suicide risk are encouraging, but it must be emphasized that such a role has not been definitively demonstrated. A major limitation of studies finding less suicidal risk during long-term treatment with lithium is that, to date, even randomized controlled treatment trials involve incidental findings (among other passively noted reports of adverse effects) and were not designed to test for suicidal behavior as an explicit outcome. An additional limitation – indeed, of all studies of therapeutic effects – is that patients who accept, tolerate, and adhere to long-term treatment with lithium may, to some extent, be self-selected and not entirely representative of the full spectrum of clinically encountered mood disorder patients. Moreover, factors such as female sex, being married, having more education and employment, the presence of certain personality traits, relative improvement of depressive versus other symptoms with treatment, and the occurrence of adverse effects, as well as being less severely ill or ill for less time, all are likely to affect suicidal risk and so tend to confound interpretation of observed effects of treatment, especially in the absence of randomized study designs and explicit outcome measures. Whether the same patients were assessed with and without lithium, or whether subjects were randomly assigned to particular treatments in parallel groups, those who accept and continue the treatment may differ from others who fail to accept lithium treatment, tolerate it poorly, or discontinue early. Nevertheless, in order to test for long-term effects of *any* treatment, only patients who accept and tolerate it are available for analysis. Since a growing number of bipolar disorder and other mood disorder patients are reluctant to be treated with lithium or to accept it for prolonged periods (Baldessarini, 2013), it is increasingly important to identify alternative treatments that can reduce suicidal risk, particularly among agents with commercial backing to support the challenging and expensive trials required to test for antisuicidal effects.

Ideal studies of such treatments would involve randomized assignment to specific and clinically plausible treatment options for prolonged periods, and would involve primary outcome measures specific to suicidal behavior. However, use of a placebo-control condition is unlikely to be feasible owing to ethical constraints when death is a possible outcome, and due to difficulties of recruiting patients into placebo-controlled treatment trials and retaining them for a long time (Baldessarini, 2013). Nevertheless, trials involving randomization to different but similarly plausible, even if unproved, treatments might be ethically and practically feasible, as in the InterSePT trial comparing clozapine with olanzapine in schizophrenia patients (Meltzer et al., 2003). So far, however, trials that compare, for example, lithium to an anticonvulsant or antipsychotic agent are rare and almost never continued for more than several months. Moreover, head-to-head comparisons of competing commercial products are unlikely to be favored by the pharmaceutical industry.

Finally, lithium treatment requires closer monitoring of patients than with most other mood-stabilizing agents. This added level of clinical follow-up might facilitate identification of emerging symptoms associated with suicidal behavior, including suicidal ideation, and early agitation, dysphoria, and anger, or otherwise provide supportive and protective influences. We reported previously that various measures that can be considered indices of access to clinical care were closely correlated with state suicide rates in the USA (Tondo et al., 2006). However, the value of additional clinical contact and close supervision required by lithium treatment may not be a critical factor, given experience in the InterSePT trial for schizophrenia patients, which found superior antisuicidal effects of clozapine over olanzapine, despite matching for clinician contact time (Meltzer et al., 2003).

In conclusion, major mood disorders are associated with major increases of suicidal behavior and fatalities, especially when the illnesses present as mixed, dysphoric-agitated states, sometimes accompanied by anger, aggression, or impulsivity. In such conditions, antidepressant treatments may lack a beneficial effect or even increase agitation and suicidal risk, whereas mood stabilizers, and particularly lithium salts, maintained for prolonged times may be more effective treatments as a component of comprehensive clinical management aimed at suicide prevention.

Acknowledgments

Supported in part by Aretæus Association (LT), by a grant from the Bruce J. Anderson Foundation and by the McLean Private Donors Research Fund (RJB).

References

Ahearn, E. P., Chen, P., Hertzberg, M., et al. (2013). Suicide attempts in veterans with bipolar disorder during treatment with lithium, divalproex, and atypical antipsychotics. *Journal of Affective Disorders*, **145**, 77–82.

Ahrens, B., & Müller-Oerlinghausen, B. (2001). Does lithium exert an independent antisuicidal effect? *Pharmacopsychiatry*, **34**, 132–136.

American Psychiatric Association (APA). (2013) *Diagnostic and Statistical Manual of Mental Disorders,* fifth revision (DSM-5). Washington: American Psychiatric Publishing.

Angst, J., Angst, F., Gerber-Werder, R., et al. (2005). Suicide in 406 mood-disorder patients with and without long-term medication: 40–44 years follow-up. *Archives of Suicide Research*, **9**, 279–300.

Baldessarini, R. J. (2013). *Chemotherapy in Psychiatry*, 3rd edn. New York: Springer Press.

Baldessarini, R. J., & Tondo, L. (2008). Lithium and suicidal risk. *Bipolar Disorder*, **10**, 114–115.

Baldessarini, R. J., & Tondo, L. (2009). Suicidal risks during treatment of bipolar disorder patients with lithium versus anticonvulsants. *Pharmacopsychiatry*, **42**, 72–75.

Baldessarini, R. J., Faedda, G. L., & Hennen, J. (2005). Risk of mania with serotonin reuptake inhibitors vs. tricyclic antidepressants in children, adolescents and young adults. *Archives of Pediatric and Adolescent Medicine*, **159**, 298–299.

Baldessarini, R. J., Tondo, L., Davis, P., et al. (2006). Decreased suicidal risk during long-term lithium treatment: meta-analysis. *Bipolar Disorder*, **8**, 625–639.

Baldessarini, R. J., Tondo, L., Strombom, I., et al. (2007). Analysis of ecological studies of relationships between antidepressant utilization and suicidal risk. *Harvard Review of Psychiatry*, **15**, 133–145.

Baldessarini, R. J., Salvatore, P., Khalsa, H. M., et al. (2010). Morbidity in 303 first-episode bipolar I disorder patients. *Bipolar Disorders*, **12**, 264–270.

Barbui, C., Esposito, E., & Cipriani, A. (2009). Selective serotonin reuptake inhibitors and risk of suicide: a systematic review of observational studies. *CMAJ*, **180**, 291–297.

Barraclough, B. (1972). Suicide prevention, recurrent affective disorder and lithium. *British Journal of Psychiatry*, **121**, 391–392.

Bauer, M., Forsthoff, A., Baethge, C., et al. (2003). Lithium augmentation therapy in refractory depression-update. *European Archives of Psychiatry and Clinical Neuroscience*, **253**, 132–139.

Blüml, V., Regier, M. D., Hlavin, G., et al. (2013). Lithium in the public water supply and suicide mortality in Texas. *Journal of Psychiatric Research*, **47**, 407–411.

Cipriani, A., Pretty, H., Hawton, K., et al. (2005). Lithium in the prevention of suicidal behavior and all-cause mortality in patients with mood disorders: systematic review of randomized trials. *American Journal of Psychiatry*, **162**, 1805–1819.

Cipriani, A., Hawton, K., Stockton, S., & Geddes, J. R. (2013). Lithium in the prevention of suicide in mood disorders: updated systematic review and meta-analysis. *BMJ*, **346** (Epub ahead of print, 27 Jun).

Collins, J. C., & McFarland, B. H. (2008). Divalproex, lithium and suicide among Medicaid patients with bipolar disorder. *Journal of Affective Disorders*, **107**, 23–28.

Coppen, A., & Farmer, R. (1998). Suicide mortality in patients on lithium maintenance therapy. *Journal of Affective Disorder*, **50**, 261–267.

Coppen, A., Standish-Barry, H., Bailey, J., et al. (1991). Does lithium reduce mortality of recurrent mood disorders? *Journal of Affective Disorders*, **23**, 1–7.

Dawson, E. B., Moore, T. D., & McGanity, W. J. (1972). Relationship of lithium metabolism to mental hospital admissions and homicide. *Diseases of the Nervous System*, **33**, 546–556.

De Dios, C., Ezquiaga, E., Garcia, A., Soler, B., & Vieta, E. (2010). *Journal of Affective Disorders*, **125**, 74–81.

Goodwin, F. K., Fireman, B., Simon, G. E., et al. (2003). Suicide risk in bipolar disorder during treatment with lithium and divalproex. *JAMA*, **290**, 1467–1473.

Guzzetta, F., Tondo, L., Centorrino, F., & Baldessarini, R. J. (2007). Lithium treatment reduces suicide risk in recurrent major depressive disorder. *Journal of Clinical Psychiatry*, **68**, 380–383.

Hammad, T. A., Laughren, T., & Racoosin, J. (2006). Suicidality in pediatric patients treated with antidepressant drugs. *Archives of General Psychiatry*, **63**, 332–339.

Hennen, J., & Baldessarini, R. J. (2005). Reduced suicidal risk during treatment with clozapine: meta-analysis. *Schizophrenia Research*, **73**, 139–145.

Hori, A. (1998). Pharmacotherapy for personality disorders. *Psychiatry and Clinical Neurosciences*, **52**, 13–19.

Isometsä, E. T., Henriksson, M. M., Aro, H. M., et al. (1994). Suicide in major depression. *American Journal of Psychiatry*, **151**, 530–536.

Jamison, K. R. (1986). Suicide and bipolar disorders. *Annals of the New York Academy of Sciences*, **487**, 301–315.

Kapusta, N. D., Mossaheb, N., Etzersdorfer, E., et al. (2011). Lithium in drinking water and suicide mortality. *British Journal of Psychiatry*, **198**, 346–350.

Kay, D. W. K., & Petterson, U. (1977) Manic-depressive illness. *Acta Psychiatrica Scandinavica (Suppl)*, **269**, 55–60.

Kessing, L. V., Søndergard, L., Kvist, K., et al. (2005). Suicide risk in patients treated with lithium. *Archives of General Psychiatry*, **62**, 860–866.

Kessler, R. C., Berglund, P., Borges, G., et al. (2005). Trends in suicide ideation, plans, gestures, and attempts in the United States, 1990–1992 to 2001–2003. *JAMA*, **293**, 2487–2495.

Khan, A., Khan, S. R., Hobus, J., et al. (2011). Differential pattern of response in mood symptoms and suicide risk measures in severely ill depressed patients assigned to citalopram with placebo or citalopram combined with lithium: role of lithium levels. *Journal of Psychiatric Research*, **45**, 1489–1496.

Koek, R. J., Yerevanian, B. I., & Mintz, J. (2012). Subtypes of antipsychotics and suicidal behavior in bipolar disorder. *Journal of Affective Disorders*, **143**, 27–33.

Koukopoulos, A., & Koukopoulos, A. (1999). Agitated depression as a mixed state and the problem of melancholia. *Psychiatric Clinics of North America*, **22**, 547–564.

Kovacsics, C. E., Gottesman, I. I., & Gould, T. D. (2009). Lithium's antisuicidal efficacy: elucidation of neurobiological targets using endophenotype strategies. *Annual Review of Pharmacology and Toxicology*, **49**, 175–198.

Kutcher, S. P., Amrton, P., & Korenblum, M. (1990). Adolescent bipolar illness and personality disorder. *Journal of the American Academy of Child and Adolescent Psychiatry*, **29**, 355–358.

Lauterbach, E., Felber, W., Müller-Oerlinghausen, B., et al. (2008) Adjunctive lithium treatment in the prevention of suicidal behaviour in depressive disorders: a randomised, placebo-controlled, 1-year trial. *Acta Psychiatrica Scandinavica*, **118**, 469–479.

Lenz, G., Ahrens, B., & Denk, E. (1994). Mortalität nach Ausschneiden aus der Lithiumambulanz. In B. Müller-Oerlinghausen & A. Berghöfer (Eds.) *Ziele und Ergebnisse der medicamentösen Prophylaxe affecktiver Psychosen* (pp. 49–52). Stuttgart: G. Theme Verlag.

Lepkifker, E., Horesh, N., & Floru, S. (1985). Long-term lithium prophylaxis in recurrent unipolar depression. *Acta Psychiatrica Belgica*, **85**, 434–443.

Lewitzka, U., Bauer, M., Felber, W., et al. (2013). Anti-suicidal effect of lithium: current state of research and its clinical implications for the long-term treatment of affective disorders. *Nervenärzt*, **84**, 294–306.

Maes, M., Scharpé, S., Verkerk, R., et al. (1995). Seasonal variation in plasma L-Tryptophan availability in healthy volunteers: relationships to violent suicide occurrence. *Archives of General Psychiatry*, **52**, 937–946.

Maj, M., Pirozzi, R., Magliano, L., et al. (2006). Agitated "unipolar" major depression: prevalence, phenomenology, and outcome. *Journal of Clinical Psychiatry*, **67**, 712–719.

Malhi, G. S., Tanious, M., Das, P., Coulston, C. M., & Berk, M. (2013). Potential mechanisms of action of lithium in bipolar disorder. Current understanding. *CNS Drugs*, **27**, 135–153.

Manchia, M., Hajek, T., O'Donovan, C., et al. (2013). Genetic risk of suicidal behavior in bipolar spectrum disorder: analysis of 737 pedigrees. *Bipolar Disorder* (Epub ahead of print, 5 Jun)].

Mann, J. J., Stanley, M., McBride, P. A., & McEwen, B. S. (1986). Increased serotonin-2 and beta-adrenergic receptor binding in the frontal cortices of suicide victims. *Archives of General Psychiatry*, **43**, 954–959.

Meltzer, H. Y., Alphs, L., Green, A. I., et al. International Suicide Prevention Trial Study Group. (2003). Clozapine treatment for suicidality in schizophrenia: International Suicide Prevention Trial (InterSePT). *Archives of General Psychiatry*, **60**, 82–91.

Moberg, T., Nordström, P., Forslund, K., et al. (2011). CSF 5-HIAA and exposure to and expression of interpersonal violence in suicide attempters. *Journal of Affective Disorders*, **132**, 173–178.

Müller-Oerlinghausen, B. (1985). Lithium long-term treatment: does it act via serotonin? *Pharmacopsychiatry*, **18**, 214–217.

Müller-Oerlinghausen, B., & Lewitzka, U. (2010) Lithium reduces pathological aggression and suicidality: a mini-review. *Neuropsychobiology*, **62**, 43–49.

Müller-Oerlinghausen, B., Müser-Causemann, B., & Volk, J. (1992). Suicides and parasuicides in a high-risk patient group on and off lithium long-term medication. *Journal of Affective Disorders*, **25**, 261–270.

Müller-Oerlinghausen, B., Ahrens, B., & Felber, W. (2006). The suicide-preventive and mortality-reducing effect of lithium. In M. Bauer, P. Grof, & B. Müller-Oerlinghausen (Eds.) *Lithium in Neuropsychiatry* (pp. 179–192). London: Informa Healthcare.

Nilsson, A. (1999). Lithium therapy and suicide risk. *Journal of Clinical Psychiatry*, **60** (Suppl 2), 85–88.

Novick, D. M., Swartz, H. A., & Frank, E. (2010). Suicide attempts in bipolar I and bipolar II disorder: review and meta-analysis of the evidence. *Bipolar Disorder*, **12**, 1–9.

Ohgami, H., Terao, T., Shiotsuki, I., et al. (2009). Lithium levels in drinking water and risk of suicide. *British Journal of Psychiatry*, **194**, 464–465.

Oquendo, M. A., Galfalvy, H. C., Currier, D., et al. (2011). Treatment of suicide attempters with bipolar disorder: a randomized clinical trial comparing lithium and valproate in the prevention of suicidal behavior. *American Journal of Psychiatry*, **168**, 1050–1056.

Pacchiarotti, I., Bond, D. J., Baldessarini, R. J., et al. (2013). International Society for Bipolar Disorders (ISBD) Task-Force report on antidepressant use in bipolar disorders. *American Journal of Psychiatry*, **170**(11), 1249–1262.

Pandey, G. N., Pandey, S. C., Ren, X., et al. (2003). Serotonin receptors in platelets of bipolar and schizoaffective patients: effect of lithium treatment. *Psychopharmacology*, **170**, 115–123.

Poole, A. J., James, H. D., & Hughes, W. C. (1978). Treatment experiences in the lithium clinic at St Thomas' Hospital. *Journal of the Royal Society of Medicine*, **71**, 890–894.

Price, L. H., Charney, D. S., Delgado, P. L., et al. (1990). Lithium and serotonin function: implications for the serotonin hypothesis of depression. *Psychopharmacology*, **100**, 3–12.

Prien, R. F., Klett, C. J., & Caffey, C. M. (1974). Lithium prophylaxis in recurrent affective illness. *American Journal of Psychiatry*, **131**, 198–203.

Rothenhäusler, H. B., & Kapfhammer, H. P. (1999). Outcome in borderline disorders: literature review. *Fortschritte der Neurologie-Psychiatrie*, **67**, 200–217.

Saunders, K. E., & Hawton, K. (2009). Role of psychopharmacology in suicide prevention. *Epidemiologia e Psichiatria Sociale*, **18**, 172–178.

Savitz, J., Lucki, I., & Drevets, W. C. (2009). 5-HT(1A) receptor function in major depressive disorder. *Progress in Neurobiology*, **88**, 17–31.

Schrauzer, G. N., & Shrestha, K. P. (1990). Lithium in drinking water and the incidences of crimes, suicides, and arrests related to drug addictions. *Biological Trace Element Research*, **25**, 105–113.

Simon, R. I., & Hales, R. E. (2012). *Textbook of Suicide Assessment and Management*, 2nd edn. Washington, DC: American Psychiatric Press.

Smith, E. G., Søndergård, L., Lopez, A. G., et al. (2009). Association between consistent purchase of anticonvulsants or lithium and suicide risk: longitudinal cohort study from Denmark, 1995–2001. *Journal of Affective Disorders*, **117**, 162–167.

Swann, A. C., Lafer, B., Perugi, G., et al. (2013). Bipolar mixed states: an International Society for Bipolar Disorders task force report of symptom structure, course of illness, and diagnosis. *American Journal of Psychiatry*, **170**, 31–42.

Teicher, M. H., Glod, C. A., & Cole, J. O. (1993). Antidepressant drugs and the emergence of suicidal tendencies. *Drug Safety*, **8**, 186–212.

Tharoor, H., Kotambail, A., Jain, S., et al. (2013). Study of the association of serotonin transporter triallelic 5-HTTLPR and STin2 VNTR polymorphisms with lithium prophylaxis response in bipolar disorder. *Psychiatric Genetics*, **23**, 77–81.

Thies-Flechtner, K., Müller-Oerlinghausen, B., Seibert, W., et al. (1996). Effect of prophylactic treatment on suicide risk in patients with major affective disorders: data from a randomized prospective trial. *Pharmacopsychiatry*, **29**, 103–107.

Tondo, L., & Baldessarini, R. J. (2007). Suicidal risks among 2826 Sardinian major affective disorder patients. *Acta Psychiatrica Scandinavica*, **116**, 419–428.

Tondo, L., Baldessarini, R. J., Hennen, J., et al. (1998). Lithium treatment and risk of suicidal behavior in bipolar disorder patients. *Journal of Clinical Psychiatry*, **59**, 405–414.

Tondo, L., Hennen, J., & Baldessarini, R. J. (2001). Reduced suicide risk with long-term lithium treatment in major affective illness: A meta-analysis. *Acta Psychiatrica Scandinavica*, **104**, 163–172.

Tondo, L., Isacsson, G., & Baldessarini, R. J. (2003). Suicide in bipolar disorder: risk and prevention. *CNS Drugs*, **17**, 491–511.

Tondo, L., Albert, M. J., & Baldessarini, R. J. (2006). Suicide rates in relation to health-care access in the United States: an ecological study. *Journal of Clinical Psychiatry*, **67**, 517–523.

Tondo, L., Vázquez, G. H., & Baldessarini, R. J. (2010). Mania associated with antidepressant-treatment: comprehensive meta-analytic review. *Acta Psychiatrica Scandinavica*, **121**, 404–414.

Tondo, L. Visioli C, Baldessarini, R. J. (2013). Long-term morbidity in clinically treated bipolar I disorder patients in a Sardinian mood disorder center. *Previously unpublished observations.*

Vázquez, G. H., Tondo L., & Undurraga, J., et al. (2013). Overview of antidepressant treatment in bipolar depression: critical commentary. *International Journal of Neuropsychopharmacology*, **22**, 1–13.

Vergunst, F. K., Fekadu, A., Wooderson, S. C., et al. (2013). Longitudinal course of symptom severity and fluctuation in patients with treatment-resistant unipolar and bipolar depression. *Psychiatry Research*, **207**(3), 143–149.

Waddington, D., & McKensie, I. P. (1994). Overdose rates in lithium-treated vs. antidepressant-treated outpatients. *Acta Psychiatrica Scandinavica*, **90**, 50–52.

Wasserman, D., Rihmer, Z., Rujescu, D., et al. (2012). European Psychiatric Association (EPA) guidance on suicide treatment and prevention. *European Journal of Psychiatry*, **27**, 129–141.

Watson, W. A., Litovitz, T. L., Klein-Schwartz, W., et al. (2004). Annual report of the American Association of Poison Control Centers toxic exposure surveillance system. *American Journal of Emergency Medicine*, **22**, 335–404.

Yatham, L. N., Kennedy, S. H., Parikh, S. V., et al. (2013). Canadian Network for Mood and Anxiety Treatments (CANMAT) and International Society for Bipolar Disorders (ISBD) collaborative update for the management of patients with bipolar disorder. *Bipolar Disorder*, **15**, 1–44.

Yerevanian, B. I., Koek, R. J., & Mintz, J. (2003). Lithium, anticonvulsants and suicidal behavior in bipolar disorder. *Journal of Affective Disorders*, **73**, 223–228.

Chapter 27

Clozapine

David W. Ayer and Herbert Y. Meltzer

Introduction

Clozapine, the first atypical antipsychotic drug, has been shown to be an effective antipsychotic in the majority of patients with treatment-resistant schizophrenia and to be of exceptional benefit to reduce the risk for suicide in schizophrenia (Kane et al., 1988; Meltzer et al., 2003). As will be discussed, clozapine is underutilized for both indications. There are many factors which drive this, but one is most certainly the difficulty some have in acknowledging that progress has been made in the treatment of schizophrenia beyond that to be expected from the typical antipsychotic drugs, sometimes called first-generation antipsychotics. Some experts in the field state as fact on public television, in newspapers and magazines, scientific journals, at national and international scientific meetings, and as guest lecturers at academic medical centers, and also vitally interested groups, such as the National Alliance for the Mentally Ill, that there have been no advances in the treatment of schizophrenia since the discovery of chlorpromazine in 1952. If clozapine is mentioned as a therapeutic advance, it is only in its ability to treat delusions and hallucinations in patients who fail to respond to adequate trials of typical antipsychotics, which are known to act through blockade of dopamine (DA) D_2 receptors. The established ability of clozapine to profoundly reduce the risk for suicide in schizophrenia (Meltzer et al., 2003; Hennen & Baldessarini, 2005) is, in particular, rarely mentioned. This lack of knowledge, or the failure to implement that knowledge, by a clinician, can and does lead to preventable death. The purpose of this chapter is to summarize the data concerning the risk for suicide in schizophrenia, discuss the ability of clozapine to reduce that risk, and discuss some of the issues involved in the optimal use of clozapine.

The risk of suicide in schizophrenia and recognition of that risk

A fairly recent review of the suicide rate in schizophrenia concluded that 5% of a cohort of patients with schizophrenia followed from onset to death from any cause will die due to suicide (Palmer et al., 2005). The 5% risk rate is highly likely to be an underestimate because of the reluctance of medical examiners to list suicide as a cause of death. Second, suicide may occur during the prodromal period in individuals who have not yet been diagnosed and, thus, would not be counted as a death related to the schizophrenia syndrome (Knittel et al., 2008). Between 25% and 50% of patients with schizophrenia or schizoaffective disorder will make a suicide attempt in their lifetime, with attempts being most common during the first decade of the illness, making suicide the leading cause of early mortality in schizophrenia (Bushe et al., 2010). In addition to the enormous loss and sadness to the families of those who die or make an attempt, recent analysis shows the annual fiscal cost for a patient who has attempted suicide is $46 000 (Zhu et al., 2008).

As discussed by Harvey and Fawcett in other chapters in this volume, the risk factors for suicide in schizophrenia are well established and, not surprisingly, are shared by many other clinical groups (Caldwell & Gottesman, 1990; Axelsson & Lagerkvist-Briggs, 1992). They are enumerated in Table 27.1 and should be well known to all clinicians because they affect the timing of when to consider initiation of clozapine treatment.

The number one predictor of a forthcoming suicide attempt is a prior suicide attempt. Hospitalization to prevent an attempt, or following an attempt, and discharge from hospital are highly informative because so little can be accomplished during brief hospitalizations that are currently the norm in the

A Concise Guide to Understanding Suicide, ed. Stephen H. Koslow, Pedro Ruiz, and Charles B. Nemeroff. Published by Cambridge University Press.

Table 27.1. Factors associated with suicide risk in schizophrenia

Previous suicide attempts
Concurrent substance abuse
Male gender
First decade of illness
Hospitalization and discharge
High symptom severity
Hopelessness and other depressive symptoms
Impulsivity
Progressive decline in work and social functioning
Akathisia
No antipsychotic medication

USA. Substance abuse, especially alcohol, male gender, first decade of illness, white ethnicity, family history of suicide, and hopelessness are the second most important risk factors that must be factored into the decision to consider the use of clozapine. Any one of the others in Table 27.1 that may be present, including acute stresses such as losing a job, failing in school or a training program, and conflicts within the family or with significant others, sometimes leading to more or less explicit suggestions that suicide may lead to resolution of the current intolerable state, may be sufficient reasons to consider clozapine in the treatment plan to attenuate the significance of these adverse developments. Recognizing that the onset of the ability of clozapine to reduce the risk for suicide may take several months (Meltzer et al., 2003) means that it will not be the source of immediate help, in the way that a course of electroconvulsive treatment (ECT) might be for someone with major depression suicidality. ECT may be used to enhance the efficacy of clozapine to reduce the risk for suicide (Masoudzadeh & Khalilian, 2007), along with hospitalization and other measures to protect a suicidal person from harming themselves, e.g., removing guns from the home, respite care, and intensive case management.

Pharmacologic interventions

There are no studies which reliably show that typical antipsychotic drugs reduce the risk for suicide (Palmer et al., 1999; Meltzer et al., 2003). Indeed, there has been a suggestion that they increase the risk for suicide because of akathisia and tardive dyskinesia, both of which are related to EPS produced by these agents. As with clozapine, many clinicians do not follow treatment guidelines and use doses of typical antipsychotic drugs which produce disabling and dispiriting EPS. The suicide rate before the introduction of neuroleptics for the treatment of schizophrenia was 9–13% (Bleuler, 1976), not different from that found after their introduction (Axelsson & Lagerkvist-Briggs, 1992). The recent epidemiologic study of Tiihonen et al. (2009), a major contribution to appreciating the efficacy of antipsychotic drugs to reduce the risk for suicide in schizophrenia, compared antipsychotic drug effects on the rate of suicide in 66 881 patients with schizophrenia, the total at risk population in Finland. The period covered was 1996 and 2006. The life expectancy of the patients with schizophrenia at age 20 was 32.5 years in 1996, 25 years less than the general population, which was 57.5 years. In 2006, the expectancies were 37.4 and 59.9 years, respectively. Forty-one hundred (6.1%) of the schizophrenia patients had died from all causes. Of these 4100 deaths, 677 (16.5%) had died as a result of suicide. Thus, 1.0% of the 66 881 patients had died from suicide. This has to be extrapolated to an expected total rate for these individuals. Based on the rate of 5.0% reported by Palmer et al. (2005), another 4.0% (approximately 2708) would be predicted to die from suicide. The rate of suicide in the 554 (13.5%) of the patients treated with haloperidol, thioridazine, or perphenazine was significantly greater than that with clozapine, but not different from that with olanzapine, quetiapine, or risperidone. The inability of typical APDs to reduce the risk for suicide, despite their expected ability to treat positive symptoms in the estimated 70% of patients with schizophrenia who are non-treatment-resistant, indicates that suicide is independent of positive symptoms and requires a unique treatment strategy (Meltzer & Okayli, 1995; Meltzer et al., 2003; Altamura et al., 2007). There is no evidence that the addition of antidepressants and mood stabilizers as adjunctive therapy to typical APDs enhanced their ability to reduce the risk for suicide (Siris et al., 1994). Electroconvulsive treatment, however, is an effective means of reducing the risk for suicide in schizophrenia, most likely for both typical and atypical APDs (Pompili et al., 2013).

Clozapine, other atypical APDs, and the risk for suicide

The first evidence that clozapine reduced suicide was provided by Meltzer and Okayli (1995). Clinical impressions of a reduction in the number of suicide attempts in a cohort treated with clozapine on an open basis stimulated a mirror-image study of 88 treatment refractory patients with schizophrenia or schizoaffective disorder. Comparison of the rates of suicide attempts 2–3 years before and after clozapine, revealed the number of patients with no suicidality increased from 53% at baseline to 88% during clozapine treatment. There were 22 suicide attempts during the 2 years before initiation of clozapine therapy and three in the following 2 years, an 88% reduction in attempts. None of the three were considered to have substantial potential for lethality. Decreased hopelessness and depressive symptoms were found after 6 weeks of clozapine treatment, as well as the rest of the 2-year follow-up period. Similar results were reported by Spivak et al. (1998) who reported fewer suicide attempts ($P < 0.05$) and decreased impulsivity ($P < 0.05$) and aggressiveness ($P < 0.01$) in clozapine-treated patients compared with those treated with traditional neuroleptics. Reviews of data from clozapine treatment registries required to assess the risk of agranulocytosis during clozapine treatment (Reid et al., 1998; Munro et al., 1999) also showed that treatment with clozapine reduced the rate of *completed* suicide by 80%. Walker et al. (1997) undertook a large-scale retrospective epidemiologic evaluation of mortality and morbidity in 67 072 current and past clozapine users included in the US Clozaril National Registry. Deaths occurring in this cohort of patients were ascertained using the Social Security Administration Death Master Files and The National Death Index. An 83% reduction in death by suicide was observed in current clozapine users compared with past users. The risk of death by suicide increased after clozapine discontinuation. Reid et al. (1998) also used the US National Clozaril Registry to conduct a retrospective analysis of completed suicide during clozapine treatment. They reported a 0.0157% per year incidence of suicide in patients receiving clozapine compared to a 0.4–0.8% per year rate reported in previous studies using typical antipsychotics (Caldwell & Gottesman, 1990), and consistent with previous estimates.

Despite the evidence in support of the Meltzer and Okayli (1995) results, the possibility that the basis for the reduction in attempts and completions in the studies mentioned above was the increased contact with patients required for monitoring for agranulocytosis, contributed to minimal impact of the InterSePT study on the use of clozapine to reduce the risk for suicide. It was thought that a prospective, randomized, study controlling for clinical contact might be helpful in this regard, even though there are no data that would suggest more frequent clinical contact has a substantial effect on suicide risk. This led the senior author to propose an investigator-initiated randomized, blinded controlled clinical trial of clozapine vs. olanzapine. Sandoz not only agreed to such a study, but upgraded it to a registration level Phase 4 study, with adequate power and other rigorous features needed to obtain US FDA approval. This is the origin of the International Suicide Prevention Trial (InterSePT; Meltzer et al., 2003). Much persuasion of the US FDA to even consider the possibility of approving clozapine for suicide risk reduction was necessary, because at that time, the FDA considered any component of the schizophrenia syndrome was unsuitable for an indication because of the concept of pseudospecificity, i.e., no separate indication for a non-independent feature of the schizophrenia syndrome as a whole. Ultimately, the FDA was persuaded that there was a possibility that suicide was an independent feature of the illness. The lack of impact of typical neuroleptic drugs on the suicide attempt and completion rates, despite their ability to improve psychosis, was one of the arguments that was persuasive. The FDA approval of the *possibility* of obtaining a suicide indication for clozapine had historic significance because other features of the illness, e.g., cognitive impairment and negative symptoms, might also be targeted for separate treatments and labeled indications. After intensive discussion with the FDA, the InterSePT study was initiated. It was an international, large-scale, prospective, randomized, open label but rater blind, parallel groups 2-year study. It compared the effectiveness of clozapine with olanzapine, a very similar molecule to clozapine, on risk of suicide, in 990 patients diagnosed with schizophrenia or schizoaffective disorder who were at high risk for suicide. The reliability of the trial depended upon a blinded Suicide Monitoring Board who decided whether each putative suicide event met criteria based upon a written, edited report to exclude drug treatment information. Clozapine proved superior to olanzapine in reducing suicidal behavior, suicide attempts, number of required hospitalizations, or urgent interventions to prevent suicide, and the use of adjunctive treatments such as antidepressants and anxiolytics (Meltzer et al., 2003). The major finding was a 25% reduction in the risk of suicide attempts in patients using clozapine compared to those using olanzapine. The two treatments differentiated at 3 months, with the number of attempts still increasing in the olanzapine-treated group during the last 3 months of the study, but not so in the clozapine-treated group. This finding led the FDA to approve an indication for clozapine to reduce the risk of suicide in patients with schizophrenia or schizoaffective disorder considered to be at high risk for suicide.

Subsequent to the InterSePT trial, Modestin et al. (2005) conducted a mirror-image design, retrospective study with data from hospitalized patients with schizophrenia which produced results nearly identical to the 85% decrease in the Meltzer and Okayli (1995) study, including a 12-fold decrease in the risk for suicidal behaviors. They also reported suicidal behaviors increased to baseline rate in those patients who discontinued clozapine. As naturalistic studies, with each patient as his or her own control, these two studies provide an estimate of the reduction in the risk of suicide that should be possible in clinical practice. A recent study of "avoidable mortality," including suicide, in the UK, estimated that the all-cause standardized mortality ratio for patients with schizophrenia would decrease from 4.23 (95% CI 3.85–4.60) to 2.38 (2.09–2.66), a nearly 50% reduction (Hoang et al., 2013).

Results from trials investigating the effects on suicide of other atypical antipsychotics, specifically risperidone (Tran et al., 1997; Muller-Siecheneder et al., 1998) and olanzapine (Beasley et al., 1997) have been mixed. A recent study reported decreased suicide attempt rates with sertindole (Thomas et al., 2010). This is promising but needs replication. There is no other evidence we are aware of that suggests olanzapine or other atypical APDs reduce the risk for suicide in schizophrenia (Meltzer, 2005; Tiihonen et al., 2009).

Reasons for underutilization of clozapine

Despite the demonstration by the InterSePT trial of a huge reduction of suicide risk in patients with schizophrenia receiving clozapine, an aggressive education campaign by the InterSePT study sponsor, Novartis, and the naturalistic studies providing real-world evidence for the validity of the InterSePT data, the rate of clozapine utilization has remained unchanged in the USA, approximately 5% (Meltzer, 2012). Horvitz-Lennon et al. (2009) lists the underutilization of clozapine as one of the two most serious examples of the lack of attention to evidence-based practices in the treatment of schizophrenia. The use of clozapine in the Scandinavian countries and China is much higher than the USA while the rate is much lower in Japan, which just approved clozapine with greatly restricted access to it. Safety and tolerability issues are considered the major reasons for this underutilization: (1) agranulocytosis; (2) metabolic side effects; and (3) cardiovascular risks. As clozapine is now generic in nearly all parts of the world, except Japan, cost is not the issue. The additional burden of approval to receive clozapine, working with pharmacies to assure blood monitoring, and drawing blood to check WBC counts, contribute to the underutilization.

The risk for developing agranulocytosis or granulocytopenia is between 0.7% and 1.0% with most cases occurring within the first 6 months of treatment initiation. The risk of development in the second 6 months of treatment falls to 0.70/1000 patient-years and, after the first year, 0.39/1000 patient-years. Data from the US Clozapine Registry covering the first 5 years of use by 99 502 patients revealed 382 (0.38%) cases of agranulocytosis and 12 deaths (0.01%). With appropriate monitoring, the rate of fatal agranulocytosis should be in the range of 1 per 10 000 patients. This low risk, when compared to the significantly reduced risk of suicide as a result of clozapine treatment, makes it imperative to increase the utilization to prevent suicide in high-risk patients.

Of note, between 4% and 8% of African Americans and people of Middle Eastern origin suffer from chronically low white blood cell counts. There have been numerous efforts to identify genetic risk markers for agranulocytosis. Our group utilized whole exon sequencing in an effort to find a genetic marker. The final results are not sufficiently robust for a laboratory test to identify those who are not at risk (Tiwari et al., 2013). Sequencing of the entire genome may be needed to accomplish this goal which would revolutionize the use of clozapine.

Clozapine, like other APDs, but more so than all but olanzapine, can induce marked weight gain, glucose dysregulation leading in some cases to type II diabetes mellitus and diabetic ketoacidosis, and lipid increases. This syndrome is related to insulin resistance. Many of the people who need clozapine to reduce suicide risk will already be obese from previous drug treatment, poor diet, and lack of exercise. Intensive counseling may be helpful to prevent further metabolic problems. However, an interesting feature of weight gain with clozapine is it predicts clinical response (Leadbetter et al., 1992; Meltzer, et al., 2003). Treatments to counteract the metabolic side effects should be strongly considered. Metformin has been shown to treat a wide range of the metabolic adverse effects of clozapine.

Clozapine is associated with a low (0.015% to 0.188%) risk of potentially fatal myocarditis or cardiomyopathy (Merrill et al., 2005). A higher rate of suspected myocarditis (0.7% and 1.2%) was identified in Australia. Clozapine is not associated with prolongation of the QTc interval or sudden death due to torsades de pointes (Warner & Hoffmann, 2002).

As previously noted, a recent major epidemiologic study revealed that clozapine markedly reduces *all-cause* mortality compared to all other antipsychotic drugs and that a major contributing factor is the reduction in death by suicide (Tiihonen et al., 2009). Clozapine was superior to all other antipsychotic drugs in reducing death due to suicide (P <0.0001). The risk for death from suicide on clozapine, adjusted for risk factors, was 0.34, compared to 1.0 for perphenazine and 1.58 for quetiapine. Also, Tiihonen et al. (2009) found there was no offsetting increase in mortality due to ischemic heart disease.

De Hert et al. (2010) challenged the all-cause mortality conclusion of the Tiihonen et al. (2009) study, but not the conclusion that clozapine reduces the risk for suicide compared to other antipsychotics. The chief objection is a survivor bias in the overall mortality rate, based on the assumption that patients early in their course of illness made a suicide attempt, and were prescribed clozapine and remained on it, noting that discontinuation from clozapine is less frequent than other drugs. However, there are no data available which indicate the proportion of patients who are treated with clozapine in Finland is due to a prior suicide attempt. Treatment resistance would be a much more common reason for prescribing clozapine.

The risk of fatal agranulocytosis has proven to be about two-thirds lower than was thought when clozapine was first introduced (Hall et al., 2003). This has led to slightly less stringent blood monitoring in the USA. Every other week after 6 months and monthly after 12 months for individuals who experience no problems is now mandated. As the risk for suicide returns when clozapine treatment is stopped, it is likely that individuals who benefit from clozapine should take it for very prolonged times, perhaps indefinitely, especially if they are treatment-resistant, and no other therapies are approved for that purpose. Lifelong blood sampling places a real burden on patient and caregiver and does lead to discontinuation. The logistics of monitoring in rural areas is a real challenge and must be addressed with better resources and perhaps modified monitoring procedures, such as telemedicine. The metabolic side effects of clozapine are another factor that causes some patients and physicians to be reluctant to use clozapine, but these side effects do not affect all patients and can be minimized by diet, exercise, and use of a statin or other anti-lipid medications. Nevertheless, it should be noted that prolonged use of clozapine is not associated with increased mortality due to cardiovascular causes (Tiihonen et al., 2009). In addition, there should be efforts by managed care and governmental agencies, including the National Institute of Mental Health and the Departments of Mental Health of the 50 states, to make clinicians aware of the evidence in support of this application of clozapine. Finally, it is essential that this information about suicide and clozapine be introduced during residency training, as there is evidence that treatment practices acquired during this time are enduring. Further education of all practicing clinicians about the benefits of clozapine to reduce suicide is essential. Evidence such as that provided by Modestin et al. (2005) will no doubt help. When it becomes widely accepted that the standard of care for patients with schizophrenia or schizoaffective disorder who are at increased risk for suicide requires discussing the option of clozapine to reduce the risk of suicide, then many clinicians will feel compelled to do so. When that happens, lives will be saved, and the cost of treating schizophrenia, in both human and monetary terms, will be significantly reduced.

Guidelines for using clozapine for suicide risk reduction

The key risk factors for suicide risk for schizophrenia are listed in Table 27.1. Clozapine should be considered for anyone determined to be at high risk for suicide. This is particularly true if they include a recent suicide attempt, early stages of the illness, substance abuse, and impulsivity. Consideration of treatment with clozapine should be one component of the effort to understand the reasons for a suicide attempt or serious contemplation, thereof. Involvement of significant others for a patient during the discussion is often helpful, and may be necessary. Patients must understand the benefits and risks of utilizing clozapine, and the commitment needed to maintain treatment because of the risk for relapse if clozapine treatment is discontinued.

The importance of initial titration, dosage, and adequate duration of treatment, and avoidance of additional add on antipsychotic drugs until monotherapy has been tried are important general principles in utilizing clozapine. It is critical at the outset of treatment with clozapine to educate patients and their significant other as to why a trial with clozapine has been suggested, whether it be for treatment resistance or suicide risk reduction, how evidence has accumulated that for the right patient, benefits outweigh risks, how the risk will be minimized with white blood cell monitoring, what will happen if the white count falls below the thresholds for granulocytopenia and agranulocytosis, and the wide range of annoying side effects, including sedation, hypersalivation, tachycardia, weight gain, lipid changes, myoclonic jerks, and seizures. This group of side effects can generally be effectively managed, although the weight gain less so. They should rarely be the cause for discontinuation in patients who require clozapine because of treatment resistance or suicide. A discussion of reduction in any current extrapyramidal side effects and reduced risk of tardive dyskinesia, the necessity for compliance, and not stopping the medication in order to avoid a relapse should also be part of this discussion.

Achieving adequate plasma levels of clozapine (≥350 ng/ml), which may require periodic measurement at the early phase of treatment, and utilization of doses up to 900 mg/day will enhance the benefit to risk ratio. If the patient is receiving another antipsychotic drug when clozapine is initiated, it should be discontinued shortly after adequate clozapine dosage has been achieved. Monotherapy trials of clozapine should last for 6 months whenever possible. As discussed above, for some patients, a second antipsychotic drug may sometimes be effective. There is controversy about the value of adding risperidone or other APDs or drugs of other classes (Yağcioğlu et al., 2005; Weiner et al., 2010). Some selective serotonin reuptake inhibitors, including paroxetine and fluoxetine, but especially fluvoxamine impair the metabolism of clozapine, so that reducing the dose of clozapine is usually required when these drugs are added. Sertraline and citalopram do not interfere with the metabolism of clozapine (Urichuk et al., 2008). Valproic acid may also increase plasma levels of clozapine, warranting reducing the dosage (Urichuk et al., 2008). Smoking leads to induction of cytochrome P450 CYP1A2 which will lead to lower plasma clozapine levels. Conversely, smoking cessation may markedly elevate clozapine plasma levels (Cormac et al., 2010). Plasma levels of clozapine should be monitored for at least 3–6 months after smoking cessation and dosage adjustments made as needed. Patients receiving clozapine will need psychosocial treatment to maximize the benefits from the improvement in psychosis, negative symptoms, and cognitive impairment which may emerge in the months after starting clozapine. Family and group therapy, cognitive behavioral treatment, supportive employment, and activity therapy have all been used with considerable success to enhance improvement with clozapine.

Summary and conclusions

There now exists an abundance of evidence supporting the consideration of and probable utilization of clozapine in the majority of patients with schizophrenia and schizoaffective disorder who have made a recent suicide attempt, been hospitalized to prevent an attempt, or have a cluster of the risk factors that demonstrate high vulnerability to make a suicide attempt. However, just as the use of clozapine for patients with persistent positive symptoms who have failed two or more trials of other antipsychotic drugs, though supported by a similar body of evidence, influences clinical practice much less than it should, the same is even more true for suicide. Yet, in light of the human burden and financial consequences of suicidal behaviors, the finality and horror of completed suicide, it is imperative that the only drug shown to significantly diminish the risk and rate of suicide be widely utilized when indicated. For this to occur, fundamental issues with regard to using clozapine need to be addressed. Specifically, appreciation of the limited frequency of agranulocytosis after 12 months of treatment should lead to changes in the US policy mandating indefinite blood monitoring, while enhancing methods to diminish metabolic and other side effects such as seizures, hypotension, and hypersalivation, need to be addressed. Policy changes in community mental health centers as part of the Affordable Care Act might be implemented to consider clozapine use for suicide as a critical quality assessment measure. Further research on the most efficient way to administer clozapine in the community is essential.

Conflicts of interest

HYM is a consultant to Teva Pharmaceuticals, which is a purveyor of clozapine. He received grant support from Novartis which first introduced clozapine in many countries. He is a consultant to and has received grant support from ACADIA, DaiNippon Sumitomo, Eli Lilly, EnVivo, Janssen, Lundbeck, and Sunovion.

References

Altamura, C., Bobo, W. V., & Meltzer, H. Y. (2007). Factors affecting outcome in schizophrenia and their relevance for psychopharmacological treatment. *International Clinical Psychopharmacology*, **22**, 249–267.

Axelsson, R., & Lagerkvist-Briggs, M. (1992). Factors predicting suicide in psychotic patients. *European Archives of Psychiatry and Clinical Neuroscience*, **241**, 259–266.

Beasley, C. M. Jr, Tollefson, G. D., & Tran, P. V. (1997). Efficacy of olanzapine: an overview of pivotal clinical trials. *Journal of Clinical Psychiatry*, **58**(Suppl 10), 7–12.

Bleuler, M. (1976). An approach to a survey of research results on schizophrenia. *Schizophrenia Bulletin*, **2**, 356–357.

Bushe, C. J., Taylor, M., & Haukka, J. (2010). Mortality in schizophrenia: a measurable clinical endpoint. *Journal of Psychopharmacology*, **24**(4 Suppl), 17–25.

Caldwell, C. B., & Gottesman, I. I. (1990). Schizophrenics kill themselves too: a review of risk factors for suicide. *Schizophrenia Bulletin*, **16**, 571–589.

Cormac, I., Brown, A., Creasey, S., Ferriter, M., & Huckstep, B. (2010).A retrospective evaluation of the impact of total smoking cessation on psychiatric inpatients taking clozapine. *Acta Psychiatrica Scandinavica*, **121**(5), 393–397.

De Hert, M., Correll, C. U., & Cohen, D. (2010). Do antipsychotic medications reduce or increase mortality in schizophrenia? A critical appraisal of the FIN-11 study. *Schizophrenia Research*, **117**(1), 68–74.

Hall, R. L., Smith, A. G., & Edwards, J. G. (2003). Haematological safety of antipsychotic drugs. *Expert Opinion on Drug Safety*, **2**, 395–399.

Hennen, J., & Baldessarini, R. J. (2005). Suicidal risk during treatment with clozapine: a meta-analysis. *Schizophrenia Research*, **73**(2–3), 139–145.

Hoang, U., Goldacre, M. J., & Stewart, R. (2013). Avoidable mortality in people with schizophrenia or bipolar disorder in England. *Acta Psychiatrica Scandinavica*, **127** (3), 195–201.

Horvitz-Lennon, M., Donohue, J. M., Domino, M. E., & Norman, S -L. T. (2009). Improving quality and diffusing best practices: The case of schizophrenia. *Health Affairs*, **28**(3), 701–712.

Kane, J., Honigfeld, G., Singer, J., & Meltzer, H. (1988). Clozapine for the treatment-resistant schizophrenic. A double-blind comparison with chlorpromazine. *Archives of General Psychiatry*, **45**(9), 789–796.

Knittel, D., Munn, G., & Simmer, E. (2008). Prodromal psychosis as an etiology of suicide: a case report and review of the literature. *American Journal of Forensic Medicine and Pathology*, **29**(3), 238–241.

Leadbetter, R., Shutty, M., Pavalonis, D., et al. (1992). Clozapine-induced weight gain: prevalence and clinical relevance. *American Journal of Psychiatry*, **149**(1), 68–72.

Masoudzadeh, A., & Khalilian, A. R. (2007). Comparative study of clozapine, electroshock and the combination of ECT with clozapine in treatment-resistant schizophrenic patients. *Pakistani Journal of Biological Sciences*, **10**(23), 4287–4290.

Meltzer, H. Y. (2005). Suicide in schizophrenia, clozapine, and adoption of evidence-based medicine. *Journal of Clinical Psychiatry*, **66**(4), 530–533.

Meltzer, H. Y. (2012). Clozapine: balancing safety with superior antipsychotic efficacy. *Clinical Schizophrenia and Related Psychoses*, **6**(3), 134–144.

Meltzer, H. Y., & Okayli, G. (1995). Reduction of suicidality during clozapine treatment of neuroleptic-resistant schizophrenia: impact on risk-benefit assessment. *American Journal of Psychiatry*, **152**, 183–190.

Meltzer, H. Y., Alphs, L., Green, A. I., et al., for the International Suicide Prevention Trial Study Group. (2003a). Clozapine treatment for suicidality in schizophrenia: International Suicide Prevention Trial (InterSePT). *Archives of General Psychiatry*, **60**, 82–89.

Meltzer, H. Y., Perry, E., & Jayathilake, K. (2003b). Clozapine-induced weight gain predicts improvement in psychopathology. *Schizophrenia Research*, **59**, 19–27.

Merrill, D. B., Dec, G. W., & Goff, D. C. (2005). Adverse cardiac effects associated with clozapine. *Journal of Clinical Psychopharmacology*, **25**(1), 32–41.

Modestin, J., Dal Pian, D., & Agarwalla, P. (2005). Clozapine diminishes suicidal behavior: a retrospective evaluation of clincial records. *Journal of Clinical Psychiatry*, **66**, 534–538.

Muller-Siecheneder, F., Muller, M. J., Hillert, A., et al. (1998). Risperidone versus haloperidol and amitriptyline in the treatment of patients with a combined psychotic and depressive syndrome. *Journal of Clinical Psychopharmacology*, **18**, 111–120.

Munro, J., O'Sullivan, D., Andrews, C., et al. (1999). Active monitoring of 12,760 clozapine recipients in the UK and Ireland. Beyond pharmacovigilance. *The British Journal of Psychiatry*, **175**, 576–580.

Palmer, D. D., Henter, I. D., & Wyatt, R. J. (1999). Do antipsychotic medications decrease the risk of suicide in patients with schizophrenia? *Journal of Clinical Psychiatry* **60**(Suppl 2): 100–103.

Palmer, B. A., Pankrantz, V. S., & Bostwick, J. M. (2005). The lifetime risk of suicide in schizophrenia. *Archives of General Psychiatry*, **62**, 247–253.

Pompili, M., Lester, D., Dominici, G., et al. (2013). Indications for electroconvulsive treatment in schizophrenia: A systematic review. *Schizophrenia Research*, **146**, 1–9.

Reid, W. H., Mason, M., & Hogan, T. (1998). Suicide prevention effects associated with clozapine therapy in schizophrenia and schizoaffective disorder. *Psychiatric Services*, **49**, 1029–1033.

Siris, S. G., Bermanzohn, P. C., Mason, E. D., & Shuwall, M. D. (1994). Maintenance imipramine therapy for secondary depression in schizophrenia. A controlled trial. *Archives of General Psychiatry*, **51**(2), 109–115.

Spivak, B., Roitman, S., Vered, Y., et al. (1998). Diminished suicidal and aggressive behavior, high plasma norepinephrine levels, and serum triglyceride levels in chronic neuroleptic-resistant schizophrenic patients maintained on clozapine. *Clinical Neuropharmacology*, **21**, 245–250.

Thomas, S. H., Drici, M. D., Hall, G. C., et al. (2010). Safety of sertindole versus risperidone in schizophrenia: principal results of the sertindole cohort prospective study (SCoP). *Acta Psychiatrica Scandinavica*, **122**(5), 345–355.

Tiihonen, J., Lönnqvist, J., Wahlbeck, K., et al. (2009). 11-year follow-up of mortality in patients with schizophrenia: a population-based cohort study (FIN11 study). *Lancet*, **374**(9690), 620–627.

Tiwari, A. K., Need, A. C., Lohoff, F. W., et al. (2013). Exome sequence analysis of Finnish patients with clozapine-induced agranulocytosis. *Molecular Psychiatry*. 2013 Jun 11. doi: 10.1038/mp.2013.74. [Epub ahead of print].

Tran, P. V., Hamilton, S. H., Kuntz, A. J., et al. (1997). Double-blind comparison of olanzapine versus risperidone in the treatment of schizophrenia and other psychotic disorders. *Journal of Clinical Psychopharmacology*, **17**, 407–418.

Urichuk, L., Prior, T. I., Dursun, S., & Baker, G. (2008). Metabolism of atypical antipsychotics: involvement of cytochrome p450 enzymes and relevance for drug-drug interactions. *Current Drug Metabolism*, **9**(5), 410–418.

Walker, A. M., Lanza, L. L., Arellano, F., & Rothman, K. J. (1997). Mortality in current and former users of clozapine. *Epidemiology*, **8**, 671–677.

Warner, B., & Hoffmann, P. (2002). Investigation of the potential of clozapine to cause torsade de pointes. *Adverse Drug Reactions Toxicology Review*, **21**(4),189–203.

Weiner, E., Conley, R. R., Ball, M. P., et al. (2010). Adjunctive risperidone for partially responsive people with schizophrenia treated with clozapine. *Neuropsychopharmacology*, **35**(11), 2274–2283.

Yağcioğlu, A. E. A., Akdede, B. B. K., Turgut, T. I., et al. (2005). A double-blind controlled study adjunctive treatment with risperidone in schizophrenic patients partially responsive to clozapine: efficacy and safety. *Journal of Clinical Psychiatry*, **66**, 63–72.

Zhu, B., Ascher-Svanum, H., Faries, D. E., et al. (2008). Costs of treating patients with schizophrenia who have illness-related crisis events. *BMC Psychiatry*, **8**, 72.

Chapter 28

Antidepressants

Molly Ryan and Charles B. Nemeroff

The subject matter of antidepressants and suicide comprise, among other components, three major areas, namely: (1) the question as to whether antidepressants individually or as a class increase the risk of suicidal behavior and suicide, especially early in the course of treatment; (2) the question of whether long-term treatment, particularly of depressed patients, reduces suicide risk, and (3) the lethality of different antidepressants in overdose.

Since the early 1980s, much controversy has surrounded the use of antidepressant medications as a potential risk factor for increasing suicidality. A combined analysis of 24 short-term placebo-controlled trials indicated that suicidal thoughts and behaviors, though very low in frequency, were doubled in the patients who were treated with antidepressants versus placebo (Hammad et al., 2006), prompting reassessment of the safety of antidepressant treatment of depression. In 2007, the FDA expanded the black box warning on these medications, in place since 2004, to include information reporting an increased risk of suicidal symptoms in young adults aged 18 to 24 years. It is important to note that in the same warning, the FDA was explicit in stating that there is no evidence of an increased risk of suicide in adults older than 24 years of age and, moreover, that the suicide risk is actually decreased, or protective, by antidepressant treatment in patients older than 65. The warning also acknowledges the fact that depression itself increases the risk of suicide. It is widely believed that this purported increased risk of suicidal behaviors is secondary to the potential "activation" or increased energy experienced during the first few weeks of antidepressant treatment before the full benefit of the medication has been achieved (Friedman & Leon, 2007). It is of paramount importance to note that no completed suicides were reported in the original FDA analysis and the average incident of treatment-emergent suicidal ideations and suicidal behaviors was approximately 4% with antidepressant treatment compared with 2% in placebo. However, it is equally important to note that in general, suicidal patients were excluded from the placebo-controlled randomized, double-blind trials that comprise the FDA database.

Subsequent research has raised serious doubts about an association between antidepressant use and suicidality; in fact antidepressant use may actually exert a protective factor (Gibbons et al., 2007; Khan et al., 2003). Khan et al. (2003) reassessed nine randomized control trials involving 48 277 patients based on exposure years and suicide rates that were included in the FDA summary reports and determined these reports did not conclusively demonstrate a difference in suicide risk between antidepressant and placebo-treated depressed patients. Additionally, patient data on 226 866 veterans determined that suicide rates were lower among patients treated with antidepressants than those who were not, with an odds ratio of 0.83 (Gibbons et al., 2007). Bridge et al. (2007) conducted a meta-analysis of 4400 depressed pediatric patients and concluded that the number-needed-to-treat was far lower than the number needed to harm, 10 vs. 142, indicating that the benefits of prescribing antidepressants to treat depression outweighed the potential risks. Additionally, Friedman and Leon (2007) examined antidepressant use in over 70 studies for conditions other than depressive episodes, including insomnia, fibromyalgia, diabetic neuropathy, and smoking cessation, and found the risk for suicidal ideation or behavior to be substantially lower in these populations, suggesting that antidepressant medications per se are not suicidogenic.

One concern that has been voiced after the issuance of the black box warning is that prescribing

A Concise Guide to Understanding Suicide, ed. Stephen H. Koslow, Pedro Ruiz, and Charles B. Nemeroff. Published by Cambridge University Press.

for those with depression who would likely greatly benefit from these medications would decrease and inadvertently result in an increase in morbidity and associated suicidality. Indeed, Nemeroff et al. (2007) followed prescription trends from 2000–2005 and found a dramatic decline in antidepressant prescriptions written for adolescents coinciding with the release of the FDA reports. Gibbons et al. (2007) found that after the FDA warnings were issued, prescriptions for antidepressants in the Netherlands dropped by 22% while youth suicide rates increased by 49%. Some have concluded that although the overall risk for suicidal intent and/or attempts is increased by antidepressants when compared to placebo, these findings are either not statistically significant or statistically significant but not clinically meaningful. Antidepressants are still considered one of the first-line treatments for depression and should be prescribed in a well-monitored, controlled, and educated environment (Bridge et al., 2007). As with any treatment option in medicine, risk and benefit must be assessed to assure safety and optimal therapeutic benefit.

Certain antidepressants, particularly the older agents, are lethal in overdose. Each antidepressant medication provides a unique profile of side effects and efficacy including the potential for increasing suicidal ideations during initiation of therapy, reducing previous suicidal ideations present prior to therapy, and the potential for toxicity in overdose. Availability of recently prescribed medications, combined with the vulnerable period early in treatment in terms of reduction in depressive symptoms, interactions with other medications, and concomitant substance and alcohol use should all be assessed and considered when choosing an antidepressant medication or determining the number of tablets to allot to the patient (Hawton et al., 2010). Beasley et al. (1991) suggest that suicidal ideations and actions can be precipitated by depression alone and vigilant monitoring when starting or continuing treatment with an antidepressant should remain a high priority on every physician's agenda. The STAR*D (Sequenced Treatment Alternative to Relieve Depression) trial and a myriad of other controlled studies additionally remind us that those who are non-responsive to one medication may benefit greatly from another, often attaining remission (Gibbons et al., 2012). An important question that must be resolved is whether individual antidepressants exert greater or lesser risk for suicide ideation or behaviors. In the space below we describe the evidence relevant to each antidepressant, including the FDA analysis.

SSRIs

The first of the SSRIs, fluoxetine, was introduced in the USA in 1987. The addition to the market of this class of medication revolutionized the treatment of depression because of its efficacy, favorable side-effect profile, and extended half-life compared to the then mainstay of somatic treatment, namely tricyclic antidepressants and monoamine oxidase inhibitors. Gibbons et al. (2007) reported that treating patients with depression with an SSRI or a newer generation non-SSRI lowers the risk of suicide attempts to nearly one-third when compared with similar untreated patients. Moreover, patients are not more likely to complete suicide if prescribed an SSRI or alternative antidepressant (Khan et al., 2003). The Centers for Disease Control and Prevention (CDC) found that after the publication of the black box warning for all SSRIs, prescribing decreased significantly and the suicide rates increased dramatically in children and young adults, suggesting a correlation between the use of SSRI antidepressants and suicide prevention. In fact, the FDA reported results from a meta-analysis showing an overall protective effect of antidepressants on suicidal ideations and behaviors in all age groups over 25 years of age. Schneeweiss et al. (2010) conducted a meta-analysis on over 250 000 patients based on dispensing data that confirmed there is no clinically meaningful variation in the risk of suicide attempts and suicide completions among the five main SSRIs, including fluoxetine, citalopram, paroxetine, fluvoxamine, and sertraline, as well as when compared to alternative antidepressant medications, including the SNRI antidepressant venlafaxine, tricyclic antidepressants, monoamine oxidase inhibitors, trazodone, and mirtazapine. This study included both patients who had previous suicide attempts or exposure to antidepressants and those who were treatment naïve (Figure 28.1).

Fluoxetine: Fluoxetine has been approved for treatment of pediatric and adult MDD, obsessive-compulsive disorder (OCD), panic disorder, bulimia nervosa, and premenstrual dysphoric disorder (PMDD). It is also approved to treat depression in children ages 8 years and older. Fluoxetine has an extended half-life of 4–6 days and its major metabolite, norfluoxetine, a half-life of 4–16 days, making this

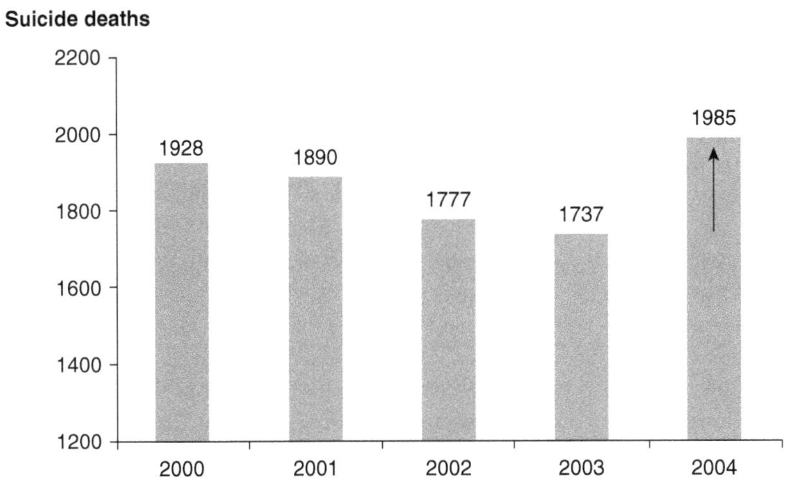

Figure 28.1. Unintended consequence of boxed warning.

the longest acting antidepressant available. As with all the SSRIs, fluoxetine is superior to placebo in treating major depressive disorder (Kasper et al., 1992). Initial case reports of six patients suggested that fluoxetine contributed or caused serious, violent suicidal ideations after an average of 4 weeks of treatment (Teicher et al., 1990). Once fluoxetine was discontinued, the suicidal ideations subsided after an average of 27 days. Larger, more comprehensive studies have determined that there is no relation between antidepressant use and suicidality, or only minimal effects on ideations or self-harm. In a comprehensive meta-analysis of clinical trial data including both patients with serious suicidal risk and those without, Beasley et al. (1991) found that fluoxetine improved suicidal ideation when compared with placebo and/or tricyclic antidepressants. The authors furthermore concluded that treatment of depression with fluoxetine did not substantially increase the risk of suicidal acts or the emergence of suicidal ideations relative to treatment with placebo and/or tricyclic antidepressants. However, should a patient ingest fluoxetine in excess of the prescribed dose, the most common side effects include tachycardia, sedation, tremor, nausea, and emesis; these symptoms are considered very minor and of short duration, thus no emergent treatment besides supportive care is warranted (Borys et al., 1992).

Citalopram and escitalopram: Citalopram and escitalopram are FDA approved to treat depression and the latter is also approved for the treatment of major depressive disorder in patients over the age of 12 years, as well as for adults with generalized anxiety disorder (GAD). In a randomized, double-blind, placebo-controlled trial, no increased risk of suicidal ideation or suicide attempts was noted in those prescribed citalopram when compared to placebo, even when accounting for duration of treatment, time of onset, or dosage (von Knorring et al., 2006). In the large STAR*D trial, a small group of males (N = 120 out of 1915) were observed to have genetic markers that predisposed to developing citalopram treatment-emergent suicidal ideation; the effect was dose related (Laje et al., 2007). Clinicians should note that many patients express suicidal ideation early in treatment, and caution must be exhibited when initiating any treatment. A review of previous studies found that the relative risk of suicide between escitalopram and placebo treatment was negligible, with no evidence suggesting an increased risk of developing suicidal ideations or actions when prescribed this SSRI (Llorca et al., 2005). In the event of overdose with citalopram or escitalopram, common side effects include nausea, vomiting, increased sweating, dry mouth, insomnia, ejaculatory dysfunction, and headaches. In March of 2012, the FDA announced that it no longer recommended prescribing citalopram in excess of 40 mg per day because higher dosages were shown to be associated with increased cardiac abnormalities, including QT interval prolongation, ventricular arrhythmias, and torsade de pointes.

Paroxetine: Paroxetine is approved by the FDA for the treatment of depression, panic disorder, OCD, PTSD, social anxiety disorder, and GAD. Paroxetine has been reported to cause an increase in suicidal ideations and attempts in children and adolescents when compared to placebo (Tiihonen et al., 2006). Carpenter et al. (2011) conducted a meta-analysis of randomized controlled trials which demonstrated an increased suicidal risk in young adults aged 18–24 years prescribed paroxetine compared to placebo when assessing age influences. This increased risk has been suggested to be secondary to medication-induced akathisia, switch of bipolar depressed patients into a mixed dysphoric mania, elevated plasma levels in individuals who possess cytochrome p450 2D6 polymorphisms rendering them slow metabolizers, or severe withdrawal effects after non-compliance. Carpenter et al. (2011) found no difference between paroxetine and placebo treatment groups in suicidal intent or actions in trials across multiple psychiatric disorders, including MDD, bipolar disorder, social anxiety disorder, panic disorder, PTSD, and OCD when including all age groups. This confirms considerable previously reported data demonstrating an overall benefit of prescribing antidepressants to treat depression and other disorders. The risk–benefit ratio would appear to be very favorable (Khan et al., 2003). Like other SSRIs, paroxetine overdose is rarely, if ever, lethal (Jenner, 1992).

Sertraline: Sertraline is currently FDA approved to treat major depressive disorder, OCD, PTSD, panic disorder, PMDD, and social anxiety disorder. As is the case with all of the SSRIs, sertraline has proven effective in treating depression both acutely and in relapse prevention, including reduced suicidality (Gibbons et al., 2007). Nelson et al. (2007) found that sertraline decreased suicidal thinking in depressed patients in an 8-week, double-blind, placebo-controlled trial of 747 patients. The authors also concluded that sertraline did not increase treatment-emergent suicidal ideations or actions during the course of the study. These results are supported by those of Vanderburg et al. (2009) who conducted a pooled analysis of suicidality in double-blind, placebo-controlled studies, reporting no statistically significant differences between sertraline and placebo in regards to increased suicidality risk in numerous individual or combined categories defined by steps toward possible suicide-related activities including self-injurious behavior, suicidal ideation, preparatory acts toward imminent suicidal behavior, suicide attempt, and completed suicide. Of note, in a review from the Department of Veterans Affairs, sertraline was found to have lower risks for suicide deaths than paroxetine; however, both of these medications posed a very low risk overall (Valenstein et al., 2012). The lethality of sertraline is similar to most other SSRIs, namely very low with minimal risk of long-term side effects.

SNRIs and other antidepressants

Newer generation medications such as non-serotonergic-specific antidepressants (non-SSRIs) or SNRIs are as effective as SSRIs in most studies, though there is some evidence for a slightly increased efficacy of SNRIs at least when compared to fluoxetine (Nemeroff et al., 2008). Many studies that focused on suicidality and antidepressants included both SSRIs and non-SSRIs with similar conclusions that both classes appear efficacious in treating depressive symptoms and preventing suicidal ideations and actions (Gibbons et al., 2005, 2007; Valenstein et al., 2012).

Venlafaxine: Introduced in 1994, this SNRI is approved to treat major depressive disorder, generalized anxiety disorder, social anxiety disorder, and panic disorder and there is evidence of efficacy in PTSD as well. Venlafaxine is thought to be comparable in efficacy to TCAs and, as noted above, is more effective than fluoxetine in treating depression (Nemeroff et al., 2008). Gibbons et al. (2012) reported that venlafaxine reduces suicidal ideations and behaviors in adult and geriatric patients, but not children and adolescents. However, there was no evidence of increased suicidal risk in children and adolescents treated with this medication. Of concern are the reports that venlafaxine has been reported to be more lethal in overdose than SSRIs after analysis of The National Health Service database in the UK; this may be due to effects on heart rate variability (Buckley & McManus, 2002). Venlafaxine is also associated with increased pulse rate and blood pressure, both dose related (Thase, 1998). Although Valenstein et al. (2012) reported venlafaxine to be comparable to SSRIs in regards to suicide death risks, Hawton et al. (2010) indicated that although venlafaxine is far less toxic than tricyclic antidepressants, it does have a relative toxicity index considerably greater than the SSRIs. In spite of the negative findings cited above in the pediatric population, an FDA analysis of clinical trials demonstrated a five-fold increase in suicidal ideation and behaviors in patients under 25 years when comparing venlafaxine to SSRIs. This suggests that venlafaxine has the highest suicide risk in children and adolescents. Emslie et al. (2007) reported an

	Increased risk
• All	1.95
• Venlafaxine XR	4.97*
• Paroxetine	2.65*
• Sertraline	1.48*
• Citalopram	1.37*
• Fluoxetine	1.52*

Figure 28.2. Suicidal behavior in children and adolescents.

increase in suicide-related events and hostility in over 300 patients aged 7–11 years treated with venlafaxine when compared to placebo (Figure 28.2).

Duloxetine: Duloxetine is an SNRI, FDA approved in 2004, to treat major depression, diabetic neuropathic pain, GAD, and fibromyalgia. As previously stated, SNRIs are comparable to SSRIs in efficacy in the treatment of depression. In a meta-analysis, Acharya et al. (2006) found an increase in suicidal ideation during initial weeks of treatment, both in the placebo and duloxetine groups. However, when compared to placebo, duloxetine both improved depressive symptom severity and prevented a worsening of suicidal ideation. The authors note that a reduction in suicidal ideations does not necessarily translate into a decrease in suicidal behaviors. Vey and Kovelman (2010) reported on the consequences of duloxetine overdose, with the most common side effects being nausea, dry mouth, constipation, somnolence, hyperhydrosis, and decreased appetite. Additional adverse effects, possibly at higher concentrations of the medication, include hepatotoxicity, orthostatic hypotension, syncope, serotonin syndrome, abnormal bleeding, seizures, hyponatremia, and elevated blood glucose levels. Hepatotoxicity appears to be the most common and potentially fatal complication, which led to labeling changes and a recommendation that duloxetine is contraindicated in patients with liver disease and hepatic impairment. Presentation of this serious side effect can include abdominal pain, hepatomegaly, and elevated transaminase levels. Vey and Kovelman (2010) additionally report that although duloxetine was involved in numerous fatal suicide acts, it was not implicated as the sole contributor to the cause of death in any of the 12 cases reported.

Bupropion: Bupropion is neither an SSRI nor an SNRI and its primary mechanism of antidepressant action remains obscure, though it is often inappropriately classified as a dual inhibitor of norepinephrine and dopamine reuptake. Bupropion is FDA approved to treat major depressive disorder, seasonal affective disorder, and smoking cessation. Bupropion is one of the top five prescribed antidepressants in the USA and is as efficacious in treating depression as TCAs and SSRIs (Grunebaum et al., 2012). A double-blind, randomized, clinical pilot study of 74 patients that did not exclude suicidal patients found bupropion in doses as high as 450 mg daily to be less efficacious for treating suicidal ideations, measured through self-report, early in treatment when compared to paroxetine 50 mg daily. Other studies have confirmed that bupropion does not increase suicidal attempts or thoughts during the course of treatment (Gibbons et al., 2007; Grunebaum et al., 2012; Valenstein et al., 2012). Common side effects of bupropion include headache, dry mouth, insomnia, nausea, constipation, and dizziness, but the dose-related lowering of seizure threshold is the most concerning in terms of overdose. This medication is safe in approved dosages but can be potentially fatal in overdose secondary to elevated blood pressure, acidosis, sinus tachycardia, cardiac toxicity with QRS widening on EKG, and seizures.

Mirtazapine: Mirtazapine is a noradrenergic and serotonergic receptor modulating antidepressant with no affinity for monoamine transporters or dopamine receptors. Mirtazapine is FDA approved to treat major depressive disorder. One study examining data from the US Department of Veteran Affairs found that mirtazapine had the highest suicide rate among newly prescribed patients, i.e., increasing rates of suicidal risk as time on the medication increased. The drug did not appear to reduce suicidal ideation when compared to bupropion. However mirtazapine was often prescribed at doses lower than those recommended to treat depression, notably as a hypnotic agent (Valenstein et al., 2012). Other reports list mirtazapine among non-SSRIs not associated with an increased risk for suicidal ideations or attempts during treatment (Gibbons et al., 2005; Gibbons et al., 2007). Kasper et al. (2010) compiled data from 15 placebo-controlled, short-term studies of mirtazapine use in the treatment of major depressive disorder and found a significantly lower suicidality risk when compared to placebo. Mirtazapine appears to be safe in overdose, with no risk of long-term side effects.

TCAs

Tricyclic antidepressants are effective medications in treating major depressive disorder and were considered the gold standard for many years prior to the introduction of the SSRIs. Numerous studies have researched the potential risk of increased suicidality after antidepressants are prescribed, and most have found no association or difference in suicidal ideations and actions after initiation of treatment of TCAs as compared to SSRIs or non-SSRIs (Beasley et al., 1991; Khan et al., 2003; Gibbons et al., 2007). Gibbons et al. (2005) did find that TCA prescriptions were positively correlated with increased suicide rates, but the effect does not appear to be causal. These authors report that low income, poor access to quality health care, lack of correct diagnoses of mental illness, poor compliance, and the increased lethality of TCAs are largely to blame. Indeed the major limitation to TCA use is their lethality in overdose. Cardiac arrhythmias, seizures, and central nervous system depression often prove fatal in overdoses even after minimal tablet ingestion. Additional concerns in toxicity include delirium, stupor, and sudden death in children and patients with prior ischemic heart disease. These concerns have appropriately resulted in a reduction in TCA prescriptions.

MAOIs

Remarkably, little research is available addressing monoamine oxidase inhibitors (MAOIs) and their effects on suicidal ideations or actions. Although MAOIs are approximately equally efficacious to TCAs in treating major depressive disorder, their side-effect profile limits their use when treating patients with a potential risk for suicide. MAOIs can cause hepatotoxicity, hypertensive crises or orthostatic hypotension, disorientation, and even coma with case reports indicating "ping-pong" eye movements. Additionally, dietary limitations involving the avoidance of tyramine-containing foods can also discourage use, because combining MAOIs with these foods intentionally could cause hypertension, occipital headache, palpitations, nausea, vomiting, chills, sweating, neck stiffness, dilated pupils, mild pyrexia, and motor agitation. These symptoms can worsen leading to altered consciousness, hyperpyrexia, cerebral hemorrhage, and death.

Discussion

Suicide continues to remain one of the leading causes of death in the USA. A diagnosis of depression is directly linked to suicidality, and therefore the use of antidepressant medications to treat this condition by shortening and preventing depressive episodes should seem intuitive. However antidepressant use has been suggested to both cause and curb suicidal ideations and actions, especially in the pediatric population. The proposed emergence of suicidal ideation when initiating treatment with certain antidepressants has clouded the benefit derived from treatment and continues to remain a focus of both the FDA and the psychiatric community. Clearly research identifying predictors of suicide risk in the small percentage of patients that exhibit increased suicidal ideation early in the course of antidepressant treatment is of paramount importance.

References

Acharya, N., Rosen, A., Polzer, J., et al (2006). Duloxetine: Meta-analysis of suicidal behaviors and ideation in clinical trials for major depressive disorder. *Journal of Clinical Psychopharmacology*, **26**, 587–594.

Beasley, C., Dornseif, B., Bosomworth, J., et al (1991). Fluoxetine and suicide: a meta-analysis of controlled trials of treatment for depression. *BMJ*, **303**, 685–692.

Borys, D. J., Setzer, S. C., Ling, L. J., et al. (1992). Acute fluoxetine overdose: a report of 234 cases. *American Journal of Emergency Medicine*, **10**, 115–120.

Bridge, J. A., Iyengar, S., Salary, C. B., et al. (2007). Clinical response and risk for reported suicidal ideation and suicide attempts in pediatric antidepressant treatment: a meta-analysis of randomized controlled trials. *JAMA*, **297**, 1683–1696.

Buckley, N. A., & McManus, P. R. (2002). Fatal toxicity of serotoninergic and other antidepressant drugs: analysis of United Kingdom mortality data. *BMJ*, **325**, 1332–1333.

Carpenter, D. J., Fong, R., Kraus, J. E., et al (2011). Meta-analysis of efficacy and treatment-emergent suicidality in adults by psychiatric indication and age subgroup following initiation of paroxetine therapy: a completed set of randomized, placebo-controlled trials. *Journal of Clinical Psychiatry*, **72**(11), 1503–1514.

Centers for Disease Control and Prevention. (2007). Suicide trends among youths and young adults aged 10–24 – United States, 1990–2004. *Morbidity and Mortality Weekly Report*, **56**, 905–908

Emslie, G. J., Findling, R. L., & Yeung, P. P. (2007). Venlafaxine ER for the treatment of pediatric subjects with depression: results of two placebo-controlled trials. *Journal of the American Academy of Child and Adolescent Psychiatry*, **46**, 479–488.

Friedman, R., & Leon, A. (2007). Expanding the black box: depression, antidepressants, and the risk of suicide. *New England Journal of Medicine*, **356**(23), 2343–2346.

Gibbons, R., Hur, K., Bhaumik, D. K., et al. (2005). The relationship between antidepressant medication use and rate of suicide. *Archives of General Psychiatry*, **62**, 165–172.

Gibbons, R., Brown, C. H., Hur, K., et al. (2007a). Relationship between antidepressants and suicide attempts: an analysis of the veterans' health administration data sets. *American Journal of Psychiatry*, **164**, 1044–1049.

Gibbons, R. D., Brown, C. H., Hur, K., et al. (2007b). Early evidence on the effects of regulators' suicidality warnings on SSRI prescriptions and suicide in children and adolescents. *American Journal of Psychiatry*, **164**(9), 1356–1363.

Gibbons, R. D., Brown, C. H., Hur, K., et al. (2012). Suicidal thoughts and behaviors with antidepressant treatment: reanalysis of the randomized placebo-controlled studies of fluoxetine and venlafaxine. *Archives of General Psychiatry*, **69**(6), 580–587.

Grunebaum, M., Ellis, S., Duan, N., et al. (2012). Pilot randomized clinical trial of an SSRI vs Bupropion: Effects on suicidal behavior, ideation and mood in major depression. *Neuropsychopharmacology*, **37**, 697–706.

Hammad, T. A., Laughren, T., & Racoosin, J. (2006). Suicidality in pediatric patients treated with antidepressant drugs. *Archives of General Psychiatry*, **63**, 332–339.

Hawton, K., Bergen, H., Simkin, S., et al. (2010). Toxicity of antidepressants: rates of suicide relative to prescribing and non-fatal overdose. *British Journal of Psychiatry*, **196**, 354–358.

Jenner, P. N. (1992). Paroxetine: an overview of dosage, tolerability and safety. *International Clinical Psychopharmacology*, **6**(4), 69–80.

Kasper, S., Fuger, J., & Moller, J. H. (1992). Comparative efficacy of antidepressants. *Drugs*, **43**, 11–23.

Kasper, S., Montgomery, S. A., Möller, H. J., et al. (2010). Longitudinal analysis of the suicidal behavior risk in short-term, placebo-controlled studies of mirtazapine in major depressive disorder. *World Journal of Biological Psychiatry*, **11**(1), 36–44.

Khan, A., Khan, S., Kolts, R., et al. (2003). Suicide rates in clinical trials of SSRIs, other antidepressants, and placebo: analysis of FDA reports. *American Journal of Psychiatry*, **160**, 790–792.

Laje, G., Paddock, S., Manji, H., et al. (2007). Genetic markers of suicidal ideation emerging during citalopram treatment of major depression. *American Journal of Psychiatry*, **164**, 1530–1538.

Llorca, P. M., Brousse, G., & Schwan, R. (2005). Escitalopram for treatment of major depressive disorder in adults. *Encephale*, **31**, 490–501.

Nelson, J. C., Delucchi, K., & Schneider, L. (2007). Suicidal thinking and behavior during treatment with sertraline in late-life depression. *American Journal of Geriatric Psychiatry*, **15**(7), 573–580.

Nemeroff, C. B., Kalali, A., & Keller, M. (2007). Impact of publicity concerning pediatric suicidality data on physician practice patterns in the United States. *Archives of General Psychiatry*, **64**(4), 466–472.

Nemeroff, C. B., Entsvah, R., & Benattia, I., et al. (2008). Comprehensive analysis of remission (COMPARE) with venlafaxine versus SSRIs. *Biological Psychiatry*, **63**(4), 424–434.

Schneeweiss, S., Patrick, A. R., Solomon, D. H., et al. (2010). Variation in the risk of suicide attempts and completed suicides by antidepressant agent in adults: a propensity score-adjusted analysis of 9 years' data. *Archives of General Psychiatry*, **67**(5), 497–506.

Teicher, M. H., Glod, C., & Cole, J. O. (1990). Emergence of intense suicidal preoccupation during fluoxetine treatment. *American Journal of Psychiatry*, **147**(2), 207–210.

Thase, M. E. (1998). Effects of venlafaxine on blood pressure: a meta-analysis of original data from 3744 depressed patients. *Journal of Clinical Psychiatry*, **59**, 502–508.

Tiihonen, J., Lonnqvist, J., Haukka, J., et al. (2006). Antidepressants and the risk of suicide, attempted suicide, and overall mortality in a nationwide cohort. *Archives of General Psychiatry*, **63**, 1358–1367.

US Food and Drug Administration: Clinical Review: relationship between antidepressant drugs and suicidality in adults. Available from: http://www.fda.gov/ohrms/dockets/ac/06/briefing/2006-4272b1-01-FDA.pdf)

Valenstein, M., Kim, H. M., Ganoczy, D., et al. (2012). Antidepressant agents and suicide death among US Department of Veterans Affairs patients in depression treatment. *Journal of Clinical Psychopharmacology*, **32**(2), 346–353.

Vanderburg, D. G., Batzer, E., Fogel, I., et al (2009). A pooled analysis of suicidality in double-blind, placebo-controlled studies of sertraline in adults. *Journal of Clinical Psychiatry*, **70**(5), 674–683.

Vey, E. L., & Kovelman, I. (2010). Adverse events, toxicology and post-mortem data on duloxetine: case reports and literature survey. *Journal of Forensic and Legal Medicine*, **17**(4), 175–185.

von Knorring, A. L., Olsson, G. I., Thomsen, P. H., et al. (2006). A randomized, double-blind, placebo-controlled study of citalopram in adolescents with major depressive disorder. *Journal of Clinical Psychopharmacology*, **26**(3), 311–315.

Chapter 29

Emergency department identification, assessment, and management of the suicidal patient

Collin L. Davidson, Jennifer H. Olson-Madden, Marian E. Betz, and Michael H. Allen

Overview of chapter

The rate of suicide attempts and self-injury has doubled in recent years and these problems now account for 0.4% of all ED visits, about 420 000 a year in the USA (Ting et al., 2012). In addition, regulators in the USA now mandate that hospitals "identify patients at risk for suicide." This has driven many to begin universal screening for suicidal ideation and behavior in their ED although the methods for doing so are only now being tested and the benefits are not yet clear. The current chapter aims to address issues surrounding the detection, assessment, and management of suicide risk in EDs, including definitions of risk stratification, the different roles of ED providers and mental health specialists, and the interactions between them. Central to the roles of ED providers are the prevalence and types of suicidal behavior, different forms of screening for suicide risk, and the expectations for immediate management. Once an at risk individual is identified, ED providers often consult mental health specialists for further assessment and recommendations for management of suicide risk. Therefore, the current chapter will also provide a brief overview of the considerations commonly made by mental health specialists in evaluating and managing risk. Given that death by suicide of a patient often results in litigation, the chapter will also address legal and ethical considerations. The chapter concludes with suggestions for future research and practice in this area.

Terminology

A major criticism of the field of suicidology is the lack of clear definitions of terms (O'Carroll et al., 1996). In practice, the use of different terms can undermine precise communication about a patient at risk for suicide. There have been several attempts at defining terms in suicidology, and this section will provide the most recent nomenclature. Table 29.1 presents the Self-Directed Violence Classification System, which is the official terminology adopted by the US Centers of Disease Control and Prevention, the Department of Defense, and the Veterans Administration (Department of Veterans Affairs, 2010). An encompassing term for thoughts or behavior related to suicide or self-harm is "self-directed violence" (SDV). As illustrated in Table 29.1, SDV can be classified into thoughts and behaviors, with varying degrees of intensity represented in both categories. For instance, an individual who thinks he/she may be better off dead but denies a specific plan and intent would be classified as someone with "suicidal ideation, without intent"; in another example, an individual who presents to the ED with a self-inflicted laceration requiring sutures with an expressed wish to die as a result would be said to have engaged in a "suicide attempt, with injury." The critical distinction between non-suicidal self-injury and suicide attempt in this case lies to some extent in the medical damage but also in the critical element of intent.

Suicidal intent can be divided into subjective intent (the self-reported intention of the SDV) and objective intent (external clues about the intention of the SDV, such as the presence of a suicide note or the lethality of an attempt). Suicidal individuals are often ambivalent about dying and there may be more or less intent to die as a result or an act of SDV. When any degree of intent to die is associated with SDV, the behavior is classified as a suicide attempt.

A Concise Guide to Understanding Suicide, ed. Stephen H. Koslow, Pedro Ruiz, and Charles B. Nemeroff. Published by Cambridge University Press.

Table 29.1. Self-Directed Violence Classification System

Type	Subtype	Definition	Modifiers	Terms
Thoughts	Non-Suicidal Self-Directed Violence Ideation	Self-reported thoughts regarding a person's desire to engage in self-inflicted potentially injurious behavior. There is no evidence of suicidal intent For example, persons engage in Non-Suicidal Self-Directed Violence Ideation in order to attain some other end (e.g., seek help, regulate negative mood, punish others, to receive attention)	N/A	• Non-Suicidal Self-Directed Violence Ideation
	Suicidal Ideation	Thoughts of engaging in suicide-related behavior For example, intrusive thoughts of suicide without the wish to die would be classified as Suicidal Ideation, Without Intent	• Suicidal Intent: – Without – Undetermined – With	• Suicidal Ideation, Without Suicidal Intent • Suicidal Ideation, With Undetermined Suicidal Intent • Suicidal Ideation, With Suicidal Intent
Behaviors	Preparatory	Acts or preparation toward engaging in Self-Directed Violence, but before potential for injury has begun. This can include anything beyond verbalization or thought, such as assembling a method (e.g., buying a gun, collecting pills) or preparing for one's death by suicide (e.g., writing a suicide note, giving things away) For example, hoarding medication for the purpose of overdosing would be classified as Suicidal Self-Directed Violence, Preparatory	• Suicidal Intent: – Without – Undetermined – With	• Non-Suicidal Self-Directed Violence, Preparatory • Undetermined Self-Directed Violence, Preparatory • Suicidal Self-Directed Violence, Preparatory
	Non-Suicidal Self-Directed Violence	Behavior that is self-directed and deliberately results in injury or the potential for injury to oneself. There is no evidence, whether implicit or explicit, of suicidal intent For example, persons engage in Non-Suicidal Self-Directed Violence in order to attain some other end (e.g., to seek help, regulate negative mood, punish others, to receive attention)	• Injury: – Without – With – Fatal • Interrupted by Self or Other	• Non-Suicidal Self-Directed Violence, Without Injury • Non-Suicidal Self-Directed Violence, Without Injury, Interrupted by Self or Other • Non-Suicidal Self-Directed Violence, With Injury • Non-Suicidal Self-Directed Violence, With Injury, Interrupted by Self or Others • Non-Suicidal Self-Directed Violence, Fatal

Table 29.1. (cont.)

Type	Subtype	Definition	Modifiers	Terms
	Undetermined Self-Directed Violence	Behavior that is self-directed and deliberately results in injury or the potential for injury to oneself. Suicidal intent is unclear based upon the available evidence For example, the person is unable to admit positively to the intent to die (e.g., unconsciousness, incapacitation, intoxication, acute psychosis, disorientation, or death); OR the person is reluctant to admit positively to the intent to die for other or unknown reasons	• Injury: – Without – With – Fatal • Interrupted by Self or Other	• Undetermined Self-Directed Violence, Without Injury • Undetermined Self-Directed Violence, Without Injury, Interrupted by Self or Other • Undetermined Self-Directed Violence, With Injury • Undetermined Self-Directed Violence, With Injury, Interrupted by Self or Other • Undetermined Self-Directed Violence, Fatal
	Suicidal Self-Directed Violence	Behavior that is self-directed and deliberately results in injury or the potential for injury to oneself. There is evidence, whether implicit or explicit, of suicidal intent For example, a person with the wish to die cutting her wrists with a knife would be classified as Suicide Attempt, With Injury	• Injury: – Without – With – Fatal • Interrupted by Self or Other	• Suicide Attempt, Without Injury • Suicide Attempt, Without Injury, Interrupted by Self or Other • Suicide Attempt, With Injury • Suicide Attempt, With Injury, Interrupted by Self or Other • Suicide

Elements of suicide assessment are divided into warning signs and risk factors. Many risk factors have been identified. Risk factors include those that are remote or distal to an episode of risk and those that are relatively current or proximal. Risk factors are often unmodifiable traits or elements of history such as age and prior attempts and tend to accumulate contributing to chronic risk which may exist for months or years. Despite a large number of such factors, risk may be low unless the risk factors are recently acquired and there are accompanying warning signs. Warning signs are elements reflecting more current or episodic states and include suicidal thinking, agitation, and sleeplessness. Warning signs appear close to an attempt and help to define an imminent risk period of usually days or weeks.

Focus of care in the emergency department

The distinction between risk factors and warning signs is important because ED providers are most interested in preventing morbidity and mortality evolving over a period of hours to, at most, several weeks. Up to 39% of people visiting an ED following a suicide attempt go on to reattempt, and those with multiple attempts are at greater than double the risk to die by suicide than those with a single attempt (Kapur et al., 2006). The conditional probability of suicidal ideation progressing to an attempt in 1 year is 7.3–9.7% in the community and it may be that this figure is higher in ED populations. Therefore, emergency providers must be concerned with protecting the individual from attempts during and following ED visits with suicidal ideation and behavior although ED providers are generally concerned primarily with proximal risk.

Identifying and assessing people at risk for suicide

The first step for ED providers in appropriately addressing suicide risk in the ED is to identify those at risk. Suicidal thoughts or behavior may be presented at triage as the reason for the visit, may be divulged only as part of another mental health complaint, or may be present incidentally along with another primary or given reason for visiting the ED. Screening methods allow for the systematic detection of risk in these different populations and follow the general schema of indicated, selective, and universal screening (Table 29.2).

Table 29.2. Definitions of types of suicide prevention interventions

Indicated	*"Targeted to high-risk individuals who are identified as having minimal but detectable signs or symptoms foreshadowing mental, emotional, or behavioral disorder, or biological markers indicating predisposition for such a disorder, but who do not meet diagnostic levels at the current time. Indicated interventions might be reasonable even if intervention costs are high and even if the intervention entails some risk."* *Example: Suicide screening of an individual patient by a clinician based on concerning symptoms or signs (e.g., patient is unusually tearful or has a flat affect).*
Selective	*"Targeted to individuals or a population subgroup whose risk of developing mental disorders is significantly higher than average. The risk may be imminent or it may be a lifetime risk. Risk groups may be identified on the basis of biological, psychological, or social risk factors that are known to be associated with the onset of a mental, emotional, or behavioral disorder. Selective interventions are most appropriate if their cost is moderate and if the risk of negative effects is minimal or nonexistent."* *Example: Suicide screening of all patients with substance abuse.*
Universal	*"Targeted to the general public or a whole population that has not been identified on the basis of individual risk. The intervention is desirable for everyone in that group. Universal interventions have advantages when their costs per individual are low, the intervention is effective and acceptable to the population, and there is a low risk from the intervention."* *Example: Suicide screening of all ED patients, regardless of presenting complaint, demographics, or presence of risk factors*

Indicated screening is targeted to individuals with apparent signs of risk or conditions associated with risk. This includes cases where further questioning is triggered by "red flag" symptoms or signs suggestive of depression or emotional distress in the ED. These "red flags" may also include other acute risk factors for suicide (Table 29.3): psychosocial stressors, impulsivity, severe anxiety or agitation, hopelessness, physical illness, aging, or substance use problems (Ronquillo et al., 2012; Bilén et al., 2013).

Selective screening includes screening all patients in a certain high-risk group for suicidal thoughts or behaviors. This would include screening patients who have lifetime (or chronic) suicide risk factors but may not have acute warning signs suggesting imminent risk. These chronic risk factors include: previous suicide attempts, a history of mental illness, a family

Table 29.3. Suicide risk factors

Acute/current	Presence of suicidal ideation Presence of a suicide plan or attempt Lethality of suicide plan or attempt Psychosocial stressors Presence of hopelessness Presence of psychosis Physical illness Male gender Age over 65 years White race
Chronic/ background	Family history of mental illness or suicide Current psychiatric diagnosis History of depression or personality disorder Prior suicide attempts Childhood traumas

Table 29.4. Modified SAD PERSONS score

Letter and meaning	Description	Points
S = Sex	Male	1
A = Age	<19 or >45 years	1
D = Depression or hopelessness	Admits to depression or decreased concentration, appetite, sleep, libido	2
P = Previous attempts or psychiatric care	Previous inpatient or outpatient psychiatric care	1
E = Excessive alcohol or drug use	Stigmata of chronic addiction or recent frequent use	1
R = Rational thinking loss	Organic brain syndrome or psychosis	2
S = Separated, divorced, or widowed		1
O = Organized or serious attempt	Well-thought-out plan or "life-threatening" presentation	2
N = No social supports	No close family, friends, job, or active religious affiliation	1
S = Stated future intent	Determined to repeat attempt, or ambivalent	2

Scoring: ≥6 requires emergent consultation with a mental health professional and possible hospitalization.

history of suicide, or alcohol or other substance abuse (Baca-Garcia et al., 2007).

Universal screening involves asking all ED patients, regardless of presenting complaint or personal history, about suicidal thoughts or behaviors. Proponents of this approach point out that many patients will be missed by current selective or indicated screening practices. A recent multicenter study of universal screening in six diverse EDs found 7.3% of non-psychiatric ED patients admitting to suicidal ideation of whom almost half, 3.3%, had a prior attempt and would be considered at least moderate risk (Allen et al., 2013) A 2010 Joint Commission national patient safety goal (15.01.01) requires "behavioral health care organizations, psychiatric hospitals, and general hospitals treating individuals for emotional or behavioral disorders, to identify patients at risk for suicide" (Joint Commission, 2011). This goal has been interpreted by some as a requirement for universal ED suicide screening. However, the practice of universal suicide screening in EDs is controversial, as there is no evidence of a mortality benefit from the practice and there are concerns about the additional burdens it could place on already busy EDs. It is unlikely that ED providers perform universal suicide screening unless there is a department protocol, and in one national survey of physicians at eight EDs, only 8% of attending physicians said they screen most or all patients for suicidal ideation (Betz et al., 2013).

Assessment instruments

To aid in further assessment of suicide risk in the ED, a few standardized measures are available. Structured approaches improve the consistency of assessment. Available measures are quite sensitive but less specific and serve primarily to document the presence or absence of selected risk factors which, if present, then require a clinical interview and risk estimation.

The Modified SAD PERSONS (MSPS) (Hockberger & Rothstein, 1988; see Table 29.4) was developed in a population of ED patients presenting for suicidal ideation or suicide attempts with a goal of predicting which patients require a mental health consultation. The tool includes 10 criteria weighted 1 or 2 points each, and a final score of ≥6 necessitates emergent consultation with a mental health professional for possible hospitalization. In the derivation sample, a score of ≥6 was 94% sensitive and 71% specific for the outcome of psychiatric hospitalization. More recently, Bolton and colleagues obtained MSPS scores and followed a large cohort of attempters for 6 months following an ED visit and used suicide attempts as the outcome (Bolton et al., 2012). Unfortunately, the MSPS proved no better than

Table 29.5. The Manchester Self-Harm Rule

Any history of self-harm
Previous psychiatric treatment
Benzodiazepine use in attempt
Any current psychiatric treatment
Scoring: ≥1 factor indicates moderate/high-risk of repeated self-harm or suicide within 6 months.

chance at positive prediction. However, a smaller set of five items accounted for most of the variance and a score of 2 or more was associated with a 5.58-fold greater odds of future attempt. Perhaps most interesting, scores of 0 or 1 had a negative predictive value of 0.993 suggesting that such patients were very unlikely to make a future attempt. This may be more important for triage in emergency settings.

Another measure is the Manchester Self-Harm Rule (Cooper et al., 2006; see Table 29.5). This measure includes four factors, is easy to score, and the presence of at least one factor was 94% sensitive and 25% specific for suicide within 6 months. In an external validation sample in Sweden, the rule had 89% sensitivity and 21% specificity for a repeated deliberate self-harm (including suicide and suicide attempts) within 6 months (Bilén et al., 2013). However, the rule includes the use of benzodiazepines as a risk factor which may not generalize to other settings.

When to make a referral to mental health specialists

This is a difficult question with little evidence to support a recommendation. Clearly most people with suicidal ideation will not make an attempt in the immediate future. Absent other warning signs or risk factors, the emergency physician may choose to release an otherwise stable patient who is not requesting or is refusing additional evaluation. The potential harms of forcing a patient to accept unwanted services must also be weighed against any putative benefits. However, as the number of warning signs and risk factors present increases, the need for a specialty assessment becomes more compelling and is probably warranted in the following circumstances:

- The individual presents with a suicide attempt or there is evidence of self-directed violent behavior including planning or preparation.
- The suicidal ideation is in the context of a significant mental disorder.
- The individual recently has been discharged from a psychiatric inpatient unit.
- The individual presents with a pattern of risky behaviors and injuries.
- The individual has a pattern of repeated, unexplained ED visits.

"Medical clearance" and the process of referral

A final important role for the ED provider is the medical assessment of the suicidal patient. Medical problems frequently cause or contribute to psychiatric disturbance or may be incidental, yet require attention during an ED visit. The scope of medical assessment required is the subject of intense debate. Mental health providers may ask for tests that do not seem indicated to ED providers. Substance use is common in such presentations and ED providers may be called on to determine whether individuals are incapacitated for the purposes of a mental health assessment and subsequently whether they are sober enough to reliably participate.

An American College of Emergency Physicians clinical policy committee has recommended that cognitive ability, rather than blood alcohol level, should inform this decision and that urine toxicology does not affect emergency management. It further recommended that in alert, cooperative patients with psychiatric complaints, the medical assessment be directed by vital signs, history and physical exam, i.e., a so-called "focused medical assessment." Routine laboratory testing was found to be of low yield and was not recommended (Lukens et al., 2006).

Once it is determined that a patient is appropriate for mental health assessment, this may occur in one of two ways with important implications. In one scenario, the patient is transferred to the care of a mental health team, perhaps in a specialized area of the ED. In the other, more common, scenario, the ED provider obtains a consultation from a mental health specialist who makes recommendations, but the patient remains under the care of the ED provider. In such cases, it is incumbent on the ED provider to accept and implement the mental health specialist's recommendations. In such cases, the ED provider and the mental health specialist share responsibility for the quality of the assessment and the outcome of the visit and the ED provider may be liable for adverse outcomes. For this reason, it is ideal for ED providers and mental health consultants to have established relationships and good communication. It is also wise for ED providers to have some independent knowledge of suicide risk assessment rather than relying exclusively on the mental health assessor. In cases where the mental health specialist and ED provider disagree, further discussion is critical.

Mental health specialists: assessment and management of suicide risk

For patients identified through brief screening as higher risk and in need of a full risk assessment, the best option is to have a dedicated multidisciplinary team with expertise in suicide and self-harm assessment (Mitchell & Dennis, 2006). This is especially true since many ED providers lack advanced training in suicide risk assessment and may not feel confident in their skills (Betz et al., 2013). However, practice patterns vary by ED size and location (Mitchell & Dennis, 2006) and mental health professionals including psychiatrists, psychologists, or trained social workers are often not available (Baraff et al., 2006). Thus, in many cases, the ED provider is responsible for the full suicide risk assessment (Ronquillo et al., 2012).

This section will detail the steps that are often undertaken by a mental health consultation team. For ED providers who have mental health specialist support, this section will be useful as it provides a comprehensive sense of the factors that mental health specialists deem important and how recommendations are made. For ED providers without mental health specialist support, this section will provide a basis for the next level of assessment.

Assessment of risk

To obtain a comprehensive assessment of suicide risk, mental health specialists generally ask questions in several different domains. As discussed above, characterization of suicidal ideation, suicide intent, and SDV behaviors such as attempts is a critical first step. A skilled interviewer will ask directly but put such questions in a context to normalize them. For instance, if there is evidence of depression, one might open with "Often when people are feeling depressed, they have suicidal thoughts. Are you currently having thoughts about wanting to kill or harm yourself?" A detailed history includes the frequency, intensity, and duration of suicidal ideation each of which helps to determine severity. Determining if an individual has a specific plan for suicide and if they have intent to die are crucial pieces of a suicide risk assessment. The more specific the plan and the greater the patient's intention to act on it, the higher the risk in most cases, although some patients will say they acted quickly with little planning.

It is also important to obtain a description of the precipitants, particularly relationship disruptions, job loss, major financial setbacks, and so forth. Particular attention to validated suicide risk factors such as hopelessness, depression, agitation, and negative life events is warranted. Further, given that one of the strongest predictors of suicidal behavior is past suicide attempts, detailed information on prior attempts is critical including actual lethality and intent to die. However, most completed suicides have no known prior attempt so the lack of an attempt is uninformative. Finally, a crucial component to suicide risk assessment is the determination of access to lethal means for suicide such as firearms or medications. Collaboratively limiting access to lethal means can drastically reduce a patient's suicide risk in the context of a comprehensive treatment plan. Practitioners are highly encouraged to collect collateral information from a knowledgeable person in the patient's life as a routine part of the suicide risk assessment. Failing to do so could result in missing vital information that the patient has withheld, missing opportunities to mitigate risk and increasing the risk for litigation (discussed further below).

Estimation of level of suicide risk

In emergency settings, the most important assessment is the level of "imminent" or "acute" risk, i.e., risk for injury or death in the near term. Many individuals will accumulate "chronic" risk factors over time and may be vulnerable to suicidal behavior under some circumstances over many decades. However, in the absence of precipitants and warning signs, their acute risk may be such that it is not a focus of emergency treatment. For individuals with warning signs, an estimate of the imminent risk of suicide is made. This is generally described as low, moderate, or high. ED providers may choose to release those at low risk without further assessment, while those at higher risk should receive a more detailed risk assessment. A more comprehensive determination of risk is presented in Table 29.6 (Joiner et al., 1999; Bryan & Rudd, 2006).

Table 29.6. Levels of imminent (i.e., acute) suicide risk

Level of risk	Low risk	Moderate risk	High risk
Patient characteristics	• Denial of thoughts, plan, intent • No or mild sadness/depression • No psychotic symptoms • Hopeful about the future • None or limited anger • No recent attempt/1 attempt of low lethality/intentionality • No or limited use of substances • Good support/connected, accepting of help	• Positive evidence of ideation, plan, intent or attempt • Moderate depression, hopelessness, anger/hostility • Frequent ideation and/or threats; low lethality attempt history • Substance abuse, dependence • Moderate support, few relationships/supporters • Access to means • Unwilling/unable to seek or obtain help	• Frequent, intense, and enduring ideation • Specific plans • Subjective or objective markers of intent (e.g., means, attempt with high lethality) • Evidence of impaired self-control, severe dysphoria, preoccupied with hopelessness/worthlessness • Poor corroborative history • Many risk factors and no/little protective factors, refusing help
Treatment recommendation	Follow-up with outpatient mental health provider	Mental health specialist consultation	Inpatient psychiatric hospitalization

Low risk

On screening, if an individual is deemed to be at "low imminent risk," there are usually no significant changes to treatment or discharge plans. Individuals described as low risk would be considered for discharge without the need to hold for further mental health evaluation. Documentation should include relevant mental health diagnoses (e.g., depression), as well as recommendations regarding appropriate outpatient treatment (e.g., referral to primary care provider or outpatient mental health providers for treatment of depression).

Moderate risk

An individual with "moderate imminent risk" would be presenting with either: (1) a recent suicide attempt; or (2) a combination of multiple risk factors and some warning signs. Such patients should be held in a safe area within the ED under observation until assessment by a mental health specialist. Requiring patients to disrobe and placing them under observation as a matter of policy may be distressing and counterproductive.

Some patients at moderate risk may be safely discharged, but this will require some planning if they are to be discharged to the community. A safety plan is a prioritized written list of coping strategies and sources of support that is developed collaboratively with the patient (Stanley & Brown, 2012). The purpose of a safety plan is to develop realistic strategies that the patient can use before or during a crisis. This plan should be brief and composed in the patient's own words. There are some necessary content areas to address, including the following:

1. Identify warning signs (e.g., thoughts, images, behaviors).
2. Determine internal coping strategies (e.g., what the individual can do for self-help).
3. Identify social contacts and supports the individual can call simply for distraction without necessarily revealing their distress (e.g., friends, family, religious leaders, or other supports).
4. Identify individuals the individual can call and tell about their distress when in crisis.
5. Identify mental health providers, medical facility-based if available, and crisis hotlines the patient can contact when in crisis (e.g., the National Suicide Prevention Lifeline (1–800–273-TALK [8255]).
6. Determine access to lethal means (e.g., firearms and medications) and develop a plan to limit access to those means.

For discharged patients, outreach has been found to be an effective means for bridging the transition to outpatient treatment, and for facilitating greater adherence with discharge plans. Such outreach could include telephone contacts or reminders to the patient or identified supports. Note that for referral to outpatient care to be successful, a first appointment needs to be scheduled within a week; blind referral, (i.e., providing a phone number and telling the patient to call on their own) is usually not effective and should not be done in cases with moderate or high risk.

High risk

When an individual presents in crisis and appears at "high imminent risk" and outpatient safety cannot be assured, holding for observation is indicated. If the condition persists, or, if necessary, transfer to a safe and stable recovery environment (e.g., crisis residence or inpatient psychiatry unit) should be completed as soon as is practicable. Prior to "hand off" to psychiatry services, it is imperative that the high-risk individual be monitored appropriately and escorted by someone at all times in order to mitigate flight risk and to ensure safety. In the case that the individual has already established mental health care and can identify this provider to ED clinicians, consultation and correspondence regarding continuity of care should be completed.

Legal considerations

This section will address important issues to consider from a legal standpoint related to assessing and managing suicide risk. Specifically the standard of care for risk assessment, intoxication and decisional capacity, voluntary and involuntary care, confidentiality and collateral informants, and documentation will be discussed.

The standard of care for risk assessment

The Emergency Medical Treatment and Active Labor Act (EMTALA) requires that patients in the midst of a medical emergency receive evaluation and treatment regardless of their ability to pay. Under this law, suicide risk qualifies as an emergency, mandating the assessment and treatment of suicidal individuals. Further, as discussed above, the NPSG.15.01.01 guidelines suggest that persons at risk for suicide should be identified in both psychiatric hospitals and general ED settings. If a patient endorses suicidal ideation, a full risk assessment should be conducted (as outlined above), the patient's immediate safety should be ensured, and resources should be provided to the patient and/or family to mitigate risk. Currently it is an open question whether ED providers are held to a different standard by courts than mental health specialists.

Intoxication and capacity

"Decisional capacity" requires the abilities to express a clear and consistent choice, to comprehend treatment information, to understand the potential medical consequences of undergoing treatment and refusal of treatment, and to reason about treatment options (Appelbaum, 2007). Mental disorders are not usually incapacitating. Intoxication and other alterations of mental status, on the other hand, are incapacitating. Individuals incapacitated by intoxication or confusion are treated under the emergency exception to the doctrine of informed consent rather than mental health laws. The provisions of mental health law should not be used to detain incapacitated individuals.

Suicide risk assessment and related interventions should be conducted with an individual deemed to have decisional capacity. If a patient is intoxicated or confused, the assessment should be delayed until intoxication or confusion subside. States of confusion may wax and wane and decisional capacity should be reassessed if acute changes in consciousness occur (Hazelton et al., 2003). Finally, it is important that the results of the decisional capacity evaluation be thoroughly documented in the medical record.

Voluntary and involuntary treatment

Voluntary treatment occurs when an individual, deemed to have decisional capacity, provides informed consent for further treatment. Involuntary civil commitment occurs only when a patient is judged to be a danger to self or others as a result of a mental disorder and refuses voluntary treatment. Failure to meet involuntary commitment standards should not prevent the clinician from offering and documenting the offer of voluntary hospitalization if appropriate. Only when a patient refuses voluntary admission and their risk rises to the level of a jurisdiction's civil commitment criteria does involuntary treatment become an issue (Simon, 2003). It is important to note that specific laws and procedures regarding involuntary admission differ by state and country (Zinkler & Priebe, 2002), so familiarity with local laws is imperative. The standard of care for an individual deemed to be at imminent suicide risk is most often specialty care to ensure adequate assessment and attention to safety. Therefore, many patients who evidence a high level of imminent risk but refuse hospitalization are involuntarily held for further assessment by a mental health specialist and transferred if necessary to obtain that level of care.

Confidentiality and collateral informants

Collateral information refers to gathering information and perspectives from family, friends, other health care providers, and any other individuals who may have contact with the patient. It is frequently important both because patients may withhold critical information and because collaterals may be resources for safety planning and continuity of care (Jacobs & Brewer, 2004). When possible, a release of information should be signed by the patient to indicate their willingness for the provider to talk with collateral informants. If a patient does not consent for collateral information gathering in a situation where there are safety concerns, confidentiality may be breached (Jacobs & Brewer, 2004). In this circumstance, the provider asks for information from informants but does not provide confidential information to informants. Sometimes patients are willing to sign consent on this condition. The reasons for any breach should be documented in the medical record. It is also important to note that failure to attempt to obtain collateral information has been linked to litigation if a patient later dies by suicide (Melonas, 2011), further underscoring the importance of collateral information.

Documentation

Documentation has been called the "cornerstone of the defense of a potential suicide case" (Simpson & Stacy, 2004). Since malpractice cases often hinge on determining if the provider acted in accordance with what other reasonable clinicians would do, it is very important to document the thought process that leads to a given clinical decision (i.e., admitting the patient versus discharging with a safety or continuity plan). It is also important to document the details of the chosen plan such as the time of a scheduled appointment, the components of a safety plan, or other factors that mitigate suicide risk.

Future directions

This is a challenging area of practice. The field has focused on predicting events that are pleomorphic and rare but occur against a backdrop of other conditions that are common such as depression. The result has been assessment methods that can be quite sensitive and yet non-specific, thereby producing many false positives. However, for the ED provider, positive prediction is not the goal. Triage really

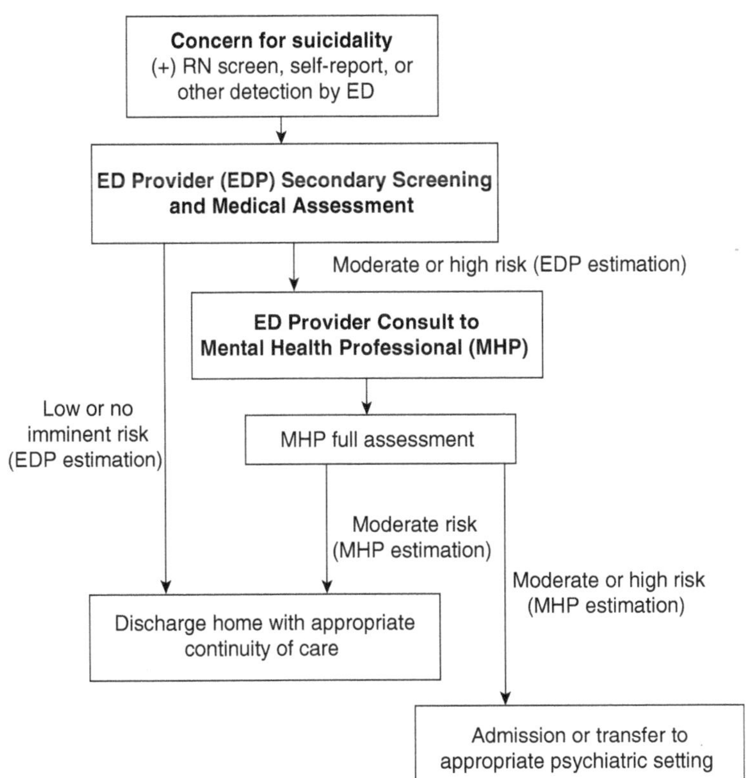

Figure 29.1. Suicide risk assessment in the emergency department (ED).

requires negative prediction, i.e., which cases are at low imminent risk of self-harm and therefore do not require a more extensive assessment and emergency treatment. Once a decision is made that a case is "not negative" or has some higher level of risk, then appropriate emergency procedures may be initiated. Other clinical decision rules in use in the ED may serve as an example. The Ottawa Ankle Rule is a list of three pieces of data from the history or physical exam; if any is present in a patient with an ankle injury, then a radiograph is indicated; if none is present, the patient is at low risk of acute fracture and does not require a radiograph. Similarly, the Pulmonary Embolism Rule-out Criteria (PERC) is a list of eight simple pieces of data which if present obviate the need for further testing. If increasing numbers of individuals are to be screened for suicide risk, similar methods will be required for distinguishing non-zero but low imminent risk patients from moderate to high imminent risk cases that require a more detailed examination and emergency mental health care.

References

Allen, M. H., Abar, B. W., McCormick, M., et al. (2013). Screening for suicidal ideation and attempts among emergency department medical patients: instrument and results from the Psychiatric Emergency Research Collaboration. *Suicide and Life-Threatening Behavior*, **43**(3), 313–323.

Appelbaum, P. S. (2007). Assessment of patients' competence to consent to treatment. *New England Journal of Medicine*, **357**, 1834–1840.

Baca-Garcia, E., Parra, C. P., Perez-Rodriguez, M. M., et al. (2007). Psychosocial stressors may be strongly associated with suicide attempts. *Stress and Health*, **23**, 191–198.

Baraff, L. J., Janowicz, N. & Asarnow, J. R. (2006). Survey of California emergency departments about practices for management of suicidal patients and resources available for their care. *Annals of Emergency Medicine*, **48**, 452–458.

Betz, M. E., Sullivan, A. F., Manton, A. P., et al. (2013). Knowledge, attitudes, and practices of emergency department providers in the care of suicidal patients. *Depression and Anxiety*. Epub Feb 20, 2013.

Bilén, K., Ponzer, S., Ottosson, C., Castrén, M., & Pettersson, H. (2013). Deliberate self-harm patients in the emergency department: who will repeat and who will not? Validation and development of clinical decision rules. *Emergency Medicine Journal*, **30**(8), 650–656.

Boltan, I. M., Spiwak, R. & Sareen, J. (2012). Predicting suicide attempts with the SAD PERSONS scale: a longitudinal analysis. *Journal of Clinical Psychiatry*, **73**(6), e735–741.

Bryan, C. J., & Rudd, M. D. (2006). Advances in the assessment of suicide risk. *Journal of Clinical Psychology*, **62**, 185–200.

Cooper, J., Kapur, N., Dunning, J., et al. (2006). A clinical tool for assessing risk after self-harm. *Annals of Emergency Medicine*, **48**, 459–466.

Department of Veterans Affairs. (2010). *Memorandum re: Standardized Suicide Nomenclature (Self-Directed Violence Classification System)*. Washington, DC: US Government Printing Office.

Hazelton, L. D., Sterns, G. L., & Chisholm, T. (2003). Decision-making capacity and alcohol abuse: clinical and ethical considerations in personal care choices. *General Hospital Psychiatry*, **25**, 130–135.

Hockberger, R. S., & Rothstein, R. J. (1988). Assessment of suicide potential by nonpsychiatrists using the SAD PERSONS score. *The Journal of Emergency Medicine*, **6**, 99–107.

Jacobs, D., & Brewer, M. (2004). APA practice guideline. *Psychiatric Annals*, **34**, 373.

Joiner, Jr, T. E., Walker, R. L., Rudd, M. D. & Jobes, D. A. (1999). Scientizing and routinizing the assessment of suicidality in outpatient practice. *Professional Psychology: Research and Practice*, **30**, 447–453.

Joint Commission. (2011). Hospital National Patient Safety Goals, 2011 (accessed 3/20/2014) http://www.jointcommission.org/assests/1/6/2011_NPSGs_HAP.pdf.

Kapur, N., Cooper, J., King-Hele, S., et al. (2006). The repetition of suicidal behavior: a multicenter cohort study. *Journal of Clinical Psychiatry*, **67**, 1599–1609.

Lukens, T. W., Wolf, S. J. J., Edlow, J. A., et al. (2006). Clinical policy: Critical issues in the diagnosis and management of the adult psychiatric patient in the emergency department. *Annals of Emergency Medicine*, **47**(1), 79–99.

Melonas, J. M. (2011). Patients at risk for suicide: risk management and patient safety considerations to protect the patient and the physician. *Innovations in Clinical Neuroscience*, **8**, 45.

Mitchell, A., & Dennis, M. (2006). Self harm and attempted suicide in adults: 10 practical questions and answers for emergency department staff. *Emergency Medicine Journal*, **23**, 251–255.

O'Carroll, P. W., Berman, A. L., Maris, R. W., et al. (1996). Beyond the Tower of Babel: a nomenclature for suicidology. *Suicide and Life-Threatening Behavior*, **26**, 237–252.

Ronquillo, L., Minassian, A., Vilke, G. M. & Wilson, M. P. (2012). Literature-based recommendations for suicide assessment in the emergency department: a review. *The Journal of Emergency Medicine*, **43**(5), 836–842.

Simon, R. I. (2003). *Clinical Psychiatry and the Law.* Washington DC: American Psychiatric Publishing.

Simpson, S., & Stacy, M. (2004). Avoiding the malpractice snare: documenting suicide risk assessment. *Journal of Psychiatric Practice*, **10**, 185–189.

Stanley, B., & Brown, G. K. (2012). Safety planning intervention: a brief intervention to mitigate suicide risk. *Cognitive and Behavioral Practice*, **19**, 256–264.

Ting, S. A., Sullivan, A. F., Boudreaux, E. D., Miller, I., & Camargo, C. A. (2012). Trends in US emergency department visits for attempted suicide andself-inflicted injury, 1993–2008. *General Hospital Psychiatry*, **34**, 557–565.

Zinkler, M., & Priebe, S. (2002). Detention of the mentally ill in Europe: a review. *Acta Psychiatrica Scandinavica*, **106**, 3–8.

Chapter 30

Psychosocial approaches to reduce suicidal behavior

Anne C. Ward, Catherine R. Glenn, Matthew K. Nock, and Michael W. Otto

Each year, nearly one million people die by suicide worldwide, and an additional 20 million people attempt suicide but survive (World Health Organization, 1996). Non-lethal suicidal behaviors (e.g., suicide attempts) are a serious public health concern in their own right and account for billions of dollars in lost productivity and health care costs annually (Center for Disease Control and Prevention, 2012). Despite advances in our understanding and treatment of major psychological disorders over the past 50 years, as well as the development of interventions to treat suicide-related behaviors specifically, rates of suicide attempts and mortalities have not declined (WHO, 1996). Thus, there is an urgent need for more effective suicide intervention and prevention strategies.

The purpose of the current chapter is to review the existing research on psychosocial approaches for reducing suicidal behavior, to summarize the limitations of current treatments, and to recommend directions for future research that could help improve the effectiveness of suicide interventions. Instead of examining treatment of specific disorders (e.g., major depression) that included a suicide-related outcome, trials in our review were devoted to the treatment of suicidal behaviors directly, either as a transdiagnostic characteristic of high-risk patients or as a primary symptom of a psychiatric disorder (e.g., BPD). We begin our review by considering some of the central targets for these treatments – identified risk factors for suicidal behaviors.

Risk factors and treatment targets

Interventions to reduce suicidal behaviors target a range of cognitive-emotional and interpersonal variables that are thought to be the most pivotal and modifiable causes of suicide risk. Central cognitive-emotional factors that have been associated with suicidal behaviors include hopelessness, anger, rumination, negative attentional bias, and low self-esteem, as well as deficient coping, emotion regulation, and problem solving skills (Rudd et al., 1994; Pietrzak et al., 2011; Hirsch et al., 2012). In addition, interpersonal concerns such as lack of meaningful relationships, deficient social skills, isolation, and attachment difficulties often drive depression and thoughts of suicide (Van Orden et al., 2010; Stepp et al., 2011).

Interventions aimed specifically at reducing suicide risk draw from several theoretical explanations for suicidal behavior that attempt to disentangle the destructive forces at work. For instance, the cognitive model of suicidal behavior highlights the difference between mood disturbances and suicide-specific concepts (e.g., wanting to die) (Wenzel & Beck, 2008). This theory proposes that dispositional factors (e.g., personality, comorbid disorders) put an individual at risk because resulting symptoms predispose them to engage in concomitant cognitive processes (e.g., attentional bias toward negative stimuli, rumination on past negative events) while at the same time lowering the threshold at which distressing events are viewed as "unbearable" (i.e., reducing distress tolerance). In this diathesis-stress model, environmental complications contribute to psychiatric symptoms, but additional psychosocial stressors are typically necessary for suicidal thoughts to be triggered. This model further assumes that once these thoughts are provoked, risk for suicide escalates as stressors intensify.

The interpersonal-psychological theory of suicidal behavior suggests that although someone may desire death, they must first acquire the capability to carry out their ideations through the experience of painful and provocative events (Joiner, 2005; Van Orden et al., 2010). Furthermore, this theory posits that thwarted

A Concise Guide to Understanding Suicide, ed. Stephen H. Koslow, Pedro Ruiz, and Charles B. Nemeroff. Published by Cambridge University Press.

belongingness (i.e. "I am alone") and perceived burdensomeness (i.e., "I burden others") contribute to desire for suicide, and that reducing these feelings is critical when treating suicidal patients (Joiner, 2005). For example, perceived burdensomeness has been shown to predict attempt severity and completed suicide above and beyond emotional pain and hopelessness, suggesting that people who score high on this construct tend to genuinely desire death (Conner et al., 2007). Additional research suggests that problem solving deficits, especially in interpersonal domains, contribute to hopelessness and risk for suicide (Dixon et al., 1994; Rudd et al., 1994).

Overview of studies and outcomes targeted

For this chapter, we searched PsycINFO, PubMed, and MEDLINE with relevant keywords (e.g., suicide, suicidal behavior, self-harm, parasuicide, and suicide ideation combined with therapy, psychosocial, treatment, intervention, and prevention) for articles published through 2012. We identified 55 RCTs in which an intervention aimed at reducing a suicide-related outcome (i.e., suicidal ideation, suicide attempts, deliberate self-harm) was compared to a control condition (e.g., community standard of care or treatment as usual [TAU]).

The identified RCTs ranged in sample size and composition, inclusion/exclusion criteria, as well as intervention modality and length (see Table 30.1). Therefore, when interpreting and comparing results, it is important to note the heterogeneity of approaches, even within categories. In addition, although all RCTs had the primary goal of reducing suicidal behaviors among high-risk populations (and most recruited only patients presenting for these behaviors), studies differed in the specific suicide-related outcomes targeted. For instance, few studies reported rates of completed suicide (CS) because suicide deaths are rare and their relative infrequency makes it difficult to detect between groups differences. In fact, of the RCTs reviewed, only eight (14%) reported the number of suicide deaths that occurred during the follow-up period, and only two found significantly fewer CSs in the treatment group. Instead of CS, most studies reported suicide-related outcomes with higher prevalence rates, including suicidal ideation (SI; thoughts about killing oneself), suicide attempts (SA; self-directed injury with suicidal intent), and deliberate self-harm (DSH; self-directed injury with or without suicidal intent). Given the current review's focus on *suicidal* behavior, DSH is not an ideal outcome variable because it combines suicidal and non-suicidal forms of self-injury (e.g., non-suicidal skin-cutting) – two distinct types of self-injurious behavior distinguished by their suicidal intent, medical severity, and function (Nock, 2010; Hamza et al., 2012). However, we chose to include DSH studies in our review given the limited treatment research in this area.

SI was evaluated as an outcome in 30 studies, SA in 22, DSH in 26, and 32 studies reported two or more suicide-related outcomes (see columns six and seven in Table 30.1). Our review below is organized by the primary intervention technique utilized; for each intervention type, we discuss the overall results and highlight studies reporting significant treatment effects.

Randomized controlled trials

Cognitive behavioral techniques

Cognitive behavioral therapy is predicated on the idea that cognitions, behaviors, and emotions are connected, and that by modifying dysfunctional thinking and behavioral patterns, individuals can change how they feel. CBT interventions are empirically supported treatments for several mental disorders that confer increased risk for suicide (Butler et al., 2006), and are typically short-term and problem-focused (Wright, 2006; Wenzel & Beck, 2008). Cognitive techniques may help patients overcome the dysfunctional cognitive processes that fuel suicidal thoughts and behaviors by teaching them to challenge and restructure beliefs related to hopelessness, shame, and guilt (Joiner & Rudd, 1996; Hastings et al., 2002). Diminished activity and anhedonia are also typical of depression; individuals are unable to experience pleasure, and therefore stop participating in the very activities that could help them break the cycle of negative affect. As such, behavioral activation may be a useful technique to help patients reengage while giving them the opportunity for enjoyment. The majority of RCTs included in our review (56%) utilized some form of CBT intervention.

Problem solving therapy

Given that negative life events (e.g., death, job loss, relationship disputes) commonly precede suicide-related behaviors (Rich et al., 1991; Pompili et al., 2011), problem solving interventions may help reduce these behaviors by teaching patients how to more

Table 30.1. Randomized controlled trials for suicidal thoughts and behaviors

Source	Sample characteristics			Experimental design	Results			
	Sample size (% female); age mean (age range)	Inclusion (In) and exclusion (Ex) criteria	Diagnoses	Experimental group vs. control group	DV: suicide ideation	Type of suicidal behavior (SA, DSH, CS)	DV: suicidal behaviors	Effect
Problem Solving Therapy (PST)								
Donaldson, et al. (2005)	N = 39 (82%); 15.0 (12–17)	In: presenting for SA; Ex: psychosis, low IQ	MDD (29%), disruptive behavior disorder (45%), alcohol (19%) or cannabis (45%) use disorders	Skills-based treatment vs. Supportive relationship treatment	3 mo. DT *ns*; 6 mo. FU *ns*	SA	6 mo. FU *ns*	E=C
Gibbons et al. (1978)	N = 400 (71%); mean not reported (≥17)	In: presenting for self-poisoning; Ex: other psychiatric illness requiring immediate psychiatric treatment, deemed an immediate suicide risk, or in continuing treatment with a session in last wk	–	PS intervention vs. TAU	–	DSH	1 yr. FU *ns*	E=C
Hatcher et al. (2011)	N = 552 (69%); 33.7 (≥16)	In: presenting for DSH; Ex: receiving DBT for BPD or management plan which precluded short-term therapy, low IQ, admitted for ≥48 hrs	–	PST vs. TAU	all FU* (3 mo., 1 yr.)	DSH	1 yr. FU *ns*	E>C
Hawton et al. (1981)	N = 96 (70%); 25.3 (≥16)	In: presenting with self-poisoning; Ex: requiring treatment for SU, high-risk for repetition	–	Domicillary problem-oriented treatment vs. Outpatient PST	–	DSH	1 yr. FU *ns*	E=C
Hawton et al. (1987)	N = 80 (66%); 29.3 (≥16)	In: recent overdose, >16, registered with GP; Ex: needing treatment for other disorder	–	PST vs. GP care	–	SA	1 yr. FU *ns*	E=C
Hvid et al. (2011)	N = 133 (71%); 37.1 (≥12)	In: recent SA; Ex: SCZ, psychosis, BD, severe or psychotic depression, low IQ, dementia	Rates not reported: psychoactive substance abuse, depression, neurotic and stress-related disorders, PDs, and some patients with no diagnosis	E :OPAC (outreach, problem solving, adherence, continuity) vs. TAU	–	SA	1 yr. FU*	E>C

Patsiokas & Clum (1985)	N = 15 (sex and age not reported)	In: admitted for SA, no intense psychiatric intervention needed; Ex: psychosis, alcoholism, or drug abuse	–	Interpersonal PS skills training (IPS) vs. Cognitive restructuring vs. Nondirective individual therapy	3 wk. FU *ns*	–	–	E=C
Rudd et al. (1996)	N = 264 (18%); 22.0 (range not reported)	In: recent SA, SI with mood or adjustment disorder, SI with alcohol abuse; Ex: psychosis, substance dependence, severe PD, thought disorder	Depressive disorders (52%), BD (20%), panic disorder (4%), phobias (71%), OCD (2%), PTSD (23%), somatoform pain disorder (24%), substance abuse (51%), no diagnosis (8%)	PSGT vs. TAU	all FU (1 mo., 6 mo., 1 yr., 18 mo., 2 yr.) *ns*	SA	all FU (6 mo., 1 yr.) *ns*	E=C
Salkovskis, Atha, & Storer (1990)	N = 20 (50%); 27.3 (16–55)	In: ≥2 SA, overdose on antidepressant, deemed likely to repeat behavior; Ex: psychosis or requiring immediate psychiatric intervention	–	PST vs. TAU	1 wk. DT *ns*; all FU* (1 mo., 3 mo., 6 mo., 1 yr.) *ns*	SA	6 mo. FU*; 18 mo. FU ns	E>C
van der Sande et al. (1997)	N = 274 (66%); 36.3 (≥15)	In: presenting for SA; Ex: habitual NSSI, excessive SU, accidental overdose, psychosis	Mood disorder (32%), adjustment disorder (14.5%)	1–4 day hospitalization followed by PST vs. TAU	–	SA	1 yr. FU *ns*	E=C
Dialectical Behavior Therapy (DBT)								
Koons et al. (2001)	N = 20 (100%); 35.0 (21–46)	In: female veterans with BPD; Ex: SCZ, BD, substance dependence, antisocial PD	BPD (100%), substance abuse (25%)	DBT vs. TAU	3 mo. DT*; 6 mo FU*	DSH	6 mo. FU *ns*	E>C
Linehan et al. (1991); Linehan et al. (1993)	N = 44 (100%); mean not reported (18–45)	In: BPD, SA in last 2 mo. and ≥2 parasuicide events in the last 5 yr.; Ex: SCZ, BD, substance dependence, or low IQ	BPD (100%)	DBT vs. TAU	1 yr. FU *ns*	DSH	all FU* (1 yr., 2 yr.)	E>C
Linehan et al. (2006)	N = 101 (100%); 29.3 (18–45)	In: SA in last 2 mo. and ≥2 DSH episodes in past 5 yr.; Ex: SCZ, schizoaffective disorder, BD, psychotic disorder, or low IQ	BPD (100%), MDD (72%), panic disorder (41%), PTSD (50%), any AD (78%), any SU disorder (30%), any ED (24%)	DBT vs. Non-behavioral psychotherapy	all FU (1 yr., 2 yr.) *ns*	SA	2 yr. FU*	E>C
McMain et al. (2009)	N = 180 (92%); 30.4 (18–60)	In: BPD, ≥2 SA or NSSI events in the last 5 yr. (one in last 3 mo.); Ex: psychotic disorder, BD, delirium, dementia, low IQ, substance dependence in past mo.	BPD (100%), MDD (49%), panic disorder (22%), PTSD (39%), any AD (75%), any SU disorder (9%), any ED (13%)	DBT vs. General psychiatric treatment	–	DSH	all DT (4 mo., 8 mo.) *ns*; 1 yr. FU *ns*	E=C

Table 30.1. (cont.)

Source	Sample characteristics			Experimental design	Results			
	Sample size (% female); age mean (age range)	Inclusion (In) and exclusion (Ex) criteria	Diagnoses	Experimental group vs. control group	DV: suicide ideation	Type of suicidal behavior (SA, DSH, CS)	DV: suicidal behaviors	Effect
Pistorello et al. (2012)	N = 63 (81%); 20.9 (18–25)	In: SI at entry, ≥1 lifetime NSSI or SA, ≥3 BPD criteria; Ex: psychosis, need for inpatient care, prior DBT	BPD (100%), MDD (81%), any SU disorder (37%), any AD (79%), any ED (16%)	DBT vs. Optimized TAU	all DT (3 mo., 6 mo., 9 mo.) *ns*; all FU* (1 yr. 18 mo.)	DSH	all DT (3 mo., 6 mo., 9 mo.) *ns*; all FU *ns* (1 yr. 18 mo.)	E>C
Turner (2000)	N = 24 (79%); 22.0 (18–27)	In: BPD and SA; Ex: SCZ, schizoaffective disorder, BD, OBS, low IQ	BPD (100%), dysthymia with GAD (71%). MDD (13%), dysthymia (13%), alcohol abuse (75%), substance abuse (83%), dependent PD (38%), antisocial (8%), compulsive PD (4%), histrionic PD (25%), narcissistic PD (25%), paranoid PD (8%), and schizotypal PD (13%)	DBT vs. CCT	6 mo. DT*; 1 yr. FU*	DSH	6 mo. DT*; 1 yr. FU*	E>C
Verheul et al. (2003); van den Bosch et al. (2005)	N = 58 (100%); 34.9 (18–70)	In: BPD, addiction treatment and psychiatric services; Ex: BD, chronic psychotic disorder, severe cognitive impairments	BPD (100%), addictive problems (54%)	DBT vs. TAU	–	SA, SA/ threats/ preparation	SA- all FU (1 yr., 18 mo.) *ns* SA/threats/ preparation- all FU (1 yr., 18 mo.) *ns*	E=C
Cognitive Behavioral Therapy (CBT)								
Asarnow et al. (2005)	N = 418 (78%); 17.2 (13–21)	In: presented for primary care visit with depressive symptoms; Ex: sibling in study	MDD (23%), dysthymia (2%), externalizing symptoms/conduct problems (28%), >2 PTSD symptoms (22%), problematic substance abuse (25%)	Quality Improvement vs. TAU	6 mo. FU *ns*	DSH	6 mo. FU *ns*	E=C

Brent et al. (1997)	N = 107 (76%); 15.6 (13–18)	In: DSM-III-R MDD, BDI score >13, living with at least one guardian, normal IQ; Ex: psychosis, BD, OCD, ED, substance abuse in previous 6 mo.	MDD (100%), dysthymia (22%), AD (32%), disruptive disorder (21%)	CBT vs. Systematic behavior family therapy (SBFT) vs. Nondirective supportive therapy (NST)	6 wk. DT *ns*; 4 mo. FU *ns*	–	Removed if SA made or no improvement by midpoint	E=C
Brown et al. (2005)	N = 120 (61%); 35.0 (18–66)	In: recent DSH; Ex: confounding medical disorder	MDD (77%), SU disorder (68%)	CBT vs. TAU	1 mo. DT *ns*; all FU (3 mo., 6 mo., 1 yr., 18 mo.) *ns*	SA	18 mo. FU*	E>C
Chanen et al. (2008)	N = 86 (sex not reported); mean not reported (15–18)	In: ≥2 BPD criteria, <9 sessions with mental health specialist in previous yr. and history of at least one of the following in childhood: PD, depressive, or disruptive behavior disorder symptoms, abuse or neglect; Ex: learning disability, psychiatric disorder attributed to general medical condition, PDD, primary Axis I disorder warranting treatment focus	>2 criteria for BPD (100%)	Cognitive analytic therapy vs. TAU	–	DSH	all FU (6 mo., 1 yr., 2 yr.) *ns*	E=C
Green et al. (2011)	N = 366 (89%); mean not reported (12–17)	In: ≥2 DSH episodes in past yr.; Ex: anorexia nervosa, psychosis, substantial learning disability, in secure care	MDD (62%), behavioral disorder (33%)	Developmental GT vs. TAU	all FU (6 mo., 1 yr.) *ns*	DSH	all FU (6 mo., 1 yr.) *ns*	E=C
Hazell et al. (2009)	N = 72 (92%); 14.5 (12–16)	In: ≥2 DSH episodes in past yr., 1 in past mo.; Ex: accidental overdose, psychosis, impending further DSH, low IQ	Depression (57%), conduct/oppositional defiant disorder (7%), alcohol problems (4%)	Developmental GT vs. TAU	all FU (2 mo., 6 mo., 1 yr.) *ns*	DSH	6 mo. FU* (E group worse); 1 yr. FU *ns*	E<C
Liberman & Eckman (1981)	N = 24 (67%); 29.7 (18–47)	In: recent SA or previous SA within 2 yr.; Ex: psychosis, OBS, substance addiction	MD episode, dysthymia, and/or adjustment disorder with depression (100%), most patients had PD	Behavior therapy vs. Insight-oriented therapy	21 wk. and 9 mo. FU*; all other FU (2 wk, 6 wk., 3 mo., 2 yr.) *ns*	SA	all FU (2 wk., 6 wk., 3 mo., 21 mo., 9 mo., 2 ys.) *ns*	E>C

Table 30.1. (cont.)

Source	Sample characteristics			Experimental design	Results			
	Sample size (% female); age mean (age range)	Inclusion (In) and exclusion (Ex) criteria	Diagnoses	Experimental group vs. control group	DV: suicide ideation	Type of suicidal behavior (SA, DSH, CS)	DV: suicidal behaviors	Effect
Raj et al. (2001)	N = 34 (68%); mean not reported (16–30)	In: first or second SA by overdose, diagnosis of anxiety, depression, or adjustment disorder; Ex: PD, <20 on MMSE, psychosis, dysthymia, bipolar affective disorder, OCD, ED, alcohol dependence or substance abuse	Current diagnoses not stated, history of psychiatric illness (23%), physical illness (13%), history of sexual abuse (13%) or physical abuse (23%)	MACT vs. TAU	3 mo. FU*	SA	3 mo. FU *ns*	E>C
Slee et al. (2008)	N = 82 (94%); 24.7 (15–35)	In: recent DSH; Ex: severe psychiatric disorder requiring intensive inpatient treatment, cognitive impairments	–	CBT vs. TAU	3 mo. DT*; all FU* (6 mo., 9 mo.)	DSH, CS	DSH- 3 mo. DT *ns*; 6 mo. FU *ns*; 9 mo. FU* CS-all FU (6 mo., 9 mo.) *ns*	E>C
Tarrier et al. (2006)	N = 278 (31%); 29.6 (range not reported)	In: first or second admission for psychosis, SCZ, schizophreniform, schizoaffective, or delusional disorder, or psychosis not otherwise specified, positive psychotic symptoms ≥4 wk., score ≥4 Positive and Negative Syndrome Scale target item either for delusions or hallucinations; Ex: psychosis not caused by substance misuse or organic disorder	SCZ, schizophreniform, schizoaffective, or delusional disorder, or psychosis not otherwise specified (100%)	CBT for psychosis vs. Supportive counseling vs. TAU	–	Severe SI/ DSH, CS	DSH- all FU (6 wk., 3 mo., 18 mo.) *ns* CS- 18 mo. FU *ns*	E=C

Tyrer et al. (2003)	N = 480 (68%); 32.0 (range not reported)	In: recent DSH, another DSH episode in previous yr.; Ex: psychotic disorders, BD, primary diagnosis of substance dependence, required inpatient psychiatric treatment	PD (42%)	MACT vs. TAU	–	DSH, CS	DSH- all FU (6 mo., 1 yr.) *ns* CS- 1 yr. FU *ns*	E=C
Weinberg et al. (2006)	N = 30 (100%); 28.2 (18–40)	In: chronic NSSI with one episode in mo. prior to enrollment, BPD diagnois; Ex: substance dependent, single NSSI episodes, previous SA, pschotic disorder, BD I, elevated suicide risk (>9 on BHS or plan for impending SA)	BPD (100%)	MACT vs. TAU	all FU (2 mo., 8 mo.) *ns*	–	–	E=C
Wood et al. (2001)	N = 63 (78%); 14.2 (12–16)	In: recent DSH plus at least 1 other instance of DSH in past yr.; Ex: psychotic disorder, impending SA, incarceration, learning impairment	MDD (84%), conduct or oppositional disorder (69%)	Developmental GT vs. TAU	7 mo. FU *ns*	DSH (multiple)	7 mo. FU*	E>C
Interpersonal Therapy								
Guthrie et al. (2001)	N = 119 (55%); 31.2 (18–65)	In: recent self-poisoning; Ex: requiring inpatient treatment	–	Psychodynamic interpersonal therapy vs. TAU	1 mo. FU *ns*; 6 mo. FU*	DSH	6 mo. FU*	E>C
McLeavey et al. (1994)	N = 39 (74%); 24.4 (15–45)	In: recent self-poisoning; Ex: low IQ, psychiatric treatment required for psychiatric illness, impending SA	Dysthymia (23%), dependent PD (15%), alcohol abuse (14%), none (44%)	Interpersonal PS Skills Training vs. Brief problem-oriented treatment control	–	DSH	1 yr. FU *ns*	E=C
Family Therapy								
Asarnow et al. (2011)	N = 181 (69%); 14.7 (10–18)	In: recent SA, SI, or both; Ex: psychosis or symptoms complicating consent and assessment	Severe depression (78%), PTSD (53%), SU disorder probable (17%)	Family intervention for suicide prevention (FISP) vs. TAU	2 mo. FU *ns*	SA	2 mo. FU *ns*	E=C
Diamond et al. (2010)	N = 66 (83%); 15.2 (12–17)	In: BDI-II>20, SIQ-JR>31; Ex: psychosis, recent discharge from or need for hospitalization, low IQ	MDD (39%), dysthymia (8%), AD (67%), externalizing disorder (56%)	Attachment-based family therapy vs. Enhanced TAU	6 wk. DT *ns*; 3 mo. FU*; 6 mo. FU ns	SA	6 mo. FU *ns*	E>C

Table 30.1. (cont.)

Source	Sample characteristics			Experimental design	Results			
	Sample size (% female); age mean (age range)	Inclusion (In) and exclusion (Ex) criteria	Diagnoses	Experimental group vs. control group	DV: suicide ideation	Type of suicidal behavior (SA, DSH, CS)	DV: suicidal behaviors	Effect
Esposito-Smythers et al. (2011)	N = 36 (67%); 15.7 (13–17)	In: alcohol or cannabis use disorder with SA in past 3 mo. or >40 on SIQ; Ex: psychosis, dependent on substance other than cannabis or alcohol, homicidal, IQ<70	Unipolar mood disorder (94%), anxiety (56%), disruptive behavior disorder (50%), alcohol (64%) or cannabis (83%) use disorder, other SU disorder (14%)	CBT for SU disorder and suicidality (I-CBT) vs. Enhanced TAU	18 mo. FU *ns*	SA	18 mo. FU*	E>C
Harrington et al. (1998)	N = 162 (90%); 14.5 (10–16)	In: recent self-poisoning; Ex: accidental overdose, psychosis	Depression (67%), conduct disorder (10.5%)	Family counseling vs. TAU	all FU (2 mo., 6 mo.) *ns*	DSH (multiple)	6 mo. FU *ns*	E=C
Huey et al. (2004)	N = 156 (35%); 12.9 (10–17)	In: recent SI/planning or SA, homicidal ideation or behavior, psychosis, threat of harm to self or others; Ex: autism	–	Multisystemic therapy vs. Psychiatric hospitalization	all FU (4 mo., 16 mo.) *ns*	SA	all FU* (4 mo., 16 mo.)	E>C
Nordentoft et al. (2002)	N = 321 (40%); 27 (18–45)	In: SCZ, schizotypal or delusional disorder, psychosis; Ex: low IQ, previous antipsychotic treatment >3 mo.	SCZ (66%), schizotypal disorder (11%), delusional disorder (6%), brief psychosis (9%), schizoaffective disorder (5%), unspecific non-organic psychosis (2%), harm or dependence syndrome (22%), depression (25%)	Integrative treatment vs. TAU	1 yr. DT *ns*	SA	1 yr. DT *ns*	E=C
Psychoanalytic Therapy								
Bateman & Fonagy (1999; 2001)	N = 38 (58%); 31.8 (16–65)	In: BPD; Ex: SCZ, BD, substance misuse, low IQ, OBS	BPD (100%), MDD (66%), dysthymia (58%), panic (34%), agoraphobia (37%), sociophobia (13%), bulimia (32%)	Psychoanalytically oriented partial hospitalization vs. TAU	–	SA	all* FU (18 mo., 3 yr.)	E>C

Intensive Intervention with Outreach								
Allard et al. (1992)	N = 150 (55%); Age not reported	In: recent SA; Ex: no fixed address, receiving adherence attention for other entity, physical handicap preventing attendance	Depression (87%), substance abuse (53%)	Intense intervention vs. TAU	–	SA	1 yr. FU *ns*	E=C
Chowdhury, Hicks, & Kreitman (1973)	N = 155 (56%); 38% <30, 46% 30–50, 16% ≥50	In: repeated DSH; Ex: deemed high-risk for repetition	No psychiatric disorder (36%), depression (14%), depression plus PD (25%), organic illness (2%), epilepsy (6%), SCZ (5%), alcohol or drug abuse (53%)	Special care treatment vs. TAU	–	DSH	6 mo. FU *ns*	E=C
Möller (1989)	N = 141 (sex not reported); 49% over 30	In: presenting for self-poisoning; Ex: none reported	Described as mostly neurosis, PD, and SU disorders	Continuity of care with individual psychotherapy vs. Hospital crisis intervention and community suicide prevention services	–	SA, CS	SA- 1 yr. FU* (E group worse) CS-1 yr. FU *ns*	E<C
van Heeringen et al. (1995)	N = 516 (57%); 34 (≥15)	In: presenting for SA, outpatient referral nonattendance; Ex: needing treatment other than in ICU	Mood disorder (15%), AD (3%)	Special care vs. TAU	–	DSH	1 yr. FU *ns*	E=C
Welu (1977)	N = 120 (sex not reported); 29 (≥16)	In: recent DSH; Ex: institutionalized	–	Special outreach program vs. TAU	–	DSH	4 mo. FU*	E>C
Contact Interventions								
Beautrais et al. (2010)	N = 327 (62%); 33.9 (≥16)	In: recent DSH/SA, >16; Ex: none stated	–	Postal contact after discharge vs. TAU	–	DSH	1 yr. FU *ns*	E=C
Bennewith et al. (2002)	N = 1932 (59%); 32.6 (16–95)	In: recent DSH; Ex: DSH in response to psychotic hallucination or delusion	–	Letter invitation from GP to schedule consultation where training would be employed vs. TAU	–	DSH	1 yr. FU *ns*	E=C

Table 30.1. (cont.)

Source	Sample characteristics			Experimental design	Results			
	Sample size (% female); age mean (age range)	Inclusion (In) and exclusion (Ex) criteria	Diagnoses	Experimental group vs. control group	DV: suicide ideation	Type of suicidal behavior (SA, DSH, CS)	DV: suicidal behaviors	Effect
Bertolote et al. (2010)	N = 1,867 (58%); median 23 (range not reported)	In: recent SA; Ex: clinical conditions not allowing interview or leaving against medical order	–	Brief intervention and contact vs. TAU	–	DSH	18 mo. FU *ns*	E=C
Carter et al. (2005); Carter et al. (2007)	N = 772 (68%); median 33 (interquartile range 24–44)	In: presenting for self-poisoning; Ex: no fixed address	Diagnoses not reported, median number of comorbid disorders (interquartile range 1–2)	Postal contact program vs. TAU	–	DSH	all FU (1 yr., 2 yr.) *ns*	E=C
Cedereke et al. (2002)	N = 216 (66%); 41.0 (range not reported)	In: recent SA; Ex: not stated	Mood disorder (42%), adjustment disorder (29%), other diagnosis (22%)	Telephone contact vs. TAU	1 mo. DT *ns*; 1 yr. FU *ns*	DSH, CS	DSH-1 yr. FU *ns* CS- 11 mo. FU *ns*	E=C
Fleischmann et al. (2008)	N = 1867 (58%); median 23.0 (range not reported)	In: recent SA; Ex: clinical conditions not allowing interview or leaving against medical order	–	Brief intervention and contact vs. TAU	–	CS	18 mo. FU*	E>C
Hassanian-Moghaddam et al. (2011)	N = 2113 (66%); 24.1 (≥12)	In: recent self-poisoning, >12; Ex: treatment only in ER, incapable of informed consent, psychosis, no fixed address	–	Postal contact after discharge vs. TAU	1 yr. FU*	SA	1 yr. FU*	E>C
Hassanzadeh et al. (2010)	N = 629 (62%); 24.5 (12–69)	In: recent SA; Ex: none stated	Chronic psychiatric illness (55%)	Brief intervention and contact vs. TAU	–	SA	6 mo. FU *ns*	E=C

Motto (1976); Motto & Bostrom (2001)	N = 843 (56%); 32.3 (range not reported)	In: hospitalization for depressive or suicidal state, refused ongoing care; Ex: none reported	–	Postal contact after discharge vs. TAU	–	CS	2 yr. DT*; 5 yr. FU *ns*	E>C
Robinson et al. (2012)	N = 164 (65%); (15–24)	In: history of suicidal threats, SI, or DSH; Ex: presenting due to organic cause, low IQ	Mood disorder (67%), AD 63%, SU (25%), no diagnosis (21%)	Postal contact program vs. TAU	all FU (1 yr., 18 mo.) *ns*	SA	all FU (1 yr., 18 mo.) *ns*	E=C
Vaiva et al. (2006)	N = 605 (73%); 35.7 (18–65)	In: presenting for SA by overdose; Ex: drug dependence, homelessness	–	Telephone contact at 1 mo. vs. telephone contact at 3 mo. vs. TAU	–	SA, CS	SA- 13 mo. FU* (Contact at 1 mo. superior) CS- 13 mo. FU *ns*	E>C

* $P < 0.05$, termination included in FU.

C=control group; CS=completed suicide; DSH=deliberate self-harm; DT=during treatment; DV=dependent variable; E=experimental group; ER=emergency room; FU=follow-up; GT=group therapy; N=no; PS=problem solving; SA=suicide attempt; SI=suicidal ideation; SSRI=selective serotonin reuptake inhibitors; TAU=Treatment as usual; Y=yes

Diagnoses: AD=anxiety disorder; ADHD=attention-deficit/hyperactivity disorder; BD=bipolar disorder; BPD=borderline personality disorder; ED=eating disorder; OCD=obsessive-compulsive disorder; OBS=organic brain syndrome; PD=personality disorder; PDD=pervasive developmental disorder; PTSD=post-traumatic stress disorder; SCZ=schizophrenia; SU=substance use.

adaptively manage and resolve acute crises. Problem solving therapy (PST) offers a systematic framework for approaching problems, testing solutions, and evaluating outcomes.

Problem-focused interventions were utilized in 10 RCTs in our review (18%), and three reported significant reductions in SA (Salkovskis et al., 1990; Hvid et al., 2011) or SI (Hatcher et al., 2011). Salkovskis and colleagues (1990) found that suicide attempters who received five sessions of PST with a home-based component made significantly fewer reattempts over a 6-month follow-up than those receiving TAU; however, treatment effects were not maintained at 1-year follow-up. Likewise, Hvid et al. (2011) focused on improving problem solving skills over eight home sessions and reported significantly fewer reattempts in the treatment group a year later, compared to usual care. Similarly, nine problem solving sessions administered over 3 months also proved more successful in reducing SI than TAU (Hatcher et al., 2011). However, the remaining seven studies (70%) failed to report significant treatment findings, suggesting PST's limited effectiveness in reducing suicidal behaviors and underscoring the need to identify why PST works in some settings, and for some individuals, but not others.

Dialectical behavior therapy

DBT was originally developed to treat BPD and was one of the first treatments to specifically target self-injurious behaviors. DBT is typically administered over the course of a year through weekly individual therapy, group skills training (i.e., mindfulness, interpersonal effectiveness, distress tolerance, and emotional regulation skills), and telephone coaching sessions (Linehan, 1993).

Seven studies in our review investigated the efficacy of DBT, five of which demonstrated significant reductions in DSH (Linehan et al., 1991, 1993; Turner, 2000), SA (Linehan et al., 2006), or SI (Turner, 2000; Koons et al., 2001; Pistorello et al., 2012). Linehan and colleagues first examined the effectiveness of DBT in a sample of female patients with BPD and a history of multiple self-harm episodes: the DBT group reported significantly greater reductions in DSH and fewer inpatient psychiatric days compared to controls, both at therapy termination (Linehan et al., 1991) and at 1-year follow-up (Linehan et al., 1993). In a replication of this work, Turner (2000) found DBT to be superior to client-centered therapy in a patient sample with BPD and a recent SA, as evidenced by fewer DSH episodes, less SI, fewer hospitalizations, and greater improvement in global functioning. Another DBT trial conducted with female veterans with BPD, reported significant reductions in SI compared to usual care (Koons et al., 2001). In addition, only patients receiving DBT reduced their self-harming behaviors, but these reductions were not greater than TAU (Koons et al., 2001). Recently, Pistorello et al. (2012) tested DBT in a college student sample and also found significant reductions in SI at therapy termination and 6-month follow-up, relative to a "supervision by experts" control condition. Finally, the single DBT study to report significant reductions in SA found that reattempts occurred half as frequently in the DBT group compared to a non-behavioral psychotherapy control group, at 1-year follow-up (Linehan et al., 2006).

It is important to note that, although there is some support for the effectiveness of DBT for reducing suicidal behaviors, most trials were conducted with female patients with BPD, and trials that did include men were at least 80% female (Turner, 2000; McMain et al., 2009; Pistorello et al., 2012). Therefore, it is not clear how these treatment effects will generalize to other clinical and sociodemographic groups. In addition, most studies (except for Linehan et al., 2006) examined DBT's effectiveness for reducing rates of DSH and not *suicidal* behaviors specifically.

General CBT

As discussed previously, CBT explores the reciprocal interactions between thoughts, affect, and behavior, with specific attention to the ways in which negative automatic cognitions drive both negative emotions and maladaptive actions. Broad-based CBT interventions (i.e., those that could not be better defined by a primary focus on problem solving or DBT) were tested in 13 studies, five of which reported significant reductions in DSH (Wood et al., 2001; Slee et al., 2008), SA (Brown et al., 2005), or SI (Liberman & Eckman, 1981; Raj et al., 2001; Slee et al., 2008).

When interpreting results, it is important to consider that many of the studies included in this broad category were multimodal, and studies were organized based on their principal focus and most distinguishing features. A prime example of this diversity is a trial conducted by Wood and colleagues (2001) that assessed the efficacy of "manualized developmental group therapy" – an integrative approach that incorporated aspects of traditional CBT, as well as DBT, PST, and psychodynamic therapy. Relative to the comparison sample, adolescents who received this intervention abstained from DSH for longer periods of time and were less likely to engage in multiple DSH episodes. Brown and colleagues' (2005) CBT trial also provides support for this approach: adult patients who received case management and 10 home-based sessions reattempted suicide less frequently over the subsequent 18 months compared to those who received TAU. Similarly, Slee and colleagues (2008) reported treatment benefits following 12 sessions of individual CBT; the CBT group exhibited significant reductions in DSH and SI, as well as reduced depression and anxiety symptoms, compared to patients who received standard care. Additional CBT studies also reported significant reductions in SI following treatment. In a small inpatient sample, Liberman and Eckman (1981) found that individual and group behavior therapy administered over 10 days was significantly more effective than insight-oriented therapy for reducing SI at 6- and 9-month follow-ups. Similarly, Raj et al. (2001) reported that 10 sessions of manual-assisted CBT was more effective than standard care in reducing SI.

Although the remaining CBT studies did not detect significant treatment effects, the majority of treatment groups trended toward greater improvements in suicide-related outcomes compared to control interventions. However, one trial reported that the treatment group had *worse* outcomes than the comparison intervention. Specifically, Hazell et al. (2009) found that patients who attended developmental group therapy engaged in significantly more DSH episodes than the routine care control group (i.e., unspecified individual and family counseling, pharmacotherapy, and care coordination) over the subsequent 6 months (Hazell et al., 2009). Although the disparity between groups dissipated by 1 year, the treatment condition still trended toward increased DSH levels.

Taken together, our review indicates that CBT interventions are one of the best-researched approaches for reducing suicidal behaviors. However, findings for the effectiveness of CBT techniques are mixed and further research is needed to identify which components of CBT are most helpful and for whom.

Interpersonal therapy (IPT)

IPT examines how interactions in current and past relationships impact an individual's emotional well-being (Weissman, 2010). IPT to reduce suicidal behaviors focuses on identifying and understanding social factors that maintain symptoms, reinforcing adaptive coping strategies, and fostering relationships. IPT was used in two RCTs in our review, one of which reported significant treatment effects: Guthrie and colleagues (2001) found that four sessions of home-based IPT with a psychodynamic component resulted in reduced DSH among patients, compared to usual care. Given the limited research using IPT, more studies are necessary to determine the efficacy of this intervention for reducing suicidal behaviors.

Family therapy

The goals of family therapy are to increase family cohesion and support, reduce stress and fears within the family, and alter the deleterious progression of negative interactions within the family system (Carr, 2012). Family therapy for reducing suicidal behaviors focuses on psychoeducation, fostering skills that promote positive interactions and familial support, recognizing suicide warning signs, and taking preventive action. In our review, family interventions to reduce suicidal behaviors ranged from multisystemic family therapy (Huey et al., 2004) to CBT for substance use and suicidal behaviors (Esposito-Smythers et al., 2011); however, each trial reviewed below included a primary family component.

Family approaches were employed by six studies in our review, three of which demonstrated significant reductions in repeated SA (Huey et al., 2004; Esposito-Smythers et al., 2011) or SI (Diamond et al., 2010) in adolescent samples. Huey et al. (2004) found that multisystemic therapy (a behaviorally oriented intervention administered in the child/adolescent's home) resulted in fewer suicide reattempts than psychiatric hospitalization alone at 1 year post-treatment. Similarly, Esposito-Smythers et al. (2011) reported that CBT for substance abuse and suicide-related behaviors was more effective in reducing reattempts over the subsequent 18 months than usual care among adolescents with alcohol or cannabis use disorders. Finally, Diamond et al. (2010) reported significantly greater improvements in SI after 10 sessions of attachment-based family therapy compared to TAU. However, the other half of RCTs in this category did not report significant results.

Despite preliminary evidence in support of family-based approaches, the effectiveness data are currently mixed. In addition, almost all studies (except

Nordentoft et al., 2002) were conducted with adolescents. Therefore, it is unclear how effective interventions involving significant others (e.g., family, friends, partners) are for reducing suicide-related behaviors in adult populations.

Psychoanalytic therapy

Psychoanalytic therapy explores how an individual's distant past influences their current situation by considering concepts like attachment, avoidance, desires, mental conflict, and defense mechanisms. From a psychoanalytic perspective, SI can be conceptualized as the manifestation of conflicts between the conscious and unconscious (Huprich, 2004). In the single psychoanalytic trial in our review, psychoanalytically oriented partial hospitalization was compared to usual care in a sample of patients with BPD. Treatment resulted in fewer SA, with significant treatment effects emerging 6 months into the 18-month treatment and lasting throughout the 18-month follow-up (Bateman & Fonagy, 1999, 2001). Given that this is the only psychoanalytic RCT to target suicidal behaviors, further research is needed before the efficacy of this approach can be firmly established.

Outreach interventions

Intensive outreach interventions

Treatment non-adherence is a limiting factor for the efficacy of both psychosocial and pharmacologic treatments. Unfortunately, an examination of treatment non-adherence for the reviewed RCTs is difficult because non-adherence definitions varied widely across studies. For example, some studies reported the percentage of their sample that missed at least one session (e.g., Harrington et al., 1998), whereas others reported the proportion that attended four or more sessions (e.g., Wood et al., 2001). Nonetheless, a number of studies, using a variety of intensive outreach techniques, have been conducted in an effort to improve treatment adherence among individuals at high risk for suicide. Five of these studies were included in our review and used the following procedures: conducted sessions in patients' homes, made contact (e.g., phone call, letter) after a missed appointment, attempted to enhance motivation, or provided crisis management over the phone (Chowdhury et al., 1973; Welu, 1977; Möller, 1989; Allard et al., 1992; van Heeringen et al., 1995).

Of these five trials, two reported significant effects on suicide-related outcomes. In an early intensive outreach study, Welu (1977) found that participants who received 4 months of home-based care (therapeutic modality and elements unspecified) and increased contact engaged in a third less DSH episodes, compared to those who received usual care. Further, Möller (1989) examined an intervention including continuity of care (i.e., continuing with the same therapist in outpatient care after hospital discharge) and additional motivational efforts. Although this approach successfully increased treatment compliance, the treatment group engaged in *more* suicidal behavior (SA) than the control group over the subsequent year. The remaining three studies in this category did not report significant treatment effects for reducing suicidal behaviors. Taken together, these results provide minimal support for existing intensive outreach interventions strategies.

Contact interventions

Eleven trials in our review attempted to prevent SA repetitions among patients presenting for self-injurious behaviors by making contact (e.g., letters, emails, phone calls) after discharge. Rather than providing treatment, the purpose of these interventions was to express concern about the patient with the goal of promoting feelings of connectedness and help seeking during future crises. Four RCTs reported significant reductions in suicide-related outcomes using contact outreach interventions: two studies reported less CS (Motto, 1976; Motto & Bostrom, 2001; Fleischmann et al., 2008), one reported fewer SA (Vaiva et al., 2006), and one demonstrated significant reductions in both SA and SI (Hassanian-Moghaddam et al., 2011).

The first of these trials sent letters expressing concern to patients who did not pursue further treatment after an index attempt (i.e., letters were sent monthly for 4 months, then every other month for 8 months, and then annually for 4 years) (Motto, 1976; Motto & Bostrom, 2001). Significant decreases in CS rates were observed over 2 years post-contact, but by 5 years meaningful differences between the contact and noncontact groups were no longer apparent. Another large trial used telephone or in-person contact over 18 months following a 1-hour informational session, and reported significantly fewer CS among the intervention group compared to TAU (Fleischmann et al., 2008). In addition, Vaiva and colleagues (2006) reported that patients who were contacted by telephone 1 month post discharge endorsed significantly fewer reattempts than controls; importantly, this effect was not observed for patients who were contacted 3 months after discharge. Finally, Hassanian-Moghaddam et al. (2011) found that patients who received notes nine times over the year following a brief psychoeducational session reattempted suicide significantly less and reported less SI, compared to those not contacted.

The remaining eight studies that focused on reducing suicidal behaviors through contact outreach strategies (i.e., without therapy) did not report significant findings. Overall, outreach strategies may be promising and cost-effective methods for reducing suicidal behavior. However, future research is needed to understand why these contact outreach strategies are effective (i.e., mechanisms of action), and to identify the dose of contact necessary for these interventions to be successful.

Hospitalization

It is standard clinical practice to hospitalize high-risk patients (e.g., those presenting with highly lethal attempts, or current suicidal intent) for monitoring, and potentially short-term treatment, until stabilized. Because patients' safety is paramount, randomizing high-risk patients to receive inpatient treatment would be unethical. Therefore, there are few existing RCTs of acute treatment that indicate whether this intervention is effective in reducing suicidal behaviors, and the studies that have been conducted do not provide convincing evidence in support of hospitalization. One study examined a very brief hospitalization (median length of 17 hours) for patients who presented to an emergency room following a self-harm episode; this intervention resulted in only a small improvement in self-harm 16 weeks later (Waterhouse & Platt, 1990; See also Gray & Otto, 2001). In contrast, van der Sande et al. (1997) found that brief hospitalization (1–4 days) was not effective in reducing reattempt rates compared to standard outpatient treatment. Taken together, there is limited research indicating that brief hospitalization is an effective strategy for preventing further suicidal behavior among patients presenting to emergency departments with self-harm.

However, it has been well established that there is an increased risk for suicide *following* hospitalization for psychiatric problems (but not self-harm specifically) (Qin & Nordentoft, 2005; Tidemalm et al., 2008). Moreover, evidence suggests that the majority of psychiatric patients who commit suicide received inpatient treatment in the year preceding their death (Yim et al., 2004). Although it is unclear whether increased risk for suicide is highest following brief (Desai et al., 2005; Qin & Nordentoft, 2005) or extended hospitalizations (Ho, 2006), retrospective studies do indicate that suicide risk is greatest in the weeks following hospital discharge and then declines over time (Qin & Nordentoft, 2005; Deisenhammer et al., 2007).

Notably, whereas the effectiveness of acute hospitalization has not been established, "green cards," which allow expedited access to care during extreme distress, may be a promising approach to reduce suicide risk. The two studies to implement green/access card interventions have reported successful reductions in suicidal or self-injurious behaviors in both adult (Morgan et al., 1993) and adolescent populations (Cotgrove et al., 1995), relative to usual care. However, because the studies above included only patients with a single SA or episode of DSH, it is unknown whether this approach would be effective for patients with more chronic self-injury.

Summary and treatment recommendations

Based on our review, no single intervention has proven to be the most efficacious for reducing suicidal behavior. Overall, most RCTs reporting significant results used CBT techniques; however, CBT was also the most commonly tested therapeutic approach. In terms of specific suicide-related outcomes, more studies using CBT approaches showed significant reductions in SI, DSH, and SA than any other intervention.

Taken together, successful trials provide support for incorporating the following elements into interventions for targeting suicidal behavior: (1) rehearsal of adaptive responses, including seeking help during times of distress, (2) problem solving training with an emphasis on interpersonal problems, (3) emotion regulation and distress tolerance skills, and (4) cognitive restructuring of hopelessness-based thoughts (see also Gray & Otto, 2001). Eclectic approaches are in order when treating this challenging population, and increasing contact and access to care (e.g., letters, phone calls, home visits, case management, green cards) as well as focusing on enhancement of reasons for living may be well advised (Malone et al., 2000).

Limitations and future directions

Several shortcomings of the controlled trial research have limited the evaluation and utilization of empirically supported treatments for reducing suicidal behavior. Addressing these limitations will be important to inform further examination of effective interventions, guide clinical risk assessment and treatment selection, as well as improve utilization of empirically supported treatments.

Generalizability

A primary limitation of the controlled trial data is that results may not be generalizable to some of the clinical groups known to be at greatest risk for suicide. For example, only three studies in our review included patients with schizophrenia/psychosis, and a single trial reported treatment with bipolar patients – a group at four times the risk for suicide compared to other clinical populations (Brown et al., 2000). Suicidal patients are often excluded from treatment studies due to ethical concerns (e.g., consider hospitalization necessary, discomfort with randomizing highest risk patients to the TAU arm of the study) or because they are often considered difficult to retain. Trials without these exclusion criteria might improve clinical decision-making in cases of acute SI or when a diagnosis confers exponential risk. In fact, high-risk individuals might benefit most from therapy, and therefore establish a stronger treatment effect with more translational value to health care providers.

In some cases, studies' specific samples also limit their generalizability. For example, across DBT trials, the vast majority of participants were female patients diagnosed with BPD. Additionally, almost every family therapy study (except Nordentoft et al., 2002) was conducted with adolescents, and all other intervention types (excluding CBT and PST) did not include any studies with an entirely adolescent sample. To address these issues, future research should examine DBT's effectiveness for men, adolescents, and diagnoses other than BPD. Further studies are also necessary to determine whether family interventions are effective for reducing suicidal behavior in adults, and whether adolescents might benefit from interventions other than family therapy and traditional CBT.

Additionally, none of the studies in our review were specific to vulnerable groups that might respond best to interventions that address their diverse needs and concerns (e.g., trauma survivors, prisoners, LGBT individuals, ethnic minorities, substance abusers, elderly populations, etc.). Relatedly, it is also unknown whether demographic factors such as gender or ethnicity may moderate treatment effects.

Dependent variables

Many of the reviewed studies vaguely defined outcome measures and failed to determine whether self-injury was performed with or without suicidal intent. Small sample sizes and low prevalence rates of suicidal behaviors also complicate the interpretation of results. Given that suicidal and non-suicidal forms of self-injury are distinct (Nock, 2010), future studies should differentiate between these behaviors since it is possible that patients who self-injure with suicidal intent might benefit from different treatments than those who habitually self-injure for non-suicidal reasons. In addition, multi-site collaborations could be used to increase sample sizes, which would improve detection of significant treatment effects, as well as enable the examination of low base rate behaviors (e.g., CS) and suicide-related outcomes among specific disordered groups (e.g., bipolar disorder, schizophrenia).

Comparison conditions

When evaluating intervention efficacy and deciding which approaches have the most support, it is important to consider variation among the comparison groups used in the reviewed RCTs. In some cases, the "control" arm of a study received treatment that resembled experimental groups of other studies (e.g., Hawton et al., 1981; Patsiokas & Clum, 1985; McLeavey et al., 1994). For example, Hawton et al. (1981) compared problem-oriented home-based therapy to an outpatient PST "control" group. This sort of comparison may limit the ability to detect significant effects of any one treatment and makes it challenging to compare findings across studies.

History of self-injury

A further confounding aspect of this research is that several of the trials required that participants have a history of multiple self-injury episodes, and the majority included only patients presenting for self-injury. Although including only participants with a habitual self-injury history increases the chances that an event will occur within the time frame of the study (i.e., improving the ability to detect a significant effect), it also makes the findings less applicable to individuals presenting with suicidal thoughts or behaviors for the first time.

Adherence

Although poor treatment adherence may reflect the true clinical picture, greater adherence might better establish the effectiveness of therapies administered at the intended dosages. Aptly, theoretical support for motivational interviewing to reduce suicide has been offered (Britton et al., 2011), and future work may benefit from further exploring this strategy in suicidal populations to increase treatment adherence.

Study duration

The reviewed studies lasted an average of 1 year. However, such abbreviated studies cannot establish the durability of treatment effects over longer time periods. Indeed, although a few studies examined suicide outcomes over longer follow-up periods (e.g., Motto & Bostrom, 2001), no study in our review found significant treatment effects for reducing suicidal behavior after 2 years. Therefore, the field would greatly benefit from longer-term longitudinal investigations of approaches for reducing suicidal behaviors.

References

Allard, R., Marshall, M., & Plante, M. C. (1992). Intensive follow-up does not decrease the risk of repeat suicide attempts. *Suicide and Life-Threatening Behavior*, **22**, 303–314.

Asarnow, J. R., Jaycox, L. H., Duan, N., et al. (2005). Effectiveness of a quality improvement intervention for adolescent depression in primary care clinics. *JAMA: the Journal of the American Medical Association*, **293**, 311–319.

Asarnow, J. R., Baraff, L. J., Berk, M., et al. (2011). An emergency department intervention for linking pediatric suicidal patients to follow-up mental health treatment. *Psychiatric Services*, **62**, 1303–1309.

Bateman, A., & Fonagy, P. (1999). Effectiveness of partial hospitalization in the treatment of borderline personality disorder: a randomized controlled trial. *American Journal of Psychiatry*, **156**, 1563–1569.

Bateman, A., & Fonagy, P. (2001). Treatment of borderline personality disorder with psychoanalytically oriented partial hospitalization: an 18-month follow-up. *American Journal of Psychiatry*, **158**, 36–42.

Beautrais, A. L., Gibb, S. J., Faulkner, A., et al. (2010). Postcard intervention for repeat self-harm: Randomized controlled trail. *The British Journal of Psychiatry*, **197**, 55–60.

Bennewith, O., Stocks, N., Gunnell, D., et al. (2002). General practice based intervention to prevent repeat episodes of deliberate self harm: cluster randomised controlled trial. *BMJ: British Medical Journal*, **324**, 1254–1257.

Bertolote, J. M., Fleischmann, A., De Leo, D., et al. (2010). Repetition of suicide attempts: Data from emergency care settings in five culturally different low- and middle-income countries participating in the WHO SUPRE-MISS study. *Crisis*, **31**, 194–201.

Brent, D. A., Holder, D., Kolko, D., et al. (1997). A clinical psychotherapy trial for adolescent depression comparing cognitive, family, and supportive therapy. *Archives of General Psychiatry*, **54**, 877–885.

Britton, P. C., Patrick, H., Wenzel, A., et al. (2011). Integrating motivational interviewing and self-determination theory with cognitive behavioral therapy to prevent suicide. *Cognitive and Behavioral Practice*, **18**, 16–27.

Brown, G. K., Beck, A. T., Steer, R. A., et al. (2000). Risk factors for suicide in psychiatric outpatients: a 20-year prospective study. *Journal of Consulting and Clinical Psychology*, **68**, 371–377.

Brown, G. K., Ten Have, T., Henriques, G. R., et al. (2005). Cognitive therapy for the prevention of suicide attempts. *JAMA: the Journal of the American Medical Association*, **294**, 563–570.

Butler, A. C., Chapman, J. E., Forman, E. M., et al. (2006). The empirical status of cognitive-behavioral therapy: a review of meta-analyses. *Clinical Psychology Review*, **26**, 17–31.

Carr, A. (2012). *Family Therapy: Concepts, Process and Practice.* Hoboken: Wiley-Blackwell.

Carter, G. L., Clover, K., Whyte, I. M., et al. (2005). Postcards from the EDge project: randomised controlled trial of an intervention using postcards to reduce repetition of hospital-treated deliberate self-poisoning. *BMJ: British Medical Journal*, **331**, 805–807.

Carter, G., Clover, K., Whyte, I., et al. (2007). Postcards from the EDge project: 24-month outcomes of a randomized controlled trial for hospital-treated self-poisoning. *The British Journal of Psychiatry*, **191**, 548–553.

Cedereke, M., Monti, K., & Ojenhagen, A. (2002). Telephone contact with patients in the year after a suicide attempt: Does it affect treatment attendance and outcome?

A randomized controlled study. *European Psychiatry*, **17**, 82–91.

Centers for Disease Control and Prevention. (2012). *Suicide Facts at a Glance*. Available at: http://www.cdc.gov/ViolencePrevention/pdf/Suicide_DataSheet-a.pdf (Accessed 1 February 2013).

Chanen, A. M., Jackson, H. J., McCutcheon, L. K., et al. (2008). Early intervention for adolescents with borderline personality disorder using cognitive analytic therapy: randomised controlled trial. *British Journal of Psychiatry*, **6**, 477–484.

Chowdhury, N., Hicks, R. C., & Kreitman, N. (1973). Evaluation of an after-care service for parasuicide (attempted suicide) patients. *Social Psychiatry and Psychiatric Epidemiology*, **8**, 67–81.

Conner, K. R., Britton, P. C., Sworts, L. M., et al. (2007). Suicide attempts among individuals with opiate dependence: The critical role of belonging. *Addictive Behaviors*, **7**, 1395–1404.

Cotgrove, A., Zirinsky, L., Black, D., et al. (1995). Secondary prevention of attempted suicide in adolescence. *Journal of Adolescence*, **18**, 569–577.

Deisenhammer, E. A., Huber, M., Kemmler, G., et al. (2007). Psychiatric hospitalizations during the last 12 months before suicide. *General Hospital Psychiatry*, **29**, 63–65.

Desai, R. A., Dausey, D. J., & Rosenheck, R. A. (2005). Mental health service delivery and suicide risk: the role of individual patient and facility factors. *American Journal of Psychiatry*, **162**, 311–318.

Diamond, G. S., Wintersteen, M. B., Brown, G. K., et al. (2010). Attachment-based family therapy for adolescents with suicidal ideation: a randomized controlled trial. *Journal of the American Academy of Child & Adolescent Psychiatry*, **49**, 122–131.

Dixon, W. A., Heppner, P. P., & Rudd, M. D. (1994). Problem solving appraisal, hopelessness, and suicide ideation: Evidence for a mediational model. *Journal of Counseling Psychology*, **41**, 91–98.

Donaldson, D., Spirito, A., & Esposito-Smythers, C. (2005). Treatment for adolescents following a SA: Results of a pilot trial. *Journal of the American Academy of Child & Adolescent Psychiatry*, **44**, 113–120.

Esposito-Smythers, C., Spirito, A., Kahler, C. W., et al. (2011). Treatment of co-occurring substance abuse and suicidality among adolescents: A randomized trial. *Journal of Consulting and Clinical Psychology*, **79**, 728–739.

Fleischmann, A., Bertolote, J. M., Wasserman, D., et al. (2008). Effectiveness of brief intervention and contact for suicide attempters: A randomized control trial in five countries. *Bulletin of the World Health Organization*, **86**, 703–709.

Gibbons, J. S., Butler, J., Urwin, P., et al. (1978). Evaluation of a social work service for self-poisoning patients. *The British Journal of Psychiatry*, **133**, 111–118.

Gray, S. M., & Otto, M. W. (2001). Psychosocial approaches to suicide prevention: applications to patients with bipolar disorder. *The Journal of Clinical Psychiatry Supplement*, **62**, 56–64.

Green, J. M., Wood, A. J., Kerfoot, M. J., et al. (2011). Group therapy for adolescents with repeated self harm: randomised controlled trial with economic evaluation. *BMJ: British Medical Journal*, **342**, 1–12.

Guthrie, E., Kapur, N., Mackway-Jones, K., et al. (2001). Randomised controlled trial of brief psychological intervention after deliberate self poisoning. *BMJ: British Medical Journal*, **323**, 135–138.

Hamza, C. A., Stewart, S. L., & Willoughby, T. (2012). Examining the link between nonsuicidal self-injury and suicidal behavior: A review of the literature and an integrated model. *Clinical Psychology Review*, **32**, 482–495.

Harrington, R., Kerfoot, M., Dyer, E., et al. (1998). Randomized trial of a home-based family intervention for children who have deliberately poisoned themselves. *Journal of the American Academy of Child and Adolescent Psychiatry*, **37**, 512–518.

Hassanian-Moghaddam, H., Saeedeh, S., Kolahi, A., et al. (2011). Postcards in Persia: Randomised controlled trial to reduce suicidal behaviors 12 months after hospital-treated self-poisoning. *British Journal of Psychiatry*, **198**, 309–316.

Hassanzadeh, M., Khajeddin, N., Nojomi, M., et al. (2010). Brief intervention and contact after deliberate self-harm: An Iranian randomized controlled trial. *Iranian Journal of Psychiatry and Behavioral Sciences*, **4**, 5–12.

Hastings, M., Northman, L., & Tangney, J. (2002). Shame, guilt, and suicide. In T. Joiner & M. D. Rudd (Eds.) *Suicide Science*, 67–79.

Hatcher, S., Sharon, C., Parag, V., et al. (2011). Problem solving therapy for people who present to hospital with self-harm: Zelen randomised controlled trial. *The British Journal of Psychiatry*, **199**, 310–316.

Hawton, K., Bancroft, J., Catalan, J., et al. (1981). Domiciliary and outpatient treatment of self-poisoning patients by medical and non-medical staff. *Psychological Medicine*, **11**, 169–177.

Hawton, K., McKeown, S., Day, A., et al. (1987). Evaluation of outpatient counselling compared with general practitioner care following overdoses. *Psychological Medicine*, **17**, 751–761.

Hazell, P. L., Martin, G., McGill, K., et al.(2009). Group therapy for repeated deliberate self-harm in adolescents: failure of replication of a randomized trial. *Journal of the*

American Academy of Child & Adolescent Psychiatry, **48**, 662–670.

Hirsch, J. K., Webb, J. R., & Jeglic, E. L. (2012). Forgiveness as a moderator of the association between anger expression and suicidal behaviour. *Mental Health, Religion & Culture*, **15**, 279–300.

Ho, T. P. (2006). Duration of hospitalization and post discharge suicide. *Suicide and Life-Threatening Behavior*, **36**, 682–686.

Huey, S. J., Henggeler, S. W., Rowland, M. D., et al. (2004). Multisystemic therapy effects on attempted suicide by youths presenting psychiatric emergencies. *Journal of the American Academy of Child & Adolescent Psychiatry*, **43**, 183–190.

Huprich, S. K. (2004). Psychodynamic conceptualization and treatment of suicidal patients. *Journal of Contemporary Psychotherapy*, **34**, 23–39.

Hvid, M., Vangborg, K., Sørensen, H. J., et al. (2011). Preventing repetition of attempted suicide-II. The Amager Project, a randomized controlled trial. *Nordic Journal of Psychiatry*, **65**, 292–298.

Joiner, T. E. (2005). *Why People Die by Suicide*. Cambridge: Harvard University Press.

Joiner, T. E., & Rudd, M. D. (1996). Disentangling the interrelations between hopelessness, loneliness, and suicidal ideation. *Suicide and Life-Threatening Behavior*, **26**, 19–26.

Koons, C. R., Robins, C. J., Lindsey Tweed, J., et al. (2001). Efficacy of dialectical behavior therapy in women veterans with borderline personality disorder. *Behavior Therapy*, **32**, 371–390.

Liberman, R. P., & Eckman, T. (1981). Behavior therapy vs insight-oriented therapy for repeated suicide attempters. *Archives of General Psychiatry*, **38**, 1126–1130.

Linehan, M. (1993). *Skills Training Manual for Treating Borderline Personality Disorder*. New York: Guilford Press.

Linehan, M. M., Armstrong, H. E., Suarez, A., et al. (1991). Cognitive-behavioral treatment of chronically parasuicidal borderline patients. *Archives of General Psychiatry*, **48**, 1060–1064.

Linehan, M. M., Heard, H. L., & Armstrong, H. E. (1993). Naturalistic follow-up of a behavioral treatment for chronically parasuicidal borderline patients. *Archives of General Psychiatry*, **50**, 971–974.

Linehan, M. M., Comtois, K. A., Murray, A. M., et al. (2006). Two-year randomized controlled trial and follow-up of dialectical behavior therapy vs therapy by experts for suicidal behaviors and borderline personality disorder. *Archives of General Psychiatry*, **63**, 757–766.

Malone, K. M., Oquendo, M. A., Haas, G. L., et al. (2000). Protective factors against suicidal acts in major depression: reasons for living. *American Journal of Psychiatry*, **157**, 1084–1088.

McLeavey, B. C., Daly, R. J., Ludgate, J. W., et al. (1994). Interpersonal problem solving skills training in the treatment of self-poisoning patients. *Suicide and Life-Threatening Behavior*, **24**, 382–394.

McMain, S., Links, P., Gnam, W., et al. (2009). A randomized trial of dialectical behavior therapy versus general psychiatric management for borderline personality disorder. *American Journal of Psychiatry*, **166**, 1365–1374.

Möller, H. J. (1989). Efficacy of different strategies of aftercare for patients who have attempted suicide. *Journal of the Royal Society of Medicine*, **82**, 643–647.

Morgan, H. G., Jones, E. M., & Owen, J. H. (1993). Secondary prevention of non-fatal deliberate self-harm. The green card study. *The British Journal of Psychiatry*, **163**, 111–112.

Motto, J. A. (1976). Suicide prevention for high-risk persons who refuse treatment. *Suicide and Life-Threatening Behavior*, **6**, 223–230.

Motto, J. A., & Bostrom, A. G. (2001). A randomized controlled trial of postcrisis suicide prevention. *Psychiatric Services*, **52**, 828–833.

Nock, M. K. (2010). Self-injury. *Annual Review of Clinical Psychology*, **6**, 339–363.

Nordentoft, M., Jeppesen, P., Abel, M., et al. (2002). OPUS study: suicidal behaviour, suicidal ideation and hopelessness among patients with first-episode psychosis. One-year follow-up of a randomised controlled trial. *The British Journal of Psychiatry*, **181**, 98–106.

Patsiokas, A. T., & Clum, G. A. (1985). Effects of psychotherapeutic strategies in the treatment of suicide attempters. *Psychotherapy: Theory, Research, Practice, Training*, **22**, 281–290.

Pietrzak, R. H., Russo, A. R., Ling, Q., et al. (2011). Suicidal ideation in treatment-seeking Veterans of Operations Enduring Freedom and Iraqi Freedom: The role of coping strategies, resilience, and social support. *Journal of Psychiatric Research*, **45**, 720.

Pistorello, J., Fruzzetti, A. E., MacLane, C., et al. (2012). Dialectical Behavior Therapy (DBT) applied to college students: a randomized clinical trial. *Journal of Consulting and Clinical Psychology*, **80**, 982–994.

Pompili, M., Innamorati, M., Szanto, K., et al. (2011). Life events as precipitants of suicide attempts among first-time suicide attempters, repeaters, and non-attempters. *Psychiatry Research*, **186**, 300–305.

Qin, P., & Nordentoft, M. (2005). Suicide risk in relation to psychiatric hospitalization: evidence based on longitudinal registers. *Archives of General Psychiatry*, **62**, 427–532.

Raj, A. J., Kumaraiah, V., & Bhide, A. V. (2001). Cognitive-behavioral intervention in deliberate self-harm. *Acta Psychiatrica Scandinavica*, **104**, 340–345.

Rich, C. L., Warsradt, G. M., Nemiroff, R. A., et al. (1991). Suicide, stressors, and the life cycle. *The American Journal of Psychiatry*, **148**, 524–527.

Robinson, J., Yuen, H. P., Gook, S., et al. (2012). Can receipt of a regular postcard reduce suicide-related behaviour in young help seekers? A randomized controlled trial. *Early Intervention in Psychiatry*, **6**, 145–152.

Rudd, M., David, M., Rajab, H., et al. (1994). Problem solving appraisal in suicide ideators and attempters. *American Journal of Orthopsychiatry*, **64**, 136–149.

Rudd, M. D., Rajab, M. H., Orman, D. T., et al. (1996). Effectiveness of an outpatient intervention targeting suicidal young adults: preliminary results. *Journal of Consulting and Clinical Psychology*, **64**, 179–190.

Salkovskis, P. M., Atha, C., & Storer, D. (1990). Cognitive-behavioural problem solving in the treatment of patients who repeatedly attempt suicide. A controlled trial. *The British Journal of Psychiatry*, **157**, 871–876.

Slee, N., Garnefski, N., van der Leeden, R., Arensman, E., et al. (2008). Cognitive–behavioural intervention for self-harm: randomised controlled trial. *The British Journal of Psychiatry*, **192**, 202–211.

Stepp, S. D., Morse, J. Q., Yaggi, K. E., et al. (2011). The role of attachment styles and interpersonal problems in suicide related behaviors. *Suicide and Life-Threatening Behavior*, **38**, 592–607.

Tarrier, N., Haddock, G., Lewis, S., et al. (2006). Suicide behaviour over 18 months in recent onset schizophrenic patients: the effects of CBT. *Schizophrenia Research*, **83**, 15–27.

Tidemalm, D., Långström, N., Lichtenstein, P., et al. (2008). Risk of suicide after suicide attempt according to coexisting psychiatric disorder: Swedish cohort study with long term follow-up. *BMJ: British Medical Journal*, **337**, 2205–2210.

Turner, R. M. (2000). Naturalistic evaluation of dialectical behavior therapy-oriented treatment for borderline personality disorder. *Cognitive and Behavioral Practice*, **7**, 413–419.

Tyrer, P., Thompson, S., Schmidt, U., et al. (2003). Randomized controlled trial of brief cognitive behaviour therapy versus treatment as usual in recurrent deliberate self-harm: the POPMACT study. *Psychological Medicine*, **33**, 969–976.

Vaiva, G., Ducrocq, F., Meyer, P., et al. (2006). Effect of telephone contact on further suicide attempts in patients discharged from an emergency department: randomised controlled study. *BMJ: British Medical Journal*, **332**, 1241–1245.

van den Bosch, L. M., Koeter, M. W., Stijen, T., et al. (2005). Sustained efficacy of dialectical behaviour therapy for borderline personality disorder. *Behaviour Research and Therapy*, **43**, 1231–1241.

van der Sande, R., van Rooijen, L., Buskens, et al. (1997). Intensive inpatient and community intervention versus routine care after attempted suicide. A randomised controlled intervention study. *The British Journal of Psychiatry*, **171**, 35–41.

van Heeringen, C., Jannes, S., Buylaert, W., et al. (1995). Management of non-compliance with referral to outpatient after-care among attempted suicide patients: A controlled intervention study. *Psychological Medicine*, **25**, 963–970.

Van Orden, K. A., Witte, T. K., Cukrowicz, K. C., et al. (2010). The interpersonal theory of suicide. *Psychological Review*, **117**, 575–600.

Verheul, R., van den bosch, L. M., Koeter, M. W., et al. (2003). Dialectical behaviour therapy for women with borderline personality disorder 12-month, randomised clinical trial in The Netherlands. *The British Journal of Psychiatry*, **182**, 135–140.

Waterhouse, J., & Platt, S. (1990). General hospital admission in the management of parasuicide: A randomised controlled trial. *The British Journal of Psychiatry*, **156**, 236–242.

Weinberg, I., Gunderson, J. G., Hennen, J., et al. (2006). Manual assisted cognitive treatment for deliberate self-harm in borderline personality disorder patients. *Journal of Personality Disorders*, **20**, 482–492.

Weissman, M. M. (2010). Interpersonal psychotherapy. In *Corsini Encyclopedia of Psychology*. Hoboken: Wiley-Blackwell.

Welu, T. C. (1977). A follow-up program for suicide attempters: Evaluation of effectiveness. *Suicide and Life-Threatening Behavior*, **7**, 17–30.

Wenzel, A., & Beck, A. T. (2008). A cognitive model of suicidal behaviors: Theory and treatment. *Applied and Preventive Psychology*, **12**, 189–201.

Wood, A., Trainor, G., Rothwell, J., et al. (2001). Randomized trial of group therapy for repeated deliberate self-harm in adolescents. *Journal of the American Academy of Child & Adolescent Psychiatry*, **40**, 1246–1253.

World Health Organization. (1996). *Prevention of Suicide: Guidelines for the Formulation and Implementation of National Strategies*. Geneva, Switzerland.

Wright, J. H. (2006). Cognitive behavior therapy: Basic principles and recent advances. *Focus*, **4**, 173–178.

Yim, P., Yip, P. S. F., Li, R., et al. (2004). Suicide after discharge from psychiatric inpatient care: a case-control study in Hong Kong. *Australian & New Zealand Journal of Psychiatry*, **38**, 65–72.

Chapter 31

Genome-wide association studies of suicidal behaviors

Marcus Sokolowski, Jerzy Wasserman, and Danuta Wasserman

Genetics of suicidality entering into the GWAS-era

A general genetic diathesis of suicidality has been shown to exist by family, adoption, and twin studies, with heritability in the range between 30 and 55% (Voracek & Loibl, 2007). Such a general genetic diathesis mainly refers to the behavioral manifestations of suicidality (i.e., suicide attempts or completed suicides), rather than suicidal thoughts or ideation alone. However, this is not clear-cut, as ideation precedes a proportion of suicide attempts or completed suicides (Baca-Garcia et al., 2011). Specific genetic components (i.e., particular candidate genes) are therefore often being studied, i.e. genes which are implicated in suicidality or its associated psychopathologies on the basis of prior biological and/or pharmacological knowledge and observations (Currier & Mann, 2008; Wasserman et al., 2009). Selected genetic variants in serotonergic system genes have been the major historic focus of such investigations during the past decades, but the polygenetic perspective is nowadays also being addressed by, for example, the study of candidate genes in other neurosystems (Wasserman et al., 2005, 2007, 2008, 2009; Ernst et al., 2009; Rujescu & Giegling, 2010; Sokolowski et al., 2010, 2012; Ben-Efraim et al., 2011, 2112, 2013). A relatively novel approach for further elucidating the polygenetic perspective, which has become available in the last years, is to conduct a Genome-Wide Association Study (GWAS).

GWAS is a concept whereby many genetic markers across the whole genome are simultaneously analyzed for association with a trait (Ikegawa, 2012). It has been termed as a hypothesis-free approach (with regard to that any of the markers/genes are being hypothesized to show association), which is in contrast to the candidate gene approach (Goldstein et al., 2003). One main goal of GWAS is to suggest novel candidate genes which could not be hypothesized a priori by current knowledge. The majority of markers analyzed in GWAS are SNPs, in addition to certain Copy Number Variants (CNVs). Technological progress of genotyping chips (with Illumina Inc leading the market) combined with the huge efforts to map all human SNPs and their patterns of linkage disequilibrium (LD) in different populations (see e.g., http://www.hapmap.org and http://www.1000genomes.org), have resulted in a continuous increase in the number of SNPs analyzed for each GWAS-era year. While initial GWAS usually covered 50–100 000 high allele-frequency SNPs, one can today analyze up to 5 million of both low and high allele-frequency SNPs on one chip (e.g., the Illumina HumanOmni5-Quad chip) in a more truly genome-wide fashion. In addition, it is now also common to impute SNPs which have not been genotyped, to increase genomic coverage further and have consistency between different genotyping platforms (Marchini & Howie, 2010). In the early stages of the GWAS-era, one hoped for a fairly straightforward resolution of the genetic architecture of many complex traits (Altshuler & Daly, 2007). Original GWAS studies have subsequently been applied to hundreds of different human traits, behaviors, diseases, and other phenotype measures, and there are now more than 1500 GWAS studies documented in the NIH GWAS catalogue (http://www.genome.gov/ gwastudies). The initial enthusiasm about GWAS has been somewhat damped (Need & Goldstein, 2010; Rowe & Tenesa, 2012), e.g., as most of the initially identified "genome-wide significant" GWAS SNP-associations were found to be of small effect and thus not directly applicable to real life, e.g., in the clinic or in public health prevention (Eichler et al., 2010). Nevertheless, GWAS data remains a rich resource for elucidating polygenetic etiology, and its success (Teslovich et al., 2010) or failure (Sebastiani

A Concise Guide to Understanding Suicide, ed. Stephen H. Koslow, Pedro Ruiz, and Charles B. Nemeroff. Published by Cambridge University Press.

et al., 2010, 2011) to generate new hypotheses and insights depend on the trait under study, the study design, analysis approaches, and avoidance of previous mistakes (Terwilliger & Goring, 2009; Need & Goldstein, 2010, Rowe & Tenesa, 2012; Lambert & Black, 2012; Califano et al., 2012). The GWAS-era can therefore currently be said to be at the "end of the beginning" (Ikegawa, 2012) or entering into a new phase, in a state of transformation into maturity. The advent of GWAS to the field of suicidality research was somewhat delayed in comparison to other phenotypes studied, but there are now seven original GWAS described in the literature which will be reviewed herein. Additional GWAS on suicidality phenotypes are expected to be published in the future.

The basic idea of GWAS is thus that one "screens" through the whole genome for associations to identify the genetic etiology. Given the multiple independent tests conducted, the control of the type I error (i.e., false positive) becomes a major statistical concern. One today usually requires a P-value in the range of 10^{-8} to declare a certain SNP significant at alpha 0.05 after accounting for LD (Li et al., 2012a). Due to poor replication history of many initial GWAS significance claims, one today usually requires also independent replication (i.e., a two-stage design) or other downstream confirmatory analyses for publication, in addition to only reporting the single SNP-associations from an initial discovery sample. On the other hand, the extensive correction for multiple tests combined with the fact that lower frequency SNPs often are expected to have higher effect sizes compared to higher frequency SNPs, contributes to the problem of type II errors (i.e., false negatives) and repeated requests for bigger sample sizes and the formation of various collaborative research group networks for sample pooling. Other promising ways to improve power are also novel analysis association testing approaches on the gene-, pathway-, or network-levels being developed and applied (complementing the classical SNP-by-SNP approach), which are (i) less penalized by multiple comparison corrections and (ii) attempt to catch the association of the underlying, polygenetic biology more efficiently.

Finally, there are many other aspects of importance to consider in any genetic study of suicidality, which are however not specific for only GWAS and therefore not the main focus herein; e.g. endophenotypes (Mann et al., 2009) and intermediate phenotypes (Meyer-Lindenberg & Weinberger, 2006); phenotypic heterogeneity, psychiatric disorder definitions, and gene–environment interactions (Kendler, 2010; Leigh, 2009); population stratification (Cardon & Palmer, 2003; Bouaziz et al., 2011), sex dimorphisms (Ober et al., 2008), epigenetics (Kofink et al., 2013), and the assumed disease vs. variant frequency models (Schork et al., 2009).

Different approaches to genetic associations in GWAS

The genetic associations observed in GWAS will depend on the underlying genetic architecture of the suicidality phenotype in question, wherein the biological processes are the intermediate phenotypes (Meyer-Lindenberg & Weinberger, 2006) which are causally linked to the genetic influences. The aim of the association testing should thus be to as well as possible capture the genetic architecture of the intermediate phenotypes, which in turn may influence the probability of the suicidality phenotype (Wasserman et al., 2010). GWAS data present special opportunities for novel analysis approaches.

Classical SNP-by-SNP GWAS

The wide majority of GWAS conducted on many complex traits up to date has mainly focused on the identification of significant, single SNP-associations. The premise is that a subset of (usually higher frequency, "common") SNPs capture the overall genetic involvement in a phenotypic effect, an effect which deviates from the rest of the genome. The associations obtained from GWAS may reflect a wide mix of corresponding biological functionality, much of which is often unknown or of incomplete meaning (e.g., "intergenic" SNPs). For comprehensive reasons, protein-coding genes rather than single SNPs are often on the wish-list. Therefore, one primarily tries to map single SNP-associations to particular gene(s), by using annotation in various manners (by location, LD, or indirect functional connections). Complex traits involve the interplay of many different genetic perturbations, whereby single SNP-associations on complex traits are perhaps best interpreted if the SNPs act as trans-acting expression quantitative trait loci (eQTLs), i.e., intergenic SNPs which regulate the expression of many different genes, rather than as acting on a single gene nearby. Indeed, this may actually be a common feature of many single SNP identified in GWAS on complex traits up to date

(Teslovich et al., 2010; Nicolae et al., 2010), thus representing genetic alterations which can cause complex gene regulatory changes across the genome that are not very well understood. For psychiatric disorders, results from single SNP-analyses have as yet resolved only a subset of consistent findings (see e.g., Bhat et al., 2012; Hamshere et al., 2013) among the presumably thousands of SNP-associations of small effect that are hypothesized to be involved (Moore et al., 2011; Binder, 2012). Together, there may therefore be advantages of genomic analysis strategies which capture multi-SNP effects (Lehner, 2013).

Gene-wide GWAS

For the case of genetic heterogeneity in a single gene, different random mutations can cause the same phenotypic (biological) effect, as simplistically exemplified by, e.g., the mendelian phenylketonuria disorder (Scriver, 2007). This causes each SNP *per se* to have a low power to be detected in a classical SNP-by-SNP GWAS as the relative importance of each SNP is diluted. Different strategies are continuously being published about how to best compile a *gene*-wide association signal from multiple SNP-signals. No golden standard exists in this domain, but the general procedure is to select the most significant SNP located within, or in LD with a gene, or to combine the signal from many different SNPs (Lehne et al., 2011; Li et al., 2012b). By doing so, the focus is explicitly shifted to association of known genes with the suicidality phenotype in question, which is necessary for downstream biological interpretations and analytical extensions (see below), as well as for reducing the multiple comparison burden.

Pathway/network GWAS

In the case of complex polygenetic traits such as suicidality phenotypes, the issue of heterogeneity becomes problematic also at the gene level. Namely, if different genes can drive the same phenotypic effect (pleiotrophy), or if multiple genes, each of small marginal effects (but with large, compounded epistatic effects) underlie the phenotype, then also gene-wide associations would have a low power to be detected in either classical SNP-by-SNP or gene-wide GWAS. It is known that genes act in functional modules (e.g., as networks of co-expression or physical protein interactions), representing functionally distinct units underlying biological processes (Lehner, 2013). Therefore, novel methods are being developed and applied to (re)analyze the associations from a SNP-GWAS in relation to gene pathways (Holmans, 2010) and/or networks (Hannum et al., 2009; Akula et al., 2011; Jia et al., 2011b). Network analyses have been applied to screen, e.g., GWAS data on Crohn's disease (Akula et al., 2011), as well as to analyze, e.g., sets of candidate genes for schizophrenia (Sun et al., 2011; Jia et al., 2012) and major depressive disorder (Jia et al., 2011a; Deo et al., 2013). Network analyses in particular capture the fact that biological processes are most often the result of co-action of multiple genes, wherein each single gene acts in a redundant, pleiotropic, and/or epistatic manner in complex interplay with many other genes (McKinney & Pajewski, 2011; Califano et al., 2012). Networks can associate many different genes with the same biological functionality by "guilt-by-association" (Lee et al., 2011), and represent an important future avenue to develop and apply for analysis of GWAS data on, e.g.. psychiatric conditions (Moore et al., 2011; Binder, 2012) as well as on suicidality.

Current state of GWAS in the literature in relation to various measures of suicidality

There are to date seven original GWAS published from different research groups/constellations in relation to different measures of suicidality (Table 31.1): treatment-emergent suicidal ideation (Laje et al., 2009; Menke et al., 2012; Perroud et al., 2012), a suicidality score ranging from suicide ideation to attempts (Schosser et al., 2011), suicide attempts in bipolar disorder (Willour et al., 2012) and mood disorder (Perlis et al., 2010) subjects, as well as completed suicides (Galfalvy et al., 2011). The analyses have mainly been conducted by the classical SNP-by-SNP approach (Table 31.1).

Treatment-emergent suicidal ideation (TESI)

Laje et al. (2009) conducted a GWAS on TESI, being the first ever GWAS conducted in relation to a suicidality measure. The subjects were non-psychotic major depressive disorders enrolled in the Sequenced Treatment Alternatives to Relieve (STAR*D) cohort. Suicide ideation cases were defined by the emergence of any "Thoughts of Death or Suicide," assessed using question 12 on a 16-item Quick Inventory of Depressive Symptomatology self-report by the end of 14 weeks of standard treatment routine with citalopram. One SNP (in *PAPLN*) was reported to associate

Table 31.1. Outline of all GWAS results published (by April 2013) in relation to various measures of suicidality

Original study	Design (name)	Phenotype	Sample size (cases)	Genotyping platform	#SNPs (incl imputed) analyzed in GWAS	Association/interpretation levels			Confirmation status
						Single SNPs (annotated gene or region)	Gene-wide	Pathway network	
Laje et al. (2009)	Case–control (STAR*D)	TESI	274 (90)	Illumina Beadstation 500	109 365 (–)	rs11628713** (*PAPLN*) rs10903034* (*IL28RA*)	–	–	n.c. in Perroud et al. n.c. in Menke et al.
Perroud et al. (2012)	Case-control (GENDEP)	TESI	706 (244)	Illumina Human610-quad BeadChip	539 199 (–)	rs11143230* (*GDA*) rs358592* (*KCNIP4*) rs4732812* (*ELP3*) *and more, see text*	–	–	rs10869127 - *GDA*, by Menke et al. (gene-wide association)
Menke et al. (2012)	Case–control (MARS)	TESI	397 (32) and 501 (25)	Illumina Human-1 100k + HumanHap300-Duo BeadChip	371 335 (–)	rs1037448* (*TMEM138*) rs10997044* (*CTNNA3*) rs1109089* (*RHEB*) rs4939517* (*CYBASC3*) rs9480684* (*AIM1*) rs1884641*, rs7788668*, rs8095186*	–	–	–
Perlis et al. (2010)	Case–control (many[a])	Suicide attempts in BPD and MDD	8737 (2805)	Multiple	($\sim 1.9 \times 10^6$)	rs2576377*** (*ABI3BP*) rs4918918* (*SORBS1*) rs10854398* (*B3GALT5*) rs1360550* (*PRKCE*)	–	–	rs2576377 n.c. in same study n.c. in Schosser et al.
Schosser et al. (2011)	Case–control (many[b])	Suicidality score and suicide attempts	2023 (251 suicide attempters)	Illumina Human610-quad BeadChip	532 774	rs4751955* (*GFRA1*) rs203136* (*KIAA1244*)	–	–	–

Galfalvy et al. (2011)	Case–control	Completed suicides	99 (68)	GeneChip Mapping 50K Xba Array	37 344 (-)	58* SNPs (19* genes)	CD44* and 6* genes[c]	4* pathways[c]	7 (out of 19) genes showed altered RNA expression in same study
Willour et al. (2012)	Case–control (NIHM-BP)	Suicide attempts in BPD	2836 (1201)	Affymetrix 6.0 / Illumina HumanHap550	~730 000/516 024 (~2.4×10^6)	rs300774*** (2p25) rs10437629* (*C11orf41*) rs7296262* (*TMEM132C*) rs10170138* (*LRRTM4*)	–	Wnt signaling and lithium*	–

BPD, borderline personality disorder; MDD, major depressive disorder; TESI, treatment-emergent suicidal ideation; SA, suicide attempts; SC completed suicides; –, not done or not available; n.c., not confirmed.

* Reported or discussed as a (suggestive) association/relationship of interest for follow-up, usually with SNPs at *P* <10–5.

** P <0.05 after experiment-wide correction.

*** P <10–7, ~ genome-wide significant at alpha 0.05.

[a] Systematic Treatment Enhancement Program for Bipolar Disorder cohort, Wellcome Trust Case Control Consortium bipolar cohort, University College London cohort, NIMH Genetic Association Information Network bipolar disorder project, Sequential Treatment Alternatives to Relieve Depression cohort and the Netherlands Study of Depression and Anxiety/Netherlands Twin Register depression cohort.

[b] RADIANT Depression Case Control and Depression Network, Bonn and Lausanne cases, GSK-Munich cohort, Munich Antidepressant Response Signature (MARS) and STAR*D.

[c] Seven (out of 19) genes showed combined association with completed suicides and altered RNA expression (CYP19A1, MBNL2, KTBBD2, CD44, FOXN3, DSC2, CD300LB), with greatest confidence presented for CD44. Concurrently, pathways were also suggested for 8 (out of 19) genes suggestively associated with completed suicides: CNS development (MBNL2), homophilic cell adhesion (CD44, DSC2 and MARCH1), regulation of cell proliferation (SFRS11, TUBGCP3), and transmission of nerve impulse (LSAMP, SPTLC1).

(corrected $P = 0.01$) and another SNP (in *IL28RA*) was reported as suggestive (Table 31.1), in this subsample of STAR*D. Analysis of these SNP *post-hoc* in the entire STAR*D sample diminished both the significance and odds ratios, indicating a limited generalizability for those single SNP-associations *per se*. However, a four-SNP multivariate model, including also previously identified SNPs in GRIA3 and GRIK2, showed reasonable fit to observed data in both genders.

Perroud et al. (2012) more recently investigated TESI, during 12-week treatment with escitalopram or nortriptylin. Suicide ideation cases were defined as an increase of 0.5 standard deviations on a computed score, based on three different items from three different questionnaires, anytime during treatment. One SNP (rs11143230) was reported to have the strongest support for association with TESI, as also background haplotypes as well as other *post-hoc* imputed SNPs showed association in the 88 kb LD-block containing the guanine deaminase (*GDA*) gene. In addition, treatment-specific SNPs (rs358592 – in *KCNIP4*, rs4732812 – near *ELP3*), drug × treatment interaction SNPs (rs1368607, rs2707159 – in *APOO* gene, rs2846685 – near *p53AIP1/RICS* genes) as well as SNPs (in *NTRK2*, *CCK*, *YWHAE*, and *CRHR2*) from a supplemental candidate gene analysis were all reported as suggestive associations. No genotype × gender effect was observed. However, the study could not confirm any association of the SNPs reported by Laje et al., which was discussed to be influenced by the difference in suicide ideation measures used.

Finally, Menke et al. (2012) also performed a GWAS on TESI, with ideation measured by item 3 on the Hamilton Depression Rating Scale, during the first 12 weeks following treatment with a variety of different SSRIs. No significant associations were observed in the discovery sample, whereby 79 suggestive SNP-associations with lowest P-values were subsequently used for testing in an independent replication sample. Fourteen SNPs were reported as suggestive associations after this two-stage analysis, of which 6 SNPs were in high LD (thus nine independent SNP-associations remained; Table 31.1). Six of those SNPs could be annotated to five different genes (*TMEM138*, *CTNNA3*, *RHEB*, *CYBASC3*, and *AIMI*) and the other three SNPs had an intergenic location (Table 31.1). A multi-SNP analysis of the 79 SNPs in the replication sample also showed a significant discriminant power for TESI. Finally, the SNP-associations reported by Laje et al. could not be re-observed with any statistical confidence. However, one SNP in *GDA* (initially suggested in the GWAS by Perroud et al.) was observed to suggestively associate with TESI by using a gene-wide approach (min-P method without correction), and gene-wide SNP-associations were additionally observed for certain candidate genes of neuropsychiatric disorders (*FKBP5*, *ABCB1*).

Suicidal behaviors

The other four published GWAS focused on suicidality in mainly the behavioral domains, i.e., attempted or completed suicides. Perlis et al. (2010) was the first in this category to investigate lifetime suicide attempts in mood disorder patients from multiple cohorts, in a two-stage design, with analysis stratified by bipolar or major depression disorders. Controls were bipolar or major depression subjects without suicide attempts. However, no consistent findings were observed in such diagnosis-adjusted suicidality. One region was observed to be genome-wide significant in the major depression discovery sample (with multiple SNPs annotated to gene *ABI3BP*), but this finding failed replication in a subsequent analysis (of note is the low power for major depression, with only 133 suicide attempt cases in the replication here). Finally, analysis was combined into one giant meta-analysis for the lifetime suicide attempt across either bipolar or depressed (n = 8737 in total, with n = 2805 suicide attempts, mainly bipolar), with four loci reported as suggestively associated. Additionally, a gene-wide association analysis was conducted for 19 candidate genes, with observed suggestive association for *FKBP5* and *NGFR*. The authors concluded that "inherited risk for suicide among mood disorder patients is unlikely to be the result of individual common variants of large effect."

Next, Schosser et al. (2011) conducted a GWAS in relation to a suicidality score (reflecting the increasing continuum from suicide ideation to attempts) as well as in relation to serious lifetime suicide attempts, among major depression subjects. Controls were major depression subjects without suicide ideation/attempts. No genome-wide significant results were observed and seven SNPs from three regions showed suggestive association (main examples in Table 31.1). Additionally, a gene-wide association analysis was conducted for 33 candidate genes, with variable suggestive associations for *HTR1A*, *CCK*, *RGS18*, *NTRK2*, and *SCN8A* across different cohorts. The authors concluded "a genetic architecture of multiple genes with small effects" for suicidal behavior in depression.

In the same year, Galfalvy et al. (2011) published what is the first and yet only available GWAS on completed suicides, using an altered approach compared to the other GWAS. Controls were sudden deaths by causes other than suicide. A low-coverage array ("pilot GWAS") was used for association testing with completed suicides, and then the top-associated SNPs (nominal $P < 0.001$) were used to suggest genes of interest for follow-up by RNA-expression analysis of prefrontal and/or anterior cingulate cortex. Out of the 58 suggestively associated SNPs (as observed independently of mood disorder diagnoses or lifetime aggression scores), 22 SNPs were located in or near 19 known genes (Table 31.1). Nine of those 19 genes also showed altered RNA expression in suicides. Thus, the final analysis was to combine evidence from SNP-associations and gene-centric expression data (Table 31.1). The findings presented were both the 58 suggestively associated SNPs, 7 genes showing combined RNA gene expression alterations and suggestive SNP-associations, as well as four different pathways for the subset of suggestive SNP-associations which were annotated in or near 19 genes (Table 31.1). The main suggestive finding discussed was the *CD44* gene, as it showed results on all the investigated parameters, as well as for its altered RNA expression in two previous studies. The authors concluded that the overall results "highlight a role for neuroimmunological effects in suicidal behavior."

Finally, Willour et al. (2012) conducted the most recently published GWAS on suicidal behavior, namely in relation to lifetime suicide attempts in bipolar subjects. Controls were bipolar subjects without suicide attempts. A two-stage analysis failed to replicate any of the 2507 SNP having $P < 0.001$ in the discovery sample, after correction for multiple testing. However, a combined analysis of discovery and replication samples yielded a genome-wide significant association for SNP rs300774, as well as two more suggestive associations (Table 31.1). LD-analysis of SNP rs300774 showed it was located in a large LD-block containing three genes (*SH3YL1*, *ACP1*, and *FAM150B*). The authors then assessed gene expression data and found RNA expression changes in the prefrontal cortex of bipolar suicides for *ACP1* (but not *SH3YL1*) and thus proposed the SNP association to be involved in ACP1 functions. Of note is that *ACP1* was not the nearest gene of the three genes in the LD-block (*ACP1* is located >100 kb away from rs300774) and with no further evidence presented as to why this SNP would be involved selectively in ACP1 function. However, given also the functional involvement of *ACP1* in the intracellular Wnt signaling cascade, a pathway regulated by lithium, this finding was flagged as being the most interesting. In addition, a sex-specific analysis showed that the most associated SNP rs10170138 in females was *LRRTM4*, which is concordant to a previously demonstrated linkage peak (at 2p11–12) for suicide attempts. Together, the authors discuss that the overall results gave support for "the existence of gene(s) influencing risk for suicidal behavior on the short arm of chromosome 2, an observation that is consistent with the linkage and association findings using pedigrees with BP, major depression and alcoholism."

Concluding remarks

When viewing the results in Table 31.1 for, e.g., the three studies on suicide attempts (Perlis et al., 2010; Schosser et al., 2011; Willour et al., 2012), it is difficult to reveal any common denominator across the studies. Clearly, the SNP-by-SNP GWAS shown for suicidality phenotypes here (Table 31.1) have a lower statistical power due to smaller sample sizes, as compared to those GWAS which analyze >100 000 cases for medical illnesses (den Hoed et al., 2013) or "epidemiological" phenotypes (Rietveld et al., 2013). It is of further interest that applying other analytical approaches which better capture a complex genetic etiology, can also result in significant (power-)benefits (Califano et al., 2012; Binder, 2012). The classical SNP-by-SNP GWAS results (Table 31.1) might have some hidden biological processes in common, which could only be revealed by joint pathway and network analyses. In these perspectives, the GWAS conducted to date for suicidality phenotypes (Table 31.1) can still be viewed as being in its preliminary stages. Indeed, most GWAS to date have suffered from two main problems: (i) that the effect sizes of higher frequency SNPs (those mainly analyzed in GWAS, in contrast to rare variants) are low; and/or (ii) that classical SNP-by-SNP GWAS are generally not optimized for capturing the complexity of polygenetic biological systems. Nevertheless, classical SNP-by-SNP GWAS have identified novel candidate genes for several complex diseases (Visscher et al., 2012), and follow-up re-sequencing has subsequently also revealed rare variants with increased effect sizes in such GWAS-associated genes (Butali et al., 2013; Diogo et al., 2013). Thus, classical SNP-by-SNP GWAS can point out a certain proportion of the genetic variance of complex traits (typically up to 5%).

Novel computer simulations of evolution have revealed that polygenetic etiology is likely to reside in the suggestively significant P-value range, and that genome-wide significant associations from a classical SNP-by-SNP GWAS can be considered as "evolutionary outliers" which only reveal the tip of the genome-wide iceberg (Thornton et al., 2013). This is also supported by analyses of liability by using suggestively associated common SNPs, showing the potential to explain up to 30–40% of the expected heritability (Purcell et al., 2009; So et al., 2011; Vinkhuyzen et al., 2012). As such suggestively significant GWAS SNPs are commonly also used as input for pathway and network analyses, this further underpins the utility of those analytical approaches. In addition, one must also invoke plausible gene–environment interactions (Ben-Efraim et al., 2011), and preferentially assemble better samples (family-based, being also phenotypically well-defined and homogeneous) for the analysis of rare variants (Wasserman et al., 2010; Binder, 2012). Taken together, the question of an SNP being genome-wide significant in a classical SNP-by-SNP GWAS is not the only objective of interest any more, due to the intrinsic limitations of classical SNP-by-SNP GWAS to capture complex genetic etiology. Rather, multi-SNP analytical approaches and integration with experimental biological data to better reveal epistatic and system level differences (Califano et al., 2012; Binder, 2012) is becoming a new objective of interest to unravel in the evolution of GWAS. Reanalysis of GWAS datasets by such new approaches have showed the discovery of many new loci which were previously not observable in the same datasets by the initial use of classical SNP-by-SNP GWAS.

Recent GWAS studies strongly suggest that many genetic susceptibility loci are *not* specific for distinct psychiatric diagnoses but rather shared across diagnostic boundaries (Schulze et al., 2012), exemplified by the recent results from the Cross-Disorder Group of the Psychiatric Genomics Consortium concerning calcium channel genes (using 5–10 000 cases per diagnostic category) (Smoller et al., 2013). GWAS on large enough samples of suicidality might help to similarly unravel if diagnostic boundaries also have diminished relevance also for the genome-wide genetics of suicidality phenotypes, as has been suggested by, e.g., our own candidate gene studies (Sokolowski et al., 2010, 2012; Wasserman et al., 2007; Ben-Efraim et al., 2011, 2012, 2013). Investigations of, e.g., suicidality phenotypes might instead be refined by invoking intermediate phenotypes (Meyer-Lindenberg & Weinberger, 2006) rather than diagnoses. Intermediate phenotypes are further wanted as biological state measures will likely anyway be required for making individualized predictions from genetic data (Lehner, 2013). Studies on *CACNA1C* demonstrate these aspects of (cross-diagnostic) intermediate phenotypes as a prototypic example for genetics underlying the pathophysiology of psychiatric disease (Bhat et al., 2012; Smoller et al., 2013), and likely for suicidality phenotypes as well. Furthermore, it is also being increasingly recognized that statistical power is not augmentable by only increasing sample sizes; increasing sample size may in fact even give the opposite effect of reduced power by increased sample heterogeneity (Moore et al., 2011;Liu et al., 2013). Instead, there is a growing trend toward analyzing the data in new, more powerful ways, which better capture complex genetic etiology (in contrast to the classical SNP-by-SNP GWAS) (Califano et al., 2012; Binder, 2012), different aspects of which have been discussed herein. This latter ongoing GWAS-development is perhaps particularly promising for suicidality, as the sample sizes which are being assembled by "mega-consortia" for classical SNP-by-SNP GWAS of non-psychiatric disorders (>100 000 cases) are not obtainable in any foreseeable future for suicidality phenotypes. In the end, there are no simple answers to the inherently complex question about the genetics of suicidality. But it is clear that GWAS have lots of potential to provide some of the answers, which can ultimately be translated into better understanding and improvement of prevention, intervention, and treatment options for suicidal behaviors.

References

Akula, N., Baranova, A., Seto, D., et al. (2011). A network-based approach to prioritize results from genome-wide association studies. *PLoS One*, **6**(9), e24220.

Altshuler, D., & Daly, M. (2007). Guilt beyond a reasonable doubt. *Nature Genetics*, **39**(7), 813–815.

Baca-Garcia, E., Perez-Rodriguez, M. M., Oquendo, M. A., et al. (2011). Estimating risk for suicide attempt: are we asking the right questions? Passive suicidal ideation as a marker for suicidal behavior. *Journal of Affective Disorders*, **134**(1–3), 327–332.

Ben-Efraim, Y. J., Wasserman, D., Wasserman, J., et al. (2011). Gene-environment interactions between CRHR1 variants and physical assault in suicide attempts. *Genes, Brain and Behavior*, **10**(6), 663–672.

Ben-Efraim, Y. J., Wasserman, D., Wasserman, J., & Sokolowski, M. (2012). Family-based study of HTR2A in suicide attempts: observed gene, gene × environment and parent-of-origin associations. *Molecular Psychiatry*, **18**(7), 758–766.

Ben-Efraim, Y. J., Wasserman, D., Wasserman, J., et al. (2013). Family-based study of AVPR1B association and interaction with stressful life events on depression and anxiety in suicide attempts. *Neuropsychopharmacology*, **38**(8), 1504–1511.

Bhat, S., Dao, D. T., Terrillion, C. E., et al. (2012). CACNA1C (Ca(v)1.2) in the pathophysiology of psychiatric disease. *Progress in Neurobiology*, **99**(1), 1–14.

Binder, E. B., (2012). The genetic basis of mood and anxiety disorders – changing paradigms. *Biology of Mood and Anxiety Disorders*, **2**(1), 17.

Bouaziz, M., Ambroise, C., & Guedj, M. (2011). Accounting for population stratification in practice: a comparison of the main strategies dedicated to genome-wide association studies. *PLoS One*, **6**(12), e28845.

Butali, A., Suzuki, D., Cooper, M. E., et al. (2013). Replication of genome wide association identified candidate genes confirm the role of common and rare variants in PAX7 and VAX1 in the etiology of nonsyndromic CL(P). *American Journal of Medical Genetics A*, **161A**(5), 965–972.

Califano, A., Butte, A. J., Friend, S., et al. (2012). Leveraging models of cell regulation and GWAS data in integrative network-based association studies. *Nature Genetics*, **44** (8), 841–847.

Cardon, L. R., & Palmer, L. J. (2003). Population stratification and spurious allelic association. *Lancet*, **361** (9357), 598–604.

Currier, D., & Mann, J. J. (2008). Stress, genes and the biology of suicidal behavior. *Psychiatric Clinics of North America*, **31**(2), 247–269.

den Hoed, M., Eijgelsheim, M., Esko, T., et al. (2013). Identification of heart rate-associated loci and their effects on cardiac conduction and rhythm disorders. *Nature Genetics*, **45**(6), 621–631.

Deo, A. J., Huang, Y. Y., Hodgkinson, C. A., et al. (2013). A large-scale candidate gene analysis of mood disorders: evidence of neurotrophic tyrosine kinase receptor and opioid receptor signaling dysfunction. *Psychiatric Genetics*, **23**(2), 47–55.

Diogo, D., Kurreeman, F., Stahl, E. A., et al. (2013). Rare, low-frequency, and common variants in the protein-coding sequence of biological candidate genes from GWASs contribute to risk of rheumatoid arthritis. *American Journal of Human Genetics*, **92**(1), 15–27.

Eichler, E. E., Flint, J., Gibson, G., et al. (2010). Missing heritability and strategies for finding the underlying causes of complex disease. *Nature Reviews Genetics*, **11** (6), 446–450.

Ernst, C., Mechawar, N., & Turecki, G. (2009). Suicide neurobiology. *Progress in Neurobiology*, **89**(4), 315–333.

Galfalvy, H., Zalsman, G., Huang, Y. Y., et al. (2011). A pilot genome wide association and gene expression array study of suicide with and without major depression. *World Journal of Biological Psychiatry*, **14**(8), 574–582.

Goldstein, D. B., Ahmadi, K. R., Weale, M. E., et al. (2003). Genome scans and candidate gene approaches in the study of common diseases and variable drug responses. *Trends in Genetics*, **19**(11), 615–622.

Hamshere, M. L., Walters, J. T., Smith, R., et al. (2013). Genome-wide significant associations in schizophrenia to ITIH3/4, CACNA1C and SDCCAG8, and extensive replication of associations reported by the Schizophrenia PGC. *Molecular Psychiatry*,**18**(6), 708–712.

Hannum, G., Srivas, R., Guenole, A., et al. (2009). Genome-wide association data reveal a global map of genetic interactions among protein complexes. *PLoS Genetics*, **5** (12), e1000782.

Holmans, P. (2010). Statistical methods for pathway analysis of genome-wide data for association with complex genetic traits. *Advances in Genetics*, **72**, 141–179.

Ikegawa, S. (2012). A short history of the genome-wide association study: where we were and where we are going. *Genomics Inform*, **10**(4), 220–225.

Jia, P., Kao, C. F., Kuo, P. H., et al. (2011a). A comprehensive network and pathway analysis of candidate genes in major depressive disorder. *BMC Systems Biology*, **5** (Suppl 3), S12.

Jia, P., Zheng, S., Long, J., et al. (2011b). dmGWAS: dense module searching for genome-wide association studies in protein-protein interaction networks. *Bioinformatics*, **27** (1), 95–102.

Jia, P., Wang, L., Fanous, A. H., et al. (2012). Network-assisted investigation of combined causal signals from genome-wide association studies in schizophrenia. *PLoS Computational Biology*, **8**(7), e1002587.

Kendler, K. S. (2010). Genetic and environmental pathways to suicidal behavior: reflections of a genetic epidemiologist. *European Psychiatry*, **25**(5), 300–303.

Kofink, D., Boks, M. P., Timmers, H. T., et al. (2013). Epigenetic dynamics in psychiatric disorders: Environmental programming of neurodevelopmental processes. *Neuroscience and Biobehavioral Reviews*, **37**(5), 831–845.

Laje, G., Allen, A. S., Akula, N., et al. (2009). Genome-wide association study of suicidal ideation emerging during citalopram treatment of depressed outpatients. *Pharmacogenetic Genomics*, **19**(9), 666–674.

Lambert, C. G., & Black, L. J. (2012). Learning from our GWAS mistakes: from experimental design to scientific method. *Biostatistics*, **13**(2), 195–203.

Lee, I., Blom, U. M., Wang, P. I., et al. (2011). Prioritizing candidate disease genes by network-based boosting of genome-wide association data. *Genome Research*, **21**(7), 1109–1121.

Lehne, B., Lewis, C. M., & Schlitt, T. (2011). From SNPs to genes: disease association at the gene level. *PLoS One*, **6**(6), e20133.

Lehner, B. (2013). Genotype to phenotype: lessons from model organisms for human genetics. *Nature Reviews Genetics*, **14**(3), 168–178.

Leigh, H. (2009). A proposal for a new multiaxial model of psychiatric diagnosis. A continuum-based patient model derived from evolutionary developmental gene-environment interaction. *Psychopathology*, **42**(1), 1–10.

Li, M. X., Yeung, J. M., Cherny, S. S., et al. (2012a). Evaluating the effective numbers of independent tests and significant p-value thresholds in commercial genotyping arrays and public imputation reference datasets. *Human Genetics*, **131**(5), 747–756.

Li, M. X., Kwan, J. S., & Sham, P. C. (2012b). HYST: a hybrid set-based test for genome-wide association studies, with application to protein-protein interaction-based association analysis. *American Journal of Human Genetics*, **91**(3), 478–488.

Liu, Y. J., Zhang, L., Pei, Y., et al. (2013). On genome-wide association studies and their meta-analyses: lessons learned from osteoporosis studies. *Journal of Clinical Endocrinology and Metabolism*, **98**(7), E1278–1282

Mann, J. J., Arango, V. A., Avenevoli, S., et al. (2009). Candidate endophenotypes for genetic studies of suicidal behavior. *Biological Psychiatry*, **65**(7), 556–563.

Marchini, J., & Howie, B. (2010). Genotype imputation for genome-wide association studies. *Nature Reviews Genetics*, **11**(7), 499–511.

McKinney, B. A., & Pajewski, N. M. (2011). Six degrees of epistasis: statistical network models for GWAS. *Frontiers in Genetics*, **2**, 109.

Menke, A., Domschke, K., Czamara, D., et al. (2012). Genome-wide association study of antidepressant treatment-emergent suicidal ideation. *Neuropsychopharmacology*, **37**(3), 797–807.

Meyer-Lindenberg, A., & Weinberger, D. R. (2006). Intermediate phenotypes and genetic mechanisms of psychiatric disorders. *Nature Reviews Neuroscience*, **7**(10), 818–827.

Moore, S., Kelleher, E., & Corvin, A. (2011). The shock of the new: progress in schizophrenia genomics. *Current Genomics*, **12**(7), 516–524.

Need, A. C., & Goldstein, D. B. (2010). Whole genome association studies in complex diseases: where do we stand? *Dialogues in Clinical Neuroscience*, **12**(1), 37–46.

Nicolae, D. L., Gamazon, E., Zhang, W., et al. (2010). Trait-associated SNPs are more likely to be eQTLs: annotation to enhance discovery from GWAS. *PLoS Genetics*, **6**(4), e1000888.

Ober, C., Loisel, D. A., & Gilad, Y. (2008). Sex-specific genetic architecture of human disease. *Nature Reviews Genetics*, **9**(12), 911–922.

Perlis, R. H., Huang, J., Purcell, S., et al. (2010). Genome-wide association study of suicide attempts in mood disorder patients. *American Journal of Psychiatry*, **167**(12), 1499–1507.

Perroud, N., Uher, R., Ng, M. Y., et al. (2012). Genome-wide association study of increasing suicidal ideation during antidepressant treatment in the GENDEP project. *Pharmacogenomics Journal*, **12**(1), 68–77.

Purcell, S. M., Wray, N. R., Stone, J. L., et al. (2009). Common polygenic variation contributes to risk of schizophrenia and bipolar disorder. *Nature*, **460**(7256), 748–752.

Rietveld, C. A., Medland, S. E., Derringer, J., et al. (2013). GWAS of 126,559 individuals identifies genetic variants associated with educational attainment. *Science*, **340**(6139), 1467–1471.

Rowe, S. J., & Tenesa, A. (2012). Human complex trait genetics: lifting the lid of the genomics toolbox – from pathways to prediction. *Current Genomics*, **13**(3), 213–224.

Rujescu, D., & Giegling, I. (2010). The genetics of neurosystems in mental ill-health and suicidality: beyond serotonin. *European Journal of Psychiatry*, **25**(5), 272–274.

Schork, N. J., Murray, S. S., Frazer, K. A., et al. (2009). Common vs. rare allele hypotheses for complex diseases. *Current Opinion in Genetic Development*, **19**(3), 212–219.

Schosser, A., Butler, A. W., Ising, M., et al. (2011). Genomewide association scan of suicidal thoughts and behaviour in major depression. *PLoS One*, **6**(7), e20690.

Schulze, T. G., Akula, N., Breuer, R., et al. (2012). Molecular genetic overlap in bipolar disorder, schizophrenia, and major depressive disorder. *World Journal of Biological Psychiatry* [Epub ahead of print].

Scriver, C. R. (2007). The PAH gene, phenylketonuria, and a paradigm shift. *Human Mutatation*, **28**(9), 831–845.

Sebastiani, P., Solovieff, N., Puca, A., et al. (2010). Genetic signatures of exceptional longevity in humans. *Science* [Epub 2010 Jul 1].

Sebastiani, P., Solovieff, N., Puca, A., et al. (2011). Retraction. *Science*, **333**(6041), 404.

Smoller, J. W., Craddock, N., Kendler, K., et al. (2013). Identification of risk loci with shared effects on five major psychiatric disorders: a genome-wide analysis. *Lancet*, **381**(9875), 1371–1379.

So, H. C., Li, M., & Sham, P. C. (2011). Uncovering the total heritability explained by all true susceptibility variants in a genome-wide association study. *Genetic Epidemiology*, **35**(6), 447–456.

Sokolowski, M., Wasserman, J., & Wasserman, D. (2010). Association of polymorphisms in the SLIT2 axonal guidance gene with anger in suicide attempters. *Molecular Psychiatry*, **15**(1), 10–11.

Sokolowski, M., Ben-Efraim, Y. J., Wasserman, J., et al. (2012). Glutamatergic GRIN2B and polyaminergic ODC1 genes in suicide attempts: associations and gene-environment interactions with childhood/adolescent physical assault. *Molecular Psychiatry*, **18**(9):985–992.

Sun, J., Wan, C., Jia, P., et al. (2011). Application of systems biology approach identifies and validates GRB2 as a risk gene for schizophrenia in the Irish Case Control Study of Schizophrenia (ICCSS) sample. *Schizophrenia Research*, **125**(2–3), 201–208.

Terwilliger, J. D., & Goring, H. H. (2009). Update to Terwilliger and Goring's "Gene mapping in the 20th and 21st centuries" (2000): gene mapping when rare variants are common and common variants are rare. *Human Biology*, **81**(5–6), 729–733.

Teslovich, T. M., Musunuru, K., Smith, A. V., et al. (2010). Biological, clinical and population relevance of 95 loci for blood lipids. *Nature*, **466**(7307), 707–713.

Thornton, K. R., Foran, A. J., & Long, A. D. (2013). Properties and modeling of GWAS when complex disease risk is due to non-complementing, deleterious mutations in genes of large effect. *PLoS Genetics*, **9**(2), e1003258.

Vinkhuyzen, A. A., Pedersen, N. L., Yang, J., et al. (2012). Common SNPs explain some of the variation in the personality dimensions of neuroticism and extraversion. *Translational Psychiatry*, **2**, e102.

Visscher, P. M., Brown, M. A., McCarthy, M. I., et al. (2012). Five years of GWAS discovery. *American Journal of Human Genetics*, **90**(1), 7–24.

Voracek, M., & Loibl, L. M. (2007). Genetics of suicide: a systematic review of twin studies. *Wiener klinische Wochenschrift*, **119**(15–16), 463–475.

Wasserman, D., Geijer, T., Rozanov, V., et al. (2005). Suicide attempt and basic mechanisms in neural conduction: relationships to the SCN8A and VAMP4 genes. *American Journal of Medical Genetics Part B: Neuropsychiatric Genetics*, **133B**(1), 116–119.

Wasserman, D., Geijer, T., Sokolowski, M., et al. (2007). Genetic variation in the hypothalamic-pituitary-adrenocortical axis regulatory factor, T-box 19, and the angry/hostility personality trait. *Genes, Brain and Behavior*, **6**(4), 321–328.

Wasserman, D., Sokolowski, M., Rozanov, V., et al. (2008). The CRHR1 gene: a marker for suicidality in depressed males exposed to low stress. *Genes, Brain and Behavior*, 7(1), 14–19.

Wasserman, D., Sokolowski, M., Wasserman, J., et al. (2009). Neurobiology and the genetics of suicide. In D. Wasserman & C. Wasserman (Eds.) *Oxford Textbook of Suicidology – The Five Continents Perspective* (pp. 165–182). Oxford, UK: Oxford University Press.

Wasserman, D., Terenius, L., Wasserman, J., et al. (2010). The 2009 Nobel conference on the role of genetics in promoting suicide prevention and the mental health of the population. *Molecular Psychiatry*, **15**(1), 12–17.

Willour, V. L., Seifuddin, F., Mahon, P. B., et al. (2012). A genome-wide association study of attempted suicide. *Molecular Psychiatry*, **17**(4), 433–444.

Chapter 32

Epigenetics

Benoit Labonté and Gustavo Turecki

The burden of early life adversity and suicide

With more than 3 million reports of child maltreatment in the USA in 2009 and similar statistics elsewhere in Western societies (Children's Bureau, 2010), and a strong association between exposure to early life maltreatment and development of negative mental health outcomes, including suicidal behaviors, early life adversity is a problem of major public health concern. From an epidemiological point of view, trauma exposure in children is estimated to range between 25% and 45%, although the rates reported vary considerably between studies and according to the definition of abuse types (Scher et al., 2004; Briere & Elliott, 2003; Gorey & Leslie, 1997; McCauley et al., 1997; Heim et al., 2010).

In addition to its psychological impact, child maltreatment and trauma has a clear economic impact, which is explained in part by its effect on behavioral development and association with psychopathology later during life. Indeed, both child sexual abuse (CSA) and child physical abuse (CPA) are associated with higher odds of psychiatric disorders including depression, anxiety, bipolar disorder, substance abuse, and suicidal behaviors (Evans et al., 2005; Molnar et al., 2001; Santa Mina & Gallop, 1998; Heim & Nemeroff, 2001; Kendler et al., 2000, 2004; Kaplan & Klinetob, 2000; Agid et al., 1999; Fergusson et al., 1996). Besides increasing the risk of psychiatric disorders, CSA and CPA also associate with earlier age of onset of psychopathology, chronic course, more severe outcomes, poorer recovery rate and more importantly, with 12 times higher odds of suicidal behaviors (Dinwiddie et al., 2000; Gladstone et al., 2004; Jaffee et al., 2002; Zlotnick et al., 2001; Brown & Moran, 1994; Tanskanen et al., 2004; Bensley et al., 1999; Molnar et al., 2001).

Epigenetics and regulation of the brain by the early life environment

While substantial theoretical and empirical work supports the relationship between early life adversity and development of negative mental health outcomes in adulthood, the critical question has been how such experiences in early life impact their lifelong risk on development of psychopathology. Similarly, more mechanistic questions, such as what stable molecular processes mediate the association between early life adversity and psychopathology, have long intrigued researchers. This is clearly a complex set of questions, which we have just begun to unravel. This chapter will review recent evidence suggesting that molecular alterations result from variation in early life environment through epigenetic processes, particularly focusing on DNA methylation. We will discuss animal studies showing an impact of early life environment on behavioral development and review studies investigating associations between methylation and suicide and related behavior in humans.

Although the same DNA is found in every cell of our body, cells differentiate into specific cell types and synthesize different proteins allowing them to evolve and adapt to specific environments. This whole process is believed to involve epigenetic mechanisms. Epigenetics refers to the study of the epigenome, which is a collection of chemical and physical modifications taking place in or around the DNA molecule and altering the capacity of a gene to be activated and to produce the mRNA it encodes. This involves several mechanisms including histone modifications (Kouzarides, 2007), DNA methylation (Klose & Bird, 2006), and hydroxymethylation (Kriaucionis &

A Concise Guide to Understanding Suicide, ed. Stephen H. Koslow, Pedro Ruiz, and Charles B. Nemeroff. Published by Cambridge University Press.

Heintz, 2009). Another mechanism, which is not a priori an epigenetic mechanism but is often classified as such, is the post-translational regulation of gene expression via non-coding RNA species like micro-RNA (He & Hannon, 2004). Given the high complexity of the DNA organization and regulation, these modifications are expected to follow a defined pattern allowing the underlying molecular mechanisms to be performed correctly and to decode DNA in the context of chromatin.

Within the cells' nucleus, DNA is packaged into a structure called chromatin, composed of nucleosomes, the fundamental unit of chromatin, around which 146 bp of DNA is wrapped. The nucleosome itself is formed by an octamer of the four core histones (H2A, H2B, H3, and H4), globular structures having a tail of amino acids which can be modified by the addition or the removal of chemical residues. Chromatin has two structures: euchromatin, the active state associated with gene transcription and its counterpart, heterochromatin, the inactive state corresponding to gene repression.

Chromatin state is dynamically regulated by the recruitment of proteins carrying intrinsic enzymatic activity to histone modifications (Clements et al., 2003; Fischle et al., 2005; Nelson et al., 2006; Pray-Grant et al., 2005; Santos-Rosa et al., 2003) which induce the opening or the closing of chromatin (Wysocka et al., 2005, 2006). Up to eight types of histone modifications have been characterized (methylation (lysine, arginine), acetylation, phosphorylation, ubiquitylation, sumoylation, deimination, ADP ribosylation, and proline isomerization), although they might not be all found in eukaryotic cells (Kouzarides, 2007). While these marks may contribute concomitantly to regulate gene expression, attention has been put mainly on lysine methylation and acetylation. For instance, methylation at the fourth lysine (K) of the third histone (H; H3K4) (Kirmizis et al., 2007; Salcedo-Amaya et al., 2009; Barrera et al., 2008; Pokholok et al., 2005; Wang et al., 2008; Xiao et al., 2007) has been associated with active transcription while methylation at H3K9, H3K27 and H4K20 often correlate with transcriptional repression (Wang et al., 2008; Barski et al., 2007; Bannister et al., 2001; Botuyan et al., 2006; Lan et al., 2007; Nielsen et al., 2001; Sanders et al., 2004; Swigut & Wysocka, 2007). Each of these modifications, most likely, have distinct signature profiles which may overlap to form what is believed to be a histone code that may control the structure of the chromatin as well as gene transcription according to cell needs. However, this code is just beginning to be cracked.

DNA methylation is a post-transcriptional modification that refers mainly to the transfer of a methyl group (CH_3) from an *S*-adenosyl-l-methionine (AdoMet) donor to the 5' carbon of the cytosine from dinucleotide CpG sequences. This process requires the enzymatic activity of DNA methyltransferase (DNMT) proteins among which DNMT3a and DNMT3b are called *de novo* methylases because they introduce methyl groups at previously unmethylated cytosines (Hata et al., 2002; Okano et al., 1998). In contrast, DNA hydroxymethylation refers to the oxidation of pre-existing 5'methylcytosine to 5' hydroxymethylation by enzymes by the TET family (Tahiliani et al., 2009; Ito et al., 2010).

In somatic cells, approximately 80% of CpGs are methylated (Tucker, 2001). The remaining unmethylated ones are grouped in CpG-enriched regions called CpG islands found in genes' 5' regulatory regions. Thus, DNA methylation in gene promoter has classically been associated with translational repression by interfering with the recruitment and the binding of the transcriptional machinery to gene regulatory regions (Klose & Bird, 2006). However, when found within the gene body, DNA methylation has been associated with transcriptional activation and alternative transcript selection (Maunakea et al., 2010). In contrast, recent findings suggest that hydroxymethylation may be enriched in the gene body of active genes (Mellen et al., 2012). Moreover, different cell types exhibit different methylation and hydroxymethylation patterns which confer a specificity of expression based on the requirement of each cell type (Mellen et al., 2012; Iwamoto et al., 2011).

In the following sections, we will review findings in gene systems that have been targeted by studies investigating epigenetic factors associated with the social environment, particularly focusing on animal and human studies relevant to understanding suicide risk. We will review animal studies using models of early life environmental variation, and studies on suicide that focus on the investigation of the effects of early life adversity. Overall we will review the evidence suggesting that epigenetic mechanisms may be involved in the modification of gene expression induced by environmental factors. While suicide is the direct result of early life adversity – and in fact, most individuals who die by suicide do not have a history of abuse during childhood – a significant minority does, and in this subgroup, the association is strong. Among the systems reviewed in this chapter, we will focus in particular on gene systems coding for components of the HPA axis, and related signaling hormones and molecules, neurotrophic factors and their receptors, as well as other signaling systems.

HPA axis alterations induced by early life adversity

Child abuse has been proposed to induce its long-term behavioral consequences partly by altering the neural circuits involved in the regulation of stress (Heim et al., 2008b). The HPA axis is the main stress regulatory system (Pariante & Lightman, 2008). Under stressful conditions, corticotropin-releasing factor (CRF) and vasopressin (AVP) are released from the hypothalamus. CRF and AVP induce the release of adrenocorticotropic hormone (ACTH) and pro-opiomelanocortin (POMC) from the pituitary gland to the blood which then travels to the adrenal cortex where they induce the release of glucocorticoids, cortisol in humans and corticosterone in rodents, to the blood. Glucocorticoids then act at each level of the HPA axis to decrease the release of CRF, AVP, POMC, and ACTH and regulate the stress response. While the HPA axis can be regulated at different levels, the main locus of regulation lies in the hippocampus where glucocorticoids bind glucocorticoid receptors (GRs) and induce an inhibitory feedback on the activation of the HPA axis to bring back to basal levels the activity of the stress response.

From a structural point of view, childhood abuse and neglect have been associated with volume loss in the hippocampus (Bremner et al., 1997; Stein et al., 1997; Driessen et al., 2000), altered cortical symmetry in the frontal lobe (Carrion et al., 2001) and superior temporal gyrus (De Bellis et al., 2002) as well as a reduced neuronal density and/or neuronal integrity in the anterior cingulated gyrus (De Bellis et al., 2002). One study also reported poorer hippocampal activation on a memory task in patients with a history of childhood abuse (Bremner et al., 2003). Importantly, the structural consequences of child abuse are thought to be time-dependent, implying that particular brain regions may have unique windows of vulnerability to the effects of child abuse (Andersen et al., 2008).

From a molecular point of view, depressed patients with a history of child abuse have been reported to exhibit higher ACTH and cortisol levels following stress and dexamethasone (DEX) challenges (Heim et al., 2000, 2008a). Interestingly, in these studies, both ACTH and cortisol levels did not differ significantly between depressed subjects without history of childhood abuse and controls (Heim et al., 2000, 2008a). Childhood abuse, and particularly physical abuse, has also been shown to increase CRH levels (Heim et al., 2008b; Carpenter et al., 2004) and to decrease CSF oxytocin levels (Heim et al., 2009). More recently, low hippocampal GR levels have been reported in suicide completers with a history of childhood abuse (McGowan et al., 2009; Labonté et al., 2012b) but not in non-abused suicide completers. Altogether, these alterations are believed to lead to important behavioral changes that may increase the predisposition toward suicidal behavior later in life.

This work is also substantiated with findings from animal work. For instance, the regulation of the activity of the HPA axis has been shown to be modulated by maternal behavior in rats. Depressive-like behaviors (Francis et al., 1999) associated with altered HPA axis feedback (Liu et al., 1997) and low GR mRNA hippocampal levels (Liu et al., 1997) are common features in rats raised by mothers providing maternal care defined by low levels of licking and grooming (LG). A comprehensive model involving modulation at numerous levels, including hormonal, synaptic and molecular changes, has been proposed in an attempt to characterize the molecular pathways involved in the modulatory effects of maternal behavior in rats. High maternal LG levels, which can also be mimicked by handling pups during early life, induces a physiological response involving the release of thyroid hormone plasma levels. This increases 5-HT activity in the raphe nuclei, and consequently, stimulates serotonin (5-HT) turnover in the hippocampus and frontal cortex (Mitchell et al., 1990; Smythe et al., 1994; Meaney et al., 1987). Via activation of the G protein-coupled 5-HT_7 receptor (Laplante et al., 2002), it is believed that 5-HT activates a cAMP/PKA-dependent intracellular cascade increasing the expression of nerve growth factor 1-A (NGFI-A) and activator protein-2 (AP-2) in the hippocampus (Meaney et al., 2000). NGFI-A and AP-2 are activating transcription factors with putative binding sites within the GR promoter region (McCormick et al., 2000) that increase GR mRNA levels in the hippocampus of the offspring. This complex process is attenuated in rats raised by low LG mothers according to the molecular and behavioral processes mentioned previously and resulting in relatively lower GR expression in the hippocampus (Weaver et al., 2004; McGowan et al., 2011). Interestingly, most of these regulatory changes are temporally stable and are maintained throughout adulthood. Moreover, cross-fostering studies report that these behavioral and molecular modifications are reversed when pups raised by low LG mothers are transferred to high LG mothers (Liu et al., 1997; Francis et al., 1999) within the first week of life.

The glucocorticoid receptor gene

As the HPA programing by maternal behavior is modified by cross-fostering and temporally stable, researchers hypothesized that the long-term effects of maternal behavior and early life environment variation on GR hippocampal expression could be due to epigenetic modifications. In rats, the GR gene is preceded by 10 non-coding exons and by 14 in humans (McCormick et al., 2000; Turner and Muller, 2005). The expression of the non-coding exon 1_7 in rats and the human homologue 1_F have been shown to be specific to the hippocampus (Turner & Muller, 2005). Each of the untranslated exon 1 variants has its own promoter and multiple transcription factor binding sites, including NGFI-A (Meaney, 2001), have been identified in GR promoter sequences (Turner et al., 2008, 2010). In offspring raised by low LG rat mothers, CpG methylation levels in the exon 1_7 promoter region are significantly increased at almost all CpGs compared to offspring raised by high LG mothers. More importantly, a CpG located in the 5' end of a NGFI-A binding site is methylated in almost 100% of offspring raised by low LG mothers whereas it is almost not methylated in offspring from high LG mothers (Weaver et al., 2004). Interestingly, follow-up studies in high and low LG rats showed that DNA methylation levels are also increased in the promoters of other non-coding first exons of the GR gene which were associated with transcriptional changes (McGowan et al., 2011) suggesting that the whole GR locus may be poised for epigenetic regulation by environmental social factors.

These findings were recently translated to humans through studies investigating hippocampal tissue from individuals who died by suicide with and without a history of childhood adversity, as well as normal controls (McGowan et al., 2009; Labonté et al., 2012b). Notably, methylation levels in the exon 1_F promoter in abused suicide completers were significantly higher than among non-abused suicides and healthy controls. In addition, similarly to what was found in rats, a significant hypermethylation in a NGFI-A binding site was found in abused suicide completers but not in the other groups. Through a series of cell functional assays, this epigenetic mark was shown to repress the binding of NGFI-A to its cognate DNA sequence and to decrease GR transcription (McGowan et al., 2009).

It is also interesting to note that these findings have been supported by other groups with different populations of individuals that suffered from early life adversity. Indeed, higher levels of methylation in the promoter of GR 1_F have been reported in the infants of mothers reporting intimate partner violence during their pregnancy compared to those born from normal mothers (Radtke et al., 2011). Another study reported significant correlations between GR 1_F promoter methylation levels and parental loss, child maltreatment, and parental care (Tyrka et al., 2012). Furthermore, DNA methylation levels in GR 1_F promoter were shown to be positively correlated with childhood sexual abuse, its severity, and the number of maltreatment types in individuals with MDD, and with repetition of severe types of abuse in patients with bipolar disorders (Perroud et al., 2011). Altogether, this suggests that early life adversity may induce specific long-lasting epigenetic alterations affecting gene expression.

In a different study assessing the expression of several GR exon 1 variants expressed in the limbic system of depressed suicide completers, $GR1_F$ and $GR1_C$ hippocampal expression were significantly decreased in depressed suicide completers (Alt et al., 2010). However, this was not associated with promoter hypermethylation although it should be noted that this study investigated methylation only in a limited region and promoter methylation levels reported were particularly low. On the other hand, NGFI-A protein levels in the hippocampus (HPC) were significantly decreased in depressed suicide completers suggesting that the decrease in GR expression found in suicide completers may be mediated by different molecular pathways depending on the presence or the absence of early life adversity.

More recently, our group pushed further the investigation of early life adversity consequences on the epigenetic regulation of GR in the HPC of abused suicide completers (Labonté et al., 2012b). Our data indicated that the expression of the non-coding exons 1_B, 1_C, and 1_H is significantly decreased in suicide completers with a history of childhood abuse compared to non-abused suicides and controls. The assessment of methylation levels in the promoter of $GR1_C$ revealed methylation differences that are inversely correlated with $GR1_C$ expression in accordance with our previous finding on 1_F variant. On the other hand, $GR1_H$ promoter showed sites specific hypomethylation that was positively correlated with $hGR1_H$ expression. In other words, less methylation significantly correlated with lower expression suggests that active demethylation is also a functional mechanism that may be affected by early life adversity. While this is a mechanism that has received less attention, more work is required in order to elucidate its potential implications in the context of early life adversity.

In addition to DNA methylation, chromatin changes have also been associated with poor maternal care. For instance, H3K9 acetylation, a marker of open euchromatin state (Kouzarides, 2007), was found to be lower in the $GR1_7$ promoter in low LG raised rats. Pharmacological challenge with the histone deacetylase inhibitor (TSA) restored methylation levels, increased NGFI-A binding to the promoter, and reinstated H3K9 acetylation and GR hippocampal levels (Weaver et al., 2004). Treated rats were also less reactive to stressful conditions. By decreasing H3K9 acetylation, DNA access to the transcriptional machinery and DNA binding proteins such as transcription factors and methylated DNA binding proteins is reduced. Functionally, these results suggest that variation in the early life environment in rats and early life adversity in humans induces a coordinated remodeling of epigenetic mechanisms involving DNA methylation and chromatin modifications in the multiple promoters of GR leading to important changes in GR expression, and consequent regulation of the HPA axis.

The vasopressin (AVP) and corticotropin-releasing factor genes

Other components of the HPA axis have also been shown to be affected by early life stress. For instance, early life infant-maternal separation in mice, inducing stress-coping behavioral alterations in pups, has been shown to be associated with a long-lasting increase in corticosterone secretion and with an increased expression of POMC and AVP in the paraventricular nucleus (PVN) of the hypothalamus (Murgatroyd et al., 2009). The AVP gene in mice is composed of three coding exons and is oriented tail-to-tail with the *oxytocin* (Oxt) gene. Interestingly, the intergenic region between the AVP and the Oxt genes has been shown to include an enhancer modulating AVP expression (Gainer et al., 2001) and itself composed of a CpG island (Murgatroyd et al., 2009).

Methylation at multiple sites within the AVP enhancer was shown to be decreased in the PVN of stressed mice 6 weeks, 3 months, and 1 year following the stress regimen (Murgatroyd et al., 2009). Consistent with the repressive role of DNA methylation on expression, this was associated with overexpression of the AVP gene. The regulatory properties of this enhancer were defined by a deletion experiment. Deleting the first part of the enhancer partially reduced transcriptional activity, while removing the entire enhancer almost completely abolished the gene's activity. Furthermore, methylation of the enhancer also significantly reduced transcriptional activity. Interestingly, AVP expression was also significantly increased in stressed mice at 10 days, although no methylation differences were observed in the AVP's enhancer. The AVP enhancer can putatively bind the methylated CpG binding protein MeCP2. However, because of the repressive role of MeCP2 on transcription, one would expect the opposite tendency concerning AVP expression. MeCP2 has nevertheless been shown to be susceptible to inactivation by neuronal depolarization-induced phosphorylation, leading to its dissociation from putative targets (Chen et al., 2003; Zhou et al., 2006). Accordingly, higher neuronal activity-induced CaMKII immunoreactivity and phosphorylated MeCP2 levels have been reported in AVP-expressing neurons in the PVN of 10-day-old stressed mice. Altogether, these results suggest that in young stressed mice, methylation patterns in AVP's enhancer allow the binding of MeCP2, which could then repress expression. However, since early life stress also increases neuronal activity in AVP-expressing neurons, MeCP2 gets phosphorylated and inactivated. Consequently, the repressive effect of MeCP2 on AVP expression is abolished. On the other hand, methylation levels in AVP enhancer decrease with time. This may decrease MeCP2 binding and allow AVP to be expressed at higher levels. Overall, these results nicely suggest that alterations in DNA methylation found outside of the promoter might also be involved in physiological and behavioral modifications induced by environmental factors.

The regulation of a related peptide, corticotropin-releasing factor, has been recently shown to be also associated with epigenetic regulation by the social environment. Accordingly, CRF expression in the PVN of chronically socially defeated mice was found to be increased (Elliott et al., 2010). Interestingly, this effect was found only in animals susceptible to social stress and showing the normal subordinated behavior following chronic exposure to aggressive littermates as opposed to the resilient mice continuing to interact with their aggressor. This was associated with lower levels of methylation as reported by a reduced number of methylated clones in the susceptible group compared to control and resilient mice. A closer look at the methylation alteration induced by chronic social stress pointed to a single site of hypomethylation in the proximal promoter flanking the first exon and known to bind the CREB response element cAMP (Aguilera et al., 2007). The importance of this site was further confirmed by luciferase assays showing that mutating a single base in the CRE binding site substantially reduced the cAMP-induced CRF promoter activity (Elliott et al., 2010). These changes in methylation and expression were also accompanied by a significant decrease in the DNA methyltransferase 3b expression and by an increase in the expression of the demethylating candidate gadd45b. Interestingly, chronic treatment with the tricyclic imipramine attenuated the changes at the DNA methylation and expression levels induced by social stress (Elliott et al., 2010). Consequently, these findings in both the AVP and the CRF genes strongly support the involvement of active demethylation in the long-term effects of early life adversity.

The brain-derived neurotrophic factor gene

Neurotrophic factors are important candidate molecules to understand the development of psychopathology because of their role in neuronal survival and plasticity, as well as their expression in brain regions from the limbic system, where emotions and related behaviors are processed. For instance, it is hypothesized that their alteration could partly underlie changes in plasticity observed in the brains of suicides as well as the mood symptoms observed in depressive patients. While the major neurotrophic factors include nerve growth factor (NGF), neurotrophin 3 and 4 (NT3/4), fibroblast growth factor (FGF), transforming growth factor (TGF), and BDNF, the latter has received most of the attention in neurobiological research of psychiatric conditions such as depressive disorders and suicide. For instance, low serum and brain BDNF expression has been reported in patients with major depression (Brunoni et al., 2008; Dwivedi et al., 2003; Pandey et al., 2008) and these alterations were reversed by antidepressant treatment (Chen et al., 2001; Sen et al., 2008; Matrisciano et al., 2009). In mice, BDNF depletion induces depressive-like behaviors (Chan et al., 2006) while in rats, chronic stress and persistent pain reduces BDNF expression in the hippocampus (Gronli et al., 2006; Duric & McCarson, 2005), and these effects are counteracted by antidepressant treatment (Duric & McCarson, 2006; Rogoz et al., 2005; Xu et al., 2006).

BDNF epigenetic regulation has recently been investigated in mice and rat models of stress-induced depressive symptoms (Tsankova et al., 2006; Roth et al., 2009), as well as in a rat model of exposure to traumatic events (Roth et al., 2011). In both species, the BDNF gene contains nine 5' non-coding first exons with their own promoter coding for the same protein (Aid et al., 2007). The alternative splicing of these exons specifies the tissue in which BDNF is expressed (Aid et al., 2007). In both species, epigenetic processes involved in the transcriptional control of BDNF have been shown to be altered by stress. For instance, chronic social stress in mice decreases the expression of two specific BDNF transcripts (III and IV) in the hippocampus (Tsankova et al., 2006), while maternal maltreatment decreases prefrontal cortex (PFC) BDNF mRNA expression in rats (Roth et al., 2009). Although similar, these transcriptional alterations were shown to be induced by different epigenetic mechanisms. Indeed, chronic stress in mice raises H3K27 dimethylation levels in transcripts III and IV promoters (Tsankova et al., 2006), while site-specific hypermethylation is found in transcripts IV and IX promoters of maltreated rats (Roth et al., 2009). In the latter study, site-specific hypermethylation seems to follow a developmental pattern, exon IX promoter hypermethylation occurring immediately after the maltreatment regimen, while promoter IV methylation increases gradually to reach significantly altered levels only at adulthood. Surprisingly, in one of these studies (Tsankova et al., 2006), no DNA methylation difference was found in association with histone modifications, while no histone modification was reported in association with DNA methylation alterations in the other study (Roth et al., 2009). These findings illustrate that early life or chronic stressors may alter different epigenetic mechanisms with common transcriptional consequences: the latter leading to the compaction of chromatin in its heterochromatic state, and the former blocking the binding of transcription factors to DNA. On the other hand, these results may also highlight the heterogeneity of stress-induced epigenetic alterations between species.

Recently, the epigenetic regulation of BDNF has been shown to be altered in a rat model of PTSD symptoms (Roth et al., 2011). Given the findings discussed above, the authors focused on exon IV. Stressed rats showed increased DNA methylation in the dorsal dentate gyrus and in the CA3 regions. Contrary to expected, a global hypomethylation was observed in the ventral CA1 region. These epigenetic alterations were accompanied by significant downregulation of BDNF exon IV expression in both the dorsal and ventral CA1 regions in the stressed rats relative to non-stressed rats. Interestingly, these alterations were restricted to the hippocampus since no alterations were found in the basolateral amygdala nor in the medial prefrontal cortex. These findings suggest that DNA methylation may be affected differently within the same structure depending on the function and the connections these regions have. Given that the expression of exon IV was decreased in the ventral CA1 without any significant changes in DNA methylation, these findings also suggest that, although DNA methylation may have an important role in the regulation of BDNF, other mechanisms are probably involved.

Pharmacological treatment with the tricyclic antidepressant imipramine was able to reverse the effect of chronic stress on BDNF transcription in mice (Tsankova et al., 2006). However, this reversal does not seem to be due to the reinstatement of altered histone modifications but rather to follow an indirect pathway. Indeed, chronic but not acute imipramine treatment did not reinstate H3K27 basal dimethylation levels, but rather decreased HDAC5 levels in the hippocampus of chronically stressed mice leading to a global hyperacetylation in transcripts III and IV promoter regions. The importance of histone acetylation in the effect of antidepressant treatment has indeed been previously reported in animal models of stress-induced depression (Sun et al., 2013). Additionally, this hyperacetylation was associated with higher hippocampal levels of H3K4 dimethylation in the area of BDNF III and IV promoters with both modifications related to transcriptional activation. Consequently, these results suggest the existence of a compensatory mechanism in the reinstatement of basal BDNF levels by chronic imipramine treatment following chronic stress and emphasize the importance of chromatin hyperacetylation induced by antidepressant treatment.

Recently, the methylation state of BDNF was also assessed in postmortem brains from suicide completers (Keller et al., 2010). The human BDNF gene is also composed of 11 exons preceded by nine non-coding first exons regulating BDNF expression in different tissue (Pruunsild et al., 2007). In Keller et al.'s study (Keller et al., 2010), three different methods were used to quantify methylation levels in a region encompassing part of non-coding exon IV and its promoter in the Wernicke area. Their results show that methylation in four CpGs located downstream to promoter IV transcription initiation site was significantly increased in suicide completers compared to controls. These differences were specific to the BDNF promoter since the investigation of genome-wide methylation in these subjects did not reveal any significant difference between groups. In addition, BDNF expression in subjects with high methylation levels was significantly lower than in subjects with low and medium methylation levels, supporting the repressive effects of methylation within promoter on transcription.

Finally, following the studies in mice reported by Tsankova and colleagues (2006) and discussed above, our group provided evidence suggesting that antidepressants promote open chromatin structure (i.e., lower H3K27me3 level) in the promoter of BDNF in the PFC (Chen et al., 2011). Follow-up studies in depressed patients also revealed higher BDNF IV non-coding exon expression in the blood of citalopram treatment responders compared to non-responders (Lopez et al., 2013). Interestingly, H3K27me3 levels were inversely correlated with both BDNF IV expression levels and with the severity of symptoms.

The tropomyosin-related kinase B (TrkB) receptor gene

The trans-membrane TrkB is the receptor for BDNF and has long been investigated in the neurobiology of mood and related disorders (Duman & Monteggia,

2006; Kim et al., 2007; Dwivedi et al., 2003; 2009). Expression microarray studies have reported lower TrkB expression in the prefrontal cortex of depressed subjects (Aston et al., 2005; Nakatani et al., 2006) and antidepressant treatment has been shown to increase its expression in cultured astrocytes (Mercier et al., 2004).

The TrkB gene is found on chromosome 9 at locus q22.1 and has five splice variants. Splice variant T1 or TrkB-T1 is an astrocytic truncated form of TrkB lacking catalytic activity (Rose et al., 2003). Recently, analysis of the methylation pattern in the promoter of a subset of suicide completers with low levels of TrkB-T1 expression revealed two sites where methylation levels were higher in suicide completers compared to controls (Ernst et al., 2009b). The methylation pattern at those two sites was negatively correlated with the expression of TrkB-T1 in suicide completers, and this effect was specific to the prefrontal cortex, since no significant difference was found in the cerebellum. Such a pattern of expression and methylation are thought to increase predispositions to suicidal behaviors. In addition, suicide completers with low TrkB-T1 expression showed enrichment of H3K27 methylation in the TrkB promoter (Ernst et al., 2009a), suggesting that the astrocytic variant of TrkB may be under the control of epigenetic mechanisms involving histone modifications and DNA methylation. Interestingly, recent data showed that mice overexpressing the TrkB-T1 variant are more susceptible to chronic social stress than wild type mice by exhibiting consistent social avoidance (Razzoli et al., 2011). Together, these data suggest that epigenetic changes in TrkB-T1 promoter inducing expression changes could define the vulnerability to chronic social stress and possibly to early life adverse experience.

The GABAergic system

The GABAergic system has been the focus of many research studies in postmortem brain samples of psychiatric patients, and particularly individuals with histories of depression (Klempan et al., 2009; Merali et al., 2004; Torrey et al., 2005), schizophrenia, or bipolar disorder, many of which died by suicide (Guidotti et al., 2000; Heckers et al., 2002; Volk et al., 2000). For instance, reductions of reelin and GAD1 (glutamate decarboxylase 1) mRNA (Guidotti et al., 2000) and an increase in DNMT1 expression (Veldic et al., 2004; Kundakovic et al., 2007) were previously reported in postmortem brains of schizophrenia and bipolar subjects who died by suicide. Consistently, promoter hypermethylation was reported for both genes in accordance with the methylating role of DNMT1 (Grayson et al., 2005; Tamura et al., 2007).

More recently, the hippocampal expression of GAD1 has been shown to be affected by maternal care in rats (Zhang et al., 2010). Indeed, pups raised by mothers providing poor maternal care characterized by low amounts of LG, have lower GAD1 hippocampal expression associated with promoter hypermethylation and lower levels of H3K9ac compared to pups raised by mothers providing high levels of maternal care. Interestingly, this is also associated with higher DNMT1 hippocampal levels. Functional assays revealed that the transcription factor NGFI-A binds the GAD1 promoter in order to increase GAD1 expression. Consequently, these results suggest that similarly to the regulation of GR in rat hippocampus, GAD1 expression is modulated by maternal behavior via epigenetic mechanisms involving DNA methylation interfering with the binding of activating transcription factors and by chromatin modifications (Zhang et al., 2010).

These findings are in accordance with the study of Poulter and colleagues (Poulter et al., 2008) that examined the expression of DNA methyltransferases as well as $GABA_A$ receptor α1 subunit in the brain of suicide completers. Three hypermethylated CpG sites within α1 subunit promoter were identified in the prefrontal cortex of suicide completers and negatively correlated with DNMT3b protein expression. Besides DNMT3b, DNMT1 and DNMT3a levels have also been reported to be altered in the limbic system and brainstem of suicide completers. However, in this study there was no report of histories of early life adversity, and thus, one cannot assume that these effects would be similar in abused suicide completers.

Other epigenetic alterations in suicide brains

In light of what was discussed above, early life adversity seems to modify epigenetic control of gene expression. These changes can take place through histone modifications and/or DNA methylation. Moreover, epigenetic changes correlate with behavioral modifications in animals and humans, thus strongly suggesting that epigenetics may act as an interface mediating the effect of environment on the genome.

In addition to the findings discussed above, studies have focused on other functional systems, which had been implicated in depression and suicide. Among these systems, the polyamine and the serotonergic systems are noteworthy.

Polyamines are ubiquitous aliphatic molecules involved in cellular functions including growth, division, and signaling cascades (Gilad & Gilad, 2003; Minguet et al., 2008). The polyamines also play a major role in the regulation of stress (Rhee et al., 2007; Fiori & Turecki, 2008), being dependent on the activation of the HPA axis and the increased concentrations in circulating glucocorticoids (Gilad & Gilad, 2003). Furthermore, the emergence of the characteristic adult polyamine stress response correlates with the cessation of the hyporesponsive period of the HPA axis system (Gilad et al., 1998). Previously, spermine synthase (SMS), spermidine/spermine N1-acetyltransferase (SAT1), and ornithine aminotransferase-like 1 (OATL1) expression have been shown to be altered in the limbic system of suicide completers with a history of depressive disorders (Sequeira et al., 2006, 2007). However, follow-up studies revealed that epigenetic alterations in the promoter region of genes involved in the polyamine synthesis do not account for these changes in expression. Up to date, significant findings explain the negative correlation existing between SAT1 expression and promoter methylation levels in BA 8/9 (Fiori et al., unpublished results). More recently, site-specific differential methylation has been found in the promoter of ARG2 and AMD1 (Gross et al., 2012) that was inversely correlated with expression in BA 44.

The serotonergic system is a neurotransmitter system of great importance in psychiatry and has been extensively investigated in depression and suicide. Lower concentration, binding, neurotransmission, and reuptake of serotonin and its metabolites are risk markers for suicidality and major depression (Cronholm et al., 1977; Bhagwagar & Cowen, 2008). Among the various serotonergic receptors, particular attention has been given to the 5-HT_{2A} and its gene, as an important candidate in association studies of suicidal behavior (Du et al., 2001: Turecki et al., 1999). One of the variants most commonly investigated was the 102 C/T polymorphism, located in exon 1 (Du et al., 2000; De Luca et al., 2007). Methylation in the C-allele variant in this polymorphism has previously been associated with higher DNMT1 expression in the brain and leukocytes of healthy subjects (Polesskaya et al., 2006). Although methylation was reported as increased in leukocytes from suicide ideators, a non-significant hypomethylation was reported in the prefrontal cortex of suicide completers carrying the C-allele (De Luca et al., 2009), suggesting that methylation levels may be different in individuals who committed suicide and those who are planning suicide. On the other hand, the functional significance of this hypermethylation in leukocytes remains to be explored, and since significance levels were not reached in brain tissue, further research is required.

Genome-wide DNA methylation alteration by early life stress

Overall, environmental factors seem to target the epigenetic regulation of genes involved in key regulatory processes such as the HPA axis, neurotrophic factors, neurotransmission, polyamines, and protein synthesis. However, while a growing body of evidence supports the contribution of epigenetic factors translating the effects of ELA on the human genome, there is a real need for large-scale comprehensive studies assessing genome-wide epigenetic patterns in the context of different environmental factors. A few of these studies recently reported interesting findings suggesting that child abuse, while targeting critical genes, may also induce genome-wide reprograming of DNA methylation patterns.

Our group recently assessed the impact of child abuse on genome-wide DNA methylation signature in gene promoters (Labonté et al., 2012a). In this study, we compared hippocampal DNA methylation patterns between suicide completers with a severe history of child abuse (sexual and/or physical) and healthy controls. We identified hundreds of sites differentially methylated, both hyper- and hypomethylated, in the hippocampus of severely abused suicide completers. Interestingly, DNA methylation levels in gene promoters were inversely correlated with gene expression at the genome-wide level, and differential methylation in abused suicides were enriched in genes involved in neuroplasticity, a finding consistent with the notion that abuse experiences during childhood lead to plastic changes in the brain as a response to these negative environmental stimuli. Similar observations have been made in suicide completers (Labonté et al., 2013) who present methylation enriched in genes related to learning and memory and in peripheral samples from PTSD patients (Uddin et al., 2010). However, Uddin and colleagues did not restrict their analysis to promoters but rather measured DNA methylation levels at 14 thousand CpGs across the genome. The analysis revealed an overrepresentation of differentially methylated CpGs in genes related to immune function. This may be translated into the development of different psychopathological processes. Furthermore, a previous study performed in the PFC of psychotic and bipolar patients reported differential methylation in numerous sites that were involved in glutamatergic and GABAergic neurotransmission, brain development, and response to stress (Mill et al., 2008). More importantly, these studies were conducted in different tissues (blood versus brain) and different brain regions (HPC versus PFC), which may account for the discrepancies between studies, as different tissues (Ladd-Acosta et al., 2007) and cell types (Deaton et al., 2011; Iwamoto et al., 2011) have been shown to exhibit specific DNA methylation signatures.

Conclusion

In light of what has been discussed, there is growing evidence suggesting that early life adversity affects molecular mechanisms involved in the regulation of behavior. These effects involve alterations in DNA methylation and histone modifications, which are believed to induce behavioral aberrations during development or later in life by affecting genes involved in crucial neuronal processes. Studies performed in postmortem brains from suicide completers with a history of childhood abuse highlighted several environmentally induced epigenetic alterations in the regulatory regions of genes involved in the response to stress. Similarly, investigating the effect of variation in early life environment in animals has revealed useful information to expand our understanding of the molecular mechanisms involved in the effect of environmental stressors on the regulation of behavior. Together, these findings suggest that epigenetics may act as a mechanism whereby environmental factors act on the long-term modulation of behavioral responses. In individuals with particular predispositions toward psychiatric disorders, these alterations may help trigger the expression of the illness. From a therapeutic point of view, it is tempting to speculate on the clinical potential these findings may provide. In the future, they could potentially lead to the development of tools for the identification of individuals at risk, and therefore, the possibility of preventive intervention. However, there are major challenges in their potential implementation, not the least of which is access to target tissue in living subjects, modification of epigenetic profiles, and appropriate delivery of such interventions. Given that this is a relatively new area of research, the current knowledge is significantly limited. Integrating genome-wide approaches will provide a more comprehensive view on the complexity of the relationship between early life adversity and the psychopathology of brain disorders. Furthermore, since these studies can provide information on the molecular nature of stress-induced psychopathologies, future work should assess whether similar alterations can be found in more accessible tissue.

Table 32.1. Summary of published studies assessing epigenetic components in suicide

Studies	Brain regions	Genes	Findings
Labonté et al., 2013	Hippocampus	Genome-wide	Genome-wide changes in DNA methylation levels in the suicide completers. Inverse correlation between genome-wide DNA methylation and gene expression levels. Enrichment of DNA methylation alterations in genes involved in learning and memory processes
Labonté et al., 2012	Hippocampus	Genome-wide	Genome-wide changes in DNA methylation levels in the abused suicide completers. Inverse correlation between genome-wide DNA methylation and gene expression levels. Enrichment of DNA methylation alterations in genes involved in cellular plasticity
Labonté et al., 2012	Hippocampus	GR	DNA methylation alterations in GR1B and 1C promoters in the suicide completers with history of abuse. ↓ methylation in GR 1H promoter in the suicide completers with history of abuse. ↓ Expression of GR 1B, 1C, and 1H in the suicide completers with history of abuse Inverse correlation between DNA methylation and expression levels of 1C and positive correlation for 1H

Table 32.1. (cont.)

Studies	Brain regions	Genes	Findings
Lopez et al., 2013	Blood	BDNF	↑ BDNF IV expression in responders to citalopram treatment compared to non-responders Inverse correlation between H3K27me3 and BDNF IV expression levels Inverse correlation between H3K27me3 levels and the severity of symptoms
Chen et al., 2011	PFC	BDNF	↓ H3K27me3 levels in promoter IV in suicide completers
McGowan et al., 2009	Hippocampus	GR	↑ Methylation in NGFI-A binding site within GR promoter in the hippocampus of suicide completers with history of abuse ↓ Expression of GR in the hippocampus of suicide completers with history of abuse
Alt et al., 2010	Amygdala Hippocampus Inf frontal gyrus Cingulate gyrus Nucleus accumbens	GR	Amy: ↓GRα protein, ↑ expression of 1J, ↓ YY1 transcription factor HPC: ↓ expression of GR1F and 1C, ↓ NGFI-A transcription factor IFG: ↓GRβ protein, ↓ YY1 and Sp1 transcription factors CG: ↓GRα protein, ↑ expression of 1D, ↓ YY1, NGFI-A and Sp1 transcription factors NaC: ↓ expression of GR1B, ↓ NGFI-A transcription factor No methylation difference in promoters
McGowan et al., 2008	Hippocampus	rRNA	Overall hypermethylation of rRNA promoter in the hippocampus of suicide completers with history of abuse ↓ expression of rRNA gene in the hippocampus of suicide completers with history of abuse
Keller et al., 2010	Wernicke area	BDNF	Hypermethylation at 4 CpGs within promoter/exon IV in suicide completers Negative correlation between BDNF promoter methylation levels and expression
Ernst et al., 2009	Frontal cortex	TrkB-T1	↑ methylation in two sites within the promoter of TrkB-T1 in the frontal cortex of suicide completers ↓ Expression of TrkB-T1 in the frontal cortex of suicide completers
Ernst et al., 2009	Frontal cortex	TrkB-T1	↑ H3K27 methylation in the frontal cortex of suicide completers Negative correlation between H3K27 methylation levels and TrkB-T1 expression in the frontal cortex of suicide completers
Poulter et al., 2008	Fronto-polar cortex (FPC) Hippocampus Amygdala Brainstem	$GABA_A$ α1 DNMT1 DNMT3a DNMT3b	FPC: ↓ expression of DNMT1 mRNA in suicide completers ↑ expression of DNMT3b mRNA and protein levels in suicide completers ↑ increased methylation at two sites in the promoter region of GABAA receptor subunit α1 in suicide completers Limbic system: ↓ expression of DNMT1 and DNMT3b mRNA levels in suicide completers Brainstem: ↓ expression of DNMT3b mRNA in suicide completers
Fiori and Turecki, 2008	PFC	SMOX, SMS	No effects of promoter's methylation in SMOX and SMS on expression levels
De Luca et al., 2009	PFC	5-HT2A	↓ methylation in the promoter region of 5-HT2A receptor associated with a C-allele (trend) in the suicide completers ↑ methylation in the promoter region of 5-HT2A receptor associated with a C-allele in leukocytes of suicide attempters

Table 32.2. Summary of published studies assessing epigenetic components in animal models of stress-induced depressive symptoms

Studies	Animal model	Brain regions	Genes	Findings
Weaver et al., 2004	Low/high licking and grooming	Hippocampus	GR	In pups raised by LG mothers Overall $GR1_7$ promoter hypermethylation ↓ H3K9 acetylation in GR 1_7 promoter ↓ binding of NGFI-A in $GR1_7$ promoter
Tsankova et al., 2006	Intruder test	Hippocampus	BDNF	In stressed mice ↓ expression of transcript III and IV ↑ H3K27dimethylation in transcript III and IV promoter No DNA methylation difference

Table 32.2. (cont.)

Studies	Animal model	Brain regions	Genes	Findings
				Chronic treatment with imipramine ↑ H3 acetylation and H3K4 dimathylationin transcript III and IV promoter ↓ HDAC5 in hippocampus of stressed mice
Roth et al., 2009	Stressed mothers	Prefrontal cortex	BDNF	In maltreated rats ↓ expression of BDNF transcript IX from childhood to adulthood ↓ expression of BDNF transcript IV at adulthood Overall hypermethylation in transcript IV promoter Transgenerational DNA methylation alterations in pups raised by abusive mothers
Roth et al., 2011	PTSD animal model	Hippocampus Basolateral Amygdala Prefrontal cortext	BDNF	In stressed rats Dorsal hippocampus ↓expression of BDNF transcript IV ↑ methylation in dentate gyrus ↑ methylation in CA1 Ventral hippocampus ↓expression of BDNF transcript IV ↓ methylation in CA3 Basolateral amygdala No change in methylation pattern in transcript IV Prefrontal cortex No change in methylation pattern in transcript IV
Murgatroyd et al., 2009	Maternal deprivation	Hypothalamic paraventricular nucleus	AVP	In stressed mice ↑ expression of AVP Site-specific hypomethylation in AVP intergenic region Phosphorylation of meCP2
Elliott et al., 2010	Intruder test	PVN	CRF	In stressed mice ↑ expression of CRF ↓ methylation in CRF promoter (CRE) ↓ expression of DNMT3b (acute), HDAC2 (long term) ↑ gadd45 (acute) In resilient mice No differential CRF expression No differential methylation Chronic treatment with imipramine Regulate behavior Regulate CRF expression Regulate CRF promoter methylation
Zhang et al., 2010	Low/high licking and grooming	Hippocampus	GAD1	In pups raised by low LG mothers ↓ expression of GAD1 ↑ methylation within GAD1 promoter ↑ expression of DNMT1 ↓ H3K9 acetylation in GAD1 promoter

References

Agid, O., Shapira, B., Zislin, J., et al. (1999). Environment and vulnerability to major psychiatric illness: a case control study of early parental loss in major depression, bipolar disorder and schizophrenia. *Molecular Psychiatry*, **4**, 163–172.

Aguilera, G., Kiss, A., Liu, Y., & Kamitakahara, A. (2007). Negative regulation of corticotropin-releasing factor expression and limitation of stress response. *Stress*, **10**, 153–161.

Aid, T., Kazantseva, A., Piirsoo, M., Palm, K., & Timmusk, T. (2007). Mouse and rat BDNF gene structure and expression revisited. *Journal of Neuroscience Research*, **85**, 525–535.

Alt, S. R., Turner, J. D., Klok, M. D., et al. (2010). Differential expression of glucocorticoid receptor transcripts in major depressive disorder is not epigenetically programmed. *Psychoneuroendocrinology*, **35**, 544–556.

Andersen, S. L., Tomada, A., Vincow, E. S., et al. (2008). Preliminary evidence for sensitive periods in the effect of childhood sexual abuse on regional brain development. *Journal of Neuropsychiatry and Clinical Neuroscience*, **20**, 292–301.

Aston, C., Jiang, L., & Sokolov, B. P. (2005). Transcriptional profiling reveals evidence for signaling and oligodendroglial abnormalities in the temporal cortex from patients with major depressive disorder. *Molecular Psychiatry*, **10**, 309–322.

Bannister, A. J., Zegerman, P., Partridge, J. F., et al. (2001). Selective recognition of methylated lysine 9 on histone H3 by the HP1 chromo domain. *Nature*, **410**, 120–124.

Barrera, L. O., Li, Z., Smith, A. D., et al. (2008). Genome-wide mapping and analysis of active promoters in mouse embryonic stem cells and adult organs. *Genome Research*, **18**, 46–59.

Barski, A., Cuddapah, S., Cui, K., et al. (2007). High-resolution profiling of histone methylations in the human genome. *Cell*, **129**, 823–837.

Bensley, L. S., Van Eenwyk, J., Spieker, S. J., & Schoder, J. (1999). Self-reported abuse history and adolescent problem behaviors. I. Antisocial and suicidal behaviors. *Journal of Adolescent Health*, **24**, 163–172.

Bhagwagar, Z. & Cowen, P. J. (2008). 'It's not over when it's over': persistent neurobiological abnormalities in recovered depressed patients. *Psychological Medicine*, **38**, 307–313.

Botuyan, M. V., Lee, J., Ward, I. M., et al. (2006). Structural basis for the methylation state-specific recognition of histone H4-K20 by 53BP1 and Crb2 in DNA repair. *Cell*, **127**, 1361–1373.

Bremner, J. D., Randall, P., Vermetten, E., et al. (1997). Magnetic resonance imaging-based measurement of hippocampal volume in posttraumatic stress disorder related to childhood physical and sexual abuse – a preliminary report. *Biological Psychiatry*, **41**, 23–32.

Bremner, J. D., Vythilingam, M., Vermetten, E., et al. (2003). MRI and PET study of deficits in hippocampal structure and function in women with childhood sexual abuse and posttraumatic stress disorder. *American Journal of Psychiatry*, **160**, 924–932.

Briere, J., & Elliott, D. M. (2003). Prevalence and psychological sequelae of self-reported childhood physical and sexual abuse in a general population sample of men and women. *Child Abuse and Neglect*, **27**, 1205–1222.

Brown, G. W., & Moran, P. (1994). Clinical and psychosocial origins of chronic depressive episodes. I: A community survey. *British Journal of Psychiatry*, **165**, 447–456.

Brunoni, A. R., Lopes, M., & Fregni, F. (2008). A systematic review and meta-analysis of clinical studies on major depression and BDNF levels: implications for the role of neuroplasticity in depression. *International Journal of Neuropsychopharmacology*, **11**, 1169–1180.

Carpenter, L. L., Tyrka, A. R., McDougle, C. J., et al. (2004). Cerebrospinal fluid corticotropin-releasing factor and perceived early life stress in depressed patients and healthy control subjects. *Neuropsychopharmacology*, **29**, 777–784.

Carrion, V. G., Weems, C. F., Eliez, S., et al. (2001). Attenuation of frontal asymmetry in pediatric posttraumatic stress disorder. *Biological Psychiatry*, **50**, 943–951.

Chan, J. P., Unger, T. J., Byrnes, J., & Rios, M. (2006). Examination of behavioral deficits triggered by targeting Bdnf in fetal or postnatal brains of mice. *Neuroscience*, **142**, 49–58.

Chen, B., Dowlatshahi, D., MacQueen, G. M., Wang, J. F., & Young, L. T. (2001). Increased hippocampal BDNF immunoreactivity in subjects treated with antidepressant medication. *Biological Psychiatry*, **50**, 260–265.

Chen, E. S., Ernst, C., & Turecki, G. (2011). The epigenetic effects of antidepressant treatment on human prefrontal cortex BDNF expression. *International Journal of Neuropsychopharmacology*, **14**, 427–429.

Chen, W. G., Chang, Q., Lin, Y., et al. (2003). Derepression of BDNF transcription involves calcium-dependent phosphorylation of MeCP2. *Science*, **302**, 885–889.

Children's Bureau. (2010). Child maltreatment 2009. In *US Department of Health and Human Services, A. O. C., Youth and Families* (Ed.). Washington DC: Government Printing Office.

Clements, A., Poux, A. N., Lo, W. S., et al. (2003). Structural basis for histone and phosphohistone binding by the GCN5 histone acetyltransferase. *Molecular Cell*, **12**, 461–473.

Cronholm, B., Asberg, M., Montgomery, S., & Schalling, D. (1977). Suicidal behaviour syndrome with low CSF 5-HIAA. *British Medical Journal*, **1**, 776.

De Bellis, M. D., Keshavan, M. S., Frustaci, K., et al. (2002). Superior temporal gyrus volumes in maltreated children and adolescents with PTSD. *Biological Psychiatry*, **51**, 544–552.

De Luca, V., Likhodi, O., Kennedy, J. L., & Wong, A. H. (2007). Differential expression and parent-of-origin effect of the 5-HT2A receptor gene C102T polymorphism: analysis of suicidality in schizophrenia and bipolar disorder. *American Journal of Medical Genetics B Neuropsychiatric Genetics*, **144B**, 370–374.

De Luca, V., Viggiano, E., Dhoot, R., Kennedy, J. L., & Wong, A. H. (2009). Methylation and QTDT analysis of the 5-HT2A receptor 102C allele: analysis of suicidality in major psychosis. *Journal of Psychiatric Research*, **43**, 532–537.

Deaton, A. M., Webb, S., Kerr, A. R., et al. (2011). Cell type-specific DNA methylation at intragenic CpG islands in the immune system. *Genome Research*, **21**, 1074–1086.

Dinwiddie, S., Heath, A. C., Dunne, M. P., et al. (2000). Early sexual abuse and lifetime psychopathology: a co-twin-control study. *Psychological Medicine*, **30**, 41–52.

Driessen, M., Herrmann, J., Stahl, K., et al. (2000). Magnetic resonance imaging volumes of the hippocampus and the amygdala in women with borderline personality disorder and early traumatization. *Archives of General Psychiatry*, **57**, 1115–1122.

Du, L., Bakish, D., Lapierre, Y. D., Ravindran, A. V., & Hrdina, P. D. (2000). Association of polymorphism of serotonin 2A receptor gene with suicidal ideation in major depressive disorder. *American Journal of Medical Genetics*, **96**, 56–60.

Du, L., Faludi, G., Palkovits, M., Bakish, D., & Hrdina, P. D. (2001). Serotonergic genes and suicidality. *Crisis*, **22**, 54–60.

Duman, R. S., & Monteggia, L. M. (2006). A neurotrophic model for stress-related mood disorders. *Biological Psychiatry*, **59**, 1116–1127.

Duric, V., & McCarson, K. E. (2005). Hippocampal neurokinin-1 receptor and brain-derived neurotrophic factor gene expression is decreased in rat models of pain and stress. *Neuroscience*, **133**, 999–1006.

Duric, V., & McCarson, K. E. (2006). Effects of analgesic or antidepressant drugs on pain- or stress-evoked hippocampal and spinal neurokinin-1 receptor and brain-derived neurotrophic factor gene expression in the rat. *Journal of Pharmacology and Experimental Therapeutics*, **319**, 1235–1243.

Dwivedi, Y., Rizavi, H. S., Conley, R. R., et al. (2003). Altered gene expression of brain-derived neurotrophic factor and receptor tyrosine kinase B in postmortem brain of suicide subjects. *Archives of General Psychiatry*, **60**, 804–815.

Dwivedi, Y., Rizavi, H. S., Zhang, H., et al. (2009). Neurotrophin receptor activation and expression in human postmortem brain: effect of suicide. *Biological Psychiatry*, **65**, 319–328.

Elliott, E., Ezra-Nevo, G., Regev, L., Neufeld-Cohen, A., & Chen, A. (2010). Resilience to social stress coincides with functional DNA methylation of the Crf gene in adult mice. *Nature Neuroscience*, **13**, 1351–1353.

Ernst, C., Chen, E. S., & Turecki, G. (2009a). Histone methylation and decreased expression of TrkB.T1 in orbital frontal cortex of suicide completers. *Molecular Psychiatry*, **14**, 830–832.

Ernst, C., Deleva, V., Deng, X., et al. (2009b). Alternative splicing, methylation state, and expression profile of tropomyosin-related kinase B in the frontal cortex of suicide completers. *Archives of General Psychiatry*, **66**, 22–32.

Evans, E., Hawton, K., & Rodham, K. (2005). Suicidal phenomena and abuse in adolescents: a review of epidemiological studies. *Child Abuse and Neglect*, **29**, 45–58.

Fergusson, D. M., Horwood, L. J., & Lynskey, M. T. (1996). Childhood sexual abuse and psychiatric disorder in young adulthood: II. Psychiatric outcomes of childhood sexual abuse. *Journal of the American Academy of Child and Adolescent Psychiatry*, **35**, 1365–74.

Fiori, L. M., & Turecki, G. (2008). Implication of the polyamine system in mental disorders. *Journal of Psychiatry and Neuroscience*, **33**, 102–110.

Fischle, W., Tseng, B. S., Dormann, H. L., et al. (2005). Regulation of HP1-chromatin binding by histone H3 methylation and phosphorylation. *Nature*, **438**, 1116–1122.

Francis, D., Diorio, J., Liu, D., & Meaney, M. J. (1999). Nongenomic transmission across generations of maternal behavior and stress responses in the rat. *Science*, **286**, 1155–1158.

Gainer, H., Fields, R. L., & House, S. B. (2001). Vasopressin gene expression: experimental models and strategies. *Experimental Neurology*, **171**, 190–199.

Gilad, G. M., & Gilad, V. H. (2003). Overview of the brain polyamine-stress-response: regulation, development, and modulation by lithium and role in cell survival. *Cellular and Molecular Neurobiology*, **23**, 637–649.

Gilad, G. M., Gilad, V. H., Eliyayev, Y., & Rabey, J. M. (1998). Developmental regulation of the brain polyamine-stress-response. *International Journal of Developmental Neuroscience*, **16**, 271–8.

Gladstone, G. L., Parker, G. B., Mitchell, P. B., et al. (2004). Implications of childhood trauma for depressed women: an analysis of pathways from childhood sexual abuse to deliberate self-harm and revictimization. *American Journal of Psychiatry*, **161**, 1417–1425.

Gorey, K. M., & Leslie, D. R. (1997). The prevalence of child sexual abuse: integrative review adjustment for potential response and measurement biases. *Child Abuse and Neglect*, **21**, 391–398.

Grayson, D. R., Jia, X., Chen, Y., et al. (2005). Reelin promoter hypermethylation in schizophrenia. *Proceedings of the National Academy of Sciences USA*, **102**, 9341–9346.

Gronli, J., Bramham, C., Murison, R., et al. (2006). Chronic mild stress inhibits BDNF protein expression and CREB activation in the dentate gyrus but not in the hippocampus proper. *Pharmacology, Biochemistry and Behavior*, **85**, 842–849.

Gross, J. A., Fiori, L. M., Labonté, B., Lopez, J. P., & Turecki, G. (2012). Effects of promoter methylation on increased expression of polyamine biosynthetic genes in suicide. *Journal of Psychiatric Research*, **47**(4), 513–519.

Guidotti, A., Auta, J., Davis, J. M., et al. (2000). Decrease in reelin and glutamic acid decarboxylase67 (GAD67) expression in schizophrenia and bipolar disorder: a postmortem brain study. *Archives of General Psychiatry*, **57**, 1061–1069.

Hata, K., Okano, M., Lei, H., & Li, E. (2002). Dnmt3L cooperates with the Dnmt3 family of de novo DNA methyltransferases to establish maternal imprints in mice. *Development*, **129**, 1983–1993.

He, L., & Hannon, G. J. (2004). MicroRNAs: small RNAs with a big role in gene regulation. *Nature Reviews Genetics*, **5**, 522–531.

Heckers, S., Stone, D., Walsh, J., et al. (2002). Differential hippocampal expression of glutamic acid decarboxylase 65 and 67 messenger RNA in bipolar disorder and schizophrenia. *Archives of General Psychiatry*, **59**, 521–529.

Heim, C., & Nemeroff, C. B. (2001). The role of childhood trauma in the neurobiology of mood and anxiety disorders: preclinical and clinical studies. *Biological Psychiatry*, **49**, 1023–1039.

Heim, C., Newport, D. J., Heit, S., et al. (2000). Pituitary-adrenal and autonomic responses to stress in women after sexual and physical abuse in childhood. *JAMA*, **284**, 592–597.

Heim, C., Mletzko, T., Purselle, D., Musselman, D. L., & Nemeroff, C. B. (2008a). The dexamethasone/corticotropin-releasing factor test in men with major depression: role of childhood trauma. *Biological Psychiatry*, **63**, 398–405.

Heim, C., Newport, D. J., Mletzko, T., Miller, A. H., & Nemeroff, C. B. (2008b). The link between childhood trauma and depression: insights from HPA axis studies in humans. *Psychoneuroendocrinology*, **33**, 693–710.

Heim, C., Young, L. J., Newport, D. J., et al. (2009). Lower CSF oxytocin concentrations in women with a history of childhood abuse. *Molecular Psychiatry*, **14**, 954–958.

Heim, C., Shugart, M., Craighead, W. E., & Nemeroff, C. B. (2010). Neurobiological and psychiatric consequences of child abuse and neglect. *Developmental Psychobiology*, **52**, 671–90.

Ito, S., D'Alessio, A. C., Taranova, O. V., et al. (2010). Role of Tet proteins in 5mC to 5hmC conversion, ES-cell self-renewal and inner cell mass specification. *Nature*, **466**, 1129–1133.

Iwamoto, K., Bundo, M., Ueda, J., et al. (2011). Neurons show distinctive DNA methylation profile and higher interindividual variations compared with non-neurons. *Genome Research*, **21**, 688–696.

Jaffee, S. R., Moffitt, T. E., Caspi, A., et al. (2002). Differences in early childhood risk factors for juvenile-onset and adult-onset depression. *Archives of General Psychiatry*, **59**, 215–222.

Kaplan, M. J., & Klinetob, N. A. (2000). Childhood emotional trauma and chronic posttraumatic stress disorder in adult outpatients with treatment-resistant depression. *Journal of Nervous and Mental Disease*, **188**, 596–601.

Keller, S., Sarchiapone, M., Zarrilli, F., et al. (2010). Increased BDNF promoter methylation in the Wernicke area of suicide subjects. *Archives of General Psychiatry*, **67**, 258–267.

Kendler, K. S., Bulik, C. M., Silberg, J., et al. (2000). Childhood sexual abuse and adult psychiatric and substance use disorders in women: an epidemiological and cotwin control analysis. *Archives of General Psychiatry*, **57**, 953–959.

Kendler, K. S., Kuhn, J. W., & Prescott, C. A. (2004). Childhood sexual abuse, stressful life events and risk for major depression in women. *Psychological Medicine*, **34**, 1475–1482.

Kim, Y. K., Lee, H. P., Won, S. D., et al. (2007). Low plasma BDNF is associated with suicidal behavior in major depression. *Progress in Neuro-Psychopharmacology & Biological Psychiatry*, **31**, 78–85.

Kirmizis, A., Santos-Rosa, H., Penkett, C. J., et al. (2007). Arginine methylation at histone H3R2 controls deposition of H3K4 trimethylation. *Nature*, **449**, 928–932.

Klempan, T. A., Sequeira, A., Canetti, L., et al. (2009). Altered expression of genes involved in ATP biosynthesis and GABAergic neurotransmission in the ventral prefrontal cortex of suicides with and without major depression. *Molecular Psychiatry*, **14**, 175–189.

Klose, R. J., & Bird, A. P. (2006). Genomic DNA methylation: the mark and its mediators. *Trends in Biochemical Sciences*, **31**, 89–97.

Kouzarides, T. (2007). Chromatin modifications and their function. *Cell*, **128**, 693–705.

Kriaucionis, S., & Heintz, N. (2009). The nuclear DNA base 5-hydroxymethylcytosine is present in Purkinje neurons and the brain. *Science*, **324**, 929–930.

Kundakovic, M., Chen, Y., Costa, E., & Grayson, D. R. (2007). DNA methyltransferase inhibitors coordinately induce expression of the human reelin and glutamic acid decarboxylase 67 genes. *Molecular Pharmacology*, **71**, 644–653.

Labonté, B., Suderman, M., Maussion, G., et al. (2012a). Genome-wide epigenetic regulation by early life trauma. *Archives of General Psychiatry*, **69**, 722–731.

Labonté, B., Yerko, V., Gross, J., et al. (2012b). Differential glucocorticoid receptor exon 1(B), 1(C), and 1(H) expression and methylation in suicide completers with a history of childhood abuse. *Biological Psychiatry*, **72**, 41–48.

Labonté, B., Suderman, M., Maussion, G., et al. (2013). Genome-wide methylation changes in the suicide brain. *American Journal of Psychiatry*, **170**, 511–520.

Ladd-Acosta, C., Pevsner, J., Sabunciyan, S., et al. (2007). DNA methylation signatures within the human brain. *American Journal of Human Genetics*, **81**, 1304–1315.

Lan, F., Bayliss, P. E., Rinn, J. L., et al. (2007). A histone H3 lysine 27 demethylase regulates animal posterior development. *Nature*, **449**, 689–694.

Laplante, P., Diorio, J. & Meaney, M. J. (2002). Serotonin regulates hippocampal glucocorticoid receptor expression via a 5-HT7 receptor. *Brain Research: Developmental Brain Research*, **139**, 199–203.

Liu, D., Diorio, J., Tannenbaum, B., et al. (1997). Maternal care, hippocampal glucocorticoid receptors, and hypothalamic-pituitary-adrenal responses to stress. *Science*, **277**, 1659–1662.

Lopez, J. P., Mamdani, F., Labonté, B., et al. (2013). Epigenetic regulation of BDNF expression according to antidepressant response. *Molecular Psychiatry*, **18**, 398–399.

Matrisciano, F., Bonaccorso, S., Ricciardi, A., et al. (2009). Changes in BDNF serum levels in patients with major depression disorder (MDD) after 6 months treatment with sertraline, escitalopram, or venlafaxine. *Journal of Psychiatric Research*, **43**, 247–254.

Maunakea, A. K., Nagarajan, R. P., Bilenky, M., et al. (2010). Conserved role of intragenic DNA methylation in regulating alternative promoters. *Nature*, **466**, 253–257.

McCauley, J., Kern, D. E., Kolodner, K., et al. (1997). Clinical characteristics of women with a history of childhood abuse: unhealed wounds. *JAMA*, **277**, 1362–1368.

McCormick, J. A., Lyons, V., Jacobson, M. D., et al. (2000). 5'-heterogeneity of glucocorticoid receptor messenger RNA is tissue specific: differential regulation of variant transcripts by early life events. *Molecular Endocrinology*, **14**, 506–517.

McGowan, P. O., Sasaki, A., Huang, T. C., et al. (2008). Promoter-wide hypermethylation of the ribosomal RNA gene promoter in the suicide brain. *PLoS One*, **3**, e2085.

McGowan, P. O., Sasaki, A., D'Alessio, A. C., et al. (2009). Epigenetic regulation of the glucocorticoid receptor in human brain associates with childhood abuse. *Nature Neuroscience*, **12**, 342–348.

McGowan, P. O., Suderman, M., Sasaki, A., et al. (2011). Broad epigenetic signature of maternal care in the brain of adult rats. *PLoS One*, **6**, e14739.

Meaney, M. J. (2001). Maternal care, gene expression, and the transmission of individual differences in stress reactivity across generations. *Annual Review of Neuroscience*, **24**, 1161–1192.

Meaney, M. J., Aitken, D. H. & Sapolsky, R. M. (1987). Thyroid hormones influence the development of hippocampal glucocorticoid receptors in the rat: a mechanism for the effects of postnatal handling on the development of the adrenocortical stress response. *Neuroendocrinology*, **45**, 278–283.

Meaney, M. J., Diorio, J., Francis, D., et al. (2000). Postnatal handling increases the expression of cAMP-inducible transcription factors in the rat hippocampus: the effects of thyroid hormones and serotonin. *Journal of Neuroscience*, **20**, 3926–3935.

Mellen, M., Ayata, P., Dewell, S., Kriaucionis, S., & Heintz, N. (2012). MeCP2 binds to 5hmC enriched within active genes and accessible chromatin in the nervous system. *Cell*, **151**, 1417–1430.

Merali, Z., Du, L., Hrdina, P., et al. (2004). Dysregulation in the suicide brain: mRNA expression of corticotropin-releasing hormone receptors and GABA(A) receptor subunits in frontal cortical brain region. *Journal of Neuroscience*, **24**, 1478–1485.

Mercier, G., Lennon, A. M., Renouf, B., et al. (2004). MAP kinase activation by fluoxetine and its relation to gene expression in cultured rat astrocytes. *Journal of Molecular Neuroscience*, **24**, 207–216.

Mill, J., Tang, T., Kaminsky, Z., et al. (2008). Epigenomic profiling reveals DNA-methylation changes associated with major psychosis. *American Journal of Human Genetics*, **82**, 696–711.

Minguet, E. G., Vera-Sirera, F., Marina, A., Carbonell, J., & Blazquez, M. A. (2008). Evolutionary diversification in polyamine biosynthesis. *Molecular Biology and Evolution*, **25**, 2119–2128.

Mitchell, J. B., Iny, L. J., & Meaney, M. J. (1990). The role of serotonin in the development and environmental regulation of type II corticosteroid receptor binding in rat hippocampus. *Brain Research. Developmental Brain Research*, **55**, 231–235.

Molnar, B. E., Berkman, L. F., & Buka, S. L. (2001). Psychopathology, childhood sexual abuse and other childhood adversities: relative links to subsequent suicidal behaviour in the US. *Psychological Medicine*, **31**, 965–977.

Murgatroyd, C., Patchev, A. V., Wu, Y., et al. (2009). Dynamic DNA methylation programs persistent adverse effects of early-life stress. *Nature Neuroscience*, **12**, 1559–1566.

Nakatani, N., Hattori, E., Ohnishi, T., et al. (2006). Genome-wide expression analysis detects eight genes with robust alterations specific to bipolar I disorder: relevance to neuronal network perturbation. *Human Molecular Genetics*, **15**, 1949–1962.

Nelson, C. J., Santos-Rosa, H., & Kouzarides, T. (2006). Proline isomerization of histone H3 regulates lysine methylation and gene expression. *Cell*, **126**, 905–916.

Nielsen, S. J., Schneider, R., Bauer, U. M., et al. (2001). Rb targets histone H3 methylation and HP1 to promoters. *Nature*, **412**, 561–565.

Okano, M., XIE, S., & Li, E. (1998). Cloning and characterization of a family of novel mammalian DNA (cytosine-5) methyltransferases. *Nature Genetics*, **19**, 219–220.

Pandey, G. N., Ren, X., Rizavi, H. S., et al. (2008). Brain-derived neurotrophic factor and tyrosine kinase B receptor signalling in postmortem brain of teenage suicide victims. *International Journal of Neuropsychopharmacology*, **11**, 1047–1061.

Pariante, C. M., & Lightman, S. L. (2008). The HPA axis in major depression: classical theories and new developments. *Trends in Neurosciences*, **31**, 464–468.

Perroud, N., Paoloni-Giacobino, A., Prada, P., et al. (2011). Increased methylation of glucocorticoid receptor gene (*NR3C1*) in adults with a history of childhood maltreatment: a link with the severity and type of trauma. *Translational Psychiatry*, **1**.

Pokholok, D. K., Harbison, C. T., Levine, S., et al. (2005). Genome-wide map of nucleosome acetylation and methylation in yeast. *Cell*, **122**, 517–527.

Polesskaya, O. O., Aston, C., & Sokolov, B. P. (2006). Allele C-specific methylation of the 5-HT2A receptor gene: evidence for correlation with its expression and expression of DNA methylase DNMT1. *Journal of Neuroscience Research*, **83**, 362–373.

Poulter, M. O., Du, L., Weaver, I. C., et al. (2008). GABAA receptor promoter hypermethylation in suicide brain: implications for the involvement of epigenetic processes. *Biological Psychiatry*, **64**, 645–652.

Pray-Grant, M. G., Daniel, J. A., Schieltz, D., Yates, J. R., 3rd & Grant, P. A. (2005). Chd1 chromodomain links histone H3 methylation with SAGA- and SLIK-dependent acetylation. *Nature*, **433**, 434–438.

Pruunsild, P., Kazantseva, A., Aid, T., Palm, K., & Timmusk, T. (2007). Dissecting the human BDNF locus: bidirectional transcription, complex splicing, and multiple promoters. *Genomics*, **90**, 397–406.

Radtke, K. M., Ruf, M., Gunter, H. M., et al. (2011). Transgenerational impact of intimate partner violence on methylation in the promoter of the glucocorticoid receptor. *Translational Psychiatry*, **1**, 1–6.

Razzoli, M., Domenici, E., Carboni, L., et al. (2011). A role for BDNF/TrkB signaling in behavioral and physiological consequences of social defeat stress. *Genes, Brain and Behavior*, **10**(4), 424–433.

Rhee, H. J., Kim, E. J., & Lee, J. K. (2007). Physiological polyamines: simple primordial stress molecules. *Journal of Cellular and Molecular Medicine*, **11**, 685–703.

Rogoz, Z., Skuza, G., & Legutko, B. (2005). Repeated treatment with mirtazepine induces brain-derived neurotrophic factor gene expression in rats. *Journal of Physiology and Pharmacology*, **56**, 661–671.

Rose, C. R., Blum, R., Pichler, B., et al. (2003). Truncated TrkB-T1 mediates neurotrophin-evoked calcium signalling in glia cells. *Nature*, **426**, 74–78.

Roth, T. L., Lubin, F. D., Funk, A. J., & Sweatt, J. D. (2009). Lasting epigenetic influence of early life adversity on the BDNF gene. *Biological Psychiatry*, **65**, 760–769.

Roth, T. L., Zoladz, P. R., Sweatt, J. D., & Diamond, D. M. (2011). Epigenetic modification of hippocampal Bdnf DNA in adult rats in an animal model of post-traumatic stress disorder. *Journal of Psychiatric Research*, **45**(7), 919–926.

Salcedo-Amaya, A. M., Van Driel, M. A., Alako, B. T., et al. (2009). Dynamic histone H3 epigenome marking during the intraerythrocytic cycle of *Plasmodium falciparum*. *Proceedings of the National Academy of Sciences U S A*, **106**(24), 9655–9660.

Sanders, S. L., Portoso, M., Mata, J., et al. (2004). Methylation of histone H4 lysine 20 controls recruitment of Crb2 to sites of DNA damage. *Cell*, **119**, 603–614.

Santa Mina, E. E., & Gallop, R. M. (1998). Childhood sexual and physical abuse and adult self-harm and suicidal behaviour: a literature review. *Canadian Journal of Psychiatry*, **43**, 793–800.

Santos-Rosa, H., Schneider, R., Bernstein, B. E., et al. (2003). Methylation of histone H3 K4 mediates association of the Isw1p ATPase with chromatin. *Molecular Cell*, **12**, 1325–1332.

Scher, C. D., Forde, D. R., Mcquaid, J. R., & Stein, M. B. (2004). Prevalence and demographic correlates of childhood maltreatment in an adult community sample. *Child Abuse and Neglect*, **28**, 167–180.

Sen, S., Duman, R., & Sanacora, G. (2008). Serum brain-derived neurotrophic factor, depression, and antidepressant medications: meta-analyses and implications. *Biological Psychiatry*, **64**, 527–532.

Sequeira, A., Gwadry, F. G., Ffrench-Mullen, J. M., et al. (2006). Implication of SSAT by gene expression and genetic variation in suicide and major depression. *Archives of General Psychiatry*, **63**, 35–48.

Sequeira, A., Klempan, T., Canetti, L., et al. (2007). Patterns of gene expression in the limbic system of suicides with and without major depression. *Molecular Psychiatry*, **12**, 640–655.

Smythe, J. W., Rowe, W. B., & Meaney, M. J. (1994). Neonatal handling alters serotonin (5-HT) turnover and 5-HT2 receptor binding in selected brain regions: relationship to the handling effect on glucocorticoid receptor expression. *Brain Research. Developmental Brain Research*, **80**, 183–189.

Stein, M. B., Koverola, C., Hanna, C., Torchia, M. G., & Mcclarty, B. (1997). Hippocampal volume in women victimized by childhood sexual abuse. *Psychological Medicine*, **27**, 951–959.

Sun, H., Kennedy, P. J., & Nestler, E. J. (2013). Epigenetics of the depressed brain: role of histone acetylation and methylation. *Neuropsychopharmacology*, **38**, 124–137.

Swigut, T., & Wysocka, J. (2007). H3K27 demethylases, at long last. *Cell*, **131**, 29–32.

Tahiliani, M., Koh, K. P., Shen, Y., et al. (2009). Conversion of 5-methylcytosine to 5-hydroxymethylcytosine in mammalian DNA by MLL partner TET1. *Science*, **324**, 930–935.

Tamura, Y., Kunugi, H., Ohashi, J., & Hohjoh, H. (2007). Epigenetic aberration of the human REELIN gene in psychiatric disorders. *Molecular Psychiatry*, **12**, 519, 593–600.

Tanskanen, A., Hintikka, J., Honkalampi, K., et al. (2004). Impact of multiple traumatic experiences on the persistence of depressive symptoms: a population-based study. *Nordic Journal of Psychiatry*, **58**, 459–464.

Torrey, E. F., Barci, B. M., Webster, M. J., et al. (2005). Neurochemical markers for schizophrenia, bipolar disorder, and major depression in postmortem brains. *Biological Psychiatry*, **57**, 252–260.

Tsankova, N. M., Berton, O., Renthal, W., et al. (2006). Sustained hippocampal chromatin regulation in a mouse model of depression and antidepressant action. *Nature Neuroscience*, **9**, 519–525.

Tucker, K. L. (2001). Methylated cytosine and the brain: a new base for neuroscience. *Neuron*, **30**, 649–652.

Turecki, G., Briere, R., Dewar, K., et al. (1999). Prediction of level of serotonin 2A receptor binding by serotonin receptor 2A genetic variation in postmortem brain samples from subjects who did or did not commit suicide. *American Journal of Psychiatry*, **156**, 1456–1458.

Turner, J. D., & Muller, C. P. (2005). Structure of the glucocorticoid receptor (NR3C1) gene 5' untranslated region: identification, and tissue distribution of multiple new human exon 1. *Journal of Molecular Endocrinology*, **35**, 283–292.

Turner, J. D., Pelascini, L. P., Macedo, J. A., & Muller, C. P. (2008). Highly individual methylation patterns of alternative glucocorticoid receptor promoters suggest individualized epigenetic regulatory mechanisms. *Nucleic Acids Research*, **36**, 7207–7218.

Turner, J. D., Alt, S. R., Cao, L., et al. (2010). Transcriptional control of the glucocorticoid receptor: CpG islands, epigenetics and more. *Biochemical Pharmacology*, **80**, 1860–1868.

Tyrka, A. R., Price, L. H., Marsit, C., Walters, O. C., & Carpenter, L. L. (2012). Childhood adversity and epigenetic modulation of the leukocyte glucocorticoid receptor: preliminary findings in healthy adults. *PLoS One*, **7**, e30148.

Uddin, M., Aiello, A. E., Wildman, D. E., et al. (2010). Epigenetic and immune function profiles associated with posttraumatic stress disorder. *Proceedings of the National Academy of Sciences U S A*, **107**, 9470–9475.

Veldic, M., Caruncho, H. J., Liu, W. S., et al. (2004). DNA-methyltransferase 1 mRNA is selectively overexpressed in telencephalic GABAergic interneurons of schizophrenia brains. *Proceedings of the National Academy of Sciences U S A*, **101**, 348–353.

Volk, D. W., Austin, M. C., Pierri, J. N., Sampson, A. R., & Lewis, D. A. (2000). Decreased glutamic acid decarboxylase67 messenger RNA expression in a subset of prefrontal cortical gamma-aminobutyric acid neurons in subjects with schizophrenia. *Archives of General Psychiatry*, **57**, 237–245.

Wang, Z., Zang, C., Rosenfeld, J. A., et al. (2008). Combinatorial patterns of histone acetylations and methylations in the human genome. *Nature Genetics*, **40**, 897–903.

Weaver, I. C., Cervoni, N., Champagne, F. A., et al. (2004). Epigenetic programming by maternal behavior. *Nature Neuroscience*, **7**, 847–854.

Wysocka, J., Swigut, T., Milne, T. A., et al. (2005). WDR5 associates with histone H3 methylated at K4 and is essential for H3 K4 methylation and vertebrate development. *Cell*, **121**, 859–872.

Wysocka, J., Swigut, T., Xiao, H., et al. (2006). A PHD finger of NURF couples histone H3 lysine 4 trimethylation with chromatin remodelling. *Nature*, **442**, 86–90.

Xiao, T., Shibata, Y., Rao, B., et al. (2007). The RNA polymerase II kinase Ctk1 regulates positioning of a 5' histone methylation boundary along genes. *Molecular and Cellular Biology*, **27**, 721–731.

Xu, H., Chen, Z., He, J., et al. (2006). Synergetic effects of quetiapine and venlafaxine in preventing the chronic restraint stress-induced decrease in cell proliferation and BDNF expression in rat hippocampus. *Hippocampus*, **16**, 551–559.

Zhang, T. Y., Hellstrom, I. C., Bagot, R. C., et al. (2010). Maternal care and DNA methylation of a glutamic acid decarboxylase 1 promoter in rat hippocampus. *Journal of Neuroscience*, **30**, 13130–13137.

Zhou, Z., Hong, E. J., Cohen, S., et al. (2006). Brain-specific phosphorylation of MeCP2 regulates activity-dependent Bdnf transcription, dendritic growth, and spine maturation. *Neuron*, **52**, 255–269.

Zlotnick, C., Mattia, J., & Zimmerman, M. (2001). Clinical features of survivors of sexual abuse with major depression. *Child Abuse and Neglect*, **25**, 357–367.

Chapter

33 The use of neuroimaging to investigate the pathophysiology of suicide

Christopher R. Bailey, Allison M. Greene, and Alexander Neumeister

Introduction

Until the advent of neuroimaging technologies, investigation of the neurologic dysfunction underlying suicidal behaviors had been relatively limited. The inability to link symptomology to neuronal function made it difficult to generate meaningful and potentially clinically relevant propositions about the etiology of suicide. Fortunately, modern imaging modalities such as magnetic resonance imaging (MRI) and positron emission tomography (PET) have allowed investigators to examine pathologic neural function and receptor expression *in vivo* during precise emotional states. As a result, contemporary research on neuronal disorders is largely dedicated to exploring relationships between symptomology and neurologic pathophysiology. In this chapter, we summarize current and notable neuroimaging findings within a variety of neurobiological systems implicated in the pathophysiology of suicide. We also aim to provide an appreciation for the unique ability of neuroimaging to shed light on the multi-faceted and perplexing nature of suicidal behavior.

Neuroimaging modalities

Neuroimaging studies of the suicidal brain can be grouped broadly into three categories: structural MRI, functional magnetic resonance imaging (fMRI), and molecular imaging, which includes autoradiography, PET, and single photon emission computed tomography (SPECT). Structural MRI studies generate an image of the brain under resting-state conditions and are used to investigate neuroanatomical differences between patient populations and healthy individuals. In contrast, fMRI studies are used to determine neural activation patterns under resting-state conditions or during specific cognitive tasks. Molecular imaging techniques are employed to produce a wide range of data. For instance, autoradiography can provide information about the post-mortem functional state of a system while PET and SPECT are used to explore differences in neurophysiology *in vivo* through determining transporter and receptor density. Here, we present neuroimaging studies of suicide by imaging modality and discuss their interpretations and implications therein.

Structural MRI findings

Several neuroanatomical abnormalities in psychiatric disorders such as MDD and schizophrenia have been linked to suicidal behavior. Suicidal individuals within these patient populations have demonstrated a reduction in cortical and subcortical brain areas including the corpus callosum (CC), regions of the prefrontal cortex (PFC), and the raphe nuclei (reviewed in Desmyter et al., 2011). Though suicide can be a component of many illnesses, patients with mood disorders like MDD tend to have noticeably higher incidences of suicidal behavior relative to other psychiatric illnesses and the general population (Kasper et al., 1996). As a result, investigators have largely focused on this subset of patients with regard to structural imaging.

A growing body of evidence has implicated a fronto-striatal network in the etiology of suicidal behavior, particularly in MDD. For instance, a landmark study in 2001 by Ahearn and colleagues demonstrated enhanced subcortical gray matter hyperintensities in MDD patients with previous suicide attempts compared to MDD patients without such histories. Subcortical areas like the basal ganglia had already been shown to comprise an emotion regulation pathway with the PFC, and disruptions within these pathways were associated with mood disorders like MDD (for example Chantiluke et al., 2012; Jiao et al., 2011;

A Concise Guide to Understanding Suicide, ed. Stephen H. Koslow, Pedro Ruiz, and Charles B. Nemeroff. Published by Cambridge University Press.

Nikolaus et al., 2012). Thus, the authors hypothesized that if disruptions in these pathways could predispose individuals to MDD, these disruptions could also reasonably lead to suicidal behavior since it is a symptom seen in severe MDD.

Nearly a decade after the study by Ahearn et al. two structural imaging studies added critical pieces of information to the understanding of suicidal behavior in relation to the fronto-striatal emotion regulation pathway. First, Vang et al. (2010) compared suicide attempters with psychiatrically healthy age- and gender-matched controls and noted a smaller right caudate nucleus and bilateral globus pallidus in the suicide attempter cohort. The authors made a thoughtful interpretation of their results predicting that this finding was related to temperament; however, they warned that their results should be interpreted with caution due to the low sample size and other limitations of this preliminary study. The second study (Wagner et al., 2011) added another dimension of understanding to the previous findings of the Ahearn and Vang groups through a larger, well-controlled cohort of individuals. Specifically, Wagner and colleagues studied structural brain abnormalities in MDD patients with a high risk for suicide (i.e., has a history of past suicide attempt or a first-degree relative with past suicidal behavior) and compared them with MDD patients with low risk for suicide and physically and psychiatrically healthy controls matched by age, gender, and education level. The authors found decreased caudate and rostral ACC volumes in suicide attempters and high-risk individuals relative to the comparison groups. Taken together, these structural alterations within the fronto-striatal network may result in a lack of behavioral or emotional control. Specifically, the ACC has been implicated in cognitive and behavioral control (Gasquoine, 2013; Fritz & Dreisbach, 2013), and structural abnormalities in the ACC have been linked to lack of impulse control, a common attribute of suicidal behavior (Crunelle et al., 2012). The caudate, which receives projections from the ACC, is implicated in dopaminergic reward processes. Decreased caudate volume could represent decreased sensitivity to rewarding stimuli or anhedonic symptomology, a key feature of MDD (Pizzagalli et al., 2009). The increased degree of reduction seen in the MDD group with a high risk of suicide compared to the MDD group with a low risk of suicide may be a correlate of disease severity since the presence of suicidal behaviors is usually an indication of more severe MDD (Wagner et al., 2011).

To further elucidate this relationship Wagner et al. continued their investigation of suicidal behavior in 2012 with a similar three-group design. The authors found significantly thinner cortical thickness in the left dorsolateral prefrontal cortex (DLPFC), ventrolateral prefrontal cortex (VLPFC), and the anterior cingulate cortex in suicide attempters/high-risk individuals (Wagner et al., 2012). The DLPFC, VLPFC, and, again, ACC have been implicated in behavioral and emotional control processes and it is possible that this lack of inhibitory control may be associated with the impulsive traits often seen in those who attempt suicide (Wagner et al., 2012; Fawcett, 2012). In sum, Wagner's group posits that the fronto-striatal alterations that they observed are a characteristic structural deficit of suicidal behavior with the frontal aspect representing altered impulse control and the striatal aspect representing diminished reward processing (Wagner et al., 2012). It seems reasonable to propose that alterations in only one of these regions alone do not result in suicidal behaviors. More likely, it is the sum of these alterations that contribute to the development of increased impulsivity and delayed reward control combined with the degree of alteration that denotes suicide. Dombrovski et al. supports this notion through their finding of decreased putamen gray matter in MDD suicide attempters compared to MDD non-suicide attempters and non-MDD controls (Dombrovski et al., 2012). Though the putamen is implicated in reward processes, this finding was associated with desire for immediate rather than larger delayed rewards on a discounting of delayed rewards task (Luo et al., 2009) leading the authors to hypothesize that this alteration may be related to increased impulsivity. But, they do acknowledge that the putamen alone would not constitute increased impulsivity leading to suicidal tendencies. Instead, it is more likely a result of multiple alterations that modulate the effect of the putamen on impulsivity (Dombrovski et al., 2012).

For the sake of completeness, it is important to note that several other structural findings outside of the fronto-striatal network have been associated with suicide and MDD. For example, Cyprien and colleagues (2011) compared suicide attempters with MDD to affective control subjects (individuals with past or current MDD or high MDD symptomology with a low risk of suicide) and healthy control subjects. Volumetric analysis revealed that those who attempted suicide possessed a significantly smaller posterior third of the corpus callosum (CC) when compared to the affective and healthy control subjects. The CC primarily serves as a bundle of neuronal fibers that allow the two hemispheres of the brain to communicate with one another; however, structural abnormalities in the CC have been implicated in a variety of psychiatric disorders (Nery-Fernandes et al., 2012; Kempton et al., 2011). One hypothesis Cyprien et al. have proposed to explain their results is that an environmental stimuli during development, such as child abuse, which was prevalent in their suicide attempters' group, could lead to reduced CC size; however, this relationship was not adequately established in their cohort (Cyprien et al., 2011).

Finally, structural alterations associated with suicidal behavior have also been noted in other disorders, although these findings have been limited. For instance, Soloff and colleagues (2012) noted that certain structural alterations distinguish suicide attempters with BPD from non-suicide attempters with BPD and, astoundingly, they also discovered alterations that distinguished high lethality attempters from low lethality within the suicide attempters BPD group. In schizophrenia, Spoletini et al. (2011) found increased right amygdala volume in schizophrenia patients with a history of suicidal behavior compared to non-suicidal individuals with schizophrenia and healthy controls. Additional studies have noted alterations associated with suicide in other neurological and psychological diseases (for example: Mahon et al., 2012; Soloff et al., 2008).

In conclusion, structural abnormalities have been noted across several brain regions. We focused upon only a few, recent structural imaging studies highlighting significant structural abnormalities associated with suicidal behavior. Structural imaging remains a powerful tool for investigating neurological and psychiatric diseases and there continues to be a growing body of evidence implicating neuroanatomical alterations in the pathophysiology of these disorders.

Functional MRI findings

Researchers frequently employ quantitative neuropsychological measures to investigate cognitive functioning related to suicidal thoughts and behaviors. For instance, Keilp et al. (2012) assessed executive function in suicidal individuals with a battery of neuropsychological tests and found that individuals with MDD and a history of attempted suicide performed worse on these measures than affective controls. Similarly, Raust et al. (2007) also found diminished executive function in suicidal individuals, compared to a control group, using a different set of neuropsychological assessments. Studies such as these are certainly useful in elucidating the cognitive correlates of suicidal thoughts and behaviors, but they do not have the capability to reveal the underlying neuronal pathophysiology. Investigators can only hypothesize where in the brain cognitive and behavioral pathologies originate. To resolve this dilemma, fMRI has been employed to establish connections between the phenotypic cognitive behavioral dysfunction seen in suicide and regional neural activation patterns.

In 2000, M.D. Rudd proposed a cognitive behavioral model of suicidality. This model focuses on a discrete psychological state called the *suicidal mode*, which he described as acute crisis defined by specific cognitive, affective, behavioral, and physiological dimensions (Figure 33.1). A decade after Rudd initially

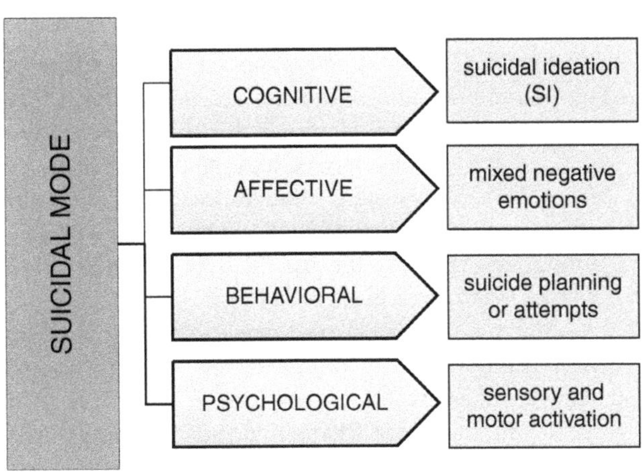

Figure 33.1. A simplified model of Rudd's suicidal mode (Rudd, 2000). See plate section for color version.

proposed his theory, Reisch and colleagues (2010) utilized fMRI to determine which brain regions are active during the suicidal mode. Using script-driven imagery, a type of cognitive activation paradigm, in female MDD suicide attempters, the authors found that recall of the mental pain with suicidal episode was associated with frontal cortical deactivation, while recall of suicidal episode alone was associated with increased activation in the medial PFC, ACC, and hippocampus, fronto-limbic structures implicated in a circuit involved in emotional/behavioral control. The authors posit that frontal deactivation in a state of mental pain inhibits the emotional control circuit, leading the individual toward suicide as a solution to their suffering. Once fixated on suicide, the mind activates regions involved in goal-directed behavior, mPFC and ACC specifically, to complete the action. Furthermore, these results suggest that activation of goal-directed behavior associated with suicide planning/action might in fact reduce the effects of mental pain. Though this group proposed an elegant discussion for their findings, they call into question the relative applicability of their findings due to the small sample size (N = 8), lack of control group, and male subjects (Reisch et al., 2010).

fMRI also has provided insight into the dysfunctional neural activation patterns related to suicidal ideation (SI). In 2012, Matthews et al. investigated the relationship between SI and self-monitoring in combat-exposed Operation Enduring Freedom-Operation Iraqi Freedom (OEF-OIF) veterans. The authors suggested that in order to cope with the internal and external stressors associated with the aforementioned *suicidal mode*, individuals must be able to self-monitor. Thus, veterans with SI may display altered self-monitoring relative to those without SI. Similar to the findings of Reisch et al., Matthews and colleagues found that, during an error-processing task, veterans with SI displayed increased activation in the ACC and PFC (emotional/behavioral control regions), suggesting greater mental effort during self-monitoring relative to the veterans without SI (Matthews et al., 2012).

Impaired decision-making neurocircuitry has also been implicated in suicidal behavior in both adolescents and adults (Clark et al., 2011; Chamberlain et al., 2013; Bridge et al., 2012; Guillaume et al., 2013). For instance, Jollant et al. (2010) found poorer performance on the Iowa Gambling Task and decreased activity in the left lateral orbitofrontal cortex, an area implicated in decision-making processes, and left occipital cortex when considering risky choices in individuals with past MDD and suicide attempt relative to affective controls. In stark contrast, Pan et al. (2013a), found that depressed adolescent individuals with a history of attempted suicide actually performed better on the Iowa Gambling Task than control subjects because they chose more low-risk choices. The authors also found that depressed individuals without suicidal behavior, but not depressed suicide attempters, demonstrated increased hippocampal activation during low-risk decision-making relative to healthy controls. These findings may indicate that altered neuronal processing associated with impaired decision-making in adolescents may be more specific to depression, without suicide attempt or SI. Of note, Jollant's group studied adults while Pan's studied adolescents. Thus, one must consider that decision-making impairments seen in suicide may have different neural correlates in different age groups. Clearly, further investigation will be needed to better characterize the neural activation patterns associated with decision-making processes in suicide.

Marchand and colleagues completed a series of studies in 2011 to discern the different activation patterns in MDD and type II bipolar depression associated with depression severity and suicidal ideation and, not included in our discussion, self-harm. In the first study, the authors studied depressed individuals with bipolar II disorder using fMRI during a motor activation task, a paradigm that the authors previously used to investigate cortico-basal ganglia activation in a variety of psychiatric disorders (for example: Marchand et al., 2009), and then correlated their imaging findings with clinical variables (i.e., depression severity and history of SI). They found a positive correlation between depression severity and left thalamus and a negative correlation between history of SI and the left putamen. For the sake of our discussion, these findings are noteworthy since this is one of the first studies to find an activation pattern that is characteristic to SI and differentiates it from severe depression. Though novel, their findings needed to be interpreted with caution due to several limitations, namely the use of only males in their cohort (Marchand et al., 2011).

Marchand's group continued their investigation into pathophysiology of suicide in 2012. Similar to their work from 2011, Marchand et al. (2012) used fMRI with the motor activation paradigm to investigate activation associated with current SI and depression symptomology but this time in a cohort of males with MDD. The findings of this study supported previous knowledge of a relationship between depressive symptomology and a circuit involving the bilateral striatum and anterior cortical midline structures (CMS) (for example, Marchand et al., 2011; Takahashi et al., 2009; Zhu et al., 2011). With regard to current SI, there was a similar association with the striatum and CMS. However, the SI specific network activation was characteristically smaller containing only the left putamen and anterior CMS. Like the results from Marchand et al. (2011), these results suggest that MDD patients with SI have a distinct pattern of neural activation; however, before this can be regarded as a potential biomarker of suicide, the authors caution, again, that these results must first be replicated in other patient populations (Marchand et al., 2012).

Most recently, Pan et al. (2013b) explored emotional processing in MDD with and without a past suicide attempt. Adolescents with MDD and past suicide attempt demonstrated increased activation in the PFC and ACC while viewing angry faces, relative to both the MDD and healthy control participants. As mentioned above, the ACC is involved in attention and emotional processing/control (for example, Wozniak et al., 2012; Kanske & Kotz, 2012), suggesting that depressed suicide attempters were more attentive to angry faces than were control groups or, more generally that this population may have impaired attention control.

Through the use of fMRI, numerous neurophysiologic alterations associated with the cognitive behavioral phenotype of suicide have already been uncovered. This important effort, however, is still at a relatively early stage. While it is not clear whether these activation patterns are the cause or effect of past suicide attempt/SI or whether they are only part of a multi-factorial neuronal dysfunction, dissecting the neuronal activity associated with cognitive behavioral processes leading to suicide is a critical step toward understanding the pathophysiology of suicide.

Molecular neuroimaging

The serotonin system plays a major role in the regulation of mood and emotion and, under the monoamine hypothesis, under-activity or reductions in the bioavailability of this transmitter may lead to MDD or other associated affective disorders (Sanacora et al., 2012; Nugent et al., 2008; Neumeister et al., 2006). Almost 40 years after a keystone study by Asberg and colleagues (1976) who discovered decreased serotonin metabolites in the cerebrospinal fluid of suicide attempters, the serotonergic system and its associated transporter (5-HTT) and receptors (5-HT1A and 5-HT2A) have assumed well-documented roles in the etiology of suicidal behavior (Desmyter et al., 2011; Meyer, 2012). In this section we focus on recent foundational PET, SPECT, and autoradiography studies investigating the serotonergic system in suicidal behavior.

The serotonin transporter (5-HTT)

5-HTT is a membrane-bound transporter that is responsible for recycling serotonin by returning it to presynaptic serotonergic neurons (reviewed in Bortolato et al., 2013). Alterations in this protein have been hypothesized to play a role in the etiology of MDD, namely through a reduction in serotonergic input to the brain leading to depressive symptoms and perhaps suicidal ideation (Figure 33.2). However, from the PET imaging literature, reports of the degree and

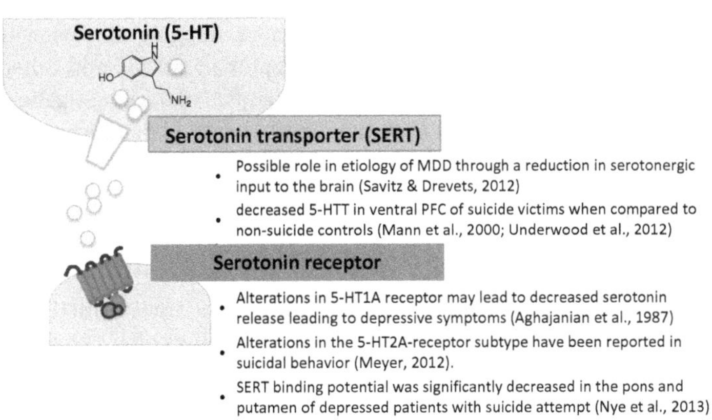

Figure 33.2. Potential role of serotonin transporter and receptor in suicide. See plate section for color version.

direction of these alterations have been inconsistent (reviewed in Savitz & Drevets, 2012). With regard to suicide, a series of landmark postmortem studies have found decreased 5-HTT in the ventral PFC of suicide victims when compared to non-suicide controls (Mann et al., 2000; Underwood et al., 2012). Though postmortem work highlights 5-HTT as a potential correlate for suicidal behavior, molecular imaging of 5-HTT in the suicidal brain has not been as productive (Desmyter et al., 2011). In 2004, Lindström et al. used SPECT and ^{123}I-beta-CIT, a cocaine analog ligand used to examine monoamine transporters to investigate 5-HTT and the dopamine transporter (DAT), in a small sample of suicide attempters (N = 12) and matched healthy control subjects. The authors reported that there was no significant difference in 5-HTT and DAT between groups; however, a correlation between low 5-HTT and impulsivity was noted (Lindström et al., 2004). The same group continued their work with ^{123}I-beta-CIT SPECT in 2006 and similarly found no significant difference between suicide attempters and healthy controls. Interestingly, some *in vivo* PET findings in MDD indicate global reductions in 5-HTT within the PFC but there were no specific alterations that characterized MDD patients who had a history of suicide attempt (Parsey et al., 2006). However, the results of a 2013 study by Nye et al. dispute those findings. Specifically, the authors used (11C)-ZIENT, a selective serotonin transporter (SERT) ligand, with PET imaging and found decreased SERT binding potential in the midbrain/pons and putamen of depressed individuals with a past suicide attempt compared to depressed patients without a past suicide attempt and healthy controls (Nye et al., 2013). These findings further implicate the serotonergic system in the pathophysiology of suicide. In the final analysis, 5-HTT remains an interesting avenue for future work and will continue to be a prevalent target for molecular studies.

The serotonin 5-HT receptors

Multiple lines of evidence link certain 5-HT receptor subtypes to suicidal behavior. In this section we will focus on associations between suicide and the 5-HT1A and 5-HT2A receptor subtypes. In animal models, 5-HT1A receptors have been hypothesized to inhibit the release of serotonin in the PFC (Aghajanian et al., 1987). Thus, alterations in this receptor may lead to decreased serotonin release in the PFC leading to depressive symptoms. A postmortem autoradiography study of suicide victims found significantly increased 5-HT1A in the dorsal and ventrolateral dorsal root nuclei compared to psychiatrically healthy control subjects (Stockmeier et al., 1998). While there have been similar reports of increased 5-HT1A in suicide victims, other studies have reported no significant differences in 5-HT1A in other brain regions (Boldrini et al., 2008). As of now, *in vivo* molecular imaging has not been able to adequately decipher the role of this receptor subtype in suicidal behavior.

Alterations in the 5-HT2A-receptor subtype have been regularly reported in suicidal behavior (reviewed in Meyer, 2012). In postmortem studies, results have generally reported increased 5-HT2A in suicide victims compared to healthy controls, although there is some degree of disagreement (reviewed in Desmyter et al., 2011). However, like work on 5-HT1A, there are also limited molecular imaging studies. In 2001, Audenaert and colleagues conducted a 123I-5-I-R91150, a 5-HT2A-specific ligand, SPECT study in medication-free recent suicide attempters, versus matched healthy controls. The authors reported that the suicide attempter group had significantly decreased 5-HT2A binding compared with healthy controls and within the suicidal group, those who were self-injurious possessed a greater decrease in 5-HT2A receptors compared with those who attempted self-poisoning (Audenaert et al., 2001). Though an elegant study, the greater applicability of these findings must be further investigated due to the small sample size of the study (suicide attempters N = 9; controls N = 12). Of note, well-conceived and executed PET studies in medication-free MDD patients, without recent suicide attempts, have found no significant differences in 5-HT2A binding between the MDD patients and healthy controls (Meyer et al., 1999; reviewed in Meyer, 2012). We believe the 5-HT2A receptor subtype is still an important target for future investigations and perhaps further molecular imaging studies will elucidate a role for this receptor in suicide and other affective disorders. In general, much of the investigation into suicide is at a preliminary stage and there are many avenues left open to explore with molecular imaging within countless neurochemical systems.

Conclusions and future directions

Neuroimaging has fundamentally transformed the way investigators study the pathophysiology of suicidal behavior. Table 33.1, which presents a summary of the findings described throughout this chapter,

Table 33.1. Summary of findings, neuroimaging in suicide

Structural MRI	
Ahearn et al. (2001)	Enhanced subcortical gray matter hyperintensities in MDD patients with previous suicide attempts
Spoletini et al. (2010)	Increased right amygdala volume in schizophrenia patients with a history of suicidal behavior
Vang et al. (2010)	Smaller right caudate nucleus and bilateral globus pallidus in individuals with past suicide attempt
Wagner et al. (2011)	Decreased caudate and rostral ACC volumes in both individuals with past suicide attempt and high-risk individuals
Cyprien et al. (2011)	Smaller posterior third of the corpus callosum in individuals with past suicide attempt
Dombrovski et al. (2012)	Decreased putamen gray matter in individuals with MDD and past suicide attempt
Soloff et al. (2012)	In BPD patients, high vs. low lethality suicide attempters display different neural alterations
Wagner et al. (2012)	Reduced cortical thickness in the left dorsolateral PFC, ventrolateral PFC, and anterior cingulate cortex in suicide attempters and high-risk individuals
Functional MRI	
Reisch et al. (2010)	Recall of mental pain with suicidal episode was associated with frontal cortical deactivation Recall of suicidal episode alone was associated with increased activation in emotional control circuit
Jollant et al. (2010)	Individuals with MDD and past suicide attempt displayed decreased activity in the left lateral orbitofrontal cortex and left occipital cortex when considering risky choices during a gambling task
Marchand et al. (2011)	Positive correlation between depression severity and left thalamus activity during a motor task Negative correlation between history of SI and left putamen activity during a motor activation task
Matthews et al. (2012)	During an error-processing task, veterans with suicidal ideation displayed increased activation in the ACC and PFC (emotional/behavioral control regions)
Pan et al. (2013a)	Depressed individuals without suicidal behavior demonstrated increased hippocampal activation during low-risk decision-making
Pan et al. (2013b)	Adolescents with MDD and past suicide attempt demonstrated increased activation in the PFC and ACC while viewing angry faces
Molecular neuroimaging	
Serotonin transporter 5-HTT	
Asberg et al. (1976)	Decreased serotonin metabolites in the cerebrospinal fluid of individuals with past suicide attempt
Lindström et al. (2004)	Using SPECT and ^{123}I-beta-CIT, found no significant difference in 5-HTT between suicide attempters and healthy controls; noted a correlation between low 5-HTT and impulsivity
Parsey et al. (2006)	MDD patients showed global reductions in 5-HTT within the PFC; no specific alterations in MDD suicide attempters
Ryding et al. (2006)	Using ^{123}I-beta-CIT and SPECT, found no significant difference between suicide attempters and healthy individuals
Mann et al. (2000); Underwood et al. (2012)	Decreased 5-HTT in the ventral PFC of suicide victims
Nye et al. (2013)	Using [^{11}C]-Zient ant PET found decreased SERT (serotonin transporter) binding in patients with depression and past suicide attempt
Serotonin 5-HT receptor	
Aghajanian et al. (1987)	5-HT1A receptors hypothesized to inhibit the release of serotonin in the PFC in animal models
Stockmeier et al. (1998)	Postmortem autoradiography study of suicide victims found significantly increased 5-HT1A in the dorsal and ventrolateral dorsal root nuclei
Audenaert et al. (2001)	Suicide attempters showed decreased 5-HT2A binding compared with healthy controls; within suicidal group, even greater decrease in 5-HT2A in self-injurious individuals
Desmyter et al. (2011)	Postmortem studies report 5-HT2A in suicide victims compared to healthy controls (although there is some degree of disagreement)
Meyer et al. (1999); Meyer (2012)	PET studies in medication-free MDD patients, without recent suicide attempts, have found no significant differences in 5-HT2A binding but alterations in the 5-HT2A-receptor subtype have been regularly reported in suicidal behavior

underscores the value of imaging in this field of research. Many of the postulated theories on neurobiological dysfunction in suicide and its related disorders can be thoroughly vetted through the use of any of the technologies highlighted above. As one can see, earlier attempts at studying suicidal behavior were largely dominated by MRI techniques. However, in recent years, the use of molecular imaging, particularly PET and SPECT, has greatly increased as a result of academic centers installing high-resolution scanners and investing greater resources into novel ligand development. Structural and functional MRI will continue to play an essential role in the investigation of all psychiatric conditions, but we strongly believe future research will be led by molecular imaging techniques due to its unique ability to study neurochemical systems with great specificity *in vivo*.

From a target standpoint, there is still a great deal of work that needs to be done within all of the systems outlined above and it is certain that we will continue to see work published on the aforementioned topics. We predict that work exploring the etiology will expand into other receptor systems that have already been implicated in MDD such as the serotonin 1B system (Murrough & Neumeister, 2011), kappa opioid system, and perhaps even systems like the endogenous cannabinoids implicated in anxiety disorders with a high potential for suicide (Neumeister, 2013). Regardless of direction, it is clear that neuroimaging will continue to play a critical role and we look forward to what future investigations will uncover.

References

Aghajanian, G. K., Sprouse, J. S., & Rasmussen, K. (1987). Physiology of the midbrain 5-HT system. In H. Y. Meltzer (Ed.) *Psychopharmacology: the Third Generation of Progress* (pp 141–148). New York: Raven.

Ahearn, E. P., Jamison, K. R., Steffens, D. C., et al. (2001). MRI correlates of suicide attempt history in unipolar depression. *Biological Psychiatry*, **50**(4), 266–270.

Asberg, M., Träskman, L., & Thorén, P. (1976). 5-HIAA in the cerebrospinal fluid: a biochemical suicide predictor? *Archives of General Psychiatry*, **33**(10), 1193–1197.

Audenaert, K., Van Laere, K., Dumont, F., et al. (2001). Decreased frontal serotonin 5-HT 2a receptor binding index in deliberate self-harm patients. *European Journal of Nuclear Medicine*, **28**(2), 175–182.

Boldrini, M., Underwood, M. D., Mann, J. J., & Arango, V. (2008). Serotonin-1A autoreceptor binding in the dorsal raphe nucleus of depressed suicides. *Journal of Psychiatric Research*, **42**(6), 433–442.

Bortolato, M., Pivac, N., Seler, D. M., et al. (2013). The role of serotonergic system at the interface of aggression and suicide. *Neuroscience*, **236**, 160–185.

Bridge, J. A., McBee-Strayer, S. M., Cannon, E. A., et al. (2012). Impaired decision-making in adolescent suicide attempters. *Journal of the American Academy of Child and Adolescent Psychiatry*, **51**(4), 394–403.

Chamberlain, S. R., Odlaug, B. L., Schreiber, L. R., & Grant, J. E. (2013). Clinical and neurocognitive markers of suicidality in young adults. *Journal of Psychiatric Research*, **47**(5), 586–591.

Chantiluke, K., Halari, R., Simic, M., et al. (2012). Fronto-striato-cerebellar dysregulation in adolescents with depression during motivated attention. *Biological Psychiatry*, **71**(1), 59–67.

Clark, L., Dombrovski, A. Y., Siegle, G. J., et al. (2011). Impairment in risk-sensitive decision-making in older suicide attempters with depression. *Psychology and Aging*, **26**(2), 321–330.

Crunelle, C. L., Veltman, D. J., Booij, J., Emmerik-van Oortmerssen, K., & van den Brink, W. (2012). Substrates of neuropsychological functioning in stimulant dependence: a review of functional neuroimaging research. *Brain Behavior*, **2**(4), 499–523.

Cyprien, F., Courtet, P., Malafosse, A., et al. (2011). Suicidal behavior is associated with reduced corpus callosum area. *Biological Psychiatry*, **70**(4), 320–326.

Desmyter, S., van Heeringen, C., & Audenaert, K. (2011). Structural and functional neuroimaging studies of the suicidal brain. *Progress in Neuropsychopharmacology and Biological Psychiatry*, **35**(4), 796–808.

Dombrovski, A. Y., Siegle, G. J., Szanto, K., et al. (2012). The temptation of suicide: striatal gray matter, discounting of delayed rewards, and suicide attempts in late-life depression. *Psychological Medicine*, **42**(6), 1203–1215.

Fawcett, J. (2012). Diagnosis, traits, states, and comorbidity in suicide. In Y. Dwivedi (Ed.) *The Neurobiological Basis of Suicide* (Chapter 1. Frontiers in Neuroscience). Boca Raton, FL: CRC Press.

Fritz, J., & Dreisbach, G. (2013). Conflicts as aversive signals: Conflict priming increases negative judgments for neutral stimuli. *Cognitive, Affective and Behavioral Neuroscience*, **13**(2), 311–317.

Gasquoine, P. G. (2013). Localization of function in anterior cingulate cortex: From psychosurgery to functional neuroimaging. *Neuroscience and Biobehavioral Reviews*, **37**(3), 340–348.

Guillaume, S., Perroud, N., Jollant, F., et al. (2013). HPA axis genes may modulate the effect of childhood adversities on decision-making in suicide attempters. *Journal of Psychiatric Research*, **47**(2), 259–265.

Jiao, Q., Ding, J., Lu, G., et al. (2011). Increased activity imbalance in fronto-subcortical circuits in adolescents with major depression. *PLoS One*, **6**(9), e25159.

Jollant, F., Lawrence, N. S., Olie, E., et al. (2010). Decreased activation of lateral orbitofrontal cortex during risky choices under uncertainty is associated with disadvantageous decision-making and suicidal behavior. *Neuroimage*, **51**(3), 1275–1281.

Kanske, P., & Kotz, S. A. (2012). Effortful control, depression, and anxiety correlate with the influence of emotion on executive attentional control. *Biological Psychology*, **91**(1), 88–95.

Kasper, S., Schindler, S., & Neumeister, A. (1996). Risk of suicide in depression and its implication for psychopharmacological treatment. *International Clinical Psychopharmacology*, **11**(2), 71–79

Keilp, J. G., Gorlyn, M., Russell, M., et al. (2012). Neuropsychological function and suicidal behavior: attention control, memory and executive dysfunction in suicide attempt. *Psychological Medicine*, **10**, 1–13.

Kempton, M. J., Salvador, Z., Munafò, M. R., et al. (2011). Structural neuroimaging studies in major depressive disorder: Meta-analysis and comparison with bipolar disorder. *Archives of General Psychiatry*, **68**(7), 675–690.

Lindström, M. B., Ryding, E., Bosson, P., et al. (2004). Impulsivity related to brain serotonin transporter binding capacity in suicide attempters. *European Neuropsychopharmacology*, **14**(4), 295–300.

Luo, S., Ainslie, G., Giragosian, L., & Monterosso, J. R. (2009). Behavioral and neural evidence of incentive bias for immediate rewards relative to preference-matched delayed rewards. *Journal of Neuroscience*, **29**(47), 14 820–14 827.

Mahon, K., Burdick, K. E., Wu, J., Ardekani, B. A., & Szeszko, P. R. (2012). Relationship between suicidality and impulsivity in bipolar I disorder: a diffusion tensor imaging study. *Bipolar Disorder*, **14**(1), 80–89.

Mann, J. J., Huang, Y. Y., Underwood, M. D., et al. (2000). A serotonin transporter gene promoter polymorphism (5-HTTLPR) and prefrontal cortical binding in major depression and suicide. *Archives of General Psychiatry*, **57**(8), 729–738.

Marchand, W. R., Lee, J. N., Healy, L., et al. (2009). An fMRI motor activation paradigm demonstrates abnormalities of putamen activation in females with panic disorder. *Journal of Affective Disorders*, **116**(1–2), 121–125.

Marchand, W. R., Lee, J. N., Garn, C., et al. (2011). Striatal and cortical midline activation and connectivity associated with suicidal ideation and depression in bipolar II disorder. *Journal of Affective Disorders*, **133**(3), 638–645.

Marchand, W. R., Lee, J. N., Johnson, S., et al. (2012). Striatal and cortical midline circuits in major depression: implications for suicide and symptom expression. *Progress in Neuropsychopharmacology and Biological Psychiatry*, **36**(2), 290–299.

Matthews, S., Spadoni, A., Knox, K., Strigo, I., & Simmons, A. (2012). Combat-exposed war veterans at risk for suicide show hyperactivation of prefrontal cortex and anterior cingulate during error processing. *Psychosomatic Medicine*, **74**(5), 471–475.

Meyer, J. H. (2012). Neuroimaging high-risk states for suicide. In Y. Diwivedi (Ed.) *The Neurobiological Basis for Suicide* (pp. 159–194). Boca Raton, FL: CRC Press.

Meyer, J. H., Kapur, S., Houle, S., et al. (1999). Prefrontal cortex 5-HT2 receptors in depression: an [18F] setoperone PET imaging study. *American Journal of Psychiatry*, **156**(7), 1029–1034.

Murrough, J. W., & Neumeister, A. (2011). The serotonin 1B receptor: a new target for depression therapeutics? *Biological Psychiatry*, **69**(8), 714–715.

Nery-Fernandes, F., Rocha, M. V., Jackowski, A., et al. (2012). Reduced posterior corpus callosum area in suicidal and non-suicidal patients with bipolar disorder. *Journal of Affective Disorders*, **142**(1–3), 150–155.

Neumeister, A. (2013). The endocannabinoid system provides an avenue for evidence-based treatment development for PTSD. *Depression and Anxiety*, **30**(2), 93–96.

Neumeister, A., Hu, X. Z., Luckenbaugh, D. A., et al. (2006). Differential effects of 5-HTTLPR genotypes on the behavioral and neural responses to tryptophan depletion in patients with major depression and controls. *Archives of General Psychiatry*, **63**(9), 978–986.

Nikolaus, S., Hautzel, H., Heinzel, A., Müller, HW. (2012). Key players in major and bipolar depression: a retrospective analysis of in vivo imaging studies. *Behavioural Brain Research*, **232**(2), 358–390.

Nugent, A. C., Neumeister, A., Goldman, D., et al. (2008). Serotonin transporter genotype and depressive phenotype determination by discriminant analysis of glucose metabolism under acute tryptophan depletion. *Neuroimage*, **43**(4), 764–774.

Nye, J. A., Purselle, D., Plisson, C., et al. (2013). Decreased brainstem and putamen SERT binding potential in depressed suicide attempters using [11C]-Zient PET imaging. *Depression and Anxiety*, **30**(10), 902–907.

Pan, L., Segreti, A., Almeida, J., et al. (2013a). Preserved hippocampal function during learning in the context of risk in adolescent suicide attempt. *Psychiatry Research*, **211**(2), 112–118.

Pan, L. A., Hassel, S., Segreti, A. M., et al. (2013b). Differential patterns of activity and functional connectivity in emotion processing neural circuitry to angry and happy faces in adolescents with and without suicide attempt. *Psychological Medicine*, **43**(10), 2129–2142.

Parsey, R. V., Hastings, R. S., Oquendo, M. A., et al. (2006). Lower serotonin transporter binding potential in the human brain during major depressive episodes. *American Journal of Psychiatry*, **163**, 52–58.

Pizzagalli, D. A., Holmes, A. J., Dillon, D. G., et al. (2009). Reduced caudate and nucleus accumbens response to rewards in unmedicated individuals with major depressive disorder. *American Journal of Psychiatry*, **166**(6), 702–710.

Raust, A., Slama, F., Mathieu, F., et al. (2007). Prefrontal cortex dysfunction in patients with suicidal behavior. *Psychological Medicine*, **37**(3), 411–419.

Reisch, T., Seifritz, E., Esposito, F., et al. (2010). An fMRI study on mental pain and suicidal behavior. *Journal of Affective Disorder*, **126**(1–2), 321–325.

Rudd, M. D. (2000). The suicidal mode: a cognitive-behavioral model of suicidality. *Suicide and Life-Threatening Behavior*, **30**(1), 18–33.

Sanacora, G., Treccani, G., & Popoli, M. (2012). Toward a glutamate hypothesis of depression: an emerging frontier of neuropsychopharmacology for mood disorders. *Neuropharmacology*, **62**(1), 63–77.

Savitz, J. B., & Drevets, W. C. (2012). Neuroreceptor imaging in depression. *Neurobiology of Disease*. Jun 9 [Epub ahead of print].

Soloff, P., Nutche, J., Goradia, D., & Diwadkar, V. (2008). Structural brain abnormalities in borderline personality disorder: a voxel-based morphometry study. *Psychiatry Research*, **164**(3), 223–236.

Soloff, P. H., Pruitt, P., Sharma, M., et al. (2012). Structural brain abnormalities and suicidal behavior in borderline personality disorder. *Journal of Psychiatric Research*, **46**(4), 516–525.

Spoletini, I., Piras, F., Fagioli, S., et al. (2011). Suicidal attempts and increased right amygdala volume in schizophrenia. *Schizophrenia Research*, **125**(1), 30–40.

Stockmeier, C. A., Shapiro, L. A., Dilley, G. E., et al. (1998). Increase in serotonin-1A autoreceptors in the midbrain of suicide victims with major depression-postmortem evidence for decreased serotonin activity. *Journal of Neuroscience*, **18**(18), 7394–7401.

Takahashi, T., Yücel, M., Lorenzetti, V., et al. (2009). Midline brain structures in patients with current and remitted major depression. *Progress in Neuropsychopharmacology and Biological Psychiatry*, **33**(6), 1058–1063.

Underwood, M. D., Kassir, S. A., Bakalian, M. J., et al. (2012). Neuron density and serotonin receptor binding in prefrontal cortex in suicide. *International Journal of Neuropsychopharmacology*, **15**(4), 435–447.

Vang, F. J., Ryding, E., Träskman-Bendz, L., van Westen, D., & Lindström, M. B. (2010). Size of basal ganglia in suicide attempters, and its association with temperament and serotonin transporter density. *Psychiatry Research*, **183**(2), 177–179.

Wagner, G., Koch, K., Schachtzabel, C., et al. (2011). Structural brain alterations in patients with major depressive disorder and high-risk for suicide: evidence for a distinct neurobiological entity? *Neuroimage*, **54**(2), 1607–1614.

Wagner, G., Schultz, C. C., Koch, K., et al. (2012). Prefrontal cortical thickness in depressed patients with high-risk for suicidal behavior. *Journal of Psychiatric Research*, **46**(11), 1449–1455.

Wozniak, J., Gonenc, A., Biederman, J., et al. (2012). A magnetic resonance spectroscopy study of the anterior cingulate cortex in youth with emotional dysregulation. *Israel Journal of Psychiatry and Related Sciences*, **49**(1), 62–69.

Zhu, X., Peng, S., Zhang, S., & Zhang, X. (2011). Stress-induced depressive behaviors are correlated with Par-4 and DRD2 expression in rat striatum. *Behavioural Brain Research*, **223**(2), 329–335.

Chapter 34

Brain serotonin in suicides with psychological autopsy

Victoria Arango and Helene Bach

Introduction

Serotonin (5-hydroxytryptamine, 5-HT) modulates many human behaviors including mood, sleep–wake cycle, memory, impulsivity, and aggressivity. Dysregulation of serotonin synthesis and serotonergic neurotransmission is implicated in the development of psychiatric illnesses including suicidal behavior. Most of the available biological evidence implicating 5-HT in suicide comes from examining the brain of suicides postmortem and examining serotonergic indices in suicide attempters, both in blood and in CSF. While evidence exists that indicates the involvement of other neurotransmitter systems, this review will focus exclusively on serotonin.

Low serotonin neurotransmission is hypothesized in the pathophysiology of suicide. Neurons synthesizing brain 5-HT are located in the brainstem raphe nuclei. From those, the dorsal and median raphe nuclei (DRN and MRN, respectively) are located in the rostral brainstem and project to the forebrain in primates. Neuronal tryptophan hydroxylase (TPH2) is the rate-limiting enzyme in the biosynthesis of 5-HT converting tryptophan to 5-hydroxytryptophan (5-HTP) on route to decarboxylation into 5-hydroxytryptamine. This chapter aims to review data that defines the neuroanatomical and neurochemical profile of serotonin-synthesizing neurons within the human DRN and MRN and relate this molecular profile to the current understanding of dysregulated 5-HT synthesis in the etiology of suicide. We will first provide a neuroanatomical description of the human DRN and MRN and will review the biochemical and immunocytochemical analyses of serotonergic neurons in suicide. We will also review the serotonergic data in the forebrain of suicides. The current understanding of the molecular underpinnings of serotonin synthesis via TPH2 and the further neurochemical characterization of 5-HT neurons by virtue of TPH2 expression will be discussed. We will then review the literature showing the deficit in serotonin in suicide as well as present a novel idea of a chemical serotonergic disconnect between the cortex and the brainstem in individuals who die by suicide.

The importance of "psychological" autopsies

In order to carry out structural or biological studies in the brain of patients with psychiatric illness that can be correlated with specific psychiatric diagnoses or at least specific symptoms or traits, it is necessary to carry out what is referred to as a "psychological autopsy." This is in lieu of the direct interview of the deceased, which is of course not possible. Interviewing individuals who were close to the deceased and administering them standardized instruments, such as the structured clinical interviews for DSM Axis I disorders (major mental disorders, SCID-I) and Axis II (personality disorders, SCID-II), enables us to collect the necessary information allowing for statements about specific correlations between behavior and biology. Families are contacted initially by a letter expressing sympathy and briefly describing the reason for contact. A phone call from the clinical evaluator follows and the "informants" (for both suicides and psychiatrically normal controls) are given the option of home, hospital, or phone interview. Written informed consent is obtained by next-of-kin for tissue use, medical and police record reviews, and interviews. In addition to Axis I and II diagnoses, information is collected regarding demographics, education, medical history, psychiatric treatment, medication use, history of suicidal behavior, family history of psychiatric disorders, aggression, early life adversity, and life events. All interviewers are experienced

A Concise Guide to Understanding Suicide, ed. Stephen H. Koslow, Pedro Ruiz, and Charles B. Nemeroff. Published by Cambridge University Press.

clinicians who have been trained in the administration of these semi-structured interviews. Adherence to DSM criteria is reviewed in diagnostic meetings attended by the interviewer as well as a group of clinicians and psychiatrists and a consensus diagnosis is reached.

In addition to the psychological autopsy, it is important to identify any medications, drugs of abuse, or alcohol present at the time of death that may interfere with the specific biochemical measure of interest. Peripheral toxicological screens of blood or other body fluids are the required minimum to indicate whether any of these substances are present. Additional toxicological assays in brain tissue offer the advantage of increased likelihood of detection since many of the psychotropic medications of interest are lipophilic, and are therefore more abundant in the fatty brain. The history of medications is also of value, especially during the recent past (3–12 months antemortem). One problem with this approach is that we can only learn about prescribed medications during that time period and not patient compliance in taking those medications. Carrying out detailed neuropathological examination is also crucial, as the aim is to find biological correlates of suicide, not of other illnesses. The manner of death is particularly important for postmortem studies, as coma or long agonal conditions with prolonged hypoxia leading to a subsequent acidosis have a major impact on RNA integrity. Sudden death cases are best suited for postmortem studies and using brains that have a pH in the physiologic range will avoid confounds not related to the study of suicide or the illness of interest.

The human dorsal and median raphe nuclei: neuroanatomical studies of serotonin-synthesizing neurons

The complexity and broad spectrum of serotonergic function is reflected in the cytoarchitectural heterogeneity and organization of serotonin-producing neurons in the DRN and MRN. The DRN and MRN are located in the ventral part of the central gray in the midbrain and in the rostral pons. In humans, Nissl-stained preparations demonstrate that the DRN extends from the caudal aspect of the oculomotor nucleus to the level of the motor trigeminal nucleus in the middle of the pons, a distance of approximately 24 mm. The DRN is cytoarchitecturally divided into five distinct subregions based on topographic and cytoarchitectonic characteristics in Nissl-stained material: the dorsal (DRd), the ventrolateral (DRvl), the ventral (DRv), the interfascicular (DRif), and the caudal (DRc) subnuclei. Immunostaining for serotonin or tryptophan hydroxylase (TPH) in postmortem human tissue has been difficult due to the rapid degradation of serotonin after death. The first anatomical studies of human DRN/MRN used an antibody developed against phenylalanine hydroxylase (PH8) which recognizes all three aromatic amino acid hydroxylases, including TPH. The cytoarchitectonic subdivisions of the DRN correspond to those observed in tissue immunoreacted with anti-PH8, but an additional component was revealed, the lateral subnucleus, not previously recognized in Nissl-stained material. The subnuclei have characteristic cellular morphometry and density. It is estimated that there are 80 000 serotonergic neurons in the DRN of normal non-psychiatric controls as determined by PH-8 immunohistochemistry (Underwood et al., 1999). Immunohistochemical studies show that most of the serotonergic neurons in the DRN are located in the rostral half, distributed among the DRd, DRv, DRif, and the DRvl subnuclei.

Cytoarchitecturally, the **interfascicular** subnucleus is described as long and dense; its cells are oriented parallel to the midline and the processes extend within the medial longitudinal fasciculi. Its rostrocaudal extent goes from the anterior pole of the DRN to the rostral fourth ventricle. Caudal to this point, all DRN neurons are on either side of the floor of the midline. The **ventrolateral** subnucleus is made up of small, multipolar neurons extending caudally from the central gray to a position just dorsal to the trochlear nuclei and the medial longitudinal fasciculus. This subdivision has no midline component and extends further caudally than the median subnucleus in the rostral pons. The **dorsal** subnucleus has loosely arranged medium-sized neurons dorsomedially flanking the dense ventrolateral subgroup. The two lateral halves are continuous in the midline. The **caudal** subnucleus is made of two dense strips of PH8-immunoreactive neurons lateral to the midline and dorsal to the medial longitudinal fasciculus. Its cells are small to medium-sized and processes are oriented parallel to the floor of the fourth ventricle. The **lateral** subdivision cannot be recognized in Nissl-stained material. It is very loosely organized and has the largest multipolar neurons of any of the DRN subdivisions. Neuronal processes extend across large fields in the central gray and axons are characteristically coiled close to the soma. The **ventral** subdivision is made up of round neurons located between the dorsal and ventrolateral subnucleus. Figure 34.1A shows PH8 immunostaining in a representative human brainstem across the anteroposterior axis of

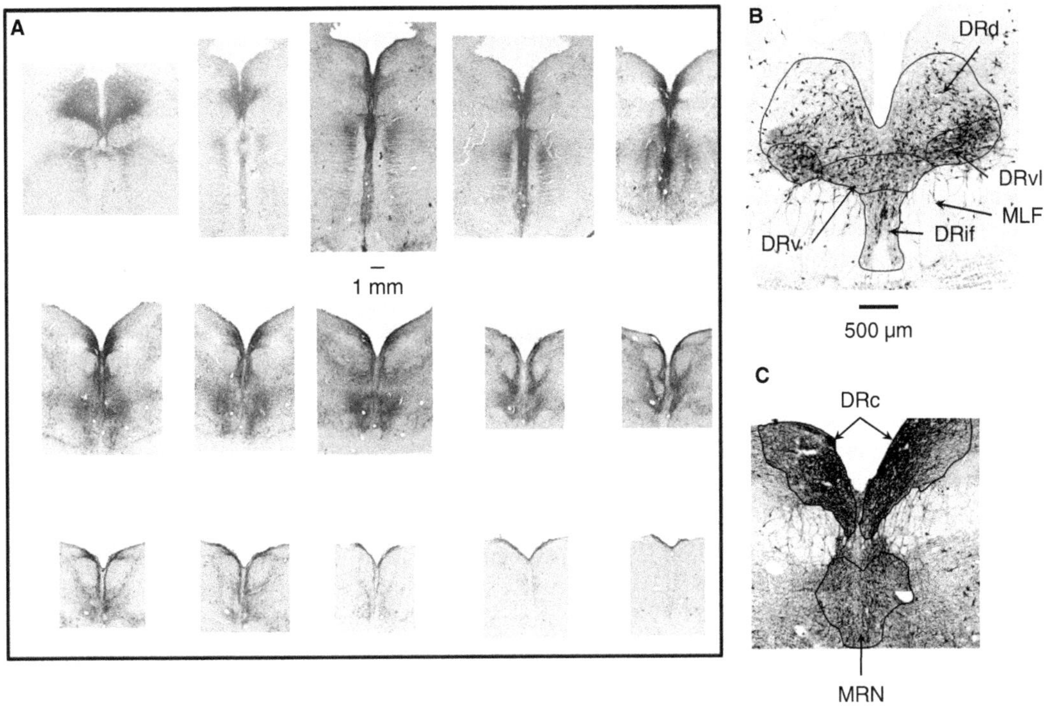

Figure 34.1. (A) Transverse sections through a representative human brainstem immunostained for PH8 that labels serotonergic neurons. The most rostral section is on the upper left-hand corner. At this level, most of the DRN subnuclei are present. The most caudal section is on the lower right-hand corner and it contains only the caudal subnucleus of the DRN. Photomicrographs are cropped, so that only the midline raphe nuclei are visible. Dorsal is to the top in all sections. (B) A higher magnification of a rostral section outlining the DRN subnuclei, which are labeled as DRd: dorsal; DRv: ventral; DRvl: ventrolateral; DRif: interfascicular. The white matter bundle of the medial longitudinal fasciculus is labeled MLF. (C) A higher magnification of a section approximately 7.5 mm caudal to B, showing only the caudal subnucleus (DRc) and the dorsal part of the median raphe nucleus (MRN).

the DRN and MRN. The rostral subnuclei are delineated in Figure 34.1B and the caudal subnucleus and MRN are indicated in Figure 34.1C.

The median raphe nucleus (MRN) extends from the decussation of the superior cerebellar peduncles in the caudal mesencephalon to the rostral pons. At its most dorsal end, the MRN is ventral to the medial longitudinal fasciculus. Ventrally it extends to the bottom of the midline tegmental region. At rostral levels of the MRN, PH8 immunostaining reveals a group of densely packed midline cells in the caudal mesencephalon while caudally, the neurons assume a paramedial location. Most neurons in the MRN have short dendrites oriented in the rostrocaudal direction and characteristically round somata.

Evidence for the involvement of serotonin in suicide

The first neurochemical studies of suicide involved the measurement of monoamines and their metabolites in brain tissue homogenates during the 1960s and 1970s. All these early studies measuring the levels of 5-HT and its metabolite 5-hydroxyindoleacetic acid (5-HIAA) were done in the area of the brainstem thought to correspond to the location of the raphe nuclei where the serotonin neurons are located. In four out of five postmortem studies of brainstem (see Arango & Mann, 1992), suicides had less 5-HT or 5-HIAA compared to controls. In contrast to the brainstem, most postmortem studies report no differences in cortical 5-HT or 5-HIAA in suicides compared to controls (Arango & Mann, 1992). Numerous problems plagued those early studies, including the lack of psychiatric characterization of the subjects, lack of toxicology and neuropathology, very long postmortem intervals, and long agonal states with oxygen deprivation and acidosis. They also presented the problem of homogenizing portions of the brainstem that were not necessarily comparable to each other, as no direct visualization of the area of interest was possible. Following those studies, 5-HIAA was reported to be lower in the CSF of depressed suicide attempters compared to controls (Åsberg et al., 1976) and in those patients who died by suicide. This CSF finding, indicating low 5-HT neurotransmission has been replicated by several groups.

The next approach to the study of monoamines still utilized homogenates but examined the receptors, which are more stable proteins, and looked at pre- and postsynaptic markers in the cortex. Most of the studies of the serotonin transporter (SERT), indicative of serotonergic innervation, in suicides employed ^{3}H-imipramine as the ligand, and about half found a decrease in the suicide group and the other half found no change. Studies using ^{3}H-paroxetine for the most part did not show changes in neocortex but the use of ^{3}H-citalopram demonstrated a reduction in subjects diagnosed with major depressive disorder. A widely reported serotonergic abnormality in major depression is fewer platelet SERT. *In vivo* imaging (Parsey et al., 2006) and postmortem brain studies (Arango et al., 2002; Mann et al., 2000) conducted in depressed patients suggest that SERT alterations are more widespread in the brain of major depression subjects compared with suicides (Arango et al., 1995), and also includes the brainstem (reviewed in Mann et al., 2001).

Quantitative receptor autoradiography allows for a better localization of changes and offers resolution down to the level of individual cortical laminae. Reduced SERT binding was found using ^{3}H-imipramine on coronal sections from a hemicerebrum in some neocortical regions and increased binding in the hippocampal formation (reviewed in Mann et al., 2001). Other studies (Arango et al., 1995; 2002; Mann et al., 2000), which also utilized coronal sections from one hemicerebrum, used ^{3}H-cyanoimipramine as the ligand and found a 45% decrease in binding in the lateral prefrontal cortex of the suicide group. Studies in the brainstem have shown no differences (Arango et al., 2001; Bligh-Glover et al., 2000). For the 5-HT$_{2A}$ receptor, both agonists (^{125}I-LSD) and antagonists (^{3}H-ketanserin and ^{3}H-spiperone), all not specific, have been used. The original report by Stanley and Mann (Stanley & Mann, 1983) of increased 5-HT$_{2A}$ receptors in cortical homogenates from suicides has been replicated by many (Arango et al., 1990; Hrdina et al., 1993; Mann et al., 1986; Pandey et al., 2002; Turecki et al., 1999), but not all (Stockmeier et al., 1997) studies. The 5-HT$_{1A}$ receptor was found elevated in the prefrontal cortex in suicide by some (Arango et al., 1995; Underwood et al., 2012), but not others (Stockmeier et al., 1997, 2009).

Alterations in serotonin indices in the DRN of depressed suicides compared to controls

Serotonin release is regulated by 5-HT$_{1A}$ presynaptic somatodendritic autoreceptors that inhibit serotonergic firing and decrease serotonergic tone within cortical targets. We and others have mapped 5-HT$_{1A}$ receptor binding and presynaptic SERT binding in the human DRN using quantitative receptor autoradiography (Arango et al., 2001; Bligh-Glover et al., 2000; Boldrini et al., 2008). We find fewer SERT-expressing DRN neurons and less 5-HT$_{1A}$ autoreceptor binding in the DRN of depressed suicides compared to non-psychiatric controls (Arango et al., 2001; Boldrini et al., 2008), indicative of homeostatic changes in serotonergic neurons consistent with upregulatory responses that would serve to enhance serotonergic neuron firing and slow reuptake in terminal fields to amplify the 5-HT signal. 5-HT$_{1A}$ binding was shown to be higher in the rostral 5 mm of the DRN of depressed suicides by other investigators (Stockmeier et al., 1998). These apparently discrepant findings were reconciled by a study (Boldrini et al., 2008) that shows higher 5-HT$_{1A}$ binding in the rostral 5 mm of the DRN in suicides and lower binding in the remaining caudal 15 mm. Females have higher 5-HT$_{1A}$ binding than males both postmortem and *in vivo* demonstrated by PET, highlighting the importance of matching controls and patient samples for sex and other demographic traits.

Neuronal tryptophan hydroxylase (TPH2)

In an attempt to determine whether the lower 5-HT neurotransmission reported in suicide is due to fewer serotonin-synthesizing neurons, we estimated the number of phenylalanine hydroxylase-immunoreactive neurons (PH8-IR), an enzyme that cross-reacts with TPH in the raphe nuclei of suicides, and determined that suicides have more serotonergic neurons than controls and a higher optical density of PH8-IR in the DRN (Underwood et al., 1999). The finding of higher TPH optical density (more TPH enzyme) was replicated using a different cohort and the more quantitative technique of immuno-autoradiography

(Boldrini et al., 2005). Another group reported no change in TPH protein (PH8) expression in depressed suicides (Bonkale et al., 2004), but found greater expression in the dorsal subnucleus of the DRN of depressed suicides who were also alcohol-dependent. The inconsistency in immuno-autoradiography findings may be explained by differences in methodologies. Bonkale et al. (2004) sampled five representative rostral sections while our group sampled the entire DRN at 1 mm intervals, thereby increasing the possibility of detecting changes in expression in the whole nucleus.

TPH is not a single gene product and there are two isoforms: a neuronal (TPH2) and a non-neuronal (TPH1) isoform. As the rate-limiting enzyme, TPH2 determines the amount of serotonin synthesized in vivo. We developed TPH2 riboprobes for the measurement of TPH2 mRNA in the DRN and MRN of humans (Bach-Mizrachi et al., 2006) and we carried out *in situ* hybridization assays (see Figure 34.1 in Bach-Mizrachi et al., 2006). Consistent with our previous findings using different methodologies (Boldrini et al., 2005; Underwood et al., 1999), we reported that TPH2 mRNA expression was elevated in depressed suicides compared to matched non-psychiatric controls and further that the serotonin-synthesizing neurons in suicide had higher transcriptional capacity (Bach-Mizrachi et al., 2006). We further mapped TPH2 mRNA expression across the antero-posterior axis of the DRN and MRN and showed that TPH2 is elevated at all levels of the DRN but is more pronounced at caudal neuroanatomical levels including the caudal subnucleus. More TPH-IR neurons (Underwood et al., 1999), when taken together with more TPH protein (Boldrini et al., 2005; Underwood et al., 1999) and more TPH2 mRNA (Bach-Mizrachi et al., 2006), would favor higher 5-HT levels and yet, as discussed earlier in this chapter, most studies of suicide report lower serotonergic neurotransmission.

Lower 5-HT levels in depressed suicides and lower CSF 5-HIAA suggest a compensatory mechanism in which the enzyme level may be increased but catalytic activity or release of 5-HT is impaired. Inefficient catalytic activity may stem from a functional mutation in the TPH2 gene; however, to date there is only one functional yet rare SNP in the human TPH2 gene that affects TPH2 catalytic activity. While this SNP was shown to be associated with MDD in one population, the association was not found in any of the several other studies that attempted to replicate this finding. While an undiscovered functional SNP in the TPH2 gene may still remain a reasonable explanation for deficits in TPH2 catalytic activity, it should be noted that TPH2 function is dependent on a number of factors including phosphorylation state, regulation by signal transduction pathways, presence of cofactors and adapters, and potentially other regulatory TPH2 isoforms (Haghighi et al., 2008). These mechanisms likely regulate TPH2 catalytic activity by gauging brain 5-HT levels and therefore in suicides where serotonin is low, TPH2 message and protein are upregulated.

Because of the discrepancies in serotonergic findings in the brainstem *versus* the cortex, especially given the findings of increases in multiple serotonergic markers in the DRN of suicides, we thought the validation of the early findings of less 5-HT and 5-HIAA was critical. To this end, as reported recently (Bach et al., 2013), we used HPLC to measure 5-HT and 5-HIAA in 60 μm brainstem sections every 1 mm throughout the DRN. Sections were adjacent to those used for the TPH2 mRNA assays. We showed that our method reliably detects 5-HT in postmortem brain tissue and the distribution of the amounts of 5-HT are consistent with the neuroanatomical organization of the DRN and MRN where rostral sections have more 5-HT than caudal sections (See Figure 34.1A). Compared with non-psychiatric control cases, suicides had four times as much total 5-HT and one and a half times more 5-HIAA. The difference in 5-HT between controls and suicides was present throughout the rostrocaudal extent of the brainstem samples.

Environmental factors affecting TPH2

The clinical literature describes many environmental risk factors for suicide. Among them, early life neglect and cigarette smoking are strong predictors of the development of psychiatric illness and suicidal behavior. As part of the structured clinical interview that is obtained from the next-of-kin, data regarding early life stress such as divorce, death of a parent, or physical and sexual abuse, in addition to information about cigarette smoking habits, are obtained. This allows the opportunity to determine whether there is an association between biochemical changes in the serotonin system with environmental factors. TPH2 is a stress-sensitive enzyme and is upregulated in rodents in response to environmental stressors such as social defeat or maternal neglect. Further, TPH2 levels fluctuate with the diurnal changes in cortisol and are affected by stress-induced HPA axis cortisol release (Donner et al., 2012). Cigarette smoking affects the release of brain serotonin and subsequently has anxiolytic effects on behavior. Therefore we sought to determine the relationship between these factors and TPH2 expression in suicides. In suicides with reported early life neglect, TPH2 mRNA is higher in the DRN than suicides without early life neglect, similar to what is seen in rodent studies (Gardner et al., 2009). Interestingly, we found that cigarette smoking was not associated with increased TPH2 expression in suicides. Smokers, both non-psychiatric controls and suicides, had less TPH2 expression than suicide non-smokers. These data suggest that TPH2 upregulation is specifically sensitive to stressful environmental factors such as early life neglect in suicide and not cigarette smoking, which may be anxiolytic.

Regulation of TPH2

Isoforms of tryptophan hydroxylase, TPH1 and TPH2, share substantial homology, with the exception of the first 41 amino acids in the N-terminal regulatory domain which are unique in each isoform. The regulatory domains of other members of this family, such as tyrosine hydroxylase, have been shown to modulate enzymatic activity and thermostability through several mechanisms including phosphorylation by protein kinases. Several studies have shown that TPH2 is phosphorylated within its regulatory domain by protein kinase A (PKA) and that this phosphorylation increases catalytic activity. Direct phosphorylation by PKA occurs on serine-58 within the regulatory domain of TPH2 so that increases in concentrations of PKA result in increased enzymatic activity. This PKA-directed regulation of TPH2 catalytic activity, specifically at serine 19, implicates this kinase as a potential source for the deficits in serotonin seen in suicides and in other psychiatric illnesses. Post-translational phosphorylation is a critical regulator of TPH2 catalytic activity and signaling cascades involving PKA likely regulate *de novo* synthesis of serotonin. We find less PKA in the DRN/MRN of suicides compared to controls, and others find less PKA in the prefrontal cortex of suicides (Dwivedi & Pandey, 2011) suggesting less phosphorylation of TPH2 in the brainstem or locally in serotonergic terminals in the cortex.

The serotonin autoreceptors gauge synaptic serotonin levels and feedback on the firing neuron to inhibit further transmission. One of the downstream signaling pathways activated by serotonin receptor stimulation is the glycogen synthase kinase 3 (GSK 3) signaling pathway. It has recently been shown that the GSK3 signaling pathway is modulated by changes in TPH2 catalytic activity (Beaulieu et al., 2008), such that reduction in serotonin synthesis results in activation of GSK3 signaling. GSK3 is also directly inhibited *in vivo* by lithium which is often used in combination with antidepressants for the management of certain mood disorders. The neuroprotective effects of lithium involve downregulation of GSK3 activity. Consistent with this, we and others find more GSK3 protein in suicides compared to non-psychiatric controls.

Summary and conclusions

Serotonin neurons in the DRN and MRN are anatomically and neurochemically distinct. Subdivided by their cytoarchitecture, serotonin neurons in the DRN subnuclei are designed to project to specific cortical targets that will ultimately regulate complex serotonin-dependent behaviors. We propose a molecular biological model (Figure 34.2) in suicide in which there is an imbalance in select signal transduction pathways specific to the DRN that will control 5-HT synthesis *via* regulation of TPH2 protein expression and catalytic activity that will also affect serotonin release and neurotransmission in the cortex. Further studies measuring TPH2 regulation by these signaling pathways within individual DRN subnuclei will elucidate the relationship between the neuroanatomical and neurochemical profiles of serotonergic neurons. Additionally, it has become evident that the molecular pathophysiology of suicide involves a disconnect between serotonin-synthesizing neurons in the brainstem and their targets in the prefrontal cortex. This disconnect may be contributed to by environmental factors such as early life experience, cigarette smoking, and HPA axis stress response. Further studies will tease out the individual effects of these factors on the pathophysiology of suicidal behaviors either independent from or in conjunction with comorbid diagnoses such as major depressive disorder.

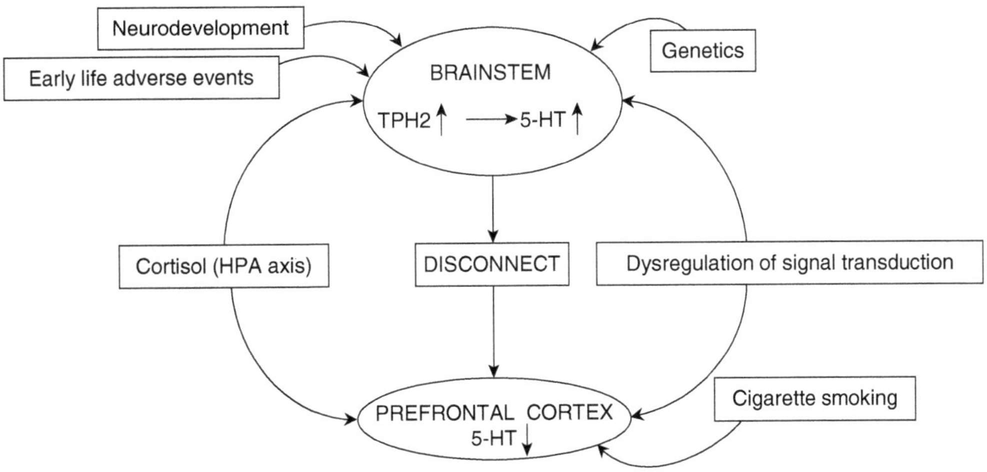

Figure 34.2. Diagram of contributors to serotonin dysregulation between the brainstem and prefrontal cortex of suicides. TPH2 and subsequent serotonin upregulation in the brainstem may be a product of neurodevelopment (more serotonin neurons), a response to early life adversity, and genetic predisposition. Additional contribution to high serotonin in the brainstem and low serotonin in the prefrontal cortex is a maladaptive stress response regulated by the HPA axis and alterations in regulatory signaling pathways. Cigarette smoking is an additional factor that contributes to low cortical serotonin but is not involved in increasing TPH2 in the brainstem. Taken together the high serotonin in the brainstem and low serotonin in the cortex in suicides suggests a disconnect (inefficient serotonin release or transport) between these two brain regions.

References

Arango, V., & Mann, J. J. (1992). Relevance of serotonergic postmortem studies to suicidal behavior. *International Review of Psychiatry*, **4**, 131–140.

Arango, V., Ernsberger, P., Marzuk, P. M., et al. (1990). Autoradiographic demonstration of increased serotonin 5-HT2 and beta-adrenergic receptor binding sites in the brain of suicide victims. *Archives of General Psychiatry*, **47**(11), 1038–1047.

Arango, V., Underwood, M. D., Gubbi, A. V., & Mann, J. J. (1995). Localized alterations in pre- and postsynaptic serotonin binding sites in the ventrolateral prefrontal cortex of suicide victims. *Brain Research*, **688**(1–2), 121–133.

Arango, V., Underwood, M. D., Boldrini, M., et al. (2001). Serotonin 1A receptors, serotonin transporter binding and serotonin transporter mRNA expression in the brainstem of depressed suicide victims. *Neuropsychopharmacology*, **25**(6), 892–903.

Arango, V., Underwood, M. D., & Mann, J. J. (2002). Serotonin brain circuits involved in major depression and suicide. *Progress in Brain Research*, **136**, 443–453.

Åsberg, M., Träskman, L., & Thorén, P. (1976). 5-HIAA in the cerebrospinal fluid: A biochemical suicide predictor? *Archives of General Psychiatry*, **33**(10), 1193–1197.

Bach, H., Huang, Y. Y., Underwood, M. D., et al. (2013). Elevated serotonin and 5-HIAA in the brainstem and lower serotonin turnover in the prefrontal cortex of suicides, *Synapse*. Jun 29. doi: 10.1002/syn.21695. [Epub ahead of print].

Bach-Mizrachi, H., Underwood, M. D., Kassir, S. A., et al. (2006). Neuronal tryptophan hydroxylase mRNA expression in the human dorsal and median raphe nuclei: major depression and suicide. *Neuropsychopharmacology*, **31**(4), 814–824.

Beaulieu, J. M., Zhang, X., Rodriguiz, R. M., et al. (2008). Role of GSK3beta in behavioral abnormalities induced by serotonin deficiency. *Proceedings of the National Academy of Sciences of the United States of America*, **105**(4), 1333–1338.

Bligh-Glover, W., Kolli, T. N., Shapiro-Kulnane, L., et al. (2000). The serotonin transporter in the midbrain of suicide victims with major depression. *Biological Psychiatry*, **47**, 1015–1024.

Boldrini, M., Underwood, M. D., Mann, J. J., & Arango, V. (2005). More tryptophan hydroxylase in the brainstem dorsal raphe nucleus in depressed suicides. *Brain Research*, **1041**(1), 19–28.

Boldrini, M., Underwood, M. D., Mann, J. J., & Arango, V. (2008). Serotonin-1A autoreceptor binding in the dorsal raphe nucleus of depressed suicides. *Journal of Psychiatric Research*, **42**(6), 433–442.

Bonkale, W. L., Murdock, S., Janosky, J. E., & Austin, M. C. (2004). Normal levels of tryptophan hydroxylase immunoreactivity in the dorsal raphe of depressed suicide victims. *Journal of Neurochemistry*, **88**(4), 958–964.

Donner, N. C., Johnson, P. L., Fitz, S. D., et al. (2012). Elevated tph2 mRNA expression in a rat model of chronic anxiety. *Depression and Anxiety*, **29**(4), 307–319.

Dwivedi, Y. & Pandey, G. N. (2011). Elucidating biological risk factors in suicide: role of protein kinase A. *Progress in Neuropsychopharmacology and Biological Psychiatry*, **35**(4), 831–841.

Gardner, K. L., Hale, M. W., Oldfield, S., et al. (2009). Adverse experience during early life and adulthood interact to elevate tph2 mRNA expression in serotonergic neurons within the dorsal raphe nucleus. *Neuroscience*, **163**(4), 991–1001.

Haghighi, F., Bach-Mizrachi, H., Huang, Y. Y., et al. (2008). Genetic architecture of the human tryptophan hydroxylase 2 gene: existence of neural isoforms and relevance for major depression. *Molecular Psychiatry*, **13**(8), 813–820.

Hrdina, P. D., Demeter, E., Vu, T. B., Sótónyi, P., & Palkovits, M. (1993). 5-HT uptake sites and 5-HT2 receptors in brain of antidepressant-free suicide victims/depressives: Increase in 5- HT2 sites in cortex and amygdala. *Brain Research*, **614**, 37–44.

Mann, J. J., Stanley, M., McBride, P. A., & McEwen, B. S. (1986). Increased serotonin2 and beta-adrenergic receptor binding in the frontal cortices of suicide victims. *Archives of General Psychiatry*, **43**(10), 954–959.

Mann, J. J., Huang, Y. Y., Underwood, M. D., et al. (2000). A serotonin transporter gene promoter polymorphism (5-HTTLPR) and prefrontal cortical binding in major depression and suicide. *Archives of General Psychiatry*, **57**(8), 729–738.

Mann, J. J., Brent, D. A., & Arango, V. (2001). The neurobiology and genetics of suicide and attempted suicide: a focus on the serotonergic system. *Neuropsychopharmacology*, **24**(5), 467–477.

Pandey, G. N., Dwivedi, Y., Rizavi, H. S., et al. (2002). Higher expression of serotonin 5-HT(2A) receptors in the postmortem brains of teenage suicide victims. *American Journal of Psychiatry*, **159**(3), 419–429.

Parsey, R. V., Hastings, R. S., Oquendo, M. A., et al. (2006). Lower serotonin transporter binding potential in the human brain during major depressive episodes. *American Journal of Psychiatry*, **163**(1), 52–58.

Stanley, M., & Mann, J. J. (1983). Increased serotonin-2 binding sites in frontal cortex of suicide victims. *Lancet*, **1**(8318), 214–216.

Stockmeier, C. A., Dilley, G. E., Shapiro, L. A., et al. (1997). Serotonin receptors in suicide victims with major depression. *Neuropsychopharmacology*, **16**(2), 162–173.

Stockmeier, C. A., Shapiro, L. A., Dilley, G. E., et al. (1998). Increase in serotonin-1A autoreceptors in the midbrain of suicide victims with major depression-postmortem evidence for decreased serotonin activity. *Journal of Neuroscience*, **18**(18), 7394–7401.

Stockmeier, C. A., Howley, E., Shi, X., et al. (2009). Antagonist but not agonist labeling of serotonin-1A receptors is decreased in major depressive disorder. *Journal of Psychiatric Research*, **43**(10), 887–894.

Turecki, G., Briere, R., Dewar, K., et al. (1999). Prediction of level of serotonin 2A receptor binding by serotonin receptor 2A genetic variation in postmortem brain samples from subjects who did or did not commit suicide. *American Journal of Psychiatry*, **156**(9), 1456–1458.

Underwood, M. D., Khaibulina, A. A., Ellis, S. P., et al. (1999). Morphometry of the dorsal raphe nucleus serotonergic neurons in suicide victims. *Biological Psychiatry*, **46**(4), 473–483.

Underwood, M. D., Kassir, S. A., Bakalian, M. J., Galfalvy, H., Mann, J. J., & Arango, V. (2012). Neuron density and serotonin receptor binding in prefrontal cortex in suicide. *International Journal of Neuropsychopharmacology*, **15**(4), 435–447.

Chapter

35 The noradrenergic system in depression and suicide

Michelle J. Chandley and Gregory A. Ordway

Introduction

Suicide is a tragic outcome that is influenced by a complex set of interactive variables such as genetics, environmental events, and developmental factors. Approximately 90% of all people who commit suicide have a diagnosable mental illness, including major depressive disorder and bipolar depression. This would suggest that the greatest hope of preventing suicide lies in improved treatment and/or management of associated psychiatric disorders. Since 80% of all suicide victims suffered premortem depressive symptoms, one critical area of research development would seem to be the search for improved antidepressant treatments. By extension, one would assume that a better understanding of the pathobiology of depression and suicide will lead to the discovery of new therapeutic targets for treatment. Currently, the most widely accepted neurobiological correlate of depression and suicide is the central monoamine theory, which implicates deficiencies of the monoamines norepinephrine (NE) and serotonin in depression and suicide. Unfortunately, this theory is based heavily on the mechanism of action of currently marketed antidepressant drugs, drugs that have far less than ideal effectiveness. Nevertheless, a vast literature demonstrates that both NE and serotonin do play a role, at least in part, in the pathology of depression and suicide. This chapter focuses on the putative role of NE in the pathobiology associated with suicide, recognizing that dysfunction in this neurotransmitter system is only one part of a complex neurobiological pathology contributing to suicide.

Brain NE is synthesized from the amino acid, tyrosine. The majority of NE synthesized in the brain occurs in neuromelanin-containing cells and their terminals. The cell bodies of these neurons are located in the locus coeruleus (LC) of the pons. The LC is found on the floor of the fourth ventricle in the brainstem. The activity of LC noradrenergic neurons is an extremely organized process that is regulated by multiple neurochemical inputs including glutamate, serotonin, GABA, substance P, corticotropin-releasing factor, glycine, orexin, dopamine, and enkephalin. Noradrenergic projections leave the LC via distinct tracts that innervate both the higher centers of the brain and spinal cord. Because NE is found in almost every region of the brain, the release of NE at neuronal terminals and en passant synapses along NE fibers influences neuronal and glial activity in target areas through noradrenergic receptors (Figure 35.1), and thereby modulates numerous cellular functions and ultimately human behaviors.

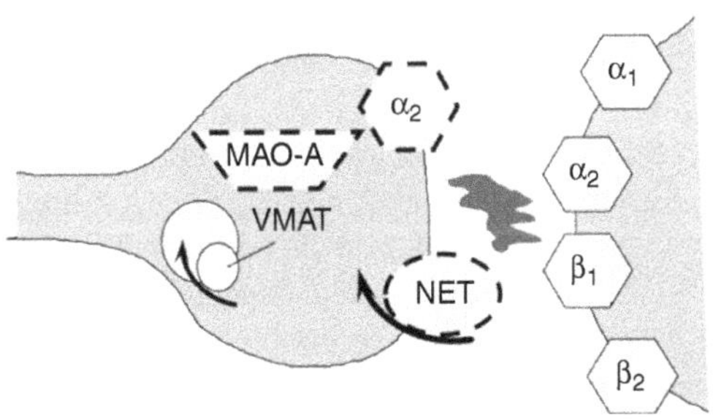

Figure 35.1. Schematic representation of a noradrenergic synapse. NE released from the presynaptic bouton enters the synapse to interact with receptors (α_1, α_2, β_1, and β_2 subtypes) that transmit information to the postsynaptic cell. Several different types of cells in the brain express noradrenergic receptors, including neurons, astrocytes, oligodendrocytes, and vascular endothelial cells. The autoreceptor on the NE neuron is the α_2 adrenergic receptor, which transmits feedback inhibition of NE neuronal firing and NE release. The action of NE is terminated by transport back into the terminal via the NE transporter (NET), where NE is further transported into storage vesicles by the vesicular monoamine transporter (VMAT). NE that does not get transported for storage into vesicles is susceptible to degradation by monoamine oxidase A (MAO-A). Proteins with dashed borders are sites of action of currently available antidepressant drugs, which antagonize the function of these proteins and thereby elevate the synaptic availability of NE.

A *Concise Guide to Understanding Suicide*, ed. Stephen H. Koslow, Pedro Ruiz, and Charles B. Nemeroff. Published by Cambridge University Press.

Behaviors modified by noradrenergic activity include stress-related behavior, cognition, arousal, memory, and sleep. Studies using laboratory animals have shown that disruptions in noradrenergic activity are associated with poor concentration, apathy, insomnia, memory deficits, and depressive symptoms – all of which are often behavioral components of suicide (Chandley & Ordway, 2012). Furthermore, depression and suicide are strongly linked to psychological stress, and stress has robust effects on brain NE. Stress elevates the firing of noradrenergic LC neurons via a variety of stress-sensitive neurotransmitter inputs to the LC, particularly CRF, glutamate, and substance P. Sustained activation of the LC as a result of chronic stress can result in a depletion of NE. Since neuronal release and firing of noradrenergic neurons is reduced by activation of presynaptic α_2 adrenergic receptors (autoreceptors) by NE, depletion of NE contributes further to elevated LC activity and further elevated demand for synaptic NE. Hence, it seems reasonable that chronic stress experienced by humans may result in NE depletion, which may in turn contribute to depression and ultimately to elevated risk of suicide. The results of decades of research on NE in depression and suicide implies that multiple biological, genetic, environmental, and/or developmental factors converge to raise vulnerability to depression and suicide, with NE being one of the key contributory factors (see Figure 35.1).

The following chapter provides insight into the pathological changes of the noradrenergic system associated with suicide and how therapeutically modulating levels of NE can have beneficial effects in treating those patients with an underlying mood disorder that may lead to suicide.

Noradrenergic neurochemistry in depression and suicide

NE

Pharmacological depletion of NE in humans does not cause the development of depressive behaviors in antidepressant drug-free psychiatrically normal subjects lacking a history of depression, nor in patients with other diagnosed mental illnesses, and it does not worsen the depressive state of depressed patients. Nevertheless, depletion of NE in antidepressant-free patients that are euthymic but have a history of depression induces depressive relapse (Berman et al., 1999). This observation demonstrates the direct link of NE depletion with depression, but simultaneously indicates that other biological factors are likely to play a contributory role in making patients susceptible to NE depletion-induced depression. By extension, since stress induces NE depletion, it is reasonable to speculate that stress-induced NE depletion will result in depression in individuals who are behaviorally, biologically, and/or genetically susceptible. Consistent with a link to suicide is the finding that low CSF levels of the NE metabolite, MHPG, were observed in patients with higher risk of suicide attempts and with greater lethality of suicide attempts (Galfalvy et al., 2009). While the link between NE and depression is strong, further research is needed to investigate the link between low brain NE and suicide or suicidal behavior.

Tyrosine hydroxylase

Tyrosine hydroxylase (TH) is the rate-limiting enzyme in the biosynthesis of NE. A variety of biological factors and drugs regulate TH at the level of gene expression and post-translational modifications. Factors that increase TH expression and/or TH activity include stress hormones such as CRF and glucocorticoids. In addition, depletion of NE as a result of chronic stress or administration of NE-depleting pharmacological agents results in an elevation of TH activity and protein. It is presumed that the elevation of TH following depletion of NE is an adaptive mechanism to overcome the neurotransmitter deficit. Reduced TH expression occurs after repeated treatment of rats with antidepressant drugs, regardless of the pharmacological class. The mechanism for this effect is not fully understood but is likely to be related to a reduced need for NE since these drugs, including SSRIs, selective NE reuptake inhibitors (SNRIs), and NE reuptake inhibitors (NRIs), reduce noradrenergic neuron activity in the LC and/or elevate the synaptic availability of NE in LC projection areas (as reviewed by Ordway, 1997).

Given the pivotal role of TH regulation in noradrenergic transmission, TH has been of interest to researchers studying the neuropathology of depression and suicide. For example, our laboratory demonstrated elevated TH protein levels in LC tissue collected from postmortem brains of antidepressant-free victims of suicide when compared to that from control subjects (Ordway, 1997). In a later study, we found elevated TH in the LC of subjects with a psychiatric diagnosis of major depression at the time of death (and without antidepressant drugs) when comparing these subjects to psychiatrically normal control subjects (Zhu et al., 1999), demonstrating that elevated TH is associated with both suicide and major depressive disorder. More recently, Gos et al. reported elevated TH in the LC of violent suicide victims compared to control subjects (Gos et al., 2008). A logical interpretation of these human postmortem studies is that there is an increased premortem demand for NE (perhaps unmet) in depression and suicide, possibly as a result of a stress-induced increase in central noradrenergic neuronal activity and local depletion of NE in the LC. This interpretation is supported by laboratory animal experimentation demonstrating that chronic stress produces a robust local depletion of NE in the LC.

Monoamine oxidases

Another mechanism at play that determines the relative availability of NE in the synapse is the enzymatic degradation of NE. Monoamine oxidase (MAO-A) in noradrenergic neurons converts cytosolic NE to an inactive metabolite, a reaction that does not occur if NE is protected by uptake into synaptic vesicles. It seems conceivable that elevated levels of MAO-A could result in reduced NE in the brain. As for TH, the role of MAO-A in the catabolism of NE has made it a target of investigation with respect to depression and suicide particularly because serotonin is also a substrate of MAO-A. The promoter region of MAO-A has multiple glucocorticoid response elements that interact with transcriptional activators and repressors making MAO-A susceptible to stress-induced changes. As shown in both animals and cell models, the synthetic glucocorticoid, dexamethasone, can increase MAO-A levels (Duncan et al., 2012). However, examination of MAO-A protein expression levels in postmortem brain tissues from depressed subjects or suicide victims has yielded inconsistent findings of decreased or unchanged levels, while PET imaging of MAO-A has indicated elevated levels in depression (Meyer, 2012). Treatment with MAO inhibitors is effective for depression even if alterations of MAO are not a core pathophysiological feature (see below).

Norepinephrine transporter

Almost 90% of all synaptic NE undergoes reuptake by the NE transporter. The NE transporter is a single unit protein found in the cellular membrane of presynaptic nerve terminals, dendrites, and the cell body of only noradrenergic neurons. Early reports indicate that both restraint stress and pharmacological depletion of NE in rats decreased NE transporter binding and presumably decreased NE transporter protein (as reviewed by Mandela & Ordway, 2006). This information suggests that a decrease in NE transporter expression is a compensatory action designed to enhance NE signaling during stress-induced depressive behaviors. In a study of major depressive disorder using postmortem LC tissue, where 13 of the 15 depressive subjects died by suicide, binding to the NE transporter was significantly reduced by approximately 25% (Mandela & Ordway, 2006). Based on depletion and stress studies in rodents, the postmortem human studies again suggest that depression and suicide are associated with a depletion of NE. Interestingly, NE transporter knockout mice demonstrate fewer depressive-like behaviors than control mice, and NE transporter knockout mice exhibit more resiliency during stress (Mandela & Ordway, 2006). This latter finding is not unexpected since drugs that block the function of the NE transporter have antidepressant properties (see below).

α_1 adrenergic receptors

There are three subtypes of α_1 adrenergic receptors, α_{1A}, α_{1B}, and α_{1D}. α_{1B} adrenergic receptors have been identified in the human cerebral cortex, while α_{1A} and α_{1D} have been shown in cortex, hippocampus, thalamus, caudate, and amygdala (De Paermentier et al., 1997). As a subclass, the α-adrenergic receptors directly activate calcium channels or can act through phospholipase C to catalyze downstream events thought to participate in a variety of behaviors including motor control and cognition (Stone et al., 2009). No differences in the levels of protein expression of α_{1A} and α_{1D} adrenergic receptors have been observed in postmortem brain tissues comparing depressed suicide subjects to psychiatrically normal controls (De Paermentier et al., 1997). Our laboratory has also measured binding to α_1 adrenergic receptors in brains from depressed suicide victims and have observed no differences relative to normal control subjects (unpublished findings). Although postmortem findings do not demonstrate evidence of involvement of α_1 adrenergic receptors in depression and suicide, animal studies have demonstrated a distinct role of these receptors in the inhibition of stress-induced activation of the LC (Stone et al., 2009). This latter finding demonstrates the need for more research on the putative role of α_1 adrenergic receptors in the neurobiology of depression and suicide, and the potential to utilize these receptors in the pharmacological management of mood disorders associated with suicide.

α_2 adrenergic receptors

α_2 adrenergic receptors are found throughout the human brain with both human and animal studies demonstrating cellular localization in multiple cell types, including postsynaptic neurons, presynaptic noradrenergic neurons, and glia. There are three subtypes of α_2 adrenergic receptors (α_{2A}, α_{2B}, and α_{2C}) in the human brain with the α_{2A} subtype being the most abundant and the α_{2B} being the least abundant. α_2 adrenergic receptors occurring on noradrenergic neurons are considered autoreceptors because their activation by NE inhibits further release of NE or inhibits noradrenergic neuronal firing. Both α_{2A} and α_{2C} adrenergic receptors occur on axons, dendrites, and cell bodies of NE-containing neurons; all three subtypes occur postsynaptically on other neurons and cells of the brain.

Given their important role in regulating NE release, α_2 adrenergic receptors have been studied extensively with respect to the biology of depression and suicide. Numerous researchers have measured radioligand binding to α_2 adrenergic receptors in postmortem brain tissues from suicide victims. It has been attractive to assume that binding to α_2 adrenergic receptors in human postmortem tissue represents binding to the presynaptic α_2 autoreceptor. However, our research has shown that when one measures radioligand binding to α_2 adrenergic receptors in a projection area of the LC, most of that binding is to α_2 adrenergic receptors on postsynaptic cells (probably neurons as well as glia). In contrast, radioligand binding to α_2 adrenergic receptors in the immediate region of the LC is most likely to receptors that are on noradrenergic neurons. With this in mind, elevated radioligand binding to α_2 adrenergic receptors has been found in the LC, as well as in LC projection areas (presumably reflecting increased presynaptic and postsynaptic receptor binding).

Regardless of the cellular location, elevations in radioligand binding to α_2 adrenergic receptors (reflecting more receptors or higher activity of these receptors) have been reported in brain tissues from depressed suicide victims when compared to that from control subjects. These findings have been interpreted as evidence of premortem enhanced inhibition of NE release (resulting in less synaptic NE), or alternatively, adaptive upregulation of α_2 adrenergic receptors (as a result of less synaptic NE). With regard to the latter, depletion of NE results in an upregulation of α_2 adrenergic receptors. Hence, elevated brain α_2 adrenergic receptors in suicide victims and depressed subjects may be reflective of a premortem depletion of NE. The regulation of α_2 adrenergic receptors as an adaptation to stress may play a role in behavioral deficits since these receptors in the LC are regulated differently in rodents resilient to stress-induced behavioral depression as compared to rats that develop stress-induced behavioral depression (Taneja et al., 2011).

It is interesting to note that functional genetic polymorphisms of α_2 adrenergic receptors have been identified. A recent study reported an association between a four consecutive amino acid deletion in the coding region of the α_{2C} adrenergic receptor and hyperactivity in the amygdala and anterior cingulate cortex in depressed patients examined during facial expression tests (Neumeister et al., 2006). Interestingly, one genomic study has identified a polymorphism that involves an amino acid switch in the α_{2A} adrenergic receptor that exists in a small population of suicide victims (Sequeira et al., 2004).

β-adrenergic receptors

There are three β adrenergic receptor subtypes (β_1, β_2, and β_3) that couple to adenylyl cyclase via G proteins to produce intracellular cAMP. In the CNS, only β_1 and β_2 receptor subtypes have been identified where both receptor subtypes are found widespread throughout the brain with the β_2 adrenergic receptor expressed more densely in the cerebellum. β adrenergic receptors have been one of the most studied proteins in research using postmortem brain tissues from victims of suicide to unearth potential pathology of the central noradrenergic system. However, the results of these findings have yielded no firm conclusions. Early binding studies reported increases and decreases of β adrenergic binding using postmortem tissue from suicide victims with later studies failing to identify any changes in postmortem tissue (Ordway, 2007). Animal studies involving β adrenergic receptor expression in response to stress have not clarified the pathophysiology of these receptors in behaviors associated with depression and suicide.

Therapeutic management of depression and suicide by manipulating NE signaling

An effective treatment modality to prevent suicide is pharmacological management of associated psychiatric disorders. Currently available antidepressant drugs are compounds that primarily modulate serotonergic and/or noradrenergic transmission. These drugs include MAOIs, tricyclic antidepressants (TCAs), SSRIs, SNRIs, NRIs, and α_2 adrenergic receptor antagonists. In addition to these drug classes, some atypical antipsychotics have also recently been approved for management of mood disorders including bipolar and major depressive disorder. The most simplistic mechanism of action described for these drugs is that they work to increase the synaptic availability of NE (Figure 35.1) and/or serotonin. These actions are acute, i.e., occur after a single dose, but therapeutic benefit does not occur until the drugs are taken for several days to weeks. Some have argued that the delayed therapeutic effect of antidepressant drugs indicates that it is not the elevation of synaptic neurotransmitter that is critical to the mechanism of action of the drugs. Since the discovery that repeated, but not acute, treatment of rats with imipramine (Frazer et al., 1978) desensitizes β adrenergic receptor-activated adenylyl cyclase, a vast array of downstream events have been identified that occur following repeated antidepressant treatment of rodents (Frazer, 2000). Many of these downstream events have been proposed to be the "final common pathway" of antidepressant drug action.

Given the vast literature indicating that NE plays a role in pathophysiology of depression, it is interesting to consider how drugs with proven antidepressant efficacy modulate brain NE. With enhanced synaptic NE signaling as a shared effect of all classes of antidepressants, central noradrenergic function should be strongly considered when therapeutically modifying behaviors that may lead to suicide. The following discussion considers how several classes of antidepressants affect noradrenergic function.

MAO inhibitors

These drugs, which include phenylzine, tranylcypromine, and selegiline, inhibit the catabolic oxidation of NE (and other monoamines). The use of MAO inhibitors as antidepressants began in the 1950s when patients taking isoniazid for tuberculosis experienced a reduction of depressive symptoms. Evidence indicating that these drugs enhance noradrenergic transmission derives from studies in rodents demonstrating regulation of noradrenergic proteins following MAO inhibitor treatment that is typical of sustained elevated NE receptor signaling, such as adaptive downregulations of β and α_2 adrenergic receptors and downregulation of TH (Rovin et al., 2012). At least in part due to an elevation of synaptic NE and feedback inhibition through α_2 adrenergic receptors on NE neurons, treatment of rodents with MAO inhibitors reduces noradrenergic LC activity similar to other antidepressants. Many clinicians are hesitant to prescribe MAO inhibitors due to the possible induction of hypertensive events and interaction with other medications; however, their efficacy is well established in the treatment of depressive disorders.

Tricyclic antidepressants

Tricyclic antidepressants (TCAs) were also discovered in the 1950s. Most of these compounds block uptake or transport of NE from the synapse to the cytosol by binding to and inhibiting the function of NE transporters on noradrenergic neurons. As a subclass, TCAs with a secondary, rather than tertiary, nitrogen group on the side chain of the molecule have a higher affinity for NE transporters than serotonin transporters. As a result of sustained elevation of synaptic NE, repeated treatment with TCAs (e.g., desipramine) downregulates postsynaptic NE receptors in many brain regions, and reduces TH protein in LC neurons. Like other antidepressants, TCAs reduce the activity of noradrenergic LC neurons. In addition, TCAs also downregulate the NE transporter itself, contributing to further reduced NE uptake and presumably facilitating antidepressant drug action. If NE is depleted prior to or during administration of a TCA, the downregulation of NE receptors does not occur. NE depletion also blocks TCA-induced antidepressant-like effects on rodent behaviors that model human depression (Zhao et al., 2008), and NE depletion in humans causes rapid relapse into depression in patients taking noradrenergic enhancing antidepressants (Booij et al., 2003). Interestingly, treatment with desipramine is associated with lower suicide scale scores in a subpopulation of patients (Sharma et al., 2007), suggesting that these drugs may have direct anti-suicide effects.

Selective reuptake inhibitors

Reuptake inhibitors, or transporter inhibitors, that selectively bind NE and/or serotonin transporters are currently the first choice of drugs for the treatment of depression. This is not due to a higher efficacy of these newer uptake inhibitors, but instead because these drugs are safer and lack complicated side effects associated with MAO inhibitors and TCAs. The selective reuptake inhibitors range from selective for NE, varying relative selectivity for NE and serotonin transporters, and selectivity for serotonin transporters. NE transporter-selective drugs produce similar effects on NE neurons as TCAs that have selectivity for NE transporters, including downregulating NE receptors and TH, and reduction of noradrenergic LC activity. Interestingly, the serotonin selective drugs also have profound effects on NE neurons. The mechanism by which this occurs is not entirely understood, although there is a dense innervation of the noradrenergic LC by serotonergic neurons of the raphe nuclei. Serotonin has complex acute effects on the LC activity, mediated in part by serotonergic modulation of excitatory afferents projecting to the LC, such as excitatory glutamatergic neurons. As a result, repeated treatment of rodents with all classes of reuptake inhibitors including mixed NE/serotonin uptake inhibitors and SSRIs reduce the firing of noradrenergic LC neurons (Grant & Weiss, 2001). Hence, these drugs, like TCAs and MAO inhibitors, reduce the activity of the LC.

A reasonable interpretation of the literature regarding the mechanism of action of uptake inhibitor antidepressants is that these drugs stabilize noradrenergic neuronal activity, especially during periods of stress that might normally result in sustained increases or over-activation of the LC and ultimately depletion of NE. It may sound contradictory that depression is associated with fewer NE transporters as noted above while an effective treatment for depression is to block the NE transporter. We believe the reduced NE transporter binding that is found in depressed suicides is adaptive to the depletion of NE and that this reduction is inadequate to compensate and protect the individual from the dire behavioral consequences of NE depletion. Treatment with NET inhibitor antidepressants produces a much higher (~90%) reduction in the function of the NE transporter, ultimately resulting in a therapeutic effect.

α_2 receptor antagonists

Treatment with reuptake inhibitors is the first line of defense in pharmacologically treating depression. Yet 60–70% of depressed patients will not reach full remission following initiation of treatment or will require many treatment changes and augmentations throughout the course of therapy. Early clinical trials indicated that an α_2 antagonist, mirtazapine, alone was efficacious in the treatment of depression. Particularly appealing was the ability of mirtazapine to reduce recurrence of depression during long-term treatment and it seemingly had an earlier onset of antidepressant action (Schatzberg et al., 2002). In a double-blind placebo study, Blier and colleagues found that augmenting an SSRI, SNRI, or NE/dopamine reuptake inhibitor (NDRI) with mirtazapine doubled the likelihood of achieving remission and the addition of mirtazapine to the venlafaxine and bupropion treatment groups had higher remission rates than adding mirtazapine to fluoxetine (Blier et al., 2010). It is also worth noting that the previous group and others have found that mirtazapine treatment was sufficient to significantly reduce suicidal behavior when compared to placebo (Blier et al., 2010; Kasper et al., 2010).

The mechanism of action of mirtazapine is not unlike uptake inhibitors and MAO inhibition, i.e., elevation of the synaptic availability of NE through inhibition of presynaptic α_2 autoreceptors (blocking feedback inhibition of NE release). α_2 adrenergic receptors are also located on serotonergic neurons and their activation reduces serotonin release. Hence, mirtazapine can simultaneously increase the synaptic availability of serotonin by blocking inhibitory α_2 adrenergic receptors on serotonergic terminals. The major side effect of mirtazapine, sedation, is also likely to be a result of α_2 adrenergic receptor blockade, although the location of this α_2 receptor is expected to be postsynaptic to noradrenergic terminals. Interestingly, although α_2 antagonism with mirtazapine would be expected to increase LC activity (by removing autoreceptor feedback inhibition), chronic treatment of rodents with mirtazapine reduces LC activity (West et al., 2009). Hence, mirtazapine is similar to reuptake inhibitors and MAO inhibitors in this pharmacological effect.

Atypical antipsychotics

The atypical antipsychotics are sometimes used as adjunctive therapy when traditional antidepressants fail or produce an inadequate response. In schizophrenia, clozapine carries an FDA approval to treat suicidal behavior. The biological mechanisms by which antipsychotic drugs reduce suicidal behavior and reduce depression are not well understood. Nevertheless, quetiapine, aripiprazole, and olanzapine are FDA-approved to treat depressive disorders. It has been argued that the combination of an atypical antipsychotic with an SSRI accelerates antidepressant response. It is especially noteworthy that these antipsychotic drugs have antagonist actions at α_2 adrenergic receptors and may produce effects on NE that overlap with mirtazapine. Interestingly, atypical antipsychotic drugs have paradoxical effects on noradrenergic LC activity when compared to traditional antidepressant compounds. That is, repeated treatment of rats with the atypical antipsychotic olanzapine increases LC activity, the opposite effect of traditional antidepressant drugs and an effect that is also seen after a single dose of olanzapine (Dawe et al., 2001). Since atypical antipsychotics are used for patients who are relatively unresponsive to traditional antidepressants, this odd effect of atypical antipsychotics on LC activity implies that the pathobiology of treatment-resistant depression may be distinct from antidepressant treatment-responsive depression. Certainly, these patients typically have more complex symptoms and often have other Axis I, II, and III diagnoses. Since atypical antipsychotic drugs have many other pharmacological actions, one would not expect behavioral responses to these drugs to mirror those of antidepressant drugs.

Future of noradrenergic studies

While drug development research has yielded antidepressant drugs with much more tolerable side effects, it has not yielded faster or more efficacious treatments than the first antidepressants discovered over 60 years ago. Since NE and serotonin are the primary sites of action of most if not all currently available antidepressant drugs, the lack of significant improvements in efficacy of these drugs as a class over the years has contributed to a loss of interest in the pathophysiology of the noradrenergic and serotonergic systems in depression and suicide. Instead, research has focused on identifying novel therapeutic targets based on signaling pathways downstream to noradrenergic and serotonergic receptors that may be reached by neurotransmitter or cellular systems other than the monoamines, and on systems found to be pathological in the postmortem brain from major depressive donors or suicide victims. The following examines two novel targets of tremendous interest to the field and considers the relationship of these systems to noradrenergic signaling in the brain.

Glutamate

Glutamate is an excitatory neurotransmitter in the brain. A growing body of physiological, pathological, and pharmacological evidence indicates abnormal glutamatergic neuronal activity in depression and suicide. Elevated glutamate/glutamine levels have been reported in blood, cerebral spinal fluid, and postmortem tissue of patients with mood disorders including depression and bipolar disorder (as reviewed by Machado-Vieira et al., 2012). In humans, single infusions of the glutamatergic NMDA receptor antagonist ketamine induced a positive antisuicidal behavioral response within hours with subsequent studies demonstrating that ketamine is both tolerable and effective in the treatment of depressive disorders (Machado-Vieira et al., 2012). The rapid antidepressant response of ketamine was reported to sustain for 1 to 2 weeks. The neurobiology underlying this antidepressant effect is poorly understood, but it is noteworthy that antidepressant action occurs after a single administration of ketamine, as opposed to traditional antidepressants that require repeated administration for days to weeks before efficacy can be significantly demonstrated. It is also interesting that the antidepressant effect of ketamine, as assessed in the laboratory, is negated when rats are pretreated with a glutamatergic AMPA receptor antagonist, suggesting a major role of the AMPA receptor in ketamine's action (Zamalloa et al., 2009).

Glutamate is the major excitatory input into the noradrenergic LC and noradrenergic activity is driven by activation of a variety of glutamate receptors including NMDA and AMPA receptors. Glutamate activation of the LC is stimulated by stress and several abnormalities of glutamate signaling at the level of the LC have been identified in depressed suicide victims by our laboratory (Chandley et al., 2013; Karolewicz et al., 2005). It seems reasonable to suggest that at least some of the antidepressant effects of ketamine may be mediated by an immediate blockade of glutamatergic activation of the noradrenergic LC. That is, NMDA receptor antagonism reduces LC activity after acute administration, similar to the effect on LC activity observed after chronic treatment with traditional antidepressants. The effects of ketamine infusion on noradrenergic activity or NE levels in LC projection areas at times following the initial acute inhibition of LC activity are unknown presently. It is conceivable that NMDA receptor blockade could result in elevated synaptic NE through glutamatergic effects mediated in terminal fields (e.g., prefrontal cortex and amygdala) of LC projections.

Glia

As discussed above, both experimental animal and human studies indicate that depression is associated with elevated glutamatergic neurotransmission. Glia, including astrocytes and oligodendrocytes, are responsible for removing extracellular glutamate from the glutamatergic synapse throughout the entire brain. Astrocytes in particular play a major role in terminating the action of glutamate. Astrocytes transport glutamate from the synaptic region through excitatory amino acid transporters (EAATs) located on their plasma membrane. In depression and suicide, a reduction in the number of glia cells and altered morphology has been demonstrated in a number of brain areas including the prefrontal cortex, cingulate cortex, hippocampus, and amygdala (as reviewed by Banasr et al., 2011). It seems logical that lower glia cell numbers in depression would contribute to elevated glutamatergic activity since a loss of EAATs would accompany the loss of the cells that express these transporters.

The findings of abnormal glia in depression would seem to be entirely separated from a role of NE in depression. However, both astrocytes and oligodendrocytes express noradrenergic receptors on their cell surface and these cells respond to NE when it is released in LC projection areas. The glial cell response to NE is complex but involves a number of cellular processes including calcium release, glycogenolysis, and synaptic remodeling (Bekar et al., 2008). Also, the transport of glutamate via EAATs is modulated by NE through NE receptors on glia. Hence, it is conceivable that the reported pathology of glia and NE in depression and suicide are linked. Evidence in support of this includes recent findings from our laboratory that demonstrate abnormal gene expressions in astrocytes in the region of the LC from suicide victims with major depressive disorder as compared to psychiatrically normal control subjects. In fact, a reduction in the expression of EAATs on astrocytes in the vicinity of noradrenergic neurons of the LC was observed in depressed suicide victims (Chandley et al., 2013). Reduced glutamate transport in the LC would result in increased glutamatergic activation of the LC. These findings further support the hypothesis that at least one major therapeutic effect of traditional antidepressants and glutamate antagonists is reduction in the activity of the LC.

At present, drugs that target specific glial function are few in number. The drug riluzole binds to glutamate transporters, increases glutamate uptake, and eventually stimulates glutamate release from glia cells. Riluzole has been FDA approved for the treatment of ALS and Huntington's disease. Riluzole was first identified as a potential antidepressant when the first open-label trial in 2004 indicated that some patients with treatment-resistant depression successfully responded to the drug (Machado-Vieira et al., 2012). Since then, there have been multiple trials of riluzole as augmentation therapy in the treatment of major depressive disorder that have exhibited some success, but riluzole has yet to undergo double-blind placebo-controlled clinical trials. Given that glutamate transporter blockade by dihydrokainic acid is sufficient to induce anhedonia-like behaviors in mice, it is conceivable that future antidepressant development will focus on specific glial glutamate transporters as well as other glial targets.

Conclusion

There is overwhelming evidence that brain NE plays a major role in the pathology of depression and suicide. While NE depletion does not produce depression in everyone, it does induce depression in those specifically predisposed to depression (e.g., as a result of previous depressive episodes) and in individuals whose mental healthiness is being maintained by treatment with noradrenergic-selective antidepressant drugs. In addition, there is a vast literature demonstrating specific abnormalities in the brain noradrenergic system in depression and suicide. The overriding commonality of the findings from research using postmortem brain tissues from suicide victims is that there are pathological abnormalities highly suggestive of adaptations in protein and gene expression that would be expected to occur in the condition of depleted NE, or prolonged elevation of central noradrenergic activity. Hence it seems reasonable to conclude that in susceptible individuals, chronic exposure to stress results in chronic elevation of central noradrenergic neuronal firing leading to depletion of brain NE stores. Resilience to stress, as determined genetically or through early life learning, would be expected to be accompanied by reduced negative impact of stress on noradrenergic homeostasis (Figure 35.2)

TCAs, MAO inhibitors, NRIs, and mirtazapine reduce LC activity as a result of a local increase in synaptic NE in the region of the LC where NE is released from LC neuronal dendrites, recurring collaterals, and noradrenergic terminals projecting from lower brainstem regions. The local elevation of synaptic NE in the region of the LC reduces LC neuronal activity by activating inhibitory α_2 adrenergic receptors on dendrites and cell bodies of LC neurons. However, this event in the LC likely does not override

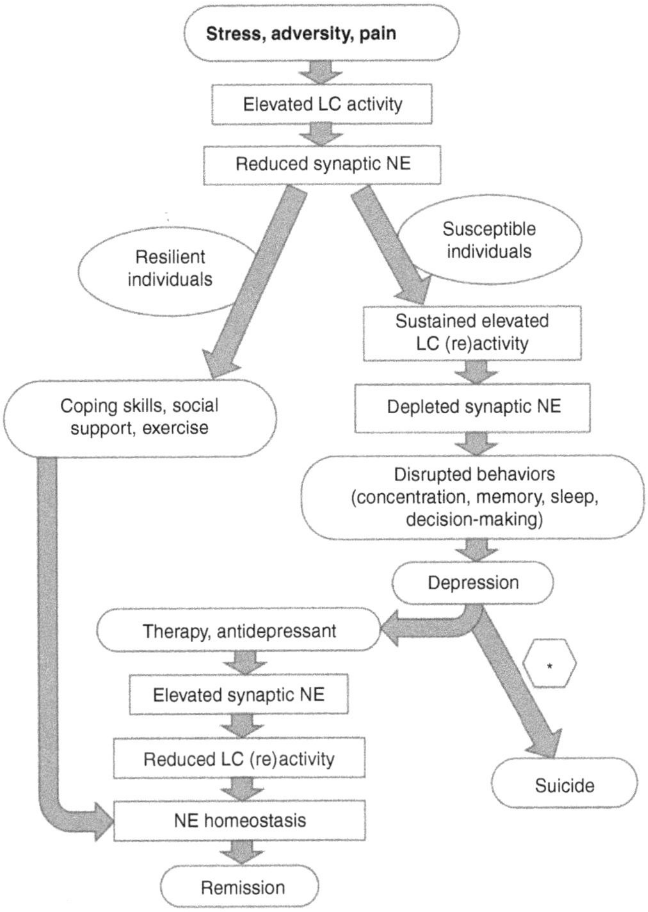

Figure 35.2. Proposed role of NE in the brain biology of stress and the pathobiology of depression and suicide. Stress elevates the activity of the noradrenergic LC as a result of activation of stress-sensitive excitatory inputs (glutamate, substance P, corticotropin-releasing factor) to the LC. Elevated LC activity results in increased release of NE in terminal projection areas (e.g., prefrontal cortex, hippocampus, amygdala) resulting in a temporary reduction in the stores of NE. In resilient individuals, learned coping skills and other factors provide protection from persistent stress-induced elevation of LC activity. In susceptible individuals, stress-induced activation of the LC persists and is accompanied by increased responsiveness or reactivity to stress, leading to depleted NE in the brain. Disruption in behaviors supported by NE ensues, resulting in specific symptoms of the behavioral spectrum of depression. Antidepressant treatments reduce LC activity and reactivity to stress (regardless of their acute mechanism of action), restoring noradrenergic transmission homeostasis and thereby mitigating disrupted behaviors. The asterisk indicates additional factors (developmental insults, adversity, genetic, etc.) that raise the risk of suicide in untreated depressed subjects. While other transmitters, such as serotonin and glutamate, are involved in the pathobiology of depression and suicide, this figure illustrates only the role of NE pathology in the development and treatment of depression.

the elevation of the synaptic availability of NE in LC projection areas (e.g., cerebral cortical regions) where NE catabolism, NE reuptake, or the α_2 adrenergic receptor is simultaneously being blocked by the antidepressant. Hence, while inhibiting LC activity, there remains an elevation of the synaptic availability of NE in LC projection areas. Antidepressants may simply restrict the activity of the LC to a level of neuronal activity and terminal NE release that is optimal for recovery in critical LC projection areas. In that regard, atypical antipsychotics produce an elevation of synaptic NE availability in LC projection areas similar to traditional antidepressant drugs, but through a different mechanism, i.e., by increasing the firing of LC neurons and increasing NE release in projection areas of the LC. Besides reducing LC activity, treatment with traditional antidepressants decreases sensory-evoked increases in LC activity. The presumed behavioral consequence of this effect would be reduced reactivity to stress-induced increases in LC firing (Figure 35.2). It is currently unknown whether atypical antipsychotics also decrease sensory-evoked increases in LC activity, while simultaneously increasing activity.

The discovery of the many post-receptor signaling effects of repeated antidepressant drug administration initiated drug development research decades ago aimed at producing the same end effect without working through NE and serotonin. Early attempts were made to bypass NE itself and activate beta-adrenergic receptors (for example) directly. Direct acting β-adrenergic agonists were developed but these never reached FDA approval. Later, downstream signaling molecules were targeted. For example, BDNF is upregulated in the hippocampus by traditional antidepressants. If this is indeed a critical effect of antidepressant drugs that imparts their therapeutic activity, one might find other non-noradrenergic or non-serotonergic pathways to increase BDNF in the brain, or administer BDNF itself. It is worth noting at this point in time that antidepressant drugs prescribed today remain nearly exclusively drugs that elevate NE and/or serotonin. An important issue to remember is that the currently popular downstream effects of traditional antidepressant drugs, often considered future antidepressant targets, occur as a result of the sustenance of the initial effects of traditional antidepressants on synaptic NE and/or serotonin that occurs with continued antidepressant administration. In fact, numerous studies in rodents and humans have demonstrated that when NE and/or serotonin is/are experimentally depleted, antidepressant drugs cease to work. As noted above, depletion of NE in patients that are being successfully treated with noradrenergic antidepressants results in a rapid relapse of depressive symptoms. It remains possible that using drugs to directly target some of the downstream biochemical events of traditional antidepressants may ultimately result in the discovery of a new type of antidepressant. However, it is also conceivable that this approach may be unsuccessful because traditional antidepressants modulate those downstream events in a neuroanatomically- and cellular-specific manner as a result of anatomically selective innervation patterns of noradrenergic and serotonergic neurons in the brain. This innervation-related specificity and complexity may be necessary for the behavior-modifying effects of antidepressants that promote recovery. Hence, future development efforts may be more productive if they are focused on adjunctive treatments that facilitate the therapeutic actions of existing antidepressant drugs.

References

Banasr, M., Dwyer, J. M., & Duman, R. S. (2011). Cell atrophy and loss in depression: reversal by antidepressant treatment. *Current Opinion in Cell Biology*, **23**, 730–737.

Bekar, L. K., He, W., & Nedergaard, M. (2008). Locus coeruleus alpha-adrenergic-mediated activation of cortical astrocytes in vivo. *Cerebral Cortex*, **18**, 2789–2795.

Berman, R. M., Narasimhan, M., Miller, H. L., et al. (1999). Transient depressive relapse induced by catecholamine depletion: potential phenotypic vulnerability marker? *Archives of General Psychiatry*, **56**, 395–403.

Blier, P., Ward, H. E., Tremblay, P., et al. (2010). Combination of antidepressant medications from treatment initiation for major depressive disorder: a double-blind randomized study. *The American Journal of Psychiatry*, **167**, 281–288.

Booij, L., Van der Does, A. J., & Riedel, W. J. (2003). Monoamine depletion in psychiatric and healthy populations: review. *Molecular Psychiatry*, **8**, 951–973.

Chandley, M., & Ordway, G. (2012). Noradrenergic function in suicide. In Y. Dwivedi (Ed) *Neurobiology of Suicide* (pp. 29–63). Boca Raton, FL: CRC Press.

Chandley, M. J., Szebeni, K., Szebeni, A., et al. (2013). Gene expression deficits in pontine locus coeruleus astrocytes in men with major depressive disorder. *Journal of Psychiatry & Neuroscience*, **38**, 276–284.

Dawe, G. S., Huff, K. D., Vandergriff, J. L., et al. (2001). Olanzapine activates the rat locus coeruleus: in vivo electrophysiology and c-Fos immunoreactivity. *Biological Psychiatry*, **50**, 510–520.

De Paermentier, F., Mauger, J. M., Lowther, S., et al. (1997). Brain alpha-adrenoceptors in depressed suicides. *Brain Research*, **757**, 60–68.

Duncan, J., Johnson, S., & Ou, X. M. (2012). Monoamine oxidases in major depressive disorder and alcoholism. *Drug Discoveries & Therapeutics*, **6**, 112–122.

Frazer, A. (2000). Norepinephrine involvement in antidepressant action. *The Journal of Clinical Psychiatry*, **61**, 25–30.

Frazer, A., Hess, M. E., Mendels, J., et al. (1978). Influence of acute and chronic treatment with desmethylimipramine on catecholamine effects in the rat. *The Journal of Pharmacology and Experimental Therapeutics*, **206**, 311–319.

Galfalvy, H., Currier, D., Oquendo, M. A., et al. (2009). Lower CSF MHPG predicts short-term risk for suicide attempt. *International Journal of Neuropsychopharmacology*, **12**, 1327–1335.

Gos, T., Krell, D., Bielau, H., et al. (2008). Tyrosine hydroxylase immunoreactivity in the locus coeruleus is elevated in violent suicidal depressive patients. *European Archives of Psychiatry and Clinical Neuroscience*, **258**, 513–520.

Grant, M. M., & Weiss, J. M. (2001). Effects of chronic antidepressant drug administration and electroconvulsive shock on locus coeruleus electrophysiologic activity. *Biological Psychiatry*, **49**, 117–129.

Karolewicz, B., Stockmeier, C. A., & Ordway, G. A. (2005). Elevated levels of the NR2C subunit of the NMDA receptor in the locus coeruleus in depression. *Neuropsychopharmacology*, **30**, 1557–1567.

Kasper, S., Montgomery, S. A., Möller, H. J., et al. (2010). Longitudinal analysis of the suicidal behaviour risk in short-term placebo-controlled studies of mirtazapine in major depressive disorder. *The World Journal of Biological Psychiatry*, **11**, 36–44.

Machado-Vieira, R., Ibrahim, L., Henter, I. D., et al. (2012). Novel glutamatergic agents for major depressive disorder and bipolar disorder. *Pharmacology, Biochemistry, and Behavior*, **100**, 678–687.

Mandela, P., & Ordway, G. A. (2006). The norepinephrine transporter and its regulation. *Journal of Neurochemistry*, **97**, 310–333.

Meyer, J. H. (2012). Neuroimaging high-risk states for suicide. In Y. Dwivedi (Ed) *The Neurobiological Basis of Suicide* (pp. 159–194). Boca Raton, FL: CRC Press.

Neumeister, A., Drevets, W. C., Belfer, I., et al. (2006). Effects of a alpha 2C-adrenoreceptor gene polymorphism on neural responses to facial expressions in depression. *Neuropsychopharmacology*, **31**, 1750–1756.

Ordway, G. A. (1997). Pathophysiology of the locus coeruleus in suicide. *Annals of the New York Academy of Sciences*, **836**, 233–252.

Ordway, G. A. (2007). Neuropathology of central norepinephrine in psychiatric disorders: postmortem research. In G. A. Ordway, M. Schwartz, & A. Frazer (Eds.) *Brain Norepinephrine* (pp. 341–362). Cambridge, UK: Cambridge University Press.

Rovin, M. L., Boss-Williams, K. A., Alisch, R. S., et al. (2012). Influence of chronic administration of antidepressant drugs on mRNA for galanin, galanin receptors, and tyrosine hydroxylase in catecholaminergic and serotonergic cell-body regions in rat brain. *Neuropeptides*, **46**, 81–91.

Schatzberg, A. F., Kremer, C., Rodrigues, H. E., et al. (2002). Double-blind, randomized comparison of mirtazapine and paroxetine in elderly depressed patients. *The American Journal of Geriatric Psychiatry*, **10**, 541–550.

Sequeira, A., Mamdani, F., Lalovic, A., et al. (2004). Alpha 2A adrenergic receptor gene and suicide. *Psychiatry Research*, **125**, 87–93.

Sharma, A., Busnello, J. V., Ribeiro, L., et al. (2007). Suicidality scores during double-blind fluoxetine and desipramine treatment in Mexican Americans. *Journal of Clinical Psychopharmacology*, **27**, 99–101.

Stone, E. A., Lin, Y., Sarfraz, Y., et al. (2009). Marked behavioral activation from inhibitory stimulation of locus coeruleus alpha1-adrenoceptors by a full agonist. *Brain Research*, **1291**, 21–31.

Taneja, M., Salim, S., Saha, K., et al. (2011). Differential effects of inescapable stress on locus coeruleus GRK3, alpha2-adrenoceptor and CRF1 receptor levels in learned helpless and non-helpless rats: a potential link to stress resilience. *Behavioural Brain Research*, **221**, 25–33.

West, C. H., Ritchie, J. C., Boss-Williams, K. A., et al. (2009). Antidepressant drugs with differing pharmacological actions decrease activity of locus coeruleus neurons. *International Journal of Neuropsychopharmacology*, **12**, 627–641.

Zamalloa, T., Bailey, C. P., & Pineda, J. (2009). Glutamate-induced post-activation inhibition of locus coeruleus neurons is mediated by AMPA/kainate receptors and sodium-dependent potassium currents. *British Journal of Pharmacology*, **156**, 649–661.

Zhao, Z., Baros, A. M., Zhang, H. T., et al. (2008). Norepinephrine transporter regulation mediates the long-term behavioral effects of the antidepressant desipramine. *Neuropsychopharmacology*, **33**, 3190–3200.

Zhu, M. Y., Klimek, V., Dilley, G. E., et al. (1999). Elevated levels of tyrosine hydroxylase in the locus coeruleus in major depression. *Biological Psychiatry*, **46**, 1275–1286.

Chapter 36

Brain corticotropin-releasing factor and the hypothalamic–pituitary–adrenal axis in suicide

Ghanshyam N. Pandey

Introduction

Suicide is a major public health concern and approximately 30 000 people die of suicide alone each year in the USA, and about 1 million people worldwide. Suicide is a major contributor of mortality in patients suffering from mood disorders, schizophrenia, and alcoholism. It is the second or third leading cause of death in adolescents and youths. The major risk factor for suicide is the presence of mental disorders, particularly depression. Familial and environmental risk factors are also associated with suicidal behavior. However, these risk factors by themselves do not explain the risk for suicide. Recent studies suggest that abnormal neurobiology, as well as genetic and environmental factors, may play a crucial role in suicide, and stress together with the environmental factors are important in triggering suicidal behavior and suicide. Stress, either acute or chronic, which is one of the main triggers of suicidal behavior, causes a dysregulation of the HPA axis, the major endocrine system implicated in suicidal behavior. A dysregulated HPA axis is one of the most consistent findings in depression and in suicidal behavior and corticotropin-releasing factor (CRF) is the key component controlling the HPA axis and plays a central role in the response of an organism to stress, which is defined as any environmental change threatening the homeostasis of an individual. However, CRF activity is not limited to the HPA axis. CRF secretion from the central nucleus of the amygdala is also increased in response to stress and it is proposed that hypothalamic CRF secretion is most sensitive to physiological stress.

In this chapter we describe studies of CRF and related components of the HPA axis and suicidal behavior. CRF is also known as the corticotropin-releasing hormone (CRH). Although this term is used in several studies reviewed here, for the sake of consistency we will use only the term CRF in this review. Extra-hypothalamic brain areas may play an important role in the regulation of CRF, as discussed in the HPA section, and may also be crucial in mediating its role in depression or suicide. Therefore, in addition to CRF in the hypothalamus, we also describe studies conducted in other brain areas.

CRF, which was first described by Vale et al. (1981), is a 41-residue hypothalamic peptide. It mediates behavioral, cognitive, neuroendocrine, and immunologic responses to stress by activating its two receptors – CRF-R1 and CRF-R2 – in the central nervous system (CNS) and the anterior pituitary. Since the levels of CRF in the CNS may regulate the sensitivity and function of these receptors, it is important to examine their role in suicide.

CRF levels in the CNS are regulated by at least two mechanisms. One such mechanism is CRF binding to a protein known as CRF binding protein (CRF-BP). There are some studies of CRF-BP in suicide. The other mechanism involves the regulation of CRF levels in the CNS by corticoid receptors. These receptors, known as glucocorticoid receptor (GR) and mineralocorticoid receptor (MR), are involved in the feedback inhibition of CRF release and have been shown to be altered in suicide. These receptors may be important in the CRF regulation of the HPA axis and CRF release.

Thus, in this review, we describe studies and discuss the role of CRF, its receptors, CRF-BP, GR and MR, and the HPA axis in suicide.

A Concise Guide to Understanding Suicide, ed. Stephen H. Koslow, Pedro Ruiz, and Charles B. Nemeroff. Published by Cambridge University Press.

HPA axis regulation and abnormalities in suicide

As discussed before, CRF is involved in the stress response and also regulates the HPA axis (described in Figure 36.1) as follows. After immediate exposure to stress, the synthesis of CRF is increased in the peptidergic neurons of the PVN of the hypothalamus, resulting in the release and production of CRF from the median eminence. CRF is then transported through the portal vascular system to the pituitary where it stimulates the secretion of adrenocorticotropic hormone (ACTH) from the anterior pituitary cells. ACTH is then secreted into the systemic circulation leading, in humans, to the secretion of cortisol from the adrenal cortex. Thus, cortisol is the end product of the HPA axis activation. Cortisol exerts negative feedback at the pituitary and the hypothalamus via two receptors known as MR and GR, which turn off the stress responses. A diagram depicting the HPA axis and the input from other brain areas is shown in Figure 36.1.

The activity of the HPA axis is regulated by circadian rhythm and in reaction to stress, as has been discussed before. Several brain areas are involved in the stress response and also in the pathophysiology of depression and suicide. These areas are also involved in the regulation of the HPA axis as the components of the HPA axis, such as CRF, GR, and MR, are richly distributed in these areas. Brain areas especially involved in the pathophysiology of suicide and depression and the activation of the HPA axis are the prefrontal cortex (PFC), hippocampus, and amygdala. These brain areas are involved in the regulation of mood and behavior and their abnormalities have been reported in mood disorders and suicide. There are numerous reports showing the involvement of the amygdala in behavior and mental disorders. It is involved in the stress response (see review by Gold et al., 2002), in fear and anxiety, and in memory and emotions. Gold et al. (2002) have elegantly reviewed the involvement of these brain regions in mood disorders and suicide and in HPA regulation. Therefore, in addition to the hypothalamus, the CRF and other components of the HPA axis have been studied in these brain areas.

There are many studies that show a strong association between HPA axis dysfunction and suicide. Initially Yerevanian et al. (1983) found that dexamethasone suppression test (DST) non-suppressors were significantly more likely to attempt and complete suicide than DST suppressors. Other investigators have also found an association between DST non-suppression and suicide. A meta-analysis by Lester (1992) found that suicide completions, but not attempts, were associated with the DST non-suppression. This observation is consistent with several studies of HPA axis function with suicidal patients. In a large study of suicidal patients, Pfennig et al. (2005) performed DEX-CRF testing

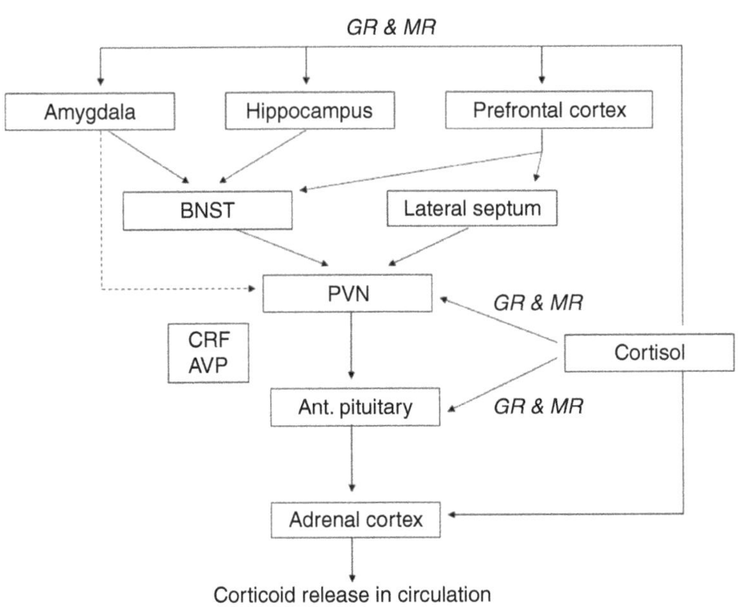

Figure 36.1. Hypothalamic–pituitary–adrenal (HPA) axis regulation. AVP, arginine vasopressin; BNST, bed nucleus of the stria terminalis; CRF, corticotropin-releasing factor; GR, glucocorticoid receptor; MR, mineralocorticoid receptor; PVN, paraventricular nucleus.

on 310 patients, including 77 patients with suicidal behavior. They found that suicidal behaviors were associated with lower ACTH and cortisol response to the DEX-CRH test. Abnormal DST has been associated with increased risk for suicide in depressed patients (Coryell & Schlesser, 2001). It may thus appear that an abnormal HPA axis is associated more with suicide completion than with suicidal behavior, although many studies link suicidal behavior with abnormal DST. Because of this observation, several investigators have studied the components of the HPA axis in the postmortem brain of depressed and suicide victims, as will be discussed in the following pages.

CRF and its receptors in suicide

The initial evidence of the involvement of CRF in depression and suicide is derived from the observation of abnormal combined dexamethasone-CRF (Dex/CRF) challenge test (Heuser et al., 1994). Abnormal Dex-CRF test results suggest specific abnormalities of CRF in depression and suicide. Further evidence supporting the CRF abnormalities in suicide is derived from the study of CRF in the CSF of depressed and suicidal subjects and of its receptors in the postmortem brain of suicide victims.

The levels of CRF in the CSF have been generally studied in depressed patients, and there are only a few studies of the CRF levels in the CSF of suicidal patients. While several studies found an increase in CSF levels of CRF in depressed patients, some studies do not find differences in the CSF between depressed and normal control subjects. In one study of suicidal patients by Arato et al. (1986), it was observed that the CRF levels in cysternal CSF from 19 suicide victims were higher than those of sudden death controls.

Nemeroff et al. (1984) have also determined the CRF immunoreactivity in the CSF of depressed patients. They found a significantly higher concentration of CRF-like immunoreactivity in 11 of 23 depressed patients they studied.

Bissette et al. (2003) determined CRF levels (CRF-like immunoreactivity) in the locus coeruleus (LC) of depressed subjects, some of whom died by suicide, and of control subjects. They found that the concentration of CRF in the anterior-posterior regions of LC of depressed subjects was significantly higher compared with control subjects. Similar results were reported by Merali et al. (2004) who also found that CRF immunoreactivity was significantly elevated in the LC and PFC of suicides compared with controls. Austin et al. (2003) determined the CRF immunoreactivity in specific pontine nuclei of subjects with major depression who died by suicide and control subjects. They found that the mean levels of CRF immunoreactivity in the depressed suicide subjects was significantly increased by about 30% in the locus coeruleus, about 40% in the caudal dorsal raphe, and 39% in the median raphe relative to the control subjects. Raadsheer et al. (1994) determined the CRF immunoreactivity in the CRF-expressing neurons in the hypothalamic PVN of depressed subjects. The total number of CRF-expressing neurons in depressed patients was significantly higher than those in the control subjects. These studies thus showed that CRF immunoreactivity is higher in the postmortem brain of depressed and/or suicidal subjects compared with normal control subjects.

As stated earlier, the receptors for CRF mediate the biological and behavioral actions of CRF. Two distinct mammalian receptor subtypes for CRF have been characterized, and these receptor subtypes display a different tissue distribution and pharmacological specificity (Steckler & Holsboer, 1999). The CRF receptor subtypes and their function have been elegantly reviewed by Steckler and Holsboer (1999). CRF-R1 is predominantly expressed in the frontal cortical areas and in the basal forebrain, in addition to the brainstem cholinergic nuclei and the basolateral nucleus of the amygdala. CRF-R2, on the other hand, is strongly expressed in the PVN and the lateral septum and the central and medial nuclei of the amygdala and the raphe nuclei. Both receptors are richly distributed in the hippocampus and entorhinal cortex, the bed nucleus of the stria terminalis (BNST), and periaqueductal gray (PAG).

It has been suggested that CRF-R1 and CRF-R2 may mediate different types of behaviors. It is reported that the action of CRF on the HPA axis is predominantly mediated by CRF-R1; whereas the central effects leading to the activation of the amygdala, PVN, and the hippocampus may involve both receptor subtypes. Both receptors may be involved in anxiety-like behaviors as it also has been shown that mice deficient for CRF-R2 may display anxiety-like behavior and are hypersensitive to stress (Steckler & Holsboer, 1999).

The role of CRF receptors in suicide was first determined by Nemeroff et al. (1988) who determined the binding of bovine CRF-125 in the frontal cortex obtained from suicide victims and control subjects. They found a significant reduction (23%) in the number of the CRF binding sites in the frontal cortex of suicide victims compared with controls. Hucks et al. (1997) also determined the CRF receptor binding sites in the prefrontal cortex as well as motor cortex of suicide victims and control subjects. They did not find, however, any significant differences in the number and affinity of CRF binding sites between the suicide and the control groups.

Hiroi et al. (2001) determined the mRNA expression and distribution of CRF-R1 and CRF-R2 in different brain regions of suicide victims and control subjects. Although they found that both CRF-R1 and CRF-R2 are expressed in high amounts in the brain (the highest expression in the pituitary), CRF-R1 was more highly expressed in the human brain compared to CRF-R2, which was predominantly expressed in the peripheral tissue. When they compared the expression of CRF-R1 and CRF-R2 in the pituitary of suicide and control subjects, they did not find any significant differences. Raadsheer et al. (1995) also determined the levels of the CRF mRNA in the PVN of patients with Alzheimer's disease and depression. They found that the mRNA levels of CRF were significantly higher in the PVN of Alzheimer's subjects compared with control subjects. However, they also found that the CRF mRNA levels were even more elevated in depressed patients compared with normal control subjects.

There are only a few genetic studies of CRH-R1 in relation to suicidal behavior. These studies have been previously conducted by Wasserman's group and reviewed by Wasserman et al. (2010). Wasserman et al. (2010) have investigated the CRF-R1 gene in relation to suicidal behavior as the main phenotype, which some others have studied as a secondary phenotype. Using a family-based sample, they found an association and linkage of an intronic SNP to suicide attempt (rs4792887). They proposed that those individuals who have been exposed to low levels of lifetime stress may carry CRF-R1 variants and are more prone to produce a dysregulated HPA-CRF system. They have confirmed and expanded these findings with more SNPs in the CRF-R1 gene and found an association of three more SNPs with increasing depression intensity among male suicide attempters. Association of the CRF-R1 gene with suicidality has also been investigated by Papiol et al. (2007), showing the association of A-allele (rs110402) with suicidality.

CRF binding protein

In addition to the two receptors of CRF, the activity of CRF is also modulated by a protein known as CRF-BP, which is a 37 kDa glycoprotein structurally unrelated to CRF receptors. CRF-BP binds to CRF with an equal or greater affinity than the CRF receptors (Herringa et al., 2006). This observation places it at an important regulatory position between CRF and its receptors. CRF-BP is expressed in many regions of the brain, including the cerebral cortex, hippocampus, amygdala, and pituitary. *In vivo* studies show that CRF-BP can block the CRF-mediated secretion of ACTH from the anterior pituitary, and thus it may act as a negative regulator for CRF activity *in vivo*.

CRF-BP is highly regulated by factors that are known to affect HPA axis activity. For example, stress and glucocorticoids, which are the major regulators of the HPA axis, also regulate CRF-BP mRNA expression in the rodent pituitary and amygdala. Adrenalectomy decreases the CRF-BP mRNA. The regulation by stress and glucocorticoids suggests that increased pituitary CRF-BP levels may provide an important negative feedback mechanism, which supports the role of CRF-BP as a regulator of HPA activity (Lombardo et al., 2001).

CRF-BP has several functions in the CNS. CRF-BP could act in an inhibitory fashion to sequester CRF and target it for degradation, thereby reducing CRF receptor activity. Some studies indicate that about 40–60% of the human CRF in the brain is bound by CRF-BP, and thus CRF-BP may have a role in limiting the bioavailability of CRF. It may also neutralize the physiological action of CRF, especially in the pituitary. CRF-BP could also bind CRF and potentiate CRF signaling by modulating its interaction with its receptor, thus delivering CRF to receptors or extending its half-life. Herringa et al. (2006) have studied the CRF-BP in the postmortem tissue from bipolar and schizophrenic subjects; they found a significant decrease in CRF-BP mRNA levels in the basolateral amygdala of male bipolar and male schizophrenic subjects and the lateral amygdala of bipolar subjects. Although some of these subjects might have died by suicide it is not clear if these changes were related to suicide or suicidal behavior.

Although CRF-BP plays an important role in the regulation of HPA axis activity and the modulation of the effects and levels of CRF, the role of CRF-BP has not been extensively studied in depression or suicide. Merali et al. (2006) did not find any significant differences in the mRNA levels of CRF-BP between suicide and control subjects.

Corticoid receptors in suicide

As discussed earlier there is ample evidence to suggest a hyperactive HPA axis and increased levels of CRF in suicide. The increased activity of the HPA axis and the increased levels of CRF are thought to be related, at least in part, to an altered feedback inhibition of CRF release by endogenous glucocorticoids. This is mediated by binding of cortisol to its receptors – GR and MR. The interaction of cortisol with its receptors GR and MR in the hippocampus and the hypothalamus or other areas of the brain induces a feedback inhibition signal that causes a reduction in the HPA axis activity, presumably by decreasing the release of CRF. It is therefore quite possible that the increased level of CRF observed in the postmortem brain of suicide victims may be related, at least in part, to altered sensitivity or the numbers of corticoid receptors GR and MR. It is therefore not surprising that both GR and MR have been studied in the postmortem brain of suicide victims.

Two types of corticoid receptors, GR and MR, have been identified in rodent and human brain. GR have a high affinity for synthetic glucocorticoid dexamethasone and a lower affinity for cortisol or corticosterone. Because of the high affinity of MR for cortisol, these receptors are generally fully occupied at basal levels. However, GR are occupied when cortisol levels are increased, for example, in stress or illness. GR get activated mostly with high concentrations of cortisol, and thus mediate the feedback effect of high cortisol levels, such as seen with stress or depression. It is therefore believed that GR are important in the regulation of the stress response when endogenous levels of cortisol are high and therefore may play a role in stress-related disorders, such as depression or suicide. Both GR and MR are present in high concentrations in different areas of human brain, including the prefrontal cortex, hippocampus, amygdala, locus coeruleus, and hypothalamus, as shown by *in situ* hybridization and autoradiography techniques.

Studies of GR and MR in human postmortem brain of subjects with mood disorders and suicide are limited to specific brain areas. Lopez et al. (1998) determined the GR and MR in various subfields of the hippocampus of six suicide victims and six controls. They found a significant decrease in mRNA in CA3 and not in other subfields; however, mRNA for GR was not significantly different between suicide and control subjects. Perlman et al. (2004) found that GR mRNA was reduced in the basolateral nuclei of amygdala in schizophrenic and bipolar subjects but not in subjects with major depression. Webster et al. (2002) found region-specific decreases in the GR mRNA in the postmortem brain of subjects with major depression, bipolar illness, and schizophrenia.

More recently, McGowan et al. (2009) observed lower expression of GR mRNA in the hippocampus of suicide victims with a history of child abuse but not in non-abused suicide victims, suggesting that lower GR mRNA may be specifically decreased in abused adult suicide victims.

There are very few studies of MR receptors in the postmortem brain. Klok et al. (2011) found lower expression levels of GR and MR in the hippocampus, inferior frontal gyrus, and cingulated gyrus tissue, but no difference in the amygdala or the nucleus accumbens of subjects with major depression compared with normal control subjects. Again, the studies of corticoid receptors GR and MR are very limited in suicide although there are some studies in depression and schizophrenia. GR and MR receptors in the postmortem brain of suicide victims need to be studied further and studied in several relevant areas of the brain, such as the PFC, hippocampus, and the amygdala nuclei.

Conclusion

There appears to be strong evidence suggesting that suicidal behavior and suicide may be associated with a disturbance in the HPA axis system, as evident by many studies of DST and Dex-CRF challenge test, and that an abnormal HPA axis may be a good predictor of completed suicide. CRF is a key component of the HPA axis and is released as a consequence of consistent stress.

CRF has many functions in the brain, besides regulating the activity of the HPA axis. It is thus not surprising the CRF has been studied both in suicidal patients and in the postmortem brains of depressed and suicide victims. Earlier studies showed increased levels of CRF in the CSF of depressed and suicidal subjects. However, the key question was whether CRF is abnormally expressed in the brain of suicidal subjects. Several studies provide some insight into the dysregulation of CRF and related neuropeptides of the HPA axis in suicide, although these studies are not comprehensive. Some investigators report increased protein and gene expression levels of CRF in several areas of the postmortem brain of suicide victims compared with controls. Since CRF produces its biological effects by acting on its two receptor subtypes, known as CRF-R1 and CRF-R2, which are also implicated in some behavioral effects, the roles of these receptors have also been studied in suicide. These studies show that CRF-R1 is altered in postmortem brain of suicide victims compared with controls. On the other hand, the other CRF receptor subtype, CRF-R2, has not been well investigated and several of the studies do not show changes in the CRF-R2 expression. Genetic studies of CRF receptors have also been performed and these studies show an association between CRF-R1 and some components of the suicidal behavior. It is suggested that the downregulation of CRF-R1 may be due to increased expression of CRF levels and this increased exposure of the CRF-R1 receptors may lead to its downregulation. The CRF levels in the brain are primarily regulated by two mechanisms. One of the mechanisms is binding to a protein known as CRF-BP and therefore it is not surprising that the role of CRF-BP has also been studied in suicide. Some studies show that the protein and gene expression of CRF-BP is decreased in the postmortem brain of depressed and suicide victims and this may be one of the reasons for the increased expression of CRF in the brain.

The levels of CRF in the brain are also regulated by the feedback mechanism mediated by the two receptor subtypes of cortisol in humans. These receptors are known as GR and MR receptors. MR receptors have a high affinity for cortisol and remain fully occupied at normal cortisol levels. On the other hand, GR respond to acute increases in cortisol levels resulting from acute stress. However, these receptors appear to be downregulated in depression and suicide victims as a result of chronic stress, and hence are unable to inhibit the release of CRF. Some studies show a downregulation of GR in the postmortem brain of depressed and suicide victims. It therefore appears that the mechanism involving the increased levels of CRF may be related to decreased expression of GR and CRF-BP.

Although CRF is primarily secreted by the PVN, the PVN also receives input from other brain areas such as PFC, hippocampus, and amygdala, and these areas have also been implicated in several forms of behavior, such as anxiety, and found to be abnormal in the brain of depressed and suicide victims. Thus, the extra-hypothalamic areas of the brain, such as PFC, hippocampus, and amygdala, may also play a crucial role in the CRF abnormalities in the brain. Therefore, several studies have reported altered levels of CRF receptors, and of GR, MR, and CRF, and CRF-BP in other areas of the brain, in addition to the PVN of the hypothalamus. However, the studies of CRF and other key components of the HPA axis in these critical brain areas are limited and need to be investigated in a more comprehensive way. In summary, therefore, the studies of CRF and related neuropeptides suggest an abnormality of the key components of the HPA axis, which in turn may be responsible for the observed dysregulation of the HPA axis in depression and suicide. Further studies may not only provide more comprehensive understanding of the role of CRF and HPA axis in suicide, but may also lead to early identification of suicidal behavior, which may be crucial in the prevention of suicide, as well as in the development of more appropriate therapeutic agents targeting these components of the HPA axis in general, and CRF and CRF receptors in particular.

References

Arato, M., Banki, C. M., Nemeroff, C. B., et al. (1986). Hypothalamic-pituitary-adrenal axis and suicide. *Annals of the New York Academy of Sciences*, **487**, 263–270.

Austin, M. C., Janosky, J. E., & Murphy, H. A. (2003). Increased corticotropin-releasing hormone immunoreactivity in monoamine-containing pontine nuclei of depressed suicide men. *Molecular Psychiatry*, **8**, 324–332.

Bissette, G., Klimek, V., Pan, J., et al. (2003). Elevated concentrations of CRF in the locus coeruleus of depressed subjects. *Neuropsychopharmacology*, **28**, 1328–1335.

Coryell, W., & Schlesser, M. (2001). The dexamethasone suppression test and suicide prediction. *American Journal of Psychiatry*, **158**, 748–753.

Gold, P. W., Drevets, W. C., & Charney, D. S. (2002). New insights into the role of cortisol and the glucocorticoid receptor in severe depression. *Biological Psychiatry*, **52**, 381–385.

Herringa, R. J., Roseboom, P. H., & Kalin, N. H. (2006). Decreased amygdala CRF-binding protein mRNA in post-mortem tissue from male but not female bipolar and schizophrenic subjects. *Neuropsychopharmacology*, **31**, 1822–1831.

Heuser, I., Yassouridis, A., & Holsboer, F. (1994). The combined dexamethasone/CRH test: a refined laboratory test for psychiatric disorders. *Journal of Psychiatric Research*, **28**, 341–356.

Hiroi, N., Wong, M. L., Licinio, J., et al. (2001). Expression of corticotropin-releasing hormone receptors type I and type II mRNA in suicide victims and controls. *Molecular Psychiatry*, **6**, 540–546.

Hucks, D., Lowther, S., Crompton, M. R., et al. (1997). Corticotropin-releasing factor binding sites in cortex of depressed suicides. *Psychopharmacology (Berlin)*, **134**, 174–178.

Klok, M. D., Alt, S. R., Irurzun Lafitte, A. J., et al. (2011). Decreased expression of mineralocorticoid receptor mRNA and its splice variants in postmortem brain regions of patients with major depressive disorder. *Journal of Psychiatric Research*, **45**, 871–878.

Lester, D. (1992). The dexamethasone suppression test as an indicator of suicide: a meta-analysis. *Pharmacopsychiatry*, **25**, 265–270.

Lombardo, K. A., Herringa, R. J., Balachandran, J. S., et al. (2001). Effects of acute and repeated restraint stress on corticotropin-releasing hormone binding protein mRNA in rat amygdala and dorsal hippocampus. *Neuroscience Letters*, **302**, 81–84.

Lopez, J. F., Chalmers, D. T., Little, K. Y., et al. (1998). A.E. Bennett Research Award. Regulation of serotonin1A, glucocorticoid, and mineralocorticoid receptor in rat and human hippocampus: implications for the neurobiology of depression. *Biological Psychiatry*, **43**, 547–573.

McGowan, P. O., Sasaki, A., D'Alessio, A. C., et al. (2009). Epigenetic regulation of the glucocorticoid receptor in human brain associates with childhood abuse. *Nature Neuroscience*, **12**, 342–348.

Merali, Z., Du, L., Hrdina, P., et al. (2004). Dysregulation in the suicide brain: mRNA expression of corticotropin-releasing hormone receptors and GABA(A) receptor subunits in frontal cortical brain region. *Journal of Neuroscience*, **24**, 1478–1485.

Merali, Z., Kent, P., Du, L., et al. (2006). Corticotropin-releasing hormone, arginine vasopressin, gastrin-releasing peptide, and neuromedin B alterations in stress-relevant brain regions of suicides and control subjects. *Biological Psychiatry*, **59**, 594–602.

Nemeroff, C. B., Widerlov, E., Bissette, G., et al. (1984). Elevated concentrations of CSF corticotropin-releasing factor-like immunoreactivity in depressed patients. *Science*, **226**, 1342–1344.

Nemeroff, C. B., Owens, M. J., Bissette, G., et al. (1988). Reduced corticotropin releasing factor binding sites in the frontal cortex of suicide victims. *Archives of General Psychiatry*, **45**, 577–579.

Papiol, S., Arias, B., Gasto, C., et al. (2007). Genetic variability at HPA axis in major depression and clinical response to antidepressant treatment. *Journal of Affective Disorders*, **104**, 83–90.

Perlman, W. R., Webster, M. J., Kleinman, J. E., et al. (2004). Reduced glucocorticoid and estrogen receptor alpha messenger ribonucleic acid levels in the amygdala of patients with major mental illness. *Biological Psychiatry*, **56**, 844–852.

Pfennig, A., Kunzel, H. E., Kern, N., et al. (2005). Hypothalamus-pituitary-adrenal system regulation and suicidal behavior in depression. *Biological Psychiatry*, **57**, 336–342.

Raadsheer, F. C., Hoogendijk, W. J., Stam, F. C., et al. (1994). Increased numbers of corticotropin-releasing hormone expressing neurons in the hypothalamic paraventricular nucleus of depressed patients. *Neuroendocrinology*, **60**, 436–444.

Raadsheer, F. C., Van Heerikhuize, J. J., Lucassen, P. J., et al. (1995). Corticotropin-releasing hormone mRNA levels in the paraventricular nucleus of patients with Alzheimer's disease and depression. *American Journal of Psychiatry*, **152**, 1372–1376.

Steckler, T., & Holsboer, F. (1999). Corticotropin-releasing hormone receptor subtypes and emotion. *Biological Psychiatry*, **46**, 1480–1508.

Vale, W., Spiess, J., Rivier, C., et al. (1981). Characterization of a 41-residue ovine hypothalamic peptide that stimulates secretion of corticotropin and beta-endorphin. *Science*, **213**, 1394–1397.

Wasserman, D., Wasserman, J., & Sokolowski, M. (2010). Genetics of HPA-axis, depression and suicidality. *European Psychiatry*, **25**, 278–280.

Webster, M. J., Knable, M. B., O'grady, J., et al. (2002). Regional specificity of brain glucocorticoid receptor mRNA alterations in subjects with schizophrenia and mood disorders. *Molecular Psychiatry*, **7**, 985–994, 924.

Yerevanian, B. I., Olafsdottir, H., Milanese, E., et al. (1983). Normalization of the dexamethasone suppression test at discharge from hospital: its prognostic value. *Journal of Affective Disorders*, **5**, 191–197.

Chapter 37

Receptor signaling in suicide

Yogesh Dwivedi

Introduction

Suicide is a major public health concern. Approximately one million people commit suicide worldwide each year and 30 000 people commit suicide in the USA alone. The lifetime suicide attempt rate among adults is approximately 10%; among adolescents, suicide is the third leading cause of death after motor vehicle crashes and homicide. Previously, most of the studies of suicidal behavior were focused on the roles of psychosocial and sociocultural factors; however, these factors are of too little predictive value to be clinically useful. Therefore, research on the biological perspective of suicide has gained a stronghold and appears to provide a promising approach for identifying biological risk factors associated with suicidal behavior.

Emerging evidence suggests that pathogenesis of mood disorders and suicide involves altered plasticity of neuronal pathways. In fact, it has been proposed that mood disorders/suicide result from an inability of the brain to make appropriate adaptive responses to environmental stimuli as a result of impaired synaptic and structural plasticity. Support for this idea comes from studies demonstrating altered brain structure during stress and depression (major components of suicidal behavior) and from suicidal patients. The alterations include reductions in cell number, density, cell body size, and neuronal and glial density in frontal cortical or hippocampal brain areas; and decreases in the parahippocampal cortex and cortical laminar thickness. In addition, changes in synaptic circuitry, synaptic connectivity, number and shape of dendritic spines, synapse formation, neuronal atrophy, and spatial cognition deficits have been reported in depression and/or during stress. The cellular mechanisms that underlie such compromised neural plasticity and structural impairments in mood disorders and suicide are not clearly understood; however, recent findings from our own laboratory and from others provide evidence that such changes may be a consequence of disruption in the cellular mechanisms governing structural/neural plasticity and cellular resilience.

Downstream signal transduction pathways are important for behavioral and environmental adaptations by regulating neural plasticity and integrating various physiological processes, including modulation of neurotransmitter synthesis and release, regulation of receptors and ion channels, neuronal excitability, gene expression, and cell proliferation. As has been discussed in the preceding chapters, a number of neurotransmitter receptors have been implicated in the pathophysiology of mood disorders and suicide, and they interact with each other in a complex fashion. Most of the interactions occur at the level of intracellular signal transduction mechanisms. Most neurotransmitter receptors regulate intracellular reactions by an indirect mechanism involving an intermediate transducing molecule known as guanosine 5'-triphosphate (GTP) binding protein, or G protein. Activated G proteins alter the functions of many downstream effectors. Also, there are receptors that contain intrinsic enzymatic properties (e.g. tyrosine receptor kinases) that initiate a cascade of events by phosphorylating themselves and further modulating the activation of effector molecules. Most of these effectors are enzymes that produce intracellular second messengers. The second messengers trigger the signaling cascade further downstream and cause a cellular response. Each signaling cascade has multiple levels of controlling mechanisms, and components of various signaling pathways interact with each other to integrate the functional response. It is the downstream intracellular signaling mediated by these neurotransmitter receptors that co-ordinates the behavior of individual cells within the brain in various physiological processes.

A Concise Guide to Understanding Suicide, ed. Stephen H. Koslow, Pedro Ruiz, and Charles B. Nemeroff. Published by Cambridge University Press.

Given the critical importance of intracellular signaling pathways, recent studies have focused on the role of various signaling molecules in the pathophysiology of mood disorders and suicide. The most studied intracellular signaling pathways in the pathophysiology of suicide are the phosphoinositide (PI) and the adenylyl cyclase-cyclic adenosine monophosphate (cAMP). In addition, recent studies have shown alterations in the components of the tyrosine receptor kinase-mediated extracellular signal-regulated kinase (ERK)/mitogen-activated protein kinase (MAP kinase) signaling. The present chapter aims to provide an insight into our understanding of the neurobiology of suicide at the levels of these signal transduction mechanisms.

Phosphoinositide (PI) and adenylyl cyclase-cAMP signaling systems in suicide

In this lipid signaling pathway, agonist binding to neurotransmitter receptors such as $5HT_{2A}$, $5HT_{2C}$, or α_1 adrenergic, causes activation of G proteins, which then activate the enzyme phosphoinositide-specific phospholipase C (PI-PLC). PI-PLC then hydrolyzes phosphatidylinositol 4,5 biphosphate (PIP_2) and generates two intracellular second messengers: inositol 1,4,5 tris phosphate (IP_3) and diacylglycerol (DAG). DAG remains within the membrane and activates phospholipid- and calcium-dependent enzyme protein kinase C (PKC), and increases its affinity for calcium. PKC phosphorylates substrate proteins in the plasma membrane and cytosol. DAG is short-lived and is rapidly phosphorylated to form phosphatidate by diacylglycerol kinase, thus causing the termination of PKC activation. The other second messenger, IP_3, leaves the cell membrane and diffuses within the cytosol. IP_3 then binds to IP_3 receptors and mobilizes Ca^{2+} from intracellular sources such as the endoplasmic reticulum. Once released, Ca^{2+} interacts with Ca^{2+}-sensitive calmodulin (CaM), which then activates calmodulin-dependent protein kinases (CaM kinases) (Fukami et al., 2010). PKC and CaM kinase can activate transcription factors, such as CREB. PKC has many substrates in cytosol where it can phosphorylate substrates, including MARCKS (Figure 37.1).

In the adenylyl cyclase-cAMP signaling system, agonist-induced modulation of G proteins causes activation of adenylyl cyclase, which converts substrate ATP to cAMP. cAMP then activates phosphorylating enzyme protein kinase A (PKA). PKA, like PKC, activates several transcription factors, resulting in the alterations in the transcription of important genes. The intracellular level of cAMP is determined by the rate of its synthesis from ATP by adenylyl cyclase and its catabolic conversion to 5'AMP by a cyclic nucleotide, phosphodiesterase (Figure 37.1). We have discussed perturbations in the critical components of PI and adenylyl cyclase-cAMP signaling pathways in suicidal behavior.

G proteins in suicide

G proteins occupy a central position and play a critical role in the transduction of extracellular signals to cellular targets, thus transmitting messages from cell surface receptors to cellular effectors (Wettschureck and Offermanns, 2005). G proteins are heterotrimers consisting of three subunits α, β, and γ, each encoded by a specific gene. β and γ subunits bind tightly to each other, whereas the β subunit also contains a common binding site for α subunit recognition. The α subunit binds to GTP and confers receptor-effector specificity to G proteins. The γ subunit has been reported to have a G protein-specific recognition site. In the resting-state, guanosine diphosphate (GDP) is bound to the α subunit, and the three subunits (α, β, and γ) are associated as a trimer. Receptor-mediated activation of G proteins causes the release of GDP from the α subunit, allowing GTP to bind to and induce the dissociation of the G protein α subunit from the βγ subunits. The α and βγ subunits can then activate various effectors to modulate cellular responses. The free α subunit has intrinsic GTPase activity, which causes the hydrolysis of bound GTP to GDP. This causes the reassociation of the α and the βγ subunits with the G protein complex and thus termination of their activity (Figure 37.1). The lifetime of the activated G protein subunit depends upon the GTPase-activating proteins (GAPs), which determine the rate at which the GTP bound to the α subunit is hydrolyzed (Hamm, 1998). The responsiveness of G protein-coupled receptors may desensitize in response to persistent stimulation. This may occur through the phosphorylation of G protein-coupled receptors by second messenger-regulated kinases, thereby blocking their interaction with G proteins. A second mechanism is through the selective phosphorylation of activated receptors by specific G protein-coupled receptor kinases. This is followed by binding of a protein of the arrestin family to the phosphorylated receptors, blocking their ability to activate G proteins, and thus results in the termination of the response (Cabrera-Vera et al., 2003).

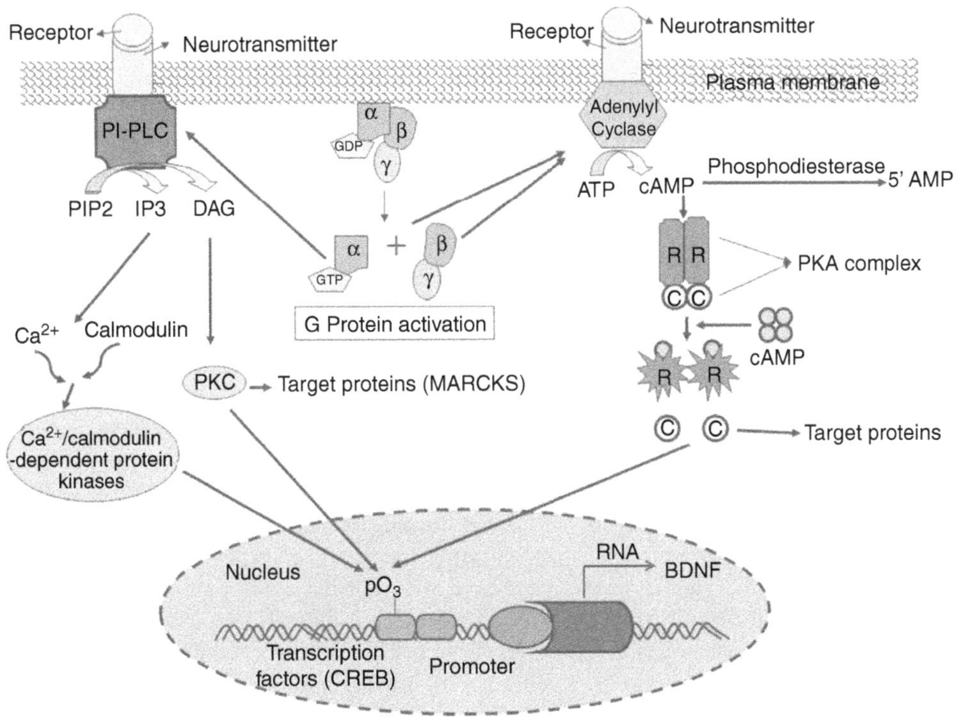

Figure 37.1. Overview of G proteins, phosphoinosite and adenylyl cyclase-cAMP signaling. In the inactive state, the α subunit of G protein is bound to guanosine diphosphate (GDP) and to βγ subunits. The binding of agonists to receptors causes an interaction of receptors with G proteins, which, in turn, releases GDP in exchange with guanosine triphosphate (GTP). This leads to generation of α-GTP and a βγ subunit dimer. Both α and βγ subunits can interact with effectors. In the phosphoinositide signaling pathway, the binding of neurotransmitter (NT) to G protein-coupled receptors leads to the activation of G proteins, which, in turn, activate enzyme phospholipase C (PLC), which then converts phosphoinositol 4, 5 bisphosphate (PIP2) into inositol tris phosphate (IP3) and diacylglycerol (DAG). DAG then activates protein kinase C (PKC) and IP3 binds to IP3 receptors and mobilizes Ca2+ from intracellular sources such as the endoplasmic reticulum. Once released, Ca2+ interacts with Ca-sensitive calmodulin (CaM), which then activates calmodulin-dependent protein kinases (CaM kinases). PKC and CaM kinases then can activate substrates such as CREB or MARCKS. In the adenylyl cyclase-cAMP signaling pathway, the binding of neurotransmitter (NT) to G protein-coupled receptors leads to the activation of G proteins, which, in turn, activate adenylyl cyclase, leading to the production of cyclic adenosine monophosphate (cAMP). Protein kinase A (PKA) is a holoenzyme composed of two subunits: regulatory (R) and catalytic (C). These regulatory and catalytic subunits form a tetrameric holoenzyme (R2C2). In the absence of cAMP, PKA exists as a stable inactive tetramer. The catalytic activity of cAMP is suppressed when the C subunits form a complex with the R subunits. Cyclic AMP, generated in response to adenylyl cyclase activation, binds to the R subunits of tetrameric PKA holoenzymes. The binding of cAMP to an R subunit lowers its affinity for the C subunit. This causes the release of free C subunits. The C subunit can catalyze phosphorylation of substrates in the cytoplasm or, after translocation of the C subunits, in the nucleus. Protein kinase A is also anchored with A kinase-anchoring proteins, causes compartmentalized localization of PKA, and initiates phosphorylation of substrates in a localized fashion. As with PKC, PKA can activate CREB, which regulates the transcription of many neuronally expressed genes, including BDNF. Deactivation of PKA is achieved through degradation of cAMP to 5'AMP by cAMP-specific phosphodiesterases. See plate section for color version.

On the basis of cDNA sequencing and the similarity of amino acid sequences, Gα subunits have been classified into four major classes: G_s, G_i, G_q, and G_{12}. More than 16 distinct genes encode the G protein α subunits, and there is a splice variant in at least two genes (Neves et al., 2002). Five distinct β subunit genes and 12 γ subunit genes have also been identified (Hildebrandt, 1997). Once activated, both α and βγ subunits can activate or inhibit multiple effectors to modulate cellular responses. $G_s\alpha$ stimulates adenylyl cyclase, whereas $G_i\alpha$ mediates the inhibition of adenylyl cyclase. $G_q\alpha$ is coupled to phospholipase C, an enzyme that is involved in PI hydrolysis. $G_s\alpha$ and $G_i\alpha$ have also been shown to be operative in gating L-type Ca^{2+} channels and K^+ channels, respectively. The G_i family includes G_t (transducin), which activates cyclic guanyl monophosphate (cGMP) phosphodiesterase and two G_o isoforms. The role of $G_{12}\alpha$ is not clear. Recent studies suggest that $G_{12}\alpha$ can stimulate GAPs and non-receptor tyrosine kinases. $G_o\alpha$ is believed to be associated with PI hydrolysis and ion channels. In addition, G proteins are also linked to effectors such as phospholipase A_2, phosphodiesterases, and phosphatidylinositol (PI)-3 kinase, and to second messengers, such as cGMP, arachidonic acid, and phosphatidic acid (Marinissen & Gutkind, 2001). A particular G protein can couple to more than one effector. Studies also demonstrate that different classes of G proteins can couple to a single effector. This occurs through the molecular switching of one G protein: effector system to a different G protein:effector system, triggered by agonist-mediated phosphorylation of receptors. Agonist-occupied receptors cannot stimulate GTP/GDP exchange on an α subunit without the presence of the βγ subunit dimer. Like the α subunit, the βγ subunit can activate different effectors and ion channels. For example, it has been shown that the βγ subunit can activate muscarinic K^+ channels and may also activate the MAP kinase pathway through Ras (a low molecular weight G protein). A few studies also suggest activation of phospholipase Cβ directly by βγ subunits.

G protein function has been studied in the postmortem brain of suicide victims by several investigators. Cowburn et al. (1994) studied adenylyl cyclase activity and expression of $G_S\alpha$ and G_i in the frontal cortex of suicide subjects and found that basal and GTPγS-stimulated adenyl-cyclase activity was significantly lower without any change in expression of $G_S\alpha$ or $G_i\alpha$. The decreased GTPγS-stimulated adenylcyclase activity was more profound in those suicide subjects who died from violence or had a history of depression. Pacheco et al. (1996) found that GTPγS-stimulated PI hydrolysis was decreased in frontal cortex of depressed suicide subjects. However, G protein-stimulated PI hydrolysis, which is a function of G protein activation, was not altered. In addition, they found increased expression of $G_S\alpha$ and decreased expression of $G_{i/2}\alpha$ in depressed suicide subjects. Gurguis et al. (1999) determined the affinity and coupling of β-adrenergic receptors to $G_S\alpha$ protein in brain of suicide subjects and found super-coupling of the receptors to the $G_S\alpha$ protein. Dowlatshahi et al. (1999) studied G proteins and the G protein-coupled cAMP signaling system in the postmortem brain of subjects with mood disorders who died of suicide and of a natural death. They did not find significant differences in the levels of $G\alpha_S$ (long or short form) or $G_i\alpha$ across-diagnostic groups in either temporal or occipital cortex. They also compared G proteins in those subjects who died as a result of suicide with the G proteins in normal control subjects. However, they did not find any significant differences in the protein expression level of $G_S\alpha$ (either long or short form) or Gi α in suicide subjects compared with control subjects.

In a large postmortem brain study, we comprehensively examined the role of G proteins in suicidal behavior by examining the gene transcription, as well as the protein levels of various α, β, and γ subunits of G proteins in the postmortem brain of suicide subjects (Dwivedi et al., 2002). We included both adult and teenage suicide subjects. This study was performed in the PFC obtained from 43 suicide subjects and 38 non-psychiatric normal control subjects. When we compared the protein levels of the various subunits of G proteins between suicide subjects and control subjects, we found that the levels of $G_{i2}\alpha$ and $G_o\alpha$ were significantly decreased and the level of $G_s\alpha_{-S}$ was significantly increased in the PFC of suicide subjects compared with normal control subjects. We did not find any significant differences in the levels of $G_S\alpha_{-L}$, $G_{i1}\alpha$, $G_{q/11}\alpha$, Gβ, or Gγ subunits between suicide subjects and normal control subjects. Since the characteristics of teenage suicide may differ from those of adult suicide, we divided the suicide subjects into subgroups of teenage suicide subjects (age <19 years) and adult suicide subjects (age >20 years), and analyzed the G protein subunits of these two populations separately (27 adult suicide subjects and 20 adult control subjects and 16 teenage suicide subjects and 16 teenage control subjects). When the suicide population was subdivided on the basis of age, we again observed that the mRNA levels of $G_{i2}\alpha$ and $G_o\alpha$ were significantly decreased and of $G_s\alpha_{-S}$ were significantly increased in PFC of adult suicide subjects compared with adult control subjects, without any change in mRNA levels of $G_{i1}\alpha$. On the other hand, there were no significant differences in mRNA levels of any of the G protein subunits between our total teenage controls and teenage suicide subjects.

More recently in brain of depressed suicide subjects, we found that Gsα is less available for adenylyl cyclase signaling because of its presence in cytoskeletal-associated lipid raft-like domains, suggesting that membrane microdomains are critical in G protein signaling and are impaired in suicide brain (Donati et al., 2008).

Overall, although there are contradictions in the studies of G protein results, our own studies indicate that the G protein-stimulated adenylyl cyclase/cAMP pathway may be activated and PI-PLC pathway may be inhibited in the brain of suicide subjects.

PI-PLC and PKC in suicide

As discussed above, PI-PLC is a critical component of the PI signaling pathway, which converts PIP2 into DAG and IP3 and thus helps to transduct signals from the receptors to the nucleus (Figure 37.1). PI-PLC is predominantly present in the cytosol but its presence in the membrane has also been demonstrated. Based on sequence homology, PI-PLC isoforms are classified into three major families: PLCβ, PLCγ, and PLCδ. The PLCβ family consists of three members that are highly expressed in brain: $PLC\beta_1$, $PLC\beta_2$, and $PLC\beta_3$. PLCγ consists of γ_1 and γ_2 subunits, whereas PLCδ is subtyped into δ_1 and δ_2. Although the involvement of receptors coupled to the PI signaling system in the pathophysiology of suicide has been studied by several investigators, studies of the other components of the PI signaling system, including PLC, have been very limited. Pacheco et al. (1996) measured the expression levels of PLCβ in the PFC of depressed suicide victims but did not find any significant differences between suicide subjects and normal control. We determined the PI-PLC activity as well as expression of PLC isozymes in membrane and cytosol fractions of postmortem brain samples obtained from Brodmann's areas 8 and 9 from teenage suicide subjects (Pandey et al., 1999). It was observed that PI-PLC activity was significantly lower in both the membrane as well as the cytosol fractions of the PFC of the teenage suicide subjects, which was associated with decreased expression of $PLC\beta_1$ isozyme. No significant differences were observed in the expression of $PLC\delta_1$ or $PLC\gamma_1$. These results suggested that adolescents who commit suicide have significantly lower than normal PI-PLC activity in the PFC and that this appears to be due to a selectively lower expression of selective $PLC\beta_1$. This could also be associated with lower Gqα protein expression.

PKC is the downstream regulatory enzyme in the PI pathway activated by DAG in response to PI-PLC activation. On the basis of molecular structure and enzymatic characterization, the PKC family has been sub-grouped into three classes, conventional (α, βI, βII, and γ), novel (δ, ε, η, and θ), and atypical (ι, κ. λ and τ). Each isozyme is encoded by a unique gene, except βI and βII, which are products of the differential splicing of the same transcript. The conventional isozymes are phospholipid- and calcium-dependent, whereas the novel PKC isozymes do not require calcium for activation. The atypical isozymes are unresponsive to phorbol esters but can be activated by phosphatidylserine. PKC isozymes are present in both the cytosol and the membrane, and activation of PKC results in its translocation from cytosol to membrane, which is required for its subsequent physiological response.

We were the first to examine PKC in brain of suicide subjects (Pandey et al., 2004) and reported that binding of $[^3H]$PDBu to regulatory regions of PKC was significantly decreased in both membrane and cytosol fractions obtained from the PFC of teenage suicide subjects, suggesting lower capability of regulatory subunits of PKC to bind its activators. Because each PKC isozyme is related to specific functions, we determined the catalytic activity of PKC and expression levels of PKC isozymes in PFC and hippocampus of teenage suicide subjects. We found that PKC activity was significantly decreased along with decreased expression of PKCα, βI, βII, and γ in both PFC and hippocampus of teenage suicide subjects. In contrast, Coull et al. (2000) did not find any change in $[^3H]$PBDu binding between antidepressant-treated suicide victims and control subjects. However, they noted increased $[^3H]$PBDu binding in antidepressant-free adult suicide victims compared with control subjects. Why there is such a discrepancy is not clear, however, this could be attributed to age-associated changes in PKC (teenage vs. adult) in suicide subjects.

As stated earlier, PKC phosphorylates not only transcription factors but also several substrates, including myristoylated alanine-rich C kinase substrate (MARCKS). MARCKS belongs to a family of homologous proteins that bind to calmodulin in a calcium-dependent manner. MARCKS has a basic binding domain for the acidic phospholipids actin and calmodulin, and this interaction can be modulated by PKC via phosphorylation. PKC-mediated phosphorylation occurs at three serine residues within the lysine-rich phosphorylation site domain and is catalyzed by a number of PKC isozymes. McNamara et al. (1999) determined MARCKS expression in the PFC and hippocampus of suicide subjects and did not observe any differences. We also did not find a change in expression of MARCKS in PFC of suicide subjects (Pandey et al., 2003); however, when suicide subjects were separated into depressed and non-depressed groups, we found that expression of MARCKS was increased in depressed suicide subjects but was decreased in suicide subjects who were not depressed. In addition, we found that PKC-mediated phosphorylation of MARCKS was significantly lower in the PFC of both depressed as well as non-depressed suicide subjects. It appears that PKC-mediated functional response at the level of MARCKS is abnormal in suicide subjects regardless of its expression levels.

PKA in suicide

In the adenylyl cyclase–cAMP pathway, the effects of cAMP are primarily mediated by its receptor PKA. Thus studying the status of PKA provides direct evidence of altered cAMP signaling. PKA is a holoenzyme composed of two subunits: regulatory (R) and catalytic (C). These subunits form a tetrameric holoenzyme (R_2C_2). In the absence of cAMP, PKA exists as a stable inactive tetramer. The catalytic activity of cAMP is suppressed when the C subunits form a complex with the R subunits. The C subunit is initially phosphorylated by phosphoinositide-dependent kinase at threonine 197 in the activation loop. This phosphorylation is necessary for the optimal biological activity of PKA. After an increase in intracellular cAMP, the regulatory PKA subunits bind to cAMP in a cooperative manner, which results in the conformational change in the regulatory subunits, leading to the dissociation of the holoenzyme into an $R_2(cAMP)_4$ dimer and two monomers of catalytically active C kinase. The R subunits remain in the cytoplasm, and the free catalytic subunits either translocate into the nucleus or remain in the cytosol. In both locations, PKA C subunits phosphorylate serine and threonine residues of specific substrates. By phosphorylating substrates, PKA can modulate neurotransmitter release; receptor desensitization; cell growth, differentiation, survival; and synaptic plasticity.

Based on the elution profile on diethylaminoethyl cellulose exchange chromatography, two major forms of PKA have been identified (i.e, types I and II). These two types differ in their structure in the regulatory subunits incorporated, termed RI or RII, whereas their catalytic subunits are either identical or very similar. Cloning studies have revealed multiple isoforms for each regulatory subunit: two RI subunits (RIα and RIβ) and two RII subunits (RIIα and RIIβ). The different PKA subtypes have different affinity for cAMP. The RI subunits have much greater affinity for cAMP than the RII subunits. The RIα-containing holoenzymes are activated at a five-fold lower concentration of cAMP than the RIβ-containing holoenzymes. Tissue distribution studies suggest that RIα is ubiquitously distributed and that RIIα is expressed in brain and testis. Similarly, RIβ is ubiquitously distributed and RIIβ is predominantly expressed in brain, adrenal, and adipose tissues and is the principal mediator of cAMP activity in the mammalian CNS. Three distinct catalytic subunits have been identified: Cα, Cβ, and Cγ. It has been shown that Cβ-containing PKA holoenzymes dissociate more easily on binding to cAMP than those containing Cα. Also, these isozymes form either homodimers or heterodimers of the R subunits, yielding holoenzyme complexes of PKA composed of a number of different combinations, including $RI\alpha_2C_2$, $RI\beta_2C_2$, $RII\alpha_2C_2$, $RII\beta_2C_2$, and $RI\alpha RI\beta C_2$. The presence of multiple C subunits adds substantial diversity to the action of PKA. Tissue distribution studies suggest that Cβ is expressed primarily in the brain, whereas Cα is ubiquitously expressed. Cγ is present only in testis.

In a comprehensive study, we examined the role of PKA in suicide. We determined cAMP binding to regulatory subunits of PKA and catalytic activity of PKA in the PFC of adult suicide subjects (Dwivedi et al., 2002, 2004). We observed that cAMP binding to regulatory subunits of PKA was significantly decreased; however, there were no significant differences in the affinity of cAMP binding to these subunits. In addition, we observed that PKA activity was decreased in the PFC of suicide subjects in both the presence and absence of cAMP. Our results suggest that decreased activation of PKA is not dependent on less availability of cAMP. This is a surprising finding given that $G_{i2}\alpha$ and $G_o\alpha$ were significantly decreased and $G_s\alpha_{-S}$ is decreased in brain of suicide subjects, suggesting greater availability of cAMP.

To examine if the decreases in PKA activity and cAMP binding in brain of suicide subjects are associated with changes in the expression of specific catalytic and/or regulatory subunits, we determined expression of all the catalytic and regulatory subunits of PKA (Dwivedi et al., 2004). We observed interesting results in both cohorts of brain samples. For example, there was a significant decrease in expression of selective regulatory RIIβ and catalytic Cβ subunits in the PFC of suicide subjects. No changes were observed in expression of RIα, RIIα, RIβ, or Cα subunits. These results suggest that decreases in cAMP binding and PKA activity could be due to decreases in the gene expression of selective RIIβ and Cβ subunits, respectively. These results have been independently confirmed by Odagaki et al. (2001).

To examine whether the changes in PKA in adult suicide are similar to those in the teenage suicide population, we conducted similar studies in brain of teenage suicide subjects. As in the adult suicide population, we found that PKA activity was decreased in the PFC of teenage suicide subjects. However, expression levels of PKA subunits showed a different pattern of changes. In contrast to adult suicide population, teenage suicide subjects showed decreased expression of RIα and RIβ. This is quite distinct from what we observed in the adult population. When teenage suicide subjects were divided into those with a history of major mental disorders and those with no such history, no significant differences in PKA activity or protein and mRNA expression of any of the subunits were noted between the two groups, suggesting that the observed changes were not related to specific mental disorders but to suicide. Certain questions remain: Why are different regulatory and catalytic subunits altered in teenage vs. adult populations? Is this related to specific behavioral characteristics, such as affective disorders or impulsive aggressive behavior? Recently, Shelton et al. (2009a) reported that PKA activity is decreased in the PFC of depressed subjects. In another study, these investigators show that melancholic depressed subjects show lower PKA RIα and Cβ expression in the frontal cortex, whereas those who died by suicide show lower PKA RIα and Cα expression (Shelton et al., 2009b). Thus, whether a decrease in specific PKA subunits is related to specific clinical phenotype needs to be further examined.

What could be the relevance of such changes in the expression of specific PKA regulatory and catalytic subunits with respect to their role in suicide? The specific functions of RIIβ and Cβ are not clearly known. However, tissue distribution studies suggest that RIIβ is predominantly expressed in brain, adrenal, and adipose tissues and is the principal mediator of cAMP activity in the mammalian CNS; whereas Cβ is expressed primarily in the brain. More specifically, RIIβ is associated with postsynaptic structures, suggesting that this subunit is involved in postsynaptic neuronal functions. Also, many studies have demonstrated that RIIβ and Cβ subunits are specifically involved in neuronal and behavioral functions. For example, the RIIβ subunit can translocate to the nucleus and phosphorylates one of the important substrates of PKA i.e., CREB. Also, RIIβ-mutant mice show defective motor behavior (Brandon et al., 1998) and increased tendency to consume ethanol (Thiele et al., 2000). The Cβ-mutant mice, on the other hand, show impaired hippocampal plasticity. Targeted disruption of the RIβ subunit gene also results in defects in long-term depression and depolarization, suggesting a deficit in a learning-related form of synaptic plasticity (Brandon et al., 1998). An RIβ deficiency produces selective defects in mossy fiber long-term potentiation (Brandon et al., 1998). Another important aspect of PKA is its involvement in the cross-talk between different signaling mechanisms. For example, PKA interferes at various levels with other signaling pathways, including: inactivation of phospholipase Cβ; phosphorylation of IP3 receptors, thereby modulating Ca^{2+} influx; phosphorylation of G proteins, with a consequent decrease in phosphoinositide hydrolysis and Ca^{2+} release; and phosphorylation of calcium-calmodulin kinase. In addition, cAMP stimulates MAP kinase activity in neurons and is required for its nuclear translocation. Furthermore, cross-talk between the cAMP/PKA and mitogen-activated protein kinase pathways is necessary to regulate gene expression. Given the significance of PKA in many biological actions in the brain, together with emerging studies demonstrating specific roles for its catalytic and regulatory subunits in physiological and behavioral manifestations, the observations of decreased catalytic and regulatory activities and the expression of specific regulatory and catalytic subunits in brain of suicide subjects suggest that abnormalities in PKA may be critically important in the pathophysiology of suicidal behavior.

CREB in suicide

The regulation of gene expression is a fundamental mechanism of brain development, homeostasis, and adaptation to the environment. Transcription factor CREB is a member of the leucine zipper family, which binds to the consensus motif 5'-TGACGTCA-3', found in the promoters of many neuronally expressed genes, and thereby activates or represses the transcription of target genes. Phosphorylation of CREB by kinases including PKA and PKC is the critical step in its activation. In its active form, CREB regulates many aspects of neuronal functioning, including excitation of nerve cells, CNS development, and long-term synaptic plasticity. One of the many important genes whose transcription is mediated through the activation of CREB is BDNF. To determine if CREB could possibly be involved in suicide, we examined the expression, and the CREB-DNA binding activity (a measure of functional characteristics), of CREB in the PFC and hippocampus of suicide subjects (Dwivedi et al., 2003a). We found that protein expression of CREB was significantly decreased in the nuclear fractions of the PFC and hippocampus obtained from suicide subjects. This decrease in protein expression levels was associated with a significant decrease in the mRNA levels of CREB, in both the PFC and hippocampus of suicide subjects. We also found decreased functional activity of CREB, such that CRE-DNA binding activity was decreased in the nuclear fractions of both the PFC and hippocampus of suicide subjects. Similar results were noted in the postmortem brain of teenage suicide subjects (Pandey et al., 2006). In addition, Young et al. (2004) reported altered levels of phosphorylated CREB in the amygdala of suicide subjects. These findings have important clinical implications. For example, all antidepressants activate CREB. Similar results have been shown in postmortem brain of depressed patients treated with antidepressants (Dowlatshahi et al., 1998). In contrast, the phosphorylation and expression of CREB are decreased in brain of depressed patients. Given the role of CREB in various physiological actions in the brain, the findings of its increased expression by antidepressants and of its decreased expression and functional characteristics in the brain of suicide subjects are quite important and implicate this gene in suicidal behavior.

BDNF in suicide

BDNF, one of the crucial neurotrophic factors, is a critical gene regulated by both PKA and PKC and participates in a wide range of physiological functions including neurite outgrowth, phenotypic maturation, morphological plasticity, and synthesis of proteins for differentiated functioning of neurons and synapses. Several studies suggest that BDNF is also involved in nerve regeneration, structural integrity, and maintenance of neuronal plasticity in the adult brain, including activity-dependent regulation of synaptic activity, and in neurotransmitter synthesis. Thus, a pathological alteration of the BDNF may lead not only to altered neural maintenance and regeneration and, therefore, structural abnormalities in the brain, but also to reduced neural plasticity. Most functions of BDNF are mediated by its receptor tropomycin receptor kinase B (TrkB), which exists in two isoforms: full-length (TrkB.FL) and truncated (TrkB.T1 and TrkB.T2). TrkB.FL contains the catalytic domain and binding of BDNF to TrkB.FL leads to the dimerization and transphosphorylation of tyrosine residues in the intracellular domain of the TrkB and subsequent activation of signaling pathways, leading to altered transcription of critical genes. These signaling pathways include ERK/MAP kinase, phosphoinositide 3-kinase, and phospholipase Cγ. Truncated TrkB lacks the signaling domain and by preventing induction of a signal transduction mechanism, it may act as a negative regulator of BDNF-mediated functioning. BDNF can also bind to pan75 neurotrophin receptor ($p75^{NTR}$), which plays an important role in neurotrophin transport, ligand-binding specificity, and Trk functioning.

We were the first to examine BDNF in brain of suicide subjects (Dwivedi et al., 2003b). We found that the mRNA level of BDNF was approximately 40–50% lower in the PFC and hippocampus of suicide subjects. By using antibody that recognizes mature BDNF, we found a significantly decreased protein level of BDNF in these areas of brain from suicide subjects. The mRNA and protein levels of BDNF were well correlated, suggesting that a decrease in BDNF is not due to unavailability but that there is a defect in the transcription of the *BDNF* gene in suicide brain. When we divided suicide subjects into those who had depression and those who had another psychiatric disorder, we found that the decrease in expression of BDNF was present in all suicide subjects regardless of psychiatric diagnosis. We also found a marginal decrease in BDNF in those suicide subjects who showed positive antidepressant toxicology. Our findings demonstrate that suicidal behavior is associated with reduced levels of BDNF. Karege et al. (2005) examined the expression of BDNF in the PFC, hippocampus, and entorhinal cortex of suicide subjects. Similar to our findings, they found lower levels of BDNF in PFC and hippocampus but not in the entorhinal cortex, suggesting that a decrease in BDNF may be specific to certain brain areas. In addition, they found that suicide subjects who were receiving antidepressants did not show any change in the level of BDNF, suggesting that psychotropic drugs normalize the decreased level of BDNF in these subjects.

Many recent studies have examined BDNF levels in the blood cells of suicidal subjects. Although the significance of BDNF in blood cells is unclear, it has been shown that BDNF may cross the blood–brain barrier and that platelet BDNF shows changes postnatally similar to brain (Karege et al., 2002), suggesting that there are parallel changes in the blood and brain levels of BDNF. Lee et al. (2007) measured plasma BDNF levels in depressed patients who had recently attempted suicide, non-suicidal depressed patients, and healthy controls. They found that BDNF levels were significantly lower in suicidal depressed patients vs. non-suicidal depressed patients or healthy controls. Interestingly, BDNF levels did not differ between fatal and non-fatal suicide attempts. Similarly, Lee et al. (2007) found that plasma BDNF level was decreased in depressed suicidal patients vs. depressed non-suicidal patients. These studies suggest that reduction of plasma BDNF levels is related to suicidal behavior in those with depression and that BDNF level may be a biological marker of suicidal depression. On the other hand, Deveci et al. (2007) reported that serum BDNF level was lower in both the attempted suicide group and the depressed group vs. the control group. Similarly, platelet BDNF levels were lower in both non-suicidal and suicidal depressed patients vs. healthy controls (Lee & Kim, 2009). Interestingly, Dawood et al. (2007) used direct internal jugular vein blood sampling methods to circumvent the issue of whether BDNF is released from sources other than the brain. They examined the relationship between brain BDNF production and suicide risk in patients with depression who were free of medication. They found that the venoarterial BDNF concentration gradient was significantly reduced in patients at medium to high suicide risk and that there was a significant negative correlation between suicide risk and BDNF concentration gradient.

TrkB in suicide

Apart from BDNF, its cognate TrkB receptors have been studied in relation to suicidal behavior. We examined the expression levels of TrkB in the same postmortem brain samples in which we determined the expression of BDNF. We found that the expression of full-length TrkB was significantly decreased in the PFC and hippocampus of suicide subjects without any changes in expression of truncated TrkB.T1 (Dwivedi et al., 2003a, 2009). Similar changes were noted in the PFC and hippocampus of teenage suicide subjects (Pandey et al., 2008). Our finding of decreased full-length TrkB expression may have serious implications as it would not only affect BDNF-induced signaling but also the supply of BDNF to neurons and, thus, the loss of trophic maintenance of neuronal types, because the catalytically active full-length TrkB is present predominantly within neuronal axons, cell soma, and dendrites. In addition, the undiminished numbers of truncated TrkB would only exacerbate any effects as a result of the loss of catalytically active full-length TrkB, because truncated TrkB inhibits BDNF-mediated neurite outgrowth via the internalization of BDNF. More recently, we examined the functionality of full-length TrkB and found that tyrosine phosphorylation of TrkB was significantly compromised in the brain of suicide subjects (Dwivedi et al., 2009). These studies suggest that not only BDNF and TrkB are less expressed, but also the functioning of TrkB is impaired in suicide brain.

Recently, Ernst et al. (2009) studied truncated TrkB.T1 in frontal cortex and cerebellum of suicide subjects. They found that about 36% of suicide completers had significant decreases in different probe sets specific to TrkB.T1 in frontal cortical areas but not the cerebellum. The decrease in TrkB expression was specific to the T1 splice variant. There was no effect of genetic variation in a 2500-base pair promoter region or at relevant splice junctions; however, an effect of methylation state at particular CpG dinucleotides on TrkB.T1 expression was noted. These results suggested a reduction in TrkB.T1 expression in suicide subjects, which was associated with the epigenetic modification of the TrkB.T1 promoter region.

p75^{NTR} in suicide

p75^{NTR}, initially discovered as a low-affinity receptor for NGF, is now known as a class of receptor that can bind to various neurotrophins, including BDNF, with equivalent nanomolar affinities. Although p75^{NTR} does not contain a catalytic motif, it interacts with Trk receptors and causes enhancement of ligand specificity and ligand affinities for Trks. Functionally, in contrast to Trk receptors, which contain autophosphorylation sites, p75^{NTR} lacks intrinsic enzymatic activity and can transmit both positive and negative signals (Meldolesi et al., 2000). When the cognate Trk receptor is less active, p75^{NTR} can mediate neuronal apoptosis. Similarly, p75^{NTR} can cause developing hippocampal neuronal death induced by neurotrophins in the absence of a Trk receptor (Friedman, 2000). In the adult CNS, excitotoxin-induced neuronal apoptosis is accompanied by the induction of p75^{NTR} in the dying neurons (Roux et al., 1999), which suggests that p75^{NTR} may represent a general stress-induced apoptotic mechanism (Miller & Kaplan, 2001). However, the apoptotic mechanisms of p75^{NTR} are active only when Trk receptors are less expressed or less active. Moreover, ectopic expression of the appropriate Trk receptor can convert a proapoptotic neurotrophin to a prosurvival neurotrophin. Thus, it appears that the ratio of expression levels and/or activation states of Trk receptors and $p75^{NTR}$ is quite relevant in neurotrophin-mediated functions. Recently, we observed that the expression ratio of $p75^{NTR}$ to Trk receptors is increased in the postmortem brain of suicide subjects (Dwivedi et al., 2009). Reduced expression of neurotrophins together with reduced expression and activation of Trk and concomitant increased expression of $p75^{NTR}$ indicate that the possible consequence is a tipping of the balance away from cell survival, which could be associated with structural abnormalities and reduced neuronal plasticity in suicide brain.

ERK1/2-MAP kinase signaling in suicide

ERK1/2-MAP kinase signaling is one of the crucial pathways by which BDNF/TrkB mediate their action in the CNS. In this pathway, dimerization and activation of Trk receptors causes activation of a small G protein, Ras, which then recruits another kinase, Raf, to the membrane, where it is phosphorylated and activated by serine/threonine/tyrosine kinases. This leads to the activation of another kinase known as ERK1/2 kinase (also known as MEK). MEK1/2 then phosphorylates and activates ERK1/2 on serine/threonine residues. The two best-characterized members of the ERK subfamily are ERK1 and ERK2. The activation of either form of MAP kinase requires dimerization of ERK and phosphorylation of the regulatory tyrosine and threonine residues of at least one of the ERKs in the dimer. Following activation, both ERK1 and ERK2 can phosphorylate regulatory targets in the cytosol or translocate to the nucleus, phosphorylate common substrates, and possess an apparently identical pattern of spatio-temporal activation. The activation of ERK1 and ERK2 also depends upon their dephosphorylation by phosphatases. For example, "dual function" MAP kinase phosphatase, (MKP)2, which specifically dephosphorylates ERK1 and ERK2, has been implicated in the inactivation of ERK1 and ERK2. The activation of ERKs leads to the phosphorylation of important extracellular proteins, effectors, and transcription factors, and results in a variety of responses, including cell proliferation and differentiation, gene expression, and cell cycle response of neurons to neural activity.

We studied the ERK1/2 signaling pathway in various prefrontal cortical areas, hippocampus, and cerebellum obtained from depressed suicide victims (Dwivedi et al., 2001). In the resting cells, ERK1/2 is primarily localized in cytosol, where a fraction is attached to cytoskeletal elements. However, this localization changes rapidly upon extracellular stimulation, which causes translocation of ERKs to the nucleus. In our study, we observed that ERK1/2 activity was significantly reduced in both nuclear and cytosol fractions of the PFC and hippocampus of depressed suicide subjects. However, the ratio of nuclear versus cytosol ERK1/2 activities was similar in all brain areas of depressed suicide subjects compared with control subjects in which we had observed changes in ERK1/2 activity. This suggests that the decrease in ERK1/2 activity is a generalized decrease and is not related to the translocation phenomenon. One of the reasons for a generalized decrease in ERK1/2 activation could be reduced expression of ERK1 and/or ERK2. To examine this, we determined protein levels of ERK1 and ERK2 using a total phosphorylation state independent antibody for ERK1/2 (Dwivedi et al., 2001). Our comparison studies showed that the immunodetectable levels of both ERK1 and ERK2 were significantly decreased in the PFC and hippocampus of depressed suicide subjects compared with control subjects. To further examine if these decreases were due to reduced gene expression, we determined individually the mRNA levels of ERK1 and ERK2. As we found in the immunolabeling studies, the mRNA levels of both ERK1 and ERK2 were significantly decreased in the PFC and hippocampus of depressed suicide subjects compared with control subjects. These results suggest that the decrease in ERK1/2 kinase activity may be due to reduced expression of ERK1 and ERK2.

In the ERK1/2 signaling cascade, other components, such as Ras, Raf, and dual function threonine/tyrosine kinases (MEK1/2) play an important role in activating ERK signaling. In addition, activation and deactivation of ERKs also depends upon their dephosphorylation, which is mediated by phosphatases. MKP2 is one of the regulatory "dual function" protein phosphatases that catalyze the dephosphorylation of ERK1 and ERK2. Interestingly, we observed that not only activation of MEK1/2 is reduced (Dwivedi et al., 2009), but also expression of B-Raf is lower (Dwivedi et al., 2006) and expression of MKP2 (Dwivedi et al., 2001) is greater in brain of depressed suicide subjects. These studies suggest that reduced activation of ERK could be associated with alterations in upstream kinases and phosphatases. At a behavioral level, ERK1 ablation in mice causes hyperactivity and resistance to behavioral despair in the forced swim test (Engel et al., 2009) and treatment of rats with MEK inhibitor induces mood disorder-related behavioral deficits (Einat et al., 2003). On the other hand, the peripheral injection of MEK inhibitors eliminates the response to antidepressants in behavioral despair (Duman et al., 2007). In a similar fashion, depressive-like behaviors in rats correlate with hypoactive ERK1/2 (Qi et al., 2008). On the other hand, fluoxetine treatment increases ERK activity and alleviates the depressive-like behavior in rats (Qi et al., 2006). A recent study suggests that a risk allele (Ser704Cyst) for depression is associated with reduced gray matter volume and lower ERK activity (Hashimoto et al., 2006). As with our findings (Dwivedi et al., 2009), it has recently been shown that not only is the expression of MAP kinase phosphatase increased in brain of depressed subjects and in brain of behavioral depressed rodents but also an increase in MKP in the hippocampus leads to depression (Duric et al., 2010). These studies suggest that ERK1/2 is impaired in mood disorders/suicide and that alteration in these signaling cascades can cause behavioral phenotypes.

To date, MAP kinases have been classified into at least six subfamilies. In addition to ERKs, the other members are stress-activated protein kinase, also known as Jun-NH_2-terminal kinase (JNK/SAPK), p38 MAP kinase, ERK5, and the recently identified ERK7 and MOK. Members of the MAP kinase family have different substrate specificities that mediate their diverse biological effects. Whether suicidal behavior is specifically related to abnormalities in ERK1/2-mediated signaling is not clear at the present time.

Conclusion

In this chapter, we have critically discussed the findings of abnormalities in signal transduction systems in suicidal behavior. We have focused primarily on PI, adenylyl cyclase, and ERK/MAP kinase signaling pathways and some of the critical substrates, whose functions are modulated in response to these signaling pathways. The results, although not always consistent, do indicate abnormalities in G proteins and of the effector molecule PLC, as well as the phosphorylating enzymes PKA and PKC. Downstream substrate CREB, which regulates transcription of important target genes including BDNF, is also altered in the postmortem brain of suicide subjects. The abnormalities in BDNF in suicide are compelling. Many postmortem brain studies in patients who complete suicide and in those with suicidal ideation or attempted suicide show decreased BDNF expression and abnormalities in its cognate TrkB/TrkB.T1 receptor. Although depression is an important factor in suicide, some studies were able to differentiate suicidal behavior vs. depressive behavior in terms of decreased level of BDNF. Not only BDNF but also TRK receptors and signaling mechanisms by which BDNF mediates its functions are impaired in the brain of suicide subjects. Interestingly, neurotrophin receptor $p75^{NTR}$, whose activity depends upon activation states of Trks, is also dysregulated in suicide brain. Overall, it appears that suicide brain is associated with abnormalities in signaling molecules that are critical in normal brain functioning.

There are many avenues that need further attention. For example, it has been shown that BDNF and TrkB regulate translational machinery in dendrites. In addition, BDNF induces the expression of Lim kinase 1, a protein kinase whose mRNA translation is inhibited by brain-specific micro-RNA-134. micro-RNA 134 is localized in dendrites and its overexpression leads to a decrease in spine size through repression of Lim kinase 1 mRNA translation. Thus, studying BDNF/TrkB and other interacting proteins in dendrites will further reveal their novel mechanistic roles in the development of depression/suicidal behavior. One of the important questions that needs to be asked is: are these abnormalities observed in suicide related to particular illnesses or risk factors, or are there common biological abnormalities in suicide across all diagnostic groups, independent of these risk factors, or related to specific diagnostic groups. For example, some of the findings observed in PKA signaling in suicide have also been found in depressed patients. Because many suicidal patients have depression, it is to be expected that such findings would also be present in depressed patients. To further relate these observed abnormalities to suicide, studies of postmortem brain samples from subjects who die of causes other than suicide need to be carried out to resolve these issues. In spite of these limitations, based on studies discussed above, a novel concept of the neurobiology of suicide is evolving, in which disruptions in cellular signaling could be seen as important biological risk factors that may be useful in delineating the etiology of suicide and could eventually result in site-specific therapeutic interventions.

References

Brandon, E. P., Logue, S. F., Adams, M. R., et al. (1998). Defective motor behavior and neural gene expression in RIIβ-protein kinase A mutant mice. *Journal of Neuroscience*, **18**, 3639–3649.

Cabrera-Vera, T. M., Vanhauwe, J., Thomas, T. O., et al. (2003). Insights into G protein structure, function, and regulation. *Endocrinology Reviews*, **24**, 765–781.

Coull, M. A., Lowther, S., Katona, C. L., et. al. (2000). Altered brain protein kinase C in depression: a post-mortem study. *European Journal of Neuropsychopharmacology*, **10**, 283–288.

Cowburn, R. F., Marcusson, J. O., Eriksson, A., et al. (1994). Adenylyl cyclase activity and G-protein subunit levels in postmortem frontal cortex of suicide victims. *Brain Research*, **633**, 297–304.

Dawood, T., Anderson. J., Barton, D., et al. (2007). Reduced overflow of BDNF from the brain is linked with suicide risk in depressive illness. *Molecular Psychiatry*, **12**, 981–983.

Deveci, A., Aydemir, O., Taskin, O., et al. (2007). Serum BDNF levels in suicide attempters related to psychosocial stressors: a comparative study with depression. *Neuropsychobiology*, **56**, 93–97.

Donati, R. J., Dwivedi, Y., Roberts, R. C., et al. (2008). Postmortem brain tissue of depressed suicides reveals increased Gs alpha localization in lipid raft domains where it is less likely to activate adenylyl cyclase. *Journal of Neuroscience*, **28**, 3042–3050.

Dowlatshahi, D., MacQueen, G. M., Wang, J. F., et al. (1998). Increased temporal cortex CREB concentrations and antidepression treatment in major depression. *Lancet*, **352**, 1754–1755.

Dowlatshahi, D., MacQueen, G. M., Wang, et al. (1999). G protein-coupled cyclic AMP signaling in postmortem brain of subjects with mood disorders: effects of diagnosis, suicide, and treatment at the time of death. *Journal of Neurochemistry*, **73**, 1121–1126.

Duman, C. H., Schlesinger, L., Kodama, M., et al. (2007). A role for MAP kinase signaling in behavioral models of depression and antidepressant treatment. *Biological Psychiatry*, **61**, 661–670.

Duric, V., Banasr, M., Licznerski, P., et al. (2010). A negative regulator of MAP kinase causes depressive behavior. *Nature Medicine*, **16**, 1328–1332.

Dwivedi, Y., Rizavi, H. S., Roberts, R. C., et al. (2001). Reduced activation and expression of ERK1/2 MAP kinase in the postmortem brain of depressed suicide subjects. *Journal of Neurochemistry*, **77**, 916–928.

Dwivedi, Y., Conley, R. R., Roberts, R. C., et al. (2002a). [3H]cAMP binding sites and protein kinase A activity in the prefrontal cortex of suicide victims. *American Journal of Psychiatry*, **159**, 66–73.

Dwivedi, Y., Rizavi, H. S., Conley, R. R., et al. (2002b). mRNA and protein expression of selective alpha subunits of G proteins are abnormal in prefrontal cortex of suicide victims. *Neuropsychopharmacology*, **27**, 499–517.

Dwivedi, Y., Rizavi, H. S., Conley, R. R., et al. (2003a). Altered gene expression of brain-derived neurotrophic factor and receptor tyrosine kinase B in postmortem brain of suicide subjects. *Archives of General Psychiatry*, **60**, 804–815.

Dwivedi, Y., Rao, J. S., Rizavi, H. S., et al. (2003b). Abnormal expression and functional characteristics of cyclic adenosine monophosphate response element-binding protein in postmortem brain of suicide subjects. *Archives of General Psychiatry*, **60**, 273–282.

Dwivedi, Y., Rizavi, H. S., Shukla, P. K., et al. (2004). Protein kinase A in postmortem brain of depressed suicide victims: altered expression of specific regulatory and catalytic subunits. *Biological Psychiatry*, **55**, 234–243.

Dwivedi, Y., Rizavi, H. S., Conley, R. R., et al. (2006). ERK MAP kinase signaling in post-mortem brain of suicide subjects: differential regulation of upstream Raf kinases Raf-1 and B-Raf. *Molecular Psychiatry*, **11**, 86–98.

Dwivedi, Y., Rizavi, H. S., Zhang, H., et al. (2009a). Aberrant extracellular signal-regulated kinase (ERK)1/2 signalling in suicide brain: role of ERK kinase 1 (MEK1). *Int J Neuropsychopharmacology*, **12**, 1337–1354.

Dwivedi, Y., Rizavi, H., Zhang, H., et al. (2009b). Neurotrophin receptor activation and expression in human postmortem brain: effect of suicide. *Biological Psychiatry*, **65**, 319–328.

Einat, H., Yuan, P., Gould, T. D., et al. (2003). The role of the extracellular signal-regulated kinase signaling pathway in mood modulation. *Journal of Neuroscience*, **23**, 7311–7316.

Engel, S. R., Creson, T. K., Hao, Y., et al. (2009). The extracellular signal-regulated kinase pathway contributes to the control of behavioral excitement. *Molecular Psychiatry*, **14**, 448–461.

Ernst, C., Deleva, V., Deng, X., et al. (2009). Alternative splicing, methylation state, and expression profile of tropomyosin-related kinase B in the frontal cortex of suicide completers. *Archives of General Psychiatry*, **66**, 22–32.

Friedman, W. (2000). Neurotrophins induce death of hippocampal neurons via the p75 receptor. *Journal of Neurosciemce*, **28**, 6340–6346.

Fukami, K., Inanobe, S., Kanemaru, K., et al. (2010). Phospholipase C is a key enzyme regulating intracellular calcium and modulating the phosphoinositide balance. *Progress in Lipid Research*, **49**, 429–437.

Gurguis, G. N., Turkka, J., Laruelle, M., et al. (1999). Coupling efficiency of brain beta-adrenergic receptors to Gs protein in suicide, alcoholism and control subjects. *Psychopharmacology (Berlin)*, **145**, 31–38.

Hamm, H. E. (1998). The many faces of G protein signaling. *Journal of Biological Chemistry*, **273**, 669–672.

Hashimoto, R., Numakawa, T., Ohnishi, T., et al. (2006). Impact of the DISC1 Ser704Cys polymorphism on risk for major depression, brain morphology and ERK signaling. *Human Molecular Genetics*, **15**, 3024–3033.

Hildebrandt, J. D. (1997). Role of subunit diversity in signaling by heterotrimeric G proteins. *Biochemical Pharmacology*, **54**, 325–339.

Karege, F., Schwald, M., & Cisse, M. (2002). Postnatal developmental profile of brain-derived neurotrophic factor in rat brain and platelets. *Neuroscience Letters*, **328**, 261–264.

Karege, F., Vaudan, G., Schwald, M., et al. (2005). Neurotrophin levels in postmortem brains of suicide victims and the effects of antemortem diagnosis and psychotropic drugs. *Brain Research. Molecular Brain Research*, **136**, 29–37.

Lee, B. H., & Kim, Y. K. (2009). Reduced platelet BDNF level in patients with depression. *Progress in Neuropsychopharmacology and Biological Psychiatry*, **33**, 849–853.

Lee, B. H., Kim, H., Park, S. H., et al. (2007). Decreased plasma BDNF level in depressive patients. *Journal of Affective Disorders*, **101**, 239–244.

Marinissen, M. J., & Gutkind, J. S. (2001). G-protein-coupled receptors and signaling networks: Emerging paradigms. *Trends in Pharmacological Sciences*, **22**, 368–376.

McNamara, R. K., Hyde, T. M., Kleinman, J. E., & Lenox, R. H. (1999). Expression of the myristoylated alanine-rich C kinase substrate (MARCKS) and MARCKS-related protein (MRP) in the prefrontal cortex and hippocampus of suicide victims. *Journal of Clinical Psychiatry*, **60**(Suppl 2), 21–26.

Meldolesi, J., Sciorati, C., & Clementi, E. (2000). The p75 receptor: first insights into the transduction mechanisms leading to either cell death or survival. *Trends in Pharmacological Sciences*, **21**, 242–243.

Miller, F. D., & Kaplan, D. R. (2001). Neurotrophin signaling pathways regulating neuronal apoptosis. *Cellular and Molecular Life Sciences*, **58**, 1045–1053.

Neves, S. R., Ram, P. T., & Iyengar, R. (2002). G protein pathways. *Science*, **296**, 1636–1639.

Odagaki, Y., Garcia-Sevilla, J. A., Huguelet. P., et al. (2001). Cyclic AMP-mediated signaling components are upregulated in the prefrontal cortex of depressed suicide victims. *Brain Research*, **898**, 224–231.

Pacheco, M. A., Stockmeier, C., Meltzer, H. Y., et al. (1996). Alterations in phosphoinositide signaling and G-protein levels in depressed suicide brain. *Brain Research*, **723**, 37–45.

Pandey, G. N., Dwivedi, Y., Pandey, S. C., et al. (1999). Low phosphoinositide-specific phospholipase C activity and expression of phospholipase C β1 protein in the PFC of teenage suicide subjects. *American Journal of Psychiatry*, **156**, 1895–1901.

Pandey, G. N., Dwivedi, Y., Ren, X., et al. (2003). Altered expression and phosphorylation of myristoylated alanine-rich C kinase substrate (MARCKS) in postmortem brain of suicide victims with or without depression. *Journal of Psychiatric Research*, **37**, 421–432.

Pandey, G. N., Dwivedi, Y., Rizavi, H. S., et al. (2004). Decreased catalytic activity and expression of protein kinase C isozymes in teenage suicide victims: a postmortem brain study. *Archives of General Psychiatry*, **61**, 685–693.

Pandey, G. N., Dwivedi, Y., Ren, X., et al. (2006). Cyclic AMP response element-binding protein in postmortem brain of teenage suicide victims: specific decrease in the prefrontal cortex but not the hippocampus. *International Journal of Neuropsychopharmacology*, **18**, 1–9.

Pandey, G. N., Ren, X., Rizavi, H. S., et al. (2008). Brain-derived neurotrophic factor and tyrosine kinase B receptor signalling in post-mortem brain of teenage suicide victims. *International Journal of Neuropsychopharmacology*, **11**, 1047–1061.

Qi, X., Lin, W., Li, J., et al. (2006). The depressive-like behaviors are correlated with decreased phosphorylation of mitogen-activated protein kinases in rat brain following chronic forced swim stress. *Behavioural Brain Research*, **175**, 233–240.

Qi, X., Lin, W., Li, J., et al. (2008). Fluoxetine increases the activity of the ERK-CREB signal system and alleviates the depressive-like behavior in rats exposed to chronic forced swim stress. *Neurobiology of Diseases*, **31**, 278–285.

Roux, P. P., Colicos, M. A., Barker, P. A., et al. (1999). p75 neurotrophin receptor expression is induced in apoptotic neurons after seizure. *Journal of Neuroscience*, **19**, 6887–6896.

Shelton, R. C., Sanders-Bush, E., Manier, D. H., et al. (2009a). Elevated 5-HT 2A receptors in postmortem prefrontal cortex in major depression is associated with reduced activity of protein kinase A. *Neuroscience*, **158**, 1406–1415.

Shelton, R. C., Hal, Manier D., & Lewis, D. A. (2009b). Protein kinases A and C in post-mortem prefrontal cortex from persons with major depression and normal controls. *International Journal of Neuropsychopharmacology*, **12**, 1223–1232.

Thiele, T. E., Willis, B., Stadler, J., et al. (2000). High ethanol consumption and low sensitivity to ethanol-induced sedation in protein kinase A-mutant mice. *Journal of Neuroscience*, **20**, RC75.

Wettschureck, N., & Offermanns, S. (2005). Mammalian G proteins and their cell type specific functions. *Physiological Reviews*, **85**, 1159–1204.

Young, L. T., Bezchlibnyk, Y. B., Chen, B., et al. (2004). Amygdala cyclic adenosine monophosphate response element-binding protein phosphorylation in patients with mood disorders: effects of diagnosis, suicide, and drug treatment. *Biological Psychiatry*, **55**, 570–577.

Funding support

The studies presented in this chapter are partly funded from NIMH R01082802 and the American Foundation for Suicide Prevention.

Chapter 38

Strategies to improve suicide prevention

Sarah A. Struthers and Robert M. A. Hirschfeld

Introduction

The most important result of improved understanding of the causes of suicide is its prevention. This chapter will review the most effective strategies to prevent suicide, summarizing the evidence supporting each strategy.

The most effective strategy to prevent suicide is to improve recognition and treatment of mood disorders by primary care providers (PCPs). Assisting PCPs in this effort are screening procedures for depression, bipolar disorder, and suicidality. Formal evaluation of suicide is the next step when suicide is suspected. If there is suicide risk, restriction of access to lethal means of committing suicide can be a lifesaver. Once suicidal risk has been established, several clinical management approaches can reduce the likelihood of suicide, including aggressive treatment of depression and bipolar disorder. Long-term management of these disorders may sustain a lower likelihood of future suicide. After a suicide attempt, appropriate clinical management may also reduce suicide in the future. Finally, public education about suicide can prevent suicide.

PCP recognition and diagnosis of mood disorders

A substantial portion of mental health care in the USA is delivered by primary care providers (Russell, 2010). Their first-line role in suicide prevention is reflected by studies showing that approximately 45% of patients completing suicide have had contact with a primary care provider within 1 month of their death, and 77% within 1 year. In contrast, only 19% of suicide completers have had contact with a mental health professional within 1 month of their death, and 32% within 1 year (Luoma et al., 2002). Unfortunately, many residents in primary care specialties receive inadequate training in the detection and management of suicidality. A 2007 study of primary care residency training directors in the USA showed that a large percentage of them lacked confidence in their resident's psychiatric evaluation skills, particularly in internal medicine and pediatrics (Sudak et al., 2007). Therefore, one strategy to improve suicide prevention would be to improve training for PCPs in the recognition and management of suicidality, and to foster incentives for PCPs to recognize and treat it (Mann et al., 2005).

It has been suggested that initiatives to improve psychiatric training of primary care residents may rest on academic psychiatry departments, rather than residents' home departments. One way of increasing residents' exposure to psychiatry is by providing them with the experience of doing a psychiatric elective in which they can learn to recognize and evaluate depression and suicidality in a hands-on setting with supervision and feedback from psychiatric attendings (Lake & Baumer, 2010).

Underlying psychopathology is a major risk factor for suicide: over 90% of patients completing suicide have been shown to have one or more psychiatric diagnoses by DSM-IV criteria. Mood disorders, particularly MDD, are present in up to 60% of suicides (Mann et al., 2005; Wasserman et al., 2012). Schizophrenia contributes to a smaller percentage of suicides; however suicide is the most frequent cause of premature death among those with schizophrenia. These disorders are frequently comorbid with alcohol or substance abuse, or presence of personality pathology, such as borderline or antisocial personality disorder (Gilbody et al., 2003). Therefore, the detection and management of mental illness by primary care and mental health providers can improve suicide

A Concise Guide to Understanding Suicide, ed. Stephen H. Koslow, Pedro Ruiz, and Charles B. Nemeroff. Published by Cambridge University Press.

prevention. Depression is the third most common reason for consultation with a primary care physician (Gilbody et al., 2003). However, many patients present with symptoms other than depression, such as fatigue, insomnia, weight loss, and difficulty with memory or concentration (WHO, 2000). Providers must become adept at identifying depression in the absence of complaints of sad mood. The provider must also recognize that general medical and psychiatric illness can coexist and that patients with certain chronic medical illnesses such as neurologic disease, neoplasm, or HIV/AIDs are at increased risk of depression and suicide (Wasserman et al., 2012; WHO, 2000).

Screening for mood disorders

A number of screening tools are available to aid primary care providers in screening for depression and other mood disorders. At minimum, patients in PCP clinics should be screened at least one time, usually upon establishing care so that a baseline can be determined. It is then up to the clinician's discretion whether to continue screening at regular intervals (US Preventive Services Task Force (USPSTF), 2009). Obtaining a brief psychiatric history, including personal and family history of psychiatric illness, on initial presentation may be helpful to evaluate a patient's risk factors for depression and devise an appropriate screening strategy.

In recent years, the PRIME-MD Patient Health Questionnaire (PHQ-9) has superseded other screening tools for depression in the primary care setting. The PHQ-9 has prevailed due to its ease of administration and interpretation. It can be completed by the patient in the waiting room in about 5–10 minutes and assesses for presence of diagnostic criteria as well as duration and degree of functional impairment. Sensitivity and specificity of the PHQ-9 have been demonstrated to be 80–90% and 70–85%, respectively. Of those patients who test positive, about 50% will meet all diagnostic criteria for depression (Nease & Malouin, 2003; USPSTF, 2009). As with other screening tools, a positive screen is not sufficient for diagnosis and warrants a more thorough clinical assessment of symptoms. This includes a diagnostic interview and consideration of the differential diagnosis, including presence of alcohol or substance abuse or any underlying medical condition.

A two-item version of the PHQ, known as the PHQ-2, has also been suggested as a suitable screening modality in primary care, with sensitivity and specificity reaching that of the PHQ-9 (Figure 38.1). It does not assess duration of symptoms or level of functional impairment, therefore patients screening positive should take the full PHQ and undergo further clinical evaluation (Nimalasuriya et al., 2009).

Patients with depression should undergo screening for bipolar disorder in addition to depression because treatment for the two disorders differs. The Mood Disorder Questionnaire (MDQ) is a 13-item yes/no inventory that screens for a lifetime history of bipolar disorder, with an additional two items assessing whether symptoms in question were experienced during the same time period and the level of functional impairment associated with the symptoms (Figure 38.2). The questionnaire is quickly and easily completed by the patient and scored by the provider, with good sensitivity (0.73) and very good specificity (0.90). As with the PHQ, patients screening positive on the MDQ should undergo clinical assessment to confirm the diagnosis (Nimalasuriya et al., 2009; Hirschfeld et al., 2000).

Screening for suicidality

A multitude of screening instruments are available to providers for evaluation of suicidality. Two of the most widely used scales with established validity include the Scale for Suicide Ideation (SSI), an interviewer-administered screening tool, and the self-report version, the Beck Scale for Suicide Ideation (BSI). Both instruments consist of 21 items evaluating the current intensity of suicidal ideation, behaviors, and plans for suicide within 1 day and 1 week of the interview, respectively. At least two items on each instrument assess the number of prior suicide attempts as well as the degree of intent associated with those attempts.

Evaluation of suicide risk should never be based upon the results of the screening instrument alone. If the patient endorses suicidal ideation or behavior, a formal suicide inquiry and comprehensive risk assessment should be undertaken (Brown, 2001).

Evaluation of suicidality

Suicide inquiry is necessary whenever a psychiatric problem is detected. The provider should ask about suicide, as patients are unlikely to volunteer information about suicidal ideation or behavior on their own volition. For example, in a study of 571 suicide completers, only 22% communicated their intent during their last appointment with a physician within 4 weeks of their death (Isometsa et al., 1995).

PATIENT HEALTH QUESTIONNAIRE-9 (PHQ-9)

Over the <u>last 2 weeks</u>, how often have you been bothered by any of the following problems? (*Use "✔" to indicate your answer*)	**Not at all**	**Several days**	**More than half the days**	**Nearly every day**
1. Little interest or pleasure in doing things	0	1	2	3
2. Feeling down, depressed, or hopeless	0	1	2	3
3. Trouble falling or staying asleep, or sleeping too much	0	1	2	3
4. Feeling tired or having little energy	0	1	2	3
5. Poor appetite or overeating	0	1	2	3
6. Feeling bad about yourself — or that you are a failure or have let yourself or your family down	0	1	2	3
7. Trouble concentrating on things, such as reading the newspaper or watching television	0	1	2	3
8. Moving or speaking so slowly that other people could have noticed? Or the opposite — being so fidgety or restless that you have been moving around a lot more than usual	0	1	2	3
9. Thoughts that you would be better off dead or of hurting yourself in some way	0	1	2	3

FOR OFFICE CODING __0__ + ______ + ______ + ______

= Total Score: ______

If you checked off <u>any</u> problems, how <u>difficult</u> have these problems made it for you to do your work, take care of things at home, or get along with other people?

Not difficult at all	**Somewhat difficult**	**Very difficult**	**Extremely difficult**
☐	☐	☐	☐

Developed by Drs. Robert L. Spitzer, Janet B.W. Williams, Kurt Kroenke and colleagues, with an educational grant from Pfizer Inc. No permission required to reproduce, translate, display or distribute.

Figure 38.1. PRIME-MD Patient Health Questionnaire (PHQ-9).

MDQ

THE MOOD DISORDER QUESTIONNAIRE

Instructions: Please answer each question as best you can.

		YES	NO
1	**Has there ever been a period of time when you were not your usual self and...**		
	... you felt so good or so hyper that other people thought you were not your normal self or you were so hyper that you got into trouble?	❍	❍
	... you were so irritable that you shouted at people or started fights or arguments?	❍	❍
	... you felt much more self-confident than usual?	❍	❍
	... you got much less sleep than usual and found you didn't really miss it?	❍	❍
	... you were much more talkative or spoke much faster than usual?	❍	❍
	... thoughts raced through your head or you couldn't slow your mind down?	❍	❍
	... you were so easily distracted by things around you that you had trouble concentrating or staying on track?	❍	❍
	... you had much more energy than usual?	❍	❍
	... you were much more active or did many more things than usual?	❍	❍
	... you were much more social or outgoing than usual, for example, you telephoned friends in the middle of the night?	❍	❍
	... you were much more interested in sex than usual?	❍	❍
	... you did things that were unusual for you or that other people might have thought were excessive, foolish or risky?	❍	❍
	... spending money got you or your family into trouble?	❍	❍
2	**If you checked YES to more than one of the above, have several of these ever happened during the same period of time?**	❍	❍
3	**How much of a problem did any of these cause you - like being unable to work; having family, money or legal troubles; getting into arguments or fights? Please circle one response only.**		
	No problem Minor problem Moderate problem Serious problem		

Figure 38.2. The Mood Disorder Questionnaire (MDQ).

In cases where suspicion is high and the patient is not forthcoming, attempts should be made to obtain collateral information from family members or close friends. Physicians should always obtain consent before contacting these people.

Suicide inquiry typically begins by asking the patient directly about the presence of suicidal thoughts. Passive suicidal ideation is characterized by the patient's having thoughts of wanting to die ("I wish I were dead"), while active suicidal ideation involves thoughts of actually killing oneself (Fiedorowicz et al., 2010). Questions are ideally posed in a straightforward, non-judgmental manner, and should avoid encouraging a negative response (e.g., "You're not thinking about suicide, are you?"). Open-ended questions that support dialogue are useful when beginning the conversation, and should be followed up with more specific questions to gain sufficient detail. Some helpful example questions for asking patients about suicidal ideation include:

- Have you ever thought about hurting or killing yourself?
- Have you ever thought that things would be better off if you were dead?
- Do you feel as if you have lost hope or that life is not worth living?
- Have you made any plans for ending your life? (WHO, 2000; Western Interstate Commission for Higher Education (WICHE) Mental Health Program and Suicide Prevention Resource Center (SPRC), 2009)

When suicidal ideation is present, the provider should assess the patient's intent to act upon the thoughts, including whether a plan has been formulated. It is important to obtain as much detail about suicide plans as possible, so that the level of intent as well as lethality can be included in the provider's final risk assessment. Actions that suggest a high level of intent include obtaining a gun or other lethal means, careful planning and rehearsal of the suicide attempt, and making preparations for death, including writing a will, giving away possessions, or saying goodbye to loved ones (Jacobs & Brewer, 2004). Patients who plan to attempt suicide when they are alone, or take precautions against possible intervention and survival, should be considered at very high risk.

Providers should assess the lethality of the patient's suicide plan in addition to the level of intent. Whether the patient has access to lethal means, including weapons or large amounts of substances that may be used to overdose, should be determined as well as the patient's understanding of the lethality of their chosen method. Generally, a highly lethal method combined with high intent signifies a high risk of completed suicide. Access to lethal means should always be carefully documented, and often a clinical decision will have to be made regarding restriction or removal of means from the patient's home environment (Jacobs & Brewer, 2004).

In addition to the presence of an underlying psychiatric disorder, a number of risk factors for elevated suicide risk have been previously identified. A history of attempted suicide is the best predictor of a future completed suicide, and as much information as possible should be obtained about prior attempts, including precipitants, level of intent, lethality of chosen methods, and aftermath (Wasserman et al., 2012). Certain demographic characteristics are also associated with an increased risk of suicide, including male gender, Caucasian ethnicity, age over 65, marital status as separated, widowed, or divorced, and unemployment or retirement (Simon, 2008).

Factors that have been cited to acutely increase the risk of suicide during a depressive episode include symptoms such as desperation, hopelessness or helplessness, anxiety, agitation, psychosis, or a history of impulsive or aggressive behaviors. In addition to depression several psychiatric disorders have been identified as risk factors for suicide. These include anxiety disorders (especially post-traumatic stress disorder), alcohol and other substance use disorders, schizophrenia, eating disorders, and trauma (Wasserman et al., 2012). Severe anxiety comorbid with depression is a particularly lethal combination which should be addressed aggressively (Fawcett, 1997, 2001).

Providers should also evaluate qualities which reduce suicide risk, known as protective factors. Often it is helpful simply to ask the patient what has prevented him/her from acting on their suicidal thoughts in the past. Certain characteristics, including good problem solving and coping skills, may help patients see beyond their current circumstances and reduce the likelihood of suicide. Strong social support from friends and family, especially if the patient is married, is an important protective factor. Having children or pets for which one is responsible also significantly reduces suicide risk. Additional protective factors include cultural, religious, or moral beliefs that discourage or disapprove of suicide, as well as fear of pain or of death itself (Simon, 2008; WICHE & SPRC, 2009).

Restriction of lethal means

One of the first things to do in assessing an individual for suicidality is to identify the individual's access to methods for suicide, and whenever possible to restrict or totally prevent access to such lethal means (Lester, 2012). Among the most lethal of suicide methods are firearms, cars, natural gas, jumping opportunities, and poisons.

The most frequently used method for completed suicide in the USA is firearms. Handguns are used in 62% of suicides among men and 39% among women (Carrigan & Lynch, 2003). Suicidal patients and their significant others should be queried about firearms and ammunition, and ease of access to them. If at all possible, firearms should be made inaccessible by encouraging a friend or family member to remove them from the patient's home. At the very least, guns should be kept locked up and stored separately from ammunition (Lester, 2012).

Access to prescription and over-the-counter medications that can be used in a potentially lethal overdose should be restricted. If the individual has a vehicle, access to this, particularly if it is housed in a garage, should be limited because of the possibility of carbon monoxide poisoning. Preventing access to bridges and buildings can be very difficult. However longer-term prevention may involve construction of fences and other barriers to jumping sites. Suicides by many of these methods have been reduced after introduction of restrictive legislation (Mann et al., 2005).

Management of suicidal patients

A comprehensive suicide risk assessment evaluation takes into account the patient's risk and protective factors in conjunction with their clinical presentation and ultimately drives treatment planning. American Psychiatric Association (APA) guidelines recommend that initial management be directed toward safety planning and treatment of modifiable risk factors, specifically psychiatric symptomatology (Jacobs & Brewer, 2004; Simon, 2008).

Patients are considered high risk and generally require admission to a psychiatric inpatient unit if they have endorsed an active suicide plan with high intent, particularly if there is access to lethal means. Hospitalization is also indicated for patients who are psychotic, agitated, or demonstrate impaired judgment or impulsivity. Patients with limited social support, or those who may be non-compliant with partial hospitalization or outpatient treatment should also be considered for inpatient treatment (Jacobs & Brewer, 2004). Whenever possible, voluntary hospitalization should be encouraged. However, in cases where the patient is not cooperative with needed treatment, involuntary commitment may be necessary.

For patients at minimal to moderate risk, the provider may initiate treatment on an outpatient basis or refer to a mental health specialist as needed. Safety planning and a strategy for frequent re-evaluation of suicide risk are crucial for patients who are to return home. Enlisting the help of close friends or family members can help insure that the patient gets adequate follow-up care.

The suicide prevention contract, also known as the no-harm, no-suicide, or safety contract, is a common practice in suicide intervention. It consists of a formal verbal or written agreement between the clinician and patient that the patient will not attempt to commit suicide over a period of time, while also providing a safety plan and list of people to contact if the patient begins to feel suicidal. Though widely used, the contract has not been shown to prevent suicide and should not replace formal suicide risk assessment (Jacobs & Brewer, 2004; Carrigan & Lynch, 2003).

Treatment of depression and bipolar disorder

It is estimated that over 80% of suicide victims with an underlying psychiatric disorder are untreated at the time of death (Wasserman et al., 2012). Even when depression is recognized and treatment initiated, the dosage and duration of pharmacotherapy, as well as frequency of follow-up, may be insufficient for proper recovery.

A number of pharmacologic agents are available for the treatment of depression and bipolar disorder. Patients suffering from MDD may be treated with antidepressants, mood stabilizers, or in some cases, antipsychotics, while bipolar disorder is typically managed with mood stabilizers or antipsychotics, as antidepressant monotherapy may destabilize bipolar patients. For depressed patients who are at minimal suicide risk, it is appropriate for the PCP to initiate antidepressant treatment in the outpatient setting. Patients with complicated psychiatric illness or those requiring polypharmacy should be managed in collaboration with a mental health provider.

There is some evidence, albeit inconclusive, demonstrating the efficacy of antidepressants in reducing suicide risk in depressed patients compared with no treatment. In patients suffering from severe depression, long-term treatment with antidepressants reduces the risk of attempted and completed suicide (Wasserman et al., 2012). Studies have also shown decreasing suicide rates in demographic groups or geographic locations with the highest prescription rates of SSRIs (Mann et al., 2005).

SSRIs reduce suicidality by decreasing depressive symptoms, but the risk for suicide still exists in the first 10–14 days of treatment due to delayed onset of action (Wasserman et al., 2012). Patients should be counseled regarding the 4- to 6-week lag time to maximal symptom relief to prevent early discontinuation of the medication. While SSRIs have largely superseded other classes of antidepressants due to their favorable safety profile, patients should be carefully monitored for increased anxiety or agitation during the initial course of treatment, as increased levels of agitation are associated with elevated suicide risk. In the case of MDD associated with anxiety or insomnia, the provider may consider short-term supplementary medication with benzodiazepines or sleep aids (Wasserman et al., 2012; Simon, 2008). In addition to counseling patients about the lag time of antidepressants, providers can attempt to increase medication adherence by addressing concerns regarding the stigma and potential side effects associated with psychotropic medications.

In 2004, the US FDA issued a black box warning for increased suicidal ideation and behavior in children and young adults actively taking antidepressants. This notion of increased suicidality with SSRIs has been challenged in a number of studies. In a meta-analysis by Robert Gibbons et al. a reduction in depressive symptoms was found in all age groups (including children and young adults) receiving antidepressants. In adults and geriatric patients, the relief of depressive symptoms correlated with decreased levels of suicidal ideation and behavior. While the same pattern was not established for youths, there was no evidence of increased suicide risk (Gibbons et al., 2012). The consensus at this time is that the benefits of antidepressant treatment significantly outweigh the risks of untreated depression.

In addition to its other therapeutic properties, lithium has been demonstrated to significantly decrease the risk of both attempted and completed suicide in patients with bipolar disorder as well as MDD. Clozapine is also FDA-approved for its suicide risk-reducing effects in patients with schizophrenia and schizoaffective disorder (Wasserman et al., 2012; Simon, 2008).

Treatment for depression is most effective when pharmacotherapy and psychotherapy are combined. The response rate of pharmacotherapy or psychotherapy alone is approximately 60%, respectively. When combined, the efficacy approaches 70% (Sudak, 2009). Cognitive behavioral therapy is an evidence-based method of treatment for suicidality in patients with MDD. A randomized controlled study of cognitive therapy versus usual care in adults who had attempted suicide found that cognitive therapy significantly reduced suicide attempts in the ensuing 18 months (Brown et al., 2005). Dialectical behavioral therapy has proven effective in preventing suicide attempts in patients with borderline personality disorder (Wasserman et al., 2012; Sudak, 2009) particularly in suicidal adolescents.

In addition to treatment of depression and bipolar disorder, attention should be given to other psychiatric disorders, including anxiety disorders, substance abuse, and schizophrenia. These disorders should be aggressively treated and managed carefully.

Follow-up care for depression and bipolar disorder

Depression and bipolar disorder are chronic illnesses and regular follow-up care is necessary to ensure medication adherence and prevent recurrent depressive or manic episodes. In a 2003 review of quality improvement initiatives and depression outcomes, successful guideline implementation and educational interventions were frequently accompanied by an organizational support system dedicated to improved patient follow-up (Gilbody et al., 2003). This was reiterated in US Preventive Services Task Force Guidelines, which cited up to 96% of successful programs involving some kind of care or case management (USPSTF, 2009). The care management team, which typically consists of a counselor, nurse, or mid-level mental health professional, assists the PCP by touching base with patients at regular intervals to monitor symptoms and provide medication counseling. This enhanced level of follow-up allows for early identification of patients in need of medication adjustments or refills and reduces non-adherence and potential for relapse.

The Care Management Model has been found to be cost effective, at least in the short term, and effective at improving outcomes for depression compared to usual care (Mann et al., 2005; Gilbody et al., 2003).

Follow-up care after suicide attempt

The risk for suicide is highest during the first year after psychiatric hospitalization for a suicide attempt (Simon, 2008). Careful discharge planning with regular follow-up is essential to monitor for risk of repeat suicidal behavior, even if the patient has appeared to improve significantly during their hospital course. Basic preventive measures should remain in effect, including involvement of family/friends and restriction of access to lethal means (Wasserman et al., 2012). Though the frequency of follow-up care may be reduced over time, the patient should be monitored for suicidality long term due to the chronic nature of psychiatric illness and the likelihood of recurrent depressive episodes.

Public education about suicide

Public education suicide prevention programs (Pompoli et al., 2012) include general education campaigns and school-based awareness programs; such programs usually focus on identification of depression and encouragement of individuals to access treatment. Such programs also seek to reduce the stigma associated with depression and its treatment. In addition there are recommendations to media on how suicide is portrayed in the media.

Programs in schools often seek to correct myths about suicide and replace them with facts. Examples of these myths are that people who talk about suicide do not actually commit suicide, or that suicide often occurs without warning. Another is that individuals who are suicidal are always fully intent on dying. An important myth is that talking with a depressed person about suicide will somehow encourage suicidal thoughts and behaviors (AFSP, 2013). No evidence has shown that talking about suicide with patients increases the risk that they will take their own life (AFSP, 2013).

An innovative school-based program has recently been introduced by the American Foundation for Suicide Prevention. This program involves an online assessment of suicidality which provides confidential feedback to the individual being assessed. This method has been shown to get people into treatment for depression.

Conclusion

This chapter has reviewed the strategies to prevent suicide. Most effective is improved recognition and treatment of depression, bipolar disorder, and suicidality by primary care providers. This goal can be achieved by better training of PCPs in these topics and implementation of appropriate screening methods. Once suicidality has been detected several strategies can be employed to prevent suicide. Finally public education can foster improved identification of those with high suicide risk and more rapid referral to professionals who can help.

References

American Foundation for Suicide Prevention (AFSP) (2013). Suicide Prevention: Saving Lives One Community at a Time. Available at: http://www.afsp.org/index.cfm?page_id=598DA610-DC4C-A681-45A4701729BA0C93 (accessed 14 January 2013).

Brown, G. K. (2001). A Review of Suicide Assessment Measures for Intervention Research with Adults and Older Adults. PhD thesis, University of Pennsylvania.

Brown, G. K., Havem, T. T., Henriques, G. R., et al. (2005). Cognitive therapy for the prevention of suicide attempts. *JAMA*, **294**, 563–570.

Carrigan, C. G., & Lynch, D. J. (2003). Managing suicide attempts: guidelines for the primary care physician. *Primary Care Companion Journal of Clinical Psychiatry*, **5**(4), 169–174.

Fawcett, J. (1997). The detection and consequences of anxiety in clinical depression. *Journal of Clinical Psychiatry*, **58**(Suppl 8), 35–40.

Fawcett, J. (2001). The anxiety disorders, anxiety symptoms and suicide. In D. Wasserman (Ed.) *Suicide: An Unnecessary Death* (pp. 59–63). London: Martin Dunitz Ltd.

Fiedorowicz, J. G., Weldon, K., & Bergus, G. (2010). Determining suicide risk (hint: a screen is not enough). *Journal of Family Practitioners*, **59**, 256–260.

Gibbons, R. D., Brown, C. H., Hur, K., et al. (2012). Suicidal thoughts and behavior with antidepressant treatment. *Archives of General Psychiatry*, **69**(6), 580–587.

Gilbody, S., Whitty, P., Grimshaw, J., et al. (2003). Educational and organizational interventions to improve the management of depression in primary care: a systematic review. *JAMA*, **289**, 3145–3151.

Hirschfeld, R. M. A., Williams, J. B. W., Spitzer, R. L., et al. (2000). Development and validation of a screening instrument for bipolar spectrum disorder: The Mood Disorder Questionnaire. *American Journal of Psychiatry*, **157**, 1873–1875.

Isometsa, E. T., Heikkinen, M. E., Marttunen, M. J., et al. (1995). The last appointment before suicide: is suicide intent communicated? *American Journal of Psychiatry*, **152**(6), 919–922.

Jacobs, D., & Brewer, M. (2004). APA Practice Guideline provides recommendations for assessing and treating patients with suicidal behaviors. *Psychiatric Annals*, **34**(5), 373–380.

Lake, C. R., & Baumer, J. (2010). Academic psychiatry's responsibility for increasing the recognition of mood disorders and risk for suicide in primary care. *Current Opinion in Psychiatry*, **23**, 157–166.

Lester, D. (2012). Suicide prevention by lethal means restriction. In R. I. Simons, R. E. Hales, & V. A. Arlington. (Eds.) *The American Psychiatric Publishing Textbook of Suicide Assessment and Management*, 2nd edn (pp. 581–592). American Psychiatric Publishing,

Luoma, J. B., Martin, C. E., & Pearson, J. L. (2002). Contact with mental health and primary care providers before suicide: a review of the evidence. *American Journal of Psychiatry*, **159**, 909–916.

Mann, J. J., Apter, A., Bertolete, J., et al. (2005). Suicide prevention strategies: a systematic review. *JAMA*, **294**, 2064–2074.

Nease, D. E., & Malouin, J. M. (2003). Depression screening: a practical strategy. *Journal of Family Practice*, **52**, 118–126.

Nimalasuriya, K., Compton, M. T., & Guillory, V. J. (2009). Screening adults for depression in primary care: A position statement of the American College of Preventive Medicine. *Journal of Family Practice*, **58**, 535–538.

Pompoli, M., Innamorati, M., & Lester, D. (2012). Suicide prevention programs. In R. I. Simons, R. E. Hales, & V. A. Arlington. (Eds.) *The American Psychiatric Publishing Textbook of Suicide Assessment and Management*, 2nd edn (pp. 593–619). American Psychiatric Publishing.

Russell, L. (2010). *Mental Health Care Services in Primary Care Tackling the Issues in the Context of Health Care Reform*. Center for American Progress. Available at: http://www.americanprogress.org/issues/healthcare/report/2010/10/04/8466/mental-health-care-services-in-primary-care/ (accessed 4 January 2013).

Simon, R. I. (2008) Suicide. In R. E. Hales, S. C. Yudofsky, G. O. Gabbards, & V. A. Arlington (Eds.) *APA Textbook of Psychiatry The American Psychiatric Publishing Textbook of Psychiatry*, 5th edn (pp. 1637–1654). American Psychiatric Publishing.

Sudak, D., Roy, A., Sudak, H., et al. (2007). Deficiencies in suicide training in primary care specialties: a survey of training directors. *Academic Psychiatry*, **31**, 345–349.

Sudak, H. S. (2009). Psychiatric emergencies. In B. J. Sadoc, V. A. Sadock, & P. Ruiz. (Eds.) *Kaplan and Sadock's Comprehensive Textbook of Psychiatry*, 9th edn (pp. 2717–2732). Philadelphia: PA Lippincott Williams & Wilkins.

US Preventive Services Task Force (USPSTF). (2009). Screening of depression in adults: US Preventive Services Task Force Recommendation Statement. *Annals of Internal Medicine*, **151**, 784–792.

Wasserman, D., Rihmer, Z., Rejescu, D., et al. (2012). The European Psychiatric Association (EPA) guidance on suicide treatment and prevention. *European Psychiatry*, **27**, 129–141.

Western Interstate Commission for Higher Education (WICHE) Mental Health Program and Suicide Prevention Resource Center (SPRC) (2009). Suicide prevention toolkit for rural primary care: The suicide Prevention Primer. Available at: http://www.sprc.org/sites/sprc.org/files/library/primer.pdf (accessed 14 January 2013).

World Health Organization, Department of Mental Health (WHO) (2000). Preventing suicide: a resource for general physicians. Available at: http://whqlibdoc.who.int/hq/2000/WHO_MNH_MBD)00.1.pdf (accessed 14 January 2013).

Chapter

39

Safety planning to prevent suicidal behavior

Barbara Stanley, Emily A. Biggs, and Gregory K. Brown

Overview

This chapter provides an overview of safety planning, its role in the care and management of suicidal patients, and how it differs from a "no-suicide contract." "Contracting for safety" is a strategy that many clinicians have used with suicidal patients in which they ask patients to promise, sometimes in the form of a written "contract," to refrain from engaging in suicidal behavior and to use emergency contacts should they become suicidal. Safety planning is an alternative to these "contracts" in which more detailed and specific strategies to manage suicidal feelings are identified with patients. We will particularly focus on one form of safety planning, the Safety Planning Intervention (SPI) for suicide prevention developed by Stanley and Brown (Stanley & Brown, 2008, 2012). SPI is a collaboratively developed document that consists of identification of warning signs, coping strategies, sources of social support, and strategies for means restriction for use as a tool to alleviate a suicidal crisis. Specifically, the basic components of the SPI include: (1) recognizing warning signs of an impending suicidal crisis; (2) employing internal coping strategies; (3) utilizing social contacts and social settings as a means of distraction from suicidal thoughts; (4) utilizing family members or friends to help resolve the crisis; (5) contacting mental health professionals or agencies; and (6) restricting access to lethal means. A detailed description of safety planning will be provided, including the components and illustration of how a safety plan may be implemented and its role in suicide prevention. We will discuss the empirical support that undergirds the Safety Planning Intervention and the populations in which safety planning can be used as well as recommended future research directions.

The need for immediate suicide interventions

Assessing suicide risk is a crucial component of evaluations used to develop treatment and disposition plans for individuals with psychiatric disorders. Although clinical practice guidelines have been published for conducting suicide risk assessments in emergency settings (American Psychiatric Association, 2003), current standards of care do not usually include providing brief psychosocial interventions for suicidal patients in the emergency department (ED), other acute care settings (Allen, et al., 2002), or even in ongoing care. Typically, when suicidal patients are evaluated in the ED or acute care settings and hospitalization is not clinically indicated, they are simply provided with a referral for outpatient mental health treatment (Allen et al., 2002) and not provided with any clinical tools to help them immediately. This approach stands in contrast to other acute problems seen in the ED. For example, fractures not requiring surgery are set; severe vomiting is medically treated in the ED and not just referred for outpatient treatment.

The current practice of conducting risk assessments and referring patients to outpatient care raises concerns about patient safety, and may cause undue anxiety and distress for the patients and their families. Unfortunately, many suicidal individuals do not attend recommended outpatient treatment following the ED visit, adding to the anxiety of discharging patients who are experiencing some measure of suicidal feelings (Rudd, 2006). According to a survey of trends in suicidal ideation, plans, gestures, and attempts in the USA, 11% and 50% of attempters refuse outpatient treatment or drop out of outpatient therapy early (Kessler et al., 2005). Given that suicidal patients who are seen in acute care do not consistently follow-up with recommended

A Concise Guide to Understanding Suicide, ed. Stephen H. Koslow, Pedro Ruiz, and Charles B. Nemeroff. Published by Cambridge University Press.

outpatient mental health treatment, brief interventions, such as completing a safety or crisis plan, could be especially useful with reducing suicide risk. SPI is an example of a brief suicide intervention that can close the gap in care between the time of discharge from the ED and outpatient care. It can also be used in ongoing care and for individuals who refuse outpatient treatment.

Similar approaches to SPI for addressing acute suicidal crisis have been developed by others, predominately in the context of ongoing outpatient or inpatient care. For example, Rudd and his colleagues developed the crisis response plan that emphasizes what patients will do during a suicidal crisis (Rudd et al., 2001). The crisis response plan is part of a cognitive behavioral therapy intervention that is aimed at reducing suicide risk. It involves helping patients to identify what triggers the crisis, to use skills to tolerate distress or regulate emotions, and, should the crisis not resolve, access emergency care. Specifically, the crisis response plan is a series of therapeutic interventions that ensures the safety of the patient by removing access to lethal means; initiating self-monitoring of the suicidal thoughts, feelings, and behaviors; identifying symptoms that are most likely to interrupt day-to-day functioning; and targeting hopelessness and sense of isolation, reinforcing the commitment to treatment and solidifying the therapeutic relationship.

Similarly, David Jobes uses a safety plan concept in the context of his approach, Collaborative Assessment and Management of Suicidality (CAMS), a psychotherapeutic approach for managing suicidal patients, in both outpatient and inpatient settings (Jobes, 2006). The CAMS safety plan focuses on whom to call during a suicidal crisis and cleansing the environment of means to commit suicide. It is a multi-faceted instrument used collaboratively with the clinician and patient to assess the patient's subjective experience of negative emotions and their view on life and reasons for living vs. dying, wish to live and die, probability of eventually dying by suicide, and identifying the "one thing" that would lead the patient to no longer be suicidal. Specifically, fives items of cognitive-emotional functioning are used and rated on a scale from 1 to 5 of negative states regarding psychological pain, stress, agitation, hopelessness, and self-hate. The responses to these items can serve as a major focus for individual therapy sessions to identify triggers for suicidal ideation and creating coping responses (Ellis et al., 2009).

No-suicide contracts

In both inpatient and outpatient settings, "safety contracts" or "no-suicide contracts" are often used by clinicians with patients who report suicidal thoughts or behaviors. These are not safety plan interventions. No-suicide contracts ask patients to stay alive without offering them strategies for how to do so. The SPI does not extract a promise to stay alive but instead focuses on strategies to fight suicidal urges. In contracting for safety, clinicians request that patients promise to refrain from engaging in suicidal behavior and then sign a no-suicide contract that memorializes this promise (Jobes, 2006). The use of no-suicide contracts may obscure the determination of the patients' actual suicide risk (Shaffer & Pfeffer, 2001; Rudd, 2006). For instance, patients may withhold information about their desire to kill themselves or lie about attempts for fear that they will disappoint their treating clinicians by violating the contract. Also, having a patient agree to and sign a no-suicide contract may provide a false sense of assurance to the clinician and institution that patients are safe once they leave the clinician's office.

Opinions differ on the utility of no-suicide contracts. According to Rudd (2006), having a patient agree to and sign a no-suicide contract can establish and maintain a healthy therapeutic relationship. On the other hand, the process can seem coercive, as the patient may fear hospitalization if they refuse to sign (Jobes, 2006). There is very little empirical evidence that speaks to the effectiveness of no-suicide contracts. Drew (2001) found that patients who signed a no-suicide contract were more likely to engage in self-injurious behavior; Kroll (2000) found that 41% of clinicians who used no-suicide contracts with their patients experienced patient suicide deaths or their patients made very serious suicide attempts while under contract. Overall, there is little empirical evidence to support the effectiveness of no-suicide contracts in preventing suicide and maintaining the safety of patients (Kelly & Knudson, 2000; Reid, 1998; Shaffer & Pfeffer, 2001; Stanford et al., 1994). Safety planning interventions may be preferable to "no-suicide contracts" because they provide strategies to reduce suicide risk instead of just asking patients to promise not to act on their suicidal feelings.

Safety planning intervention

The Stanley and Brown Safety Planning Intervention differs from other safety plan interventions in that it is a more systematic, prioritized, and comprehensive approach to maintaining safety in suicidal patients. Prior efforts have primarily focused on a single aspect of safety (e.g., means restriction or emergency contacts). Furthermore, the explicit focus on utilizing internal coping and distracting strategies as a step in an emergency plan to deal with suicidal urges is not typically an aspect of most safety plan efforts even though it is an aspect of therapies targeting suicide ideation and behavior (e.g., Cognitive Therapy and Dialectical Behavior Therapy). The intent of safety planning is to help lower patients' imminent risk of engaging in suicidal behavior by providing a predetermined set of coping strategies and a list of supportive contacts. It is a therapeutic technique that provides patients with more than just a referral at the completion of suicide risk assessment; it is an accessible tool that can be kept on the person or even memorized and used at any time. By following a predetermined set of coping strategies, social support activities, and help-seeking behaviors, patients can employ those strategies that are most personally effective (Stanley & Brown, 2008) and likely decrease their risk of suicidal behavior.

Safety planning intervention basics

The SPI consists of six steps: the first is identification of warning signs, the next four steps are coping strategies, and the sixth step is a discussion of means restriction. In developing the plan with the patient, reducing access to means is discussed after the rest of the safety plan has been completed, often with the aid of a family member or friend, for an agreed period of time.

Completing the SPI is a brief intervention and takes very little time to complete with a patient (approximately 20 to 45 minutes). Patients leave the interaction with a written document that consists of personalized warning signs, a prioritized and specific set of coping strategies and sources of support that can be used should suicidal thoughts reemerge, and ways to restrict their access to means they might use. By following a predetermined set of internal coping strategies, social support activities, and help-seeking behaviors, patients have the opportunity to evaluate those strategies that are most effective. It is recommended that the intervention be followed in a stepwise manner, going through each component of the safety plan in sequential order. It is important to note that if a patient feels at imminent risk and unable to stay safe even for a brief time to utilize the plan, then the patient should immediately go to an emergency setting. Furthermore, some patients may feel they cannot or do not wish to use one of the steps in the safety plan. In this instance, they should not feel obligated to do so, as the intent of the safety plan is to be helpful and not cause additional stress or burden for the patient.

During the risk assessment, the clinician typically obtains an accurate account of the events that transpired before, during, and after the recent suicidal crisis. Patients typically are asked to describe the suicidal crisis, including the precipitating events and their reactions to these events. This review of the crisis facilitates the identification of warning signs to be included in the safety plan and helps to build rapport. Consistent with an approach described by Jobes (2006), a collaborative stance is most effective for developing the safety plan.

The first step in developing the safety plan involves the recognition of the signs that immediately precede a suicidal crisis. These warning signs include personal situations, thoughts, images, thinking styles, moods, or behaviors. One of the most effective ways of averting a suicidal crisis is to address the problem before it fully emerges. Examples of warning signs include feeling irritable, depressed, hopeless, or having thoughts such as, "I cannot take it anymore" or behavioral changes such as increased alcohol consumption or significant change in sleeping habits. Warning signs that are more specific will cue the patient to use the safety plan, rather than vaguely described warning signs.

As a therapeutic strategy, it is useful to have patients attempt to cope on their own with their suicidal thoughts, even if it is just for a brief time. When constructing the safety plan, patients are asked to identify what they can do without the assistance of another person, should they become suicidal. Prioritizing internal strategies is important because internal strategies enhance patients' self-efficacy and can help to create a sense that suicidal urges can be mastered. This, in turn, may help them feel less vulnerable and less at the mercy of their suicidal thoughts. Once the coping strategies have been generated, the clinician may use a collaborative, problem solving approach to ensure that potential roadblocks to using these strategies are addressed and/or that alternative coping strategies are identified. Examples of internal strategies including listening to comforting music, watching television programs that are calming and distracting, and exercising.

If the internal coping strategies are ineffective and do not reduce suicidal ideation, patients can utilize two types of socialization strategies that serve as distractions: socializing with other people (e.g., family, friends) in their natural social environment who may help to distract them from their suicidal thoughts and urges or visiting healthy social settings (e.g., coffee shops, places of worship, alcoholics anonymous (AA) meetings). This strategy is not intended for the patient to seek specific help for a suicidal crisis but to distract themselves from suicidal thoughts and experience a sense of belongingness and connection with others.

If the previous two steps do not alleviate the crisis, the next step involves turning to family members or friends for support and help dealing with the suicidal crisis. In this step, patients explicitly reveal to others that they are in crisis and need support and assistance in coping. Given the complexity of deciding if patients should or should not disclose to others that they are thinking about suicide, the clinician and patient should work collaboratively to formulate an optimal plan. It is helpful for patients to let those who they wish to turn to in this way know that they are on the safety plan.

If the previous strategies are not effective for resolving the crisis, patients are instructed to contact a professional or agency. The clinicians' names and the corresponding telephone numbers and/or locations are listed on the plan and may be prioritized. For instance, the patient may feel more comfortable contacting their treating clinician before calling a national hotline. In the event their provider is not available, the safety plan should also include contact information for alternative providers as well as a local 24-hour emergency treatment facility and national support services that handle emergency calls, such as the national Suicide Prevention Lifeline: 800–273–8255 (TALK). The clinician should discuss the patients' expectations when they contact professionals and agencies for assistance and discuss any roadblocks or challenges in doing so. Patients may be reluctant, at times, to contact professionals and disclose their suicide ideation for fear of being hospitalized or being intruded upon by emergency crisis personnel. As with other components of the plan, the clinician should discuss any concerns or other obstacles that may hinder patients from contacting a professional or agency. Only those professionals whom patients are willing to be contacted during a time of crisis should be included on the safety plan (Stanley & Brown, 2011).

In developing a safety plan, means restriction is addressed after patients have identified ways of coping with suicidal feelings. Ideally, if patients feel there are other options to acting on their suicidal urges than committing suicide, they may be more likely to engage in a discussion about removing or restricting access to lethal means. The risk for suicide is amplified when patients report a specific plan to kill themselves that involves a readily available lethal method (Joiner et al., 2003). Means restriction may include safely storing and dispensing of medication, implementing firearm safety procedures, or restricting access to knives or other lethal means.

Generally, clinicians should ask patients which means they would consider using during a suicidal crisis and collaboratively identify ways to secure or limit access to these means. Clinicians should routinely ask whether patients have access to firearms, regardless of whether it is considered a "method of choice," and make arrangements for securing them. The specific behaviors necessary to make the patients' environment safer should be noted on the safety plan and the length of time (e.g., 1 week, 2 months) that this restriction should be in place. The patient's risk for suicide will increase further due to direct contact with the highly lethal method; therefore, an optimal plan would be for a designated and responsible person (e.g., friend, family member) to restrict the patient's access to the lethal means and safety storing it (Simon, 2007). Patients also may consider possession of lethal means as a safety factor and may become anxious at the thought of removing all methods. The removal of lethal means should be presented as an opportunity to give the patient more time to process their feelings of suicide (Linehan, 1993).

It is important to note that restricting access to a lethal method does not guarantee patients' safety as they may choose another method; however; studies have shown that suicidal patients typically have a preferred method of committing suicide and if that means is restricted, it is less likely they will substitute for another method. Also, suicidal crises are often short-lived (fueled by ambivalence or impulsiveness) and if their fatal outcome is prevented, it is unlikely the action will be repeated and help will more likely be made available in the meantime (Daigle, 2005).

As mentioned earlier, a safety plan should be developed in a collaborative manner with patients using a problem solving approach. To increase effectiveness, the safety plan should be written using the patient's own words so that the strategies in it are readily recognized by the patient. If, for any reason, patients are unable to follow a plan on their own, the clinician should adapt the approach to the patient needs (Stanley & Brown, 2008). Overall, the most important component of the safety plan is that it is readily accessible and easy to use. It is recommended that the clinician discuss where the safety plan will be kept and how it will be retrieved during a crisis. This may include making multiple copies of the plan to keep in various locations or changing the size or format of the plan so it could be stored in a wallet or electronic devise that is easily accessible.

Applications of SPI

The SPI has been developed for suicidal patients evaluated in the ED, trauma centers, crisis hot lines, psychiatric inpatient units, and other acute care settings (Stanley & Brown, 2008). The SPI has its roots in cognitive therapy (CT) tested by Brown et al. (2005), further expanded by Stanley & Brown (2006) and then adapted for use by high suicide risk Veterans (Stanley & Brown, 2008) and depressed suicidal adolescents in CBT for Suicide Prevention (CBT-SP). Furthermore, this intervention can be used in the context of ongoing outpatient treatment or during inpatient care of suicidal patients. It is a promising intervention used to mitigate the risk of suicide when evaluating and treating patients at risk for suicidal behaviors. Furthermore, implementing safety plans as part of ongoing mental health treatment in outpatient settings allows for revisions of coping skills or expansion of social contacts during subsequent visits, and with regular discussion and updates of the safety plan, it will be more likely that the patient will use the plan before or during a suicidal crisis.

Given that a suicidal crisis may be relatively short-lived, an intervention that assists patients in coping with such a crisis may be particularly useful, even if the intervention is only used for a brief period of time until the crisis diminishes. For example, the effectiveness of means restriction is largely based on the fact that suicidal thoughts tend to subside over time and that making it more difficult for patients to act on these thoughts would be a helpful preventive measure (Daigle, 2005). Similarly, if patients are given tools that enable them to resist or decrease suicidal urges for brief periods of time, then the risk for suicide is likely to decrease.

It is recognized that the application of the safety plan will vary depending on the population as well. For example, when developing safety plans with adolescents, it may be important to identify key adults who may become part of the plan. Adolescents are able to aid in determining which family members or other responsible adults are more likely to have a calming and positive influence. Family members can also be coached to help the adolescents use the safety plan. In addition, special care must be taken when helping the adolescent identify individuals other than family members who may offer support and distraction from the suicidal crisis (e.g., teacher, school counselor) (Stanley & Brown, 2011).

Safety plans have also been developed and implemented for populations other than suicidal patients. A computerized aid was created to assist victims of domestic violence in safety decision-making and to help generate a personalized safety plan. The authors found the majority of participants (69%) were in extreme danger in their relationship, but only 60% had made a safety plan. After using a computer program that provides feedback regarding issues such as risk for lethal violence, options for safety, and assistance with setting priorities for safety, the women felt more confident in their decisions and less conflict in their decision-making (Glass, et al., 2010).

Knox and colleagues (2012) implemented a demonstration project called Suicide Assessment Follow-up Engagement Treatment (SAFE VET) to address suicide prevention in the Veteran population who presented with suicide ideation to the several VA emergency departments but did not require hospitalization. A program evaluation found that connection to services increased following the intervention (Knox et al., 2012). Key informant interviews were conducted with veterans who were given the SPI, to assess the effectiveness of safety planning with this population. The results showed that almost all veterans (95%) reported that they found the safety planning intervention to be "helpful", "life-saving", and "supportive." Also, the majority of veterans (93%) noted that both components of the intervention were useful in keeping them safe from suicidal feelings (Stanley, 2013).

Conclusion

Safety planning is a promising intervention to mitigate risk of suicide when evaluating and treating patients who are at increased risk for suicide. It can serve as a valuable complement to risk assessment, particularly for those patients who do not require psychiatric hospitalization. The safety plan has several advantages. It is both easy to learn and utilize. Staff can be trained readily and the safety plan intervention is easier to learn than conducting a comprehensive risk assessment. Furthermore, it may be incorporated into the treatment of suicidal individuals, regardless of the clinician's theoretical perspective (Stanley & Brown, 2012). The SPI and similar interventions are easy to implement across clinical settings and easy for patients to use and should be added to the armamentarium of clinical tools clinicians use to help patients manage their suicidal feelings and to avert suicide crises.

References

Allen, M. H., Forster, P., Zealberg, J., & Currier, G. (2002). *Report and Recommendations Regarding Psychiatric Emergency and Crisis Services: A Review and Model Program Descriptions.* Washington, DC: American Psychiatric Association Task Force on Psychiatric Emergency Services.

American Psychiatric Association. (2003). *Practice Guideline for the Assessment and Treatment of Patients with Suicidal Behaviors.* Washington, DC: American Psychiatric Association.

Brown, G. K., Ten Have, T., Henriques, G. R., et al. (2005). Cognitive therapy for the prevention of suicide attempters: A randomized controlled trial. *Journal of the American Medical Association,* **294**, 563–570.

Daigle, M. S. (2005). Suicide prevention through means restriction: Assessing the risk of substitution. A critical review and synthesis. *Accident Analysis and Prevention,* **37**, 625–632.

Drew, B. L. (2001). Self-harm behavior and no-suicide contracting in psychiatric inpatient settings. *Archives of Psychiatric Nursing,* **15**, 99–106.

Ellis, T. E., Allen, J. G., Woodson, H., Frueh, B. C., & Jobes, D. A. (2009). Implementing an evidence-based approach to working with suicidal inpatients. *Bulletin of the Menninger Clinic,* **73**, 339–354.

Glass, N., Eden, K. B., Bloom, T., & Perrin, N. (2010). Computerized aid improves safety decision process for survivors of intimate partner violence. *Journal of Interpersonal Violence,* **25**, 1947–1964.

Jobes, D. A., (2006). *Managing Suicidal Risk: A Collaborative Approach.* New York: The Guilford Press.

Joiner, T. E., Steer, R. A., Brown, G., et al. (2003). Worst-point suicidal plans: A dimension of suicidality predictive of past suicide attempts and eventual death by suicide. *Behavior Research and Therapy,* **41**, 1469–1480.

Kelly, K. T., & Knudson, M. P. (2000). Are no-suicide contracts effective in preventing suicide in suicidal patients seen by primary care physicians? *Archives of Family Medicine,* **9**, 1119–1121.

Kessler, R. C., Berglund, P., Borges, G., Nock, M., & Wang, P. S. (2005). Trends in suicide ideation, plans, gestures, and attempts in the United States, 1990–1992 to 2001–2003. *Journal of the American Medical Association,* **293**, 2487–2495.

Kroll, J. (2000). Use of no-suicide contracts by psychiatrists in Minnesota. *Am J Psychiatry,* **157**, 1684–1686.

Knox, K. L., Stanley, B., Currier, G. W., et al. (2012). An Emergency Department-Based Brief Intervention for Veterans at Risk for Suicide (SAFE VET). *American Journal of Public Health,* **102** (No. S1), S33–S37.

Linehan, M. (1993). *Cognitive Behavior Therapy for Borderline Personality Disorder.* New York: Guilford.

Reid, W. H. (1998). Promises, promises: Don't rely on patients' non-suicide, no-violence 'contracts'. *Journal of Practice Psychiatry and Behavioral Health,* **4**, 316–318.

Rudd, M. D. (2006). *The Assessment and Management of Suicidality.* Sarasota, FL: Professional Resource Press.

Rudd, M. D., Joiner, T., & Rajab, M. H. (2001). *Treating Suicidal Behavior: An Effective, Time-Limited Approach.* New York: Guilford.

Shaffer, D., & Pfeffer, C. (2001). Practice parameter for the assessment and treatment of children and adolescents with suicidal behavior. *Journal of the American Academy of Child and Adolescent Psychiatry,* **40**, 24S–51S.

Simon, R. I. (2007). Gun safety management with patients at risk for suicide. *Suicide & Life-Threatening Behavior,* **37**, 518–526.

Stanford, E. J., Goetz, R. R., & Bloom, J. D. (1994). The no-harm contract in the emergency assessment of suicidal risk. *The Journal of Clinical Psychiatry,* **55**, 344–348.

Stanley, B. (2013). *Brief Interventions in the Emergency Department with Suicidal Veterans: Safety Planning and Structured Follow-up Monitoring.* Presented at the Annual Meeting of the American Psychiatric Association, San Francisco, CA, May, 2013.

Stanley, B., & Brown, G. K. (with Karlin, B., Kemp, J., Von Bergen, H.) (2008). *Safety Plan Treatment Manual to Reduce Suicide Risk: Veteran Version.* Washington, D.C.: United States Department of Veterans Affairs.

Stanley, B., & Brown, G. K. (2012). Safety planning intervention: A brief intervention to mitigate suicide risk. *Cognitive and Behavioral Practice,* **19**, 256–264.

Chapter 40 Contracting for safety

Michael Craig Miller

No-suicide contracts may have originated in the late 1960s. In the more than four decades since the strategy was first proposed as a way to manage suicide risk, no one has claimed credit for contriving the phrase, "contracting for safety."

Still, it would be hard to practice as a mental health professional in the English language world without encountering this phrase – routinely. It shows up in any setting where we expect to evaluate patients at greater than average risk for suicide.

A *contract for safety* (suicide prevention contract, no-suicide contract, or other similar term) is an agreement that a patient makes with a clinician *not* to act on the urge to commit suicide. The patient promises to contact the clinician or a surrogate before taking such action.

There is little evidence to justify the popularity of this scheme. It may have benefits for some patients, but writers mostly emphasize the technique's limits.

History of the suicide prevention contract

The idea of a suicide prevention contract may have originated with Jack Ewalt, who wrote about psychiatric emergencies in the first edition of Freedman and Kaplan's *Comprehensive Textbook of Psychiatry* (Ewalt, 1967). He described the process of negotiating with a patient who has suicidal thoughts. He suggested that such patients be invited to put off any self-destructive action until the thoughts can be discussed. Give us time, the practitioner might suggest, so that we can understand what you're going through. Let's assess the situation together before you take an irrevocable step.

Drye, Goulding, and Goulding

Whereas Ewalt's chapter may have outlined an *implicit* contract involving suicide and safety, Robert Drye, Robert Goulding, and Mary Goulding (1973) are credited as the first to *explicitly* describe no-suicide contracts as a way to manage suicide risk. They would initiate their procedure whenever they became aware that a patient had "fantasies" of suicide. They asked their patients to repeat this sentence: "No matter what happens, I will not kill myself, accidentally or on purpose, at any time" (Drye et al., 1973, p. 172). Patients were then asked to report their degree of confidence that the statement either was or was not an accurate reflection of their state of mind.

The authors believed, if the patient "reports a feeling of confidence," then suicide may be dismissed as a problem. If the patient, however, described doubts or qualifications, then the clinician could make "security arrangements."

Another theme of their paper was this simple idea:

> Since [the patient] is the one who is making the decision to kill himself or not, he has the best data – not only on how intense his urge is, but on how strong his controls are. Specifically, the patient can tell the evaluator how long, and under what conditions, he trusts himself to exercise control over his impulses.
>
> (Drye et al., 1973, p. 171).

The authors of this paper appeared to emphasize patients taking responsibility for their own decisions, for their own lives. Two of the authors of this paper, Robert and Mary Goulding, had their own ideas about how best to help patients achieve this aim. They had been developing a form of psychotherapy, an outgrowth of transactional analysis and Gestalt therapy they called "redecision therapy." The no-suicide contract strategy fitted into their model of therapy. The no-suicide statement was, essentially, a script used to assess the patient's ability to take responsibility for his or her own life and death decisions.

A Concise Guide to Understanding Suicide, ed. Stephen H. Koslow, Pedro Ruiz, and Charles B. Nemeroff. Published by Cambridge University Press.

Drye et al. based their own confidence in their method on their experience with 600 patients they evaluated over a 5-year period. None of the patients committed suicide. Additionally, the authors polled 31 therapists who used the no-suicide contract with 609 patients. Three of those patients died or made serious suicide attempts.

Statistically speaking, this paper does not prove the method's efficacy. The absence of fatalities in the authors' group and the low number among the therapists who were polled did not represent a lowering of the suicide rate. The rate of suicide in the population is low enough that the number of deaths by suicide is likely to have been at or near zero in any cohort of 600–1200 patients, no matter what the diagnosis, no matter what risk management technique was used.

So why did no-suicide contracts catch on?

The spread of the suicide prevention contract

Since the publication of Drye et al. (1973), no one has been able to demonstrate that the method contributes to lowering suicide risk. Professional guidelines in the USA (2003), UK (2012), Australia, and New Zealand (2004) uniformly advise clinicians not to rely upon such contracts.

Edwards and Harries (2007) provide a thoughtful review of the history of the no-suicide contract. They make a plausible argument for why this technique is so widely disseminated. They suggest five stages in the history:

1. rise of volunteer-based suicide crisis centers;
2. advocacy by specific professions of focused and goal-oriented treatments;
3. adoption of brief, problem-focused approaches, parallel to the ascendency of cognitive behavioral approaches to treatment;
4. adoption of the no-suicide contract by the nursing profession, because they are in the front line of managing suicide threats; and
5. routine use of no-suicide contracts to manage anxiety about being sued.

In the 1960s and 1970s, practitioners began to establish suicide crisis centers (Shneidman, 1961). Simultaneous with this development, leaders in social work were interested in developing increasingly specific goals for their interventions. Social workers made contracts with their clients in order to establish working relationships and achieve agreed upon goals. According to the theory, a good contract had elements of mutuality and accountability, with explicit responsibilities laid out for the social worker and the client. The contract was meant to be a "dynamic tool" used "to clarify objectives and encourage clients to participate in the entire process of intervention" (Maluccio & Marlow, 1974).

Thus, with all good intentions, crisis workers may have been trained to make explicit contracts with callers. No-suicide contracts may have become an entrenched part of the routine in those settings.

The effort to develop short-term treatments was reinforced by pressures to reduce cost. The no-suicide contract scheme was picked up in the nursing literature in the 1980s and became popular as nurses found themselves caring for (and making treatment decisions for) patients who expressed suicidal and other self-destructive thoughts. In the years since, there has been a steady contraction in the number of psychiatry hospital beds. Intensive outpatient treatment time is also limited. The mental health system, more and more, is staffed by health workers who have the least professional training.

The following related trends would seem to drive the popularity of the suicide prevention contract: all clinicians are under pressure to see more patients in less time. Practitioners fear being blamed or sued for devastating outcomes. The downward pressure on time limits clinicians' ability to develop working relationships with patients. The clinicians who care for the sickest patients often feel disparaged and undervalued.

No wonder so many practitioners reach for – and allow themselves to be falsely reassured by – a technique that appears to help them manage all the complexities of suicide assessment with one question, "Are you able to contract for safety?"

Contracts for safety: unintended consequences

Drye et al (1973), like Ewalt before them, were interested in helping patients talk more explicitly about their suicidal thoughts. They hoped for frank discussions about their patients' gravest concerns, so that these concerns could be understood. The ultimate goal would have been for the patient to be better able to take responsibility for the thoughts, and for staying alive.

Paradoxically, many experts and most professional organizations caution that because of the way the technique is used in most settings today, contracts for safety may do the opposite of what is intended. The emphasis on no-suicide contracts often appears to shut down conversation about suicidal thoughts, rather than encouraging it.

Although there is not a large amount of evidence to show whether no-suicide contracts help or hinder the care of suicidal patients, there is at least some data indicating that contracts do not make suicide *less* likely.

- Busch et al. (2003) reviewed the charts of 76 patients who had committed suicide while hospitalized. Seventy-eight percent denied suicidal intent and 28% had made some contract with the staff.
- Drew (2001), in a retrospective review of medical records of 650 adult inpatients, found that individuals with no-suicide contracts engaged in suicidal behavior at a rate five times greater than patients without contracts. This probably did not represent a causal relationship; rather staff were more likely to discuss suicide contracts with patients who were assessed to be at greatest risk.
- Kroll (2000) asked psychiatrists in Minnesota to respond to a postcard questionnaire. Of 267 respondents, 152 (57%) used no-suicide contracts. Of those using contracts, 62 (41%) had patients who had made serious attempts or committed suicide after entering into a no-suicide contract.

Narrative may be more telling than numbers.

Farrow and O'Brien (2003) reviewed the ethical issues surrounding no-suicide contracts, noting that patients look back on their contract discussions with some confusion. Some patients say that they doubted their own ability to have a competent conversation about a no-suicide agreement, either because of stress or because of distorted thinking caused by their underlying illness. One patient said, "My thinking was so confused [because of the life stressors] . . . I didn't understand what they were suggesting" (Farrow & O'Brien, 2003, p. 203).

Other patients raised the issue of coercion. They thought signing a contract was not truly by choice. One patient said, "I thought this [agreeing to the no-suicide contract] was the only choice . . . I didn't know I could refuse, or what other choice there was" (Farrow & O'Brien, 2003, p. 204). Patients described knowing exactly what the implications were of not agreeing, that is, involuntary hospitalization or some other undesired intrusion on autonomy: "You know what's going to happen if you say no . . . it's like they [the crisis team] pretend to give you a choice [when one doesn't exist]" (Farrow & O'Brien, 2003, p. 204). Another patient: "I think you just know just what is going to happen if you say 'no;' this is not what they want to hear, this is going to mean further trouble" (Farrow & O'Brien, 2003, p. 204).

These disclosures undermine any sense for patients that an agreement could ever be a voluntary one. In hospital, patients know that if they refuse, the staff will judge them to be a high suicide risk.

What we hear from the clinicians is no more heartening (Farrow, 2002; Edwards & Sachmann, 2010). Nurses describe feeling a high degree of personal responsibility for the safety of suicidal patients and they find caring for such patients stressful. Some report that they use no-suicide contracts as a matter of routine to protect themselves, believing that the contract shifts responsibility for staying alive back to the patients. When resources are lacking – for example, if they could not hospitalize the patient, refer them to be seen more frequently, mobilize community resources or otherwise treat them more aggressively – they may believe the no-suicide contract is the best they have to offer.

Thus, an approach initially intended to spark a detailed conversation about a patient's state of mind has become an over-simplified call and response: Will the patient contract or will he not? As it has evolved, the process of "contracting" often appears to turn clinicians and patients away from fruitful conversations about complex states of mind.

Are there advantages to using a contract for safety?

Despite the cautions of professional organizations and the reports outlined above, the no-suicide contract appears to be part of the *de facto* standard of care. In treatment settings where it is still regularly used (or required by clinical leaders), it would be useful to implement it in a way that will maximize benefit to patients.

Some suicidologists have tried to deal with the persistence of the contracting phenomenon by reframing (or renaming) it. Suggestions include a "commitment to treatment statement" (Rudd et al., 2006), an "alliance for safety" (Jacobs, 1992), or a "positive action plan" (Chiles & Strosahl, 1995). Whatever it is called, agreements with patients can help clarify treatment tasks and goals, for example, keeping appointments, removing lethal means of suicide from home, or providing specific instructions for how to get help in a crisis (from professionals or family members).

When using some form of a contract or agreement procedure, some or all of the following elements would be helpful (Miller, 1999):

- A comprehensive evaluation and treatment program.
- An established, positive treatment relationship.
- An assessment of suicide risk.
- Discussion with the patient that the risk of suicide can never be zero.
- An acknowledgment that an agreement or contract does not abolish risk.
- An evaluation of the patient's capacity to enter into a treatment agreement.
- Documentation that avoids shorthand, describes the suicide assessment, and explains the basis for clinical judgment and the plan for managing suicide risk.

Attention to these elements may actually make a contract unnecessary. Implementing a contract or agreement is not the only way or the best way of revealing information about the patient's state of mind or the strength of the alliance. Treatment plans and goals can be made explicit without a contract. Whether one frames it as a "contract" or not, writing out the elements of the treatment plan can provide additional structure and clarity for a patient to rely on, supporting the patient's adaptive defenses.

Reasons to avoid the contract for safety

The most persuasive argument against using suicide prevention contracts is that it is not the parsimonious solution for suicide risk management that Drye et al. (1973) hoped it would be and that many practitioners today may believe. There are probably better ways for clinicians and patients to spend their time.

One reason practitioners say they use contracts, following the model of Drye et al., is to help them make judgments about the level of risk and to make decisions about interventions. There is no evidence that this proposition is true. And there are currently no alternatives – no quick screening tests – that can help clinicians make such judgments. What remains is to do an evaluation and make clinical judgments about treatment options and levels of care.

Here are the potential problems:

Contracts can be a barrier to communication. They may discourage patients from talking about their painful thoughts. Patients have reported experiencing contracts as a pro forma administrative task to check off, one that is not perceived by patients to be truly helpful, and not an expression of concern.

Contracts can interfere with the working relationship. Patients are rarely if ever fooled into thinking that something meant to allay the clinicians' anxiety is actually meant to be helpful to them. Many or most suicidal patients know that their thoughts make the people around them anxious. More fitting options would be to have an open conversation about that anxiety, an explicit discussion about the risk of death, and a description of the structures that can be put in place to minimize risk. Staff can also acknowledge arrangements that are made for their own convenience or safety (e.g., locked doors, schedules, supervision).

Contracts can create a false sense of security. Many patients feel coerced by the no-suicide contract. They agree to it in order to avoid negative consequences. Many patients assent to contracts because they feel they must do so. Others feel that contracts signify that clinicians do not really want to hear what is on their mind. A no-suicide contract therefore does not reinforce safe behavior, nor is it an indicator of the strength of the therapeutic alliance.

The word "contract" is a legal term, but no-suicide contracts are not contracts in the legal sense. A legal contract should be voluntary. Since many patients feel coerced when asked to participate in a no-suicide contract, it cannot routinely be seen as voluntary. A legal contract must have mutual obligations, but clinicians are already obliged to provide care, so a no-suicide contract does not provide anything of material value to the patient.

Contracts do not provide protection against being sued. Clinicians cannot contract away the duty that they owe to patients.

Contracts do not eliminate the responsibility to exercise clinical judgment. No-suicide contracts are not simple barometers of risk. The no-suicide contract is not a substitute for clinical judgment.

Alternatives to the contract for safety

Although suicide prevention contracts continue to be widely used, there is no evidence to support their use as a suicide risk management tool. As a clinical tool, it may in fact be irrelevant. That is, it neither decreases nor increases suicide risk.

Contracts can become a problem if clinicians try to use them instead of doing a suicide risk assessment or if the term "patient contracted for safety" becomes the only documentation of that assessment in the patient's record.

Published guidelines on assessment and treatment of suicidal patients recommend avoiding using no-suicide contracts. What can clinicians do instead?

It may be enough to recommend reviewing the rest of this book closely, where the reader should find ample suggestions about how to work with patients to evaluate risk and provide helpful treatments.

Those looking for more specific guidance about alternatives to no-suicide contracts may use some or all of the following principles (Miller et al., 1998; Miller, 1999):

- Encourage the patient to communicate in detail about suicidal thoughts, impulses, or plans.
- Examine the patient's capacity to participate in the evaluation.
- Make a judgment about the state of the therapeutic alliance.
- Take an inventory of suicide risk factors; note the risk factors that may yield to treatment.
- Outline for the patient the treatments or therapy approaches that may mitigate risk factors.
- Compare the risks and benefits of the various treatment alternatives with the patient (including the alternative of no treatment).
- Discuss all risks of the illness, including risk of death by suicide as well as other risks of illness (e.g., long-term morbidity).
- Assess the patient's ability to comprehend the information.
- Assess the patient's capacity to make and be responsible for treatment decisions.
- Discuss with the patient the uncertainty that is inherent in all medical decision-making.
- Consult with a peer or supervisor if warranted.
- Make clear that the clinician and the patient (sometimes with the family's help) share responsibility for managing the risk of suicide along with other risks of treatment.

Writing good notes about these interactions is a challenge, because time is limited. Two equally important pressures compete – the pressure to be complete and the pressure to be concise. It is impossible to write lengthy notes on every encounter with every patient. It may help to keep the following outline in mind when documenting the treatment plan:

- What risks of the illness were discussed?
- What treatments were described?
- What risks and benefits of treatment were weighed?
- Was there evidence that the patient understood the discussion?
- Was the patient able to make a free choice based on an understanding of the options?

Clinicians who drop the no-suicide contract from their routine may discover more interesting and helpful ways to negotiate treatment with their patients. They are also likely to achieve more and be more effective.

References

Busch, K. A., Fawcett, J., & Jacobs, D. G. (2003). Clinical correlates of inpatient suicide. *Journal of Clinical Psychiatry*, **64**, 14–19.

Chiles, J. A., & Strosahl, K. (1995). *The Suicidal Patient: Principles of Assessment*. Washington, DC: American Psychiatric Press.

Drew, B. L. (2001). Self-harm behavior and no-suicide contracting in psychiatric inpatient settings. *Archives of Psychiatric Nursing*, **15**, 99–106.

Drye, R. C., Goulding, R. L., & Goulding, M. E. (1973). No-suicide decisions: patient monitoring of suicidal risk. *American Journal of Psychiatry*, **130**, 170–174.

Edwards, S., & Harries, M. (2007). No-suicide contracts and no-suicide agreements: a controversial life. *Australasian Psychiatry*, **15**, 484–489.

Edwards, S. J., & Sachmann, M. D. (2010). No-suicide contracts, no-suicide agreements, and no-suicide assurances: a study of their nature, utilization, perceived effectiveness, and potential to cause harm. *Crisis*, **31**, 290–302.

Ewalt, J. R. (1967). Other psychiatric emergencies. In A. M. Freedman, & H. I. Kaplan (Eds.) *Comprehensive Textbook of Psychiatry*, 1st edn (pp. 1179–1187). Baltimore, MD: Williams & Wilkins.

Farrow, T. L. (2002). Owning their expertise: why nurses use 'no suicide contracts' rather than their own assessments. *International Journal of Mental Health Nursing*, **11**, 214–219.

Farrow, T. L., & O'Brien, A. J. (2003). 'No-suicide contracts' and informed consent: an analysis of ethical issues. *Nursing Ethics*, **10**, 199–207.

Jacobs, D. (Ed.) (1992). *Suicide and Clinical Practice*. Washington, DC: American Psychiatric Press.

Jacobs, D. G., Baldessarini, R. J., Conwell, Y., et al. (2003). Practice guideline for the assessment and treatment of patients with suicidal behaviors. *American Journal of Psychiatry*, **160**, 1–60.

Kroll, J. (2000). Use of no-suicide contracts by psychiatrists in Minnesota. *American Journal of Psychiatry*, **157**, 1684–1686.

Maluccio, A., & Marlow, W. (1974). The case for contracts. *Social Work*, **19**, 28–36.

Miller, M. C. (1999). Suicide-prevention contracts: advantages, disadvantages and an alternative approach. In Jacobs, D. G. (Ed.) *The Harvard Medical School Guide to Suicide Assessment and Intervention* (pp. 463–481). San Francisco: Jossey-Bass.

Miller, M. C., Jacobs, D. G., & Gutheil, T. G. (1998). Talisman or taboo: the controversy of the suicide prevention contract. *Harvard Review of Psychiatry*, **6**, 78–87.

National Institute for Health and Clinical Excellence (Great Britain). (2012) *Self-Harm: The NICE Guideline on Longer-Term Management*. London: National Institute for Health and Clinical Excellence.

Royal Australian and New Zealand College of Psychiatrists Clinical Practice Guidelines Team for Deliberate Self-Harm. (2004). Australian and New Zealand clinical practice guidelines for the management of adult deliberate self-harm. *Australian and New Zealand Journal of Psychiatry*, **38**, 868–884.

Rudd, M. D., Mandrusiak, M., & Joiner, Jr, T. E. (2006). The case against no-suicide contracts: the commitment to treatment statement as a practice alternative. *Journal of Clinical Psychology*, **62**, 243–251.

Shneidman, E. S. (1961). The cry for help. In Farberow, N. L., & E. D. Shneidman (Eds.) *The Cry for Help* (pp. 7–33). New York: McGraw-Hill.

Chapter 41

Suicide and the media

Jane Pirkis and R. Warwick Blood

News and information media are extremely persuasive. They shape the way we view the world, and may ultimately influence our attitudes and behaviors. This is especially important in an area like suicide, where myths abound and where vulnerable people may be susceptible to influence. It is also important because the general public has a morbid fascination with suicide, so suicide stories "sell." Concerns that irresponsible reporting of suicide may lead to copycat acts have led to media guidelines being produced in many countries throughout the world. News coverage can also feed beliefs about research priorities and social policies that should be supported or opposed, and most high priority public health issues have been the focus of intensive media coverage.

There is an expanding body of research concerning suicide and the media, and this chapter provides an overview of the evidence that this research has generated. Research studies can be variously grouped. One approach is to focus on methodology. Traditional *content analysis studies*, which form part of a broader group of *textual analysis studies*, examine the nature of the content and discourses in news items on death by suicide. *Quality and accuracy studies*, which are sometimes conducted in the context of content analysis studies, investigate reportage against a priori standards of accuracy, quality, or comprehensiveness – in the case of suicide reporting, they focus on adherence to media guidelines on responsible reporting. *Audience reception studies*, using both quantitative and qualitative methodologies, examine how diverse audiences interpret, misinterpret, ignore, or even resist suicide news and information, and how risk is perceived and managed. *News production research*, using interview and observational methodologies, investigates the routine practices of news gathering and reporting on suicide, including source selection, organizational constraints on news gathering, and operational definitions of newsworthiness. *Media influence studies* examine impact that suicide-related stories potentially have on a variety of audiences. We examine content analysis studies (including quality and accuracy studies), audience reception studies, news production studies, and media influence studies in this chapter.

Two observations are important before we begin. First, the vast majority of research on suicide and the news and information media concerns traditional media such as newspapers, television, and film. Studies of newer digital media are rarer, partly because much of the research that has been done preceded the advent of the Internet, but also because newer media forms are more interactive, more volatile, and more broad-reaching and, therefore, much more difficult to study. Second, there is a significant body of literature on suicide and the entertainment media, which concerns the portrayal of suicide on stage and screen, but this is beyond the scope of the current chapter.

Content analysis studies and quality and accuracy studies

To date, the most extensive content analysis study conducted in this area is one of our own (Pirkis et al., 2009). We retrieved a comprehensive sample of media items from all television and radio stations and all national and selected regional newspapers over two 12-month periods (2000/01 and 2006/07). These periods were selected because they straddled the introduction of the first version of Australia's current guidelines on responsible reporting in 2002. These guidelines were developed through an initiative known as the *Mindframe National Media Initiative*, and suggest that reports on suicide should, for example, minimize the amount of detail provided about the method of suicide and provide helpline information.

A Concise Guide to Understanding Suicide, ed. Stephen H. Koslow, Pedro Ruiz, and Charles B. Nemeroff. Published by Cambridge University Press.

The amount of reporting almost doubled during the course of our study, with 4813 items retrieved in the period before the introduction of the guidelines, and 8363 retrieved in the period after they had been in place for some time. There was an increased emphasis on items about individuals' experiences and a reduced emphasis on policy and program initiatives. Most importantly, there was significant improvement in quality, as judged by various criteria included in the guidelines.

Others have begun to consider the content of selected media items in the context of conducting media influence studies (described below), recognizing that the influence of media reporting is almost certainly mediated by the nature of that reporting. For example, Niederkrotenthaler et al. (2010) retrieved items on suicide published in the 11 largest Austrian nationwide newspapers in the first 6 months of 2005, identifying a total of 497 relevant items. They characterized the content of these reports using a range of variables, and compared them with 15 international guidelines on responsible reporting. Using latent class analysis, they classified the items into four different groups: items on suicides by individuals; items reporting on suicide research and suicide statistics; items reporting on suicide prevention programs and expert opinion; and items reporting on potential suicides that had been averted by mastery of a crisis. Their key finding was that the last class was negatively correlated with suicide rates, suggesting that reporting alternative solutions to personal crises may have a protective effect.

The examples described above take the form of quantitative content analysis studies, and these make up the majority of pieces of work in this area. We extended our own analyses to include a qualitative component, looking at how selected stories in 2000/01 and 2006/07 were framed; that is, what aspects of complex events were given salience within the story's structure. In the former period we examined the reporting of the attempted suicide of a depressed man who had killed his wife, and found that the reporting linked his actions solely to the antidepressants that he was taking at the time (Blood et al., 2003). In the latter period we considered the case of two teenage girls who had died by hanging in a suicide pact, and identified frames related to "emo" culture and social networking (Dare et al., 2008). In both cases, these frames exaggerated the level of risk associated with the factors implicated in the stories (i.e., medication and teenage behavior/interactions).

Audience reception studies

Relatively few studies have assessed how various audiences (particularly people at risk) take in media messages about suicide, and the context within which mediated information is received and acted upon is largely unexplored (Blood & Pirkis, 2001). The paucity of studies is atypical of media audience reception studies in other areas.

A number of small-scale quantitative studies were conducted in the USA in the late 1980s and early 1990s in which people recruited through educational institutions and shopping centers were exposed to mock news items on death by suicide. The content of these items was systematically varied to determine whether particular aspects of a story influenced participants' attitudes toward suicide. For example, Range and Martin (1990) presented 180 undergraduate students with stories about a 35-year-old man who had taken his own life, and found that they were more likely to view his suicide as an acceptable response when he was described as having a terminal illness than when he was described as experiencing extreme psychological distress.

More recently, Chapple et al. (2013) conducted a qualitative study in the UK which had some elements of an audience reception study, although it dealt with the reporting of the suicide of a loved one, rather than reporting of suicide in more general terms. Chapple et al. interviewed 40 people who had been bereaved by suicide, and found that they had certain views in common. Specifically, they consistently stated that they valued accurate, compassionate, and respectful media reporting.

News production studies

Several news production studies have been undertaken in recent times. For example, Collings and Kemp (2010) and Jamieson et al. (2003) interviewed 15 New Zealand journalists and 57 US journalists who had prepared stories on suicide, respectively. The journalists involved in these studies believed that they have a role in informing the public about a range of issues, including death by suicide. They said that they balance the "public interest" of a potential story against individuals' rights to privacy, and choose to pursue a story when, for example, the person who has died is in the public eye or the circumstances of the suicide are unusual (e.g., the suicide follows an act of homicide). They were somewhat skeptical about the link between reporting of suicide and copycat acts, and were either unaware of relevant guidelines about responsible reporting or dismissed them as being too prescriptive.

The journalists' views of media guidelines are interesting in the context of some of our own work. Australia is regarded as something of a leader in the development and dissemination of these sorts of guidelines. Through *Mindframe*, our Hunter Institute of Mental Health has worked tirelessly with journalists for over a decade to produce guidelines that resonate with them and are consistent with the context in which they work (Commonwealth of Australia, 2011). Media professionals have been involved in every stage of the initial development and ongoing updating of these guidelines, and the dissemination strategy has targeted them at different career stages (e.g., presentations to undergraduate journalism students, briefing sessions with working journalists and editors). This is relatively unusual; in most other countries guidelines have been developed with minimal input from media professionals and have been provided in hard copy or online form without any personal follow-up. Our evaluation of the *Mindframe National Media Initiative*, which included follow-up surveys and interviews with journalists who had been exposed to the guidelines, suggests that under circumstances where improving media reporting of suicide is regarded as a collaborative enterprise, media professionals understand the issues related to responsible reporting of suicide and are sanguine about guidelines (Skehan et al., 2006).

Media influence studies

Numerous media influence studies have been conducted to test the hypothesis that reporting of suicide in news media or portrayal of suicide in entertainment media can lead to copycat acts. We reviewed these studies in 2001 (Pirkis & Blood, 2001) and updated our review in 2010 (Pirkis & Blood, 2010), at which time we identified almost 100 studies that considered newspapers (N = 41), television (N = 11), books (N = 5), the internet (N = 20), and mixed media (N = 20).

Twenty-nine of these studies could be characterized as *descriptive studies*. These typically present cases where an individual or a group of individuals had completed or attempted suicide and there is suggestive evidence that they had been influenced by some kind of media. For example, Lavin et al. (1992) reported the case of a 30-year-old depressed female with multiple life stressors who made a suicide attempt with guidance from the pro-suicide book, *Final Exit*. She presented to a US emergency department, where her mood became more elevated and her suicidal thoughts diminished. At follow-up after discharge, her circumstances had improved and she reported feeling much better and hopeful about the future. Similarly, Becker and colleagues described separate cases of two teenage girls, both of whom made suicide attempts following internet activity (one visited pro-suicide websites to discuss her suicidal thoughts and seek information on methods, and the other was inspired to view suicide as a problem solving strategy by these sites) (Becker et al., 2004; Becker & Schmidt, 2004). Again, both of these girls survived, but there are many other descriptive studies where the final outcome has been death.

The largest group of studies, accounting for more than half of the total (N = 53), take the form of *ecological analytical studies*. These are studies in which the outcome variable (usually, although not always, completed suicide rates) for one group or time period is compared with that for another group or time period. By way of example, a study by Yip et al. (2006) examined newspaper coverage of the suicide of Leslie Cheung, a Hong Kong singer and actor, who jumped from a height on 1 April 2003. They retrieved 1243 newspaper articles about his death published in the following 8 days, and on 6 of these 8 days there was at least one front-page newspaper report. They compared the monthly suicide rates for January–June 2003 with those for January–June in 1998–2002 and observed a significant increase in suicides in the 2003 months that was particularly evident for males and for suicides by jumping from heights.

The remaining studies (N = 15) can be described as individual-level analytical studies. Like the ecological analytical studies, these also involve a comparator. They have the advantage that they yield data that can be analyzed at an individual level, but they tend to consider attempted suicide or suicidal ideation, rather than completed suicide. As an example, Cheng, et al. (2007) examined the influence of the extensive media coverage of the suicide of Taiwanese actor, M.J. Nee, on the suicidal behavior of 461 depressed patients. These patients' psychiatrists recorded data on their suicidal thoughts and actions after the first media report of M.J. Nee's death. They also interviewed the patients about their exposure to the media reports, their history of suicidal thoughts and behaviors, and their perceptions of the influence of the media reports on these behaviors. Four hundred and thirty-eight patients were aware of the media coverage, and 38% of these claimed it had influenced subsequent suicidal behaviors. Those with severe depression and/or a recent history of suicide attempts were most susceptible to influence.

Summary and conclusions

Media influence studies dominate research in the area of suicide and the media. Collectively, these studies provide support for the hypothesis that presentations of suicide in news and information media can be associated with copycat acts. They also suggest that certain reporting may be particularly bad (e.g., reporting that emphasizes the method of suicide; Blood et al., 2007) and that other reporting may mitigate the risk (e.g., reporting that offers alternative solutions to problems). It is fair to say, however, that a relatively "black box" approach has been taken in most media influence studies, and it is not clear what mechanisms might underpin this influence. Content analysis studies, audience reception studies, and news production studies are emerging as having an important role in elucidating these mechanisms, but their potential has not yet been fully realized.

One of the reasons for the current state of play in this area of research may be the lack of cross-disciplinary collaboration. Most of the research has been conducted by suicidologists who have been trained in the fields of psychiatry, psychology, or epidemiology, and tend to take a quantitative, often fairly atheoretical approach to examining the relationship between particular exposures and particular outcomes. They tend to work in relative isolation from media academics, who draw on backgrounds in communication theory, media studies, and cultural studies, and tend to take a more qualitative approach to discovering, for example, the underlying themes in particular discourses and the way in which these themes are interpreted by readers and viewers. Our own collaboration, which has spanned more than 15 years, is unusual in its cross-disciplinary nature.

We would argue that the link between irresponsible reporting of suicide and subsequent suicidal acts is now fairly well established. We would also note, however, that there is a place for media reporting of suicide in appropriate contexts, providing it is done safely; some suicides (e.g., those by celebrities) will always be newsworthy and attract media attention, and there are instances in which the media can play a role in dispelling myths and reinforcing facts about suicide. Gaps in our knowledge remain in terms of how suicide news is generated, the form it takes, and how it is received by a range of audiences. Fostering cross-disciplinary, collaborative research may help to fill these gaps.

References

Becker, K., & Schmidt, M. (2004). Internet chat rooms and suicide. *Journal of the American Academy of Child and Adolescent Psychiatry*, **43**, 246.

Becker, K., Mayer, M., Nagenborg, M., El-Faddagh, M., & Schmidt, M. (2004). Parasuicide online: Can suicide websites trigger suicidal behaviour in predisposed adolescents? *Nordic Journal of Psychiatry*, **58**, 111–114.

Blood, R., & Pirkis, J. (2001). Suicide and the media: Part III. Theoretical issues. *Crisis*, **22**, 163–169.

Blood, R., Pirkis, J., Hickie, I., & Martin, G. (2003). The pill that killed: A case study of reporting risk knowledge. *Australian Journal of Communication*, **30**, 47–64.

Blood, R., Pirkis, J., & Holland, K. (2007). Media reporting of suicide methods: An Australian perspective. *Crisis*, **28**, 64–69.

Chapple, A., Ziebland, S., Simkin, S., & Hawton, K. (2013). How people bereaved by suicide perceive newspaper reporting: qualitative study. *British Journal of Psychiatry*, **203**, 228–232.

Cheng, A., Hawton, K., Chen, T., et al. (2007). The influence of media reporting of a celebrity suicide on suicidal behaviour in patients with a history of depressive disorder. *Journal of Affective Disorders*, **103**, 69–75.

Collings, S., & Kemp, C. (2010). Death knocks, professional practice, and the public good: The media experience of suicide reporting in New Zealand. *Social Science and Medicine*, **71**, 244–248.

Commonwealth of Australia. (2011). *Reporting Suicide and Mental Illness: A Mindframe Resource for Media Professionals*. Canberra: Commonwealth of Australia.

Dare, A., Blood, R. W., & Pirkis, J. (2008). Risk and responsibility: A qualitative analysis of newspaper coverage of deaths by suicide of two Melbourne girls. In: A. Herberth, T. Niederkrotenthaler, & B. Till (Eds.) *Suicidality in the Media: Interdisciplinary Contributions*. New Brunswick and London: Transaction Publishers.

Jamieson, P., Jamieson, K., & Romer, D. (2003). The responsible reporting of suicide in print journalism. *American Behavioral Scientist*, **46**, 1643–1660.

Lavin, M., Martin, G., & Roy, A. (1992). Final exit: the practice of self-deliverance and assisted suicide for the dying: comment. *New England Journal of Medicine*, **326**, 890.

Niederkrotenthaler, T., Voracek, M., Herberth, A., et al. (2010). Role of media reports in completed and prevented suicide: Werther v. Papageno effects. *British Journal of Psychiatry*, **197**, 234–243.

Pirkis, J., & Blood, R. (2001). Suicide and the media: Part I. Reportage in nonfictional media. *Crisis*, **22**, 146–154.

Pirkis, J., & Blood, R. (2010). *Suicide and the News and Information Media: A Critical Review*. Canberra: Commonwealth of Australia.

Pirkis, J., Dare, A., Blood, R., et al. (2009). Changes in media reporting of suicide in Australia between 2000/01 and 2006/07. *Crisis*, **30**, 25–33.

Range, L., & Martin, S. (1990). How knowledge of extenuating circumstances influences community reactions toward suicide victims and their bereaved families. *Omega: Journal of Death and Dying*, **21**, 191–198.

Skehan, J., Greenhalgh, S., Hazell, T., & Pirkis, J. (2006). Reach, awareness and uptake of media guidelines for reporting suicide and mental illness: an Australian perspective. *International Journal of Mental Health Promotion*, **8**, 29–35.

Yip, P., Fu, K., Yang, K., et al. (2006). The effects of a celebrity suicide on suicide rates in Hong Kong. *Journal of Affective Disorders*, **93**, 245–252.

Index

Note: page numbers in *italics* refer to figures; those with suffix 'n' refer to notes

Printed in the USA
CPSIA information can be obtained
at www.ICGtesting.com
CBHW081453260724
12241CB00008B/418